BATES'
Guide to
Physical
Examination
AND HISTORY TAKING

BATES'
Guide to
Physical
Examination
AND HISTORY TAKING

TENTH EDITION

Lynn S. Bickley, MD
Professor of Internal Medicine
School of Medicine
Texas Tech University Health Sciences Center
Lubbock, Texas

Peter G. Szilagyi, MD, MPH
Professor of Pediatrics
Chief, Division of General Pediatrics
University of Rochester School of Medicine and Dentistry
Rochester, New York

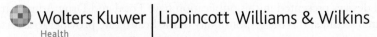
Wolters Kluwer | Lippincott Williams & Wilkins
Health
Philadelphia • Baltimore • New York • London
Buenos Aires • Hong Kong • Sydney • Tokyo

Acquisitions Editor: Peter Darcy
Development Editor: Renee Gagliardi
Senior Production Editor: Sandra Cherrey Scheinin
Director of Nursing Production: Helen Ewan
Senior Managing Editor/Production: Erika Kors
Design Coordinator: Joan Wendt
Art Director, Illustration: Brett MacNaughton
Manufacturing Coordinator: Karin Duffield
Indexer: Angie Allen
Compositor: Circle Graphics

10th Edition

9 8 7 6 5 4 3

Printed in China

Library of Congress Cataloging-in-Publication Data

Bickley, Lynn S.
    Bates' guide to physical examination and history taking. — 10th ed. / Lynn S. Bickley, Peter G. Szilagyi.
        p. ; cm.
    Includes bibliographical references and index.
    ISBN 978-0-7817-8058-2 (alk. paper)
    1. Physical diagnosis. 2.   Medical history taking.   I. Szilagyi, Peter G. II. Bates, Barbara, 1928- III. Title.
IV. Title: Guide to physical examination and history taking.
    [DNLM: 1.   Physical Examination—methods. 2.   Medical History Taking—methods.   WB 205 B583b 2009]
    RC76.B38 2009
    616.07'54—dc22
                                                                  2008030391

To Robert A. Hoekelman, master pediatrician, whose legacy of blending science with humanism for faculty, students, and patients lives on in this book, which he helped pioneer.

ACKNOWLEDGMENTS

For his expertise and thoughtful revisions of *Chapter 18, Assessing Children: Infancy Through Adolescence*, we highlight the important contribution of Peter Szilagyi, MD, MPH, our pediatrics editor, to this tenth edition *of Bates' Guide to Physical Examination and History Taking*. We appreciate the helpful suggestions of Christine Matson, MD, from East Virginia Medical School, for *Chapter 3, Interviewing and the Health History*. For special editing and updating, we are grateful to Rajat Bhatt, MD; Harry Davis, MD, FACP; Kenn Freedman, MD; Cynthia Jumper, MD, MPH; and Randolph Schiffer, MD, from Texas Tech University Health Sciences Center School of Medicine; and to Rainier Soriano, MD, from the Mt. Sinai School of Medicine and Gary Sutkin, MD, from the University of Pittsburgh School of Medicine.

It has been a pleasure to work with the talented and hard-working acquisitions, development, and production teams at Lippincott Williams & Wilkins. Peter Darcy, Publisher, has handled technical matters with courtesy and panache. Renee Gagliardi, Senior Developmental Editor, remains a pillar of dedication to excellence in the content and quality of both the tenth edition and *Bates Pocket Guide to Physical Examination and History Taking*, 6th edition. Her rare blend of flexibility, innovation, and attention to detail has been invaluable. Sandy Cherrey Scheinin, Senior Production Editor, has again brought meticulous care to every aspect of the book's production, ensuring its polished appearance and easy-to-follow format for students and teachers. Brett MacNaughton, Associate Art Director, has ensured the valued integration of both photographs and illustrations with layout and text. We remain grateful to these editors, as well as to the many other members of Lippincott Williams & Wilkins who have contributed so much to this edition.

For the many small and large tasks that accompany manuscript preparation and submission, we commend Sophia Pena and Colleen Sims, and for invaluable computer expertise, Victor Gonzales.

CONTENTS

LIST OF TABLES

INTRODUCTION

Bates' Guide to Physical Examination and History Taking is designed for students of health professions who are learning to talk with patients, to perform their physical examinations, and to apply clinical reasoning to understanding and assessing patient concerns. The tenth edition has many new features to facilitate student learning, detailed in the paragraphs to follow. As with previous editions, these changes spring from three sources: the queries of teachers and students; the goal of making the book easier to read and more efficient to use; and the abundant new evidence that underpins the techniques of interviewing, examination, and promoting health.

Bates' tenth helps students build on basic knowledge of human anatomy and physiology as they acquire the lifelong and timeless skills of patient assessment. Throughout the book, we emphasize common or important problems rather than the rare and esoteric. Occasionally, physical signs of rare disorders are included if they hold a solid niche in classic physical diagnosis or represent a disorder that is critical to the life of the patient. Each chapter explicitly reflects a strong *evidence-based perspective*, listing key citations that closely align content with new evidence from the health care literature. Color helps readers find chapter sections and tables more easily, and it highlights insets of key material and special tips for challenging aspects of examination such as examining the eye or assessing the jugular venous pressure. More than 85 new and revised photographs and drawings have been added to better illustrate key points in the accompanying text. All tables remain vertical so readers can page through the chapters more easily without turning the book to its side.

Bates Tenth Edition: Special Highlights

Continuing from the ninth edition, the tenth edition again contains three units: *Foundations of Health Assessment, Regional Examinations,* and *Special Populations.*

● *Unit 1, Foundations of Health Assessment. Chapter 1, Overview: Physical Examination and History Taking,* and *Clinical Reasoning, Assessment, and Recording Your Findings,* now *Chapter 2,* follow a new more logical sequence that introduces students to the overall process of history taking and physical examination, with a case study example of the written record for a comprehensive assessment and an office progress note. There are guidelines for ensuring a succinct and well-organized clinical record and new features describing the cardinal techniques of examination, commonly used equipment, and standard and universal precautions. New content expands the process of clinical reasoning and methods for assessing clinical data. *Chapter 3, Interviewing and the Health History,* leads students through the techniques of skilled interviewing, with a special focus on empathic interviewing, the emerging concept of cultural humility, and ethics.

- *Unit 2, Regional Examinations.* This Unit, spanning Chapters 4 through 17, again begins with the important general survey of the patient and techniques for accurate measurement of the vital signs in *Chapter 4, Beginning the Physical Examination: General Survey, Vital Signs, and Pain.* This chapter includes a new section on assessing acute and chronic pain, with evidence-based discussions relating to pain scales, types of pain, and pain management. Because assessment of mood, affect, and mental health begins at the outset of every patient encounter, *Chapter 5, Behavior and Mental Status* follows (unlike the ninth edition where it was incorporated into the chapters on the nervous system).

Subsequent chapters are devoted to the techniques of regional examination for each of the body systems. These chapters are arranged in a "head-to-toe" sequence, just as you would examine the patient. Each of these chapters contains:

- A review of relevant anatomy and physiology
- Key questions for pertinent health history
- Updated information useful for health promotion and counseling
- Well-described and well-illustrated techniques of examination
- Examples of the written record for the physical examination of that system
- Extensive citations from the clinical literature
- Tables to help students recognize and compare abnormalities in selected clinical conditions

Substantial revisions and updates appear in *Chapter 11, The Abdomen,* and *Chapter 12, The Peripheral Vascular System,* based on new criteria for assessing and defining abdominal symptoms and recent guideline revisions for identifying peripheral vascular disease. *Chapter 12, The Peripheral Vascular System,* is now positioned earlier in the book to bring it in closer proximity to content on examination of the arteries and veins in *Chapter 9, The Cardiovascular System* and *Chapter 11, The Abdomen. Chapter 16, The Musculoskeletal System,* features significantly expanded Techniques of Examination and more than 30 new illustrations of maneuvers for examining joints.

- *Unit 3, Special Populations.* In this Unit, Chapters 18 through 20, readers will again find chapters relating to special stages in the life cycle: infancy through adolescence, pregnancy, and aging.

The Tenth Edition: A Closer Look

The 10th edition features extensive new content, substantial revisions, and 85 new photos and illustrations to help students master the important skills of patient assessment. Here we describe key changes and updates. Close reading of the 20 chapters to follow will reveal many additional details that enhance student learning.

- In *Chapter 5, Behavior and Mental Status,* readers will find a new discussion of the often perplexing *Medically Unexplained Symptoms* with suggestions for recommended clinical approaches. There are new tables on the incidence of common psychiatric disorders in primary care, character disorders, and clinical identifiers that prompt mental health screening.

● In *Chapter 7, The Head and Neck,* readers will discover that Anatomy and Physiology and Techniques of Examination for each of the component examinations for the Head, the Eyes, the Ears, the Nose, the Throat, and the Neck are now combined to facilitate student learning of the complex examination techniques involved. Many new photographs of the optic disc improve visualization of the important structures of the eye.

● In *Chapter 8, The Thorax and Lungs,* and *Chapter 9, The Cardiovascular System,* there are fully updated evidence-based sections on Health Promotion and Counseling that address tobacco cessation; adult immunizations for influenza and pneumonia; hypertension screening; and risk factor screening for heart disease, stroke, dyslipidemia, and metabolic syndrome. Likewise, in *Chapter 10, The Breasts and Axillae,* look for similar updates on risk assessment for breast cancer, the Gail and Claus models for risk screening, BRCA1 and 2 mutations, and recommendations about mammography and clinical and self-breast examination.

● Other notable features include screening guidelines from the American College of Cardiology and the American Heart Association and new assessment methods for the ankle–brachial index in *Chapter 12, The Peripheral Vascular System;* a new table on Sexually Transmitted Diseases and the Male Genitalia in *Chapter 13, Male Genitalia and Hernias;* the American Urological Association symptom index for benign prostatic hyperplasia in *Chapter 15, The Anus, Rectum, and Prostate;* new guidelines for the screening neurologic examination from the American Academy of Neurology and new tables on types of stroke in *Chapter 17, The Nervous System;* updated content throughout *Chapter 18, Assessing Children: Infancy Through Adolescence;* and in *Chapter 20, The Older Adult,* expanded discussion of geriatric syndromes and measures for health promotion, along with new tables on minimum geriatric competencies for students, the "mini-cog" for mental status screening, and a management framework for managing older adult health care.

Suggestions for Students Using the Book

Although the health history and the physical examination are both essential for patient assessment and care, students often learn them separately, sometimes even from different faculty members. Students learning interviewing are advised to return to *Chapter 3, Interviewing and the Health History,* as they gain experience talking with patients of different temperaments and ages. As they begin developing a smooth sequence of examination, students may wish to review the sequence of examination outlined in *Chapter 1, Overview: Physical Examination and History Taking.*

As students begin learning how to integrate the patient's story and the patient's physical findings, we suggest that they study the related portions of the Health History as they learn successive areas of the regional physical examination. Often, symptom clusters prompt examination of more than one body system. For example, chest pain prompts evaluation of both the thorax and lungs and the cardiovascular system. The symptoms of the urinary tract are relevant to the chapters on the abdomen, the prostate, and male and female genitalia.

Students may study or review the Anatomy and Physiology sections according to their individual needs. They can study Techniques of Examination to learn how to perform the relevant examination, practice it under faculty guidance, and review the Techniques section again afterward to consolidate their learning. Students and faculty will benefit from identifying common abnormal findings, which appear in two places. The right-hand column of the Techniques of Examination sections presents possible abnormal findings. These are highlighted in red and placed directly adjacent to the relevant text. Distinguishing these findings from the normal improves learners' observations and clinical acumen. For further information on abnormalities, readers also can turn to the Tables of Abnormalities at the end of each of the regional examination chapters. These tables display or describe various abnormal conditions in a convenient format that allows students to compare and contrast related abnormalities in a single table.

As students progress through the body systems and regions, they should study the write-ups of the sample patient, Mrs. N, found in *Chapter 2, Clinical Reasoning, Assessment, and Recording Your Findings*. Students should make frequent reference to the sections in each of the regional examination chapters titled "Recording Your Findings" that display samples of the patient record. This cross-checking will help students learn how to describe and organize information from the interview and physical examination into an understandable written format. Further, studying *Chapter 2* will help students to select and analyze the data they are learning to collect.

Close scrutiny of the Tables of Abnormalities deepens student understanding of important clinical conditions, what they should be looking for, and why they are asking certain questions. However, they should not try to memorize all the detail that is presented. As students work to master the skills of clinical assessment, they should return to the related physical signs and abnormalities whenever a patient, real or described, appears with a problem. Students should use this book to try to analyze the concern or finding, and make use of other clinical texts or journals to pursue the patient's problems in as much depth as necessary. The Citations and Additional References at the end of each chapter provide many additional relevant sources for further study.

Related Learning Material

As a companion to the 10th edition, we recommend *Bates' Pocket Guide to Physical Examination and History Taking, 6th edition*, 2008 by Lynn Bickley and Peter Szilagyi. The pocket guide is an updated, abbreviated version of this text, designed for portability, review, and convenience. The pocket guide does not stand alone; readers should refer to the text and illustrations of *Bates' Guide to Physical Examination and History Taking* whenever more comprehensive study and understanding is needed. *Bates' Video Guide to Physical Examination,* 4th edition, is a completely revised, comprehensive, highly informative series of 18 videos keyed to this text. Individual and sets of modules in VHS, DVD, and streaming formats are available from Lippincott Williams and Wilkins.

The accompanying back-of-book CD-ROM includes footage from these series, focusing on "Head-to-Toe Examination" and "Approach to the Patient." Faculty and teachers can again turn to resources available on Lippincott's ThePoint Web site, including an instructor's manual and a test bank of questions, and an online course covering the basic principles of Physical Examination and History Taking.

Foundations of Health Assessment

1

Overview: Physical Examination and History Taking

The techniques of physical examination and history taking that you are about to learn embody time-honored skills of healing and patient care. Your ability to gather a sensitive and nuanced history and to perform a thorough and accurate examination deepens your relationships with patients, focuses your assessment, and sets the direction of your clinical thinking. The quality of your history and physical examination governs your next steps with patients and guides your choices from among the initially bewildering array of secondary testing and technology. Over the course of becoming an accomplished clinician, you will polish these important relational and clinical skills for a lifetime.

As you enter the realm of patient assessment, you begin integrating the essential elements of clinical care: empathic listening; the ability to interview patients of all ages, moods, and backgrounds; the techniques for examining the different body systems; and, finally, the process of clinical reasoning. Your experience with history taking and physical examination will grow and expand, and will trigger the steps of clinical reasoning from the first moments of the patient encounter: identifying problem symptoms and abnormal findings; linking findings to an underlying process of pathophysiology or psychopathology; and establishing and testing a set of explanatory hypotheses. Working through these steps will reveal the multifaceted profile of the patient before you. Paradoxically, the very skills that allow you to assess all patients also shape the image of the unique human being entrusted to your care.

This chapter provides a road map to clinical proficiency in two critical areas: the *Health History* and the *Physical Examination*. It describes the components of the health history and how to organize the patient's story; it gives an overview of the physical examination with a sequence for ensuring patient comfort; and it provides brief descriptions of techniques of examination for each component of the physical examination, from the General Survey through the Nervous System. *Chapter 2, Clinical Reasoning, Assessment, and Recording Your Findings,* immediately follows with the third area for proficiency—the written record, or "write-up," which contains the all-important *Assessment and Plan.* In Chapter 2 you will find an example of an actual write-up and learn how clinical reasoning informs your assessment and plan, the critical action steps of your patient evaluations. By studying the subsequent chapters and perfecting the skills of examination and history taking described, you will cross into the world of active patient assessment—gradually at first, but then with growing confidence and expertise.

As you study this chapter and chart the tasks ahead, subsequent chapters will guide your journey to clinical competence. Citations from the medical literature and pertinent further readings enrich each chapter so that you can continue to expand your knowledge. Further, beginning with Chapter 4, sections on Health Promotion and Counseling provide updated guidelines to help you promote and protect your patients' health and well-being.

● *Chapter 2, Clinical Reasoning, Assessment, and Recording Your Findings,* explores the steps of clinical reasoning and how to document your evaluations, diagnoses, and plans for patient care clearly and effectively. After all, your record sets the guideposts for the many members of the health care team!

● *Chapter 3, Interviewing and the Health History,* expands on the essential, varied, and often challenging skills of building patient rapport and eliciting the patient's story.

● *Chapters 4 to 17* detail the anatomy and physiology, health history, guidelines for health promotion and counseling, techniques of examination, and examples of the written record relevant to specific body systems and regions.

● *Chapters 18 to 20* extend and adapt the elements of the adult history and physical examination to special populations: newborns, infants, children, and adolescents; pregnant women; and older adults.

From mastery of these skills and the mutual trust and respect of caring relationships with your patients emerge the timeless rewards of the clinical professions.

PATIENT ASSESSMENT: COMPREHENSIVE OR FOCUSED

Determining the Scope of Your Assessment. As you build your skills in taking the health history and performing the physical examination, almost immediately you will face the question "How much should I do?" and ask "Should my assessment be comprehensive or focused?" For patients you are seeing for the first time in the office or hospital, you will usually choose to conduct a *comprehensive assessment*, which includes all the elements of the health history and the complete physical examination. Nevertheless, in many situations, a more flexible *focused* or *problem-oriented assessment* is appropriate, particularly for patients you know well who are returning for routine office follow-up care or for patients with specific "urgent care" concerns like sore throat or knee pain. Like a tailor fitting a special garment, you will adjust the scope of the history and physical examination to the situation at hand, keeping several factors in mind: the magnitude and severity of the patient's problems; your need for thoroughness; the clinical setting—inpatient or outpatient, primary or subspecialty care; and the time available. Mastery of all the components of a comprehensive assessment allows you to select the elements that are most pertinent to the patient's concerns yet meet clinical standards for best practice and diagnostic accuracy.

● The History and Physical Examination: Comprehensive or Focused?

Comprehensive Assessment	Focused Assessment
• Is appropriate for new patients in the office or hospital • Provides fundamental and personalized knowledge about the patient • Strengthens the clinician–patient relationship • Helps identify or rule out physical causes related to patient concerns • Provides baselines for future assessments • Creates platform for health promotion through education and counseling • Develops proficiency in the essential skills of physical examination	• Is appropriate for established patients, especially during routine or urgent care visits • Addresses focused concerns or symptoms • Assesses symptoms restricted to a specific body system • Applies examination methods relevant to assessing the concern or problem as precisely and carefully as possible

---

As you can see, the *comprehensive examination* does more than assess body systems. It is a source of fundamental and personalized knowledge about the patient that strengthens the clinician–patient relationship. Most people seeking your care have specific worries or symptoms. The comprehensive examination provides a more complete basis for assessing patient concerns and answering patient questions.

For the focused examination, you will select the methods relevant to thorough assessment of the targeted problem. The patient's symptoms, age, and health history help determine the scope of the focused examination, as does your knowledge of disease patterns. Of all the patients with sore throat, for example, you will need to decide who may have infectious mononucleosis and warrants careful palpation of the liver and spleen and who, in contrast, has a common cold and does not need this examination. The clinical thinking that underlies and guides such decisions is discussed in Chapter 2.

What about the *routine clinical check-up,* or *periodic physical examination?* Several studies have scrutinized the usefulness of the comprehensive physical examination for the purposes of screening and prevention of illness, in contrast to evaluation of symptoms.[1-6] Findings have validated the importance of physical examination techniques: blood pressure measurement, assessment of central venous pressure from the jugular venous pulse, listening to the heart for evidence of valvular disease, the clinical breast examination, detection of hepatic and splenic enlargement, and the pelvic examination with Papanicolaou smears. Various consensus panels and expert advisory groups have further expanded recommendations for examination and screening. A growing body of evidence documents the utility of many features of clinical assessment and techniques of examination.[7-9]

Subjective vs. Objective Data.   As you acquire the techniques of history taking and physical examination, remember the important differences between *subjective information* and ***objective information,*** as summarized in the table below. Knowing these differences helps you cluster patient information. These distinctions are equally important for organizing written and oral presentations about patients into a logical and understandable format.

● **Differences Between Subjective and Objective Data**	
Subjective Data	**Objective Data**
What the patient tells you	What you detect during the examination
The history, from Chief Complaint through Review of Systems	All physical examination findings
Example: Mrs. G is a 54-year-old hairdresser who reports pressure over her left chest "like an elephant sitting there," which goes into her left neck and arm.	*Example:* Mrs. G is an older, overweight white female, who is pleasant and cooperative. Height 5'4", weight 150 lbs, BMI 26, BP 160/ 80, HR 96 and regular, respiratory rate 24, temperature 97.5°F

COMPREHENSIVE ASSESSMENT OF THE ADULT

THE COMPREHENSIVE ADULT HEALTH HISTORY

Overview.   Here we describe the seven components of the *Comprehensive Adult Health History:*

● Identifying Data and Source of the History

● Chief Complaint(s)

● Present Illness

● Past History

● Family History

● Personal and Social History

● Review of Systems

See Chapter 18, Assessing Children: Infancy Through Adolescence, for *comprehensive pediatric health histories.*

As you will learn in Chapter 3, Interviewing and the Health History, as you talk with the patient the health history hardly springs forth in this order! The interview is more fluid . . . you will closely follow the *patient's* cues to elicit the patient's narrative of illness, provide empathy, and strengthen rapport. You will quickly learn, however, where to fit different aspects of the patient's story into the more formal format of the oral presentation and written record. You will transform the patient's language and story into the seven elements of clinical interchange so familiar to all members of the health care team. This restructuring organizes your clinical reasoning and provides a template for your expanding clinical expertise.

As you begin your clinical journey, review the features of the components of the adult health history described below, then study the more detailed explanations that follow.

● Overview: Components of the Adult Health History

Identifying Data	• *Identifying data*—such as age, gender, occupation, marital status • *Source of the history*—usually the patient, but can be a family member or friend, letter of referral, or the medical record • If appropriate, establish *source of referral*, because a written report may be needed.
Reliability	Varies according to the patient's memory, trust, and mood
Chief Complaint(s)	The one or more symptoms or concerns causing the patient to seek care
Present Illness	• Amplifies the *Chief Complaint*; describes how each symptom developed • Includes patient's thoughts and feelings about the illness • Pulls in relevant portions of the *Review of Systems*, called "pertinent positives and negatives" (see p. 10) • May include *medications, allergies,* habits of *smoking* and *alcohol*, which are frequently pertinent to the present illness
Past History	• Lists childhood illnesses • Lists adult illnesses with dates for at least four categories: medical; surgical; obstetric/gynecologic; and psychiatric • Includes health maintenance practices such as immunizations, screening tests, lifestyle issues, and home safety
Family History	• Outlines or diagrams age and health, or age and cause of death, of siblings, parents, and grandparents • Documents presence or absence of specific illnesses in family, such as hypertension, coronary artery disease, etc.
Personal and Social History	Describes educational level, family of origin, current household, personal interests, and lifestyle
Review of Systems	Documents presence or absence of common symptoms related to each major body system

Initial Information

Date and Time of History.   The date is always important. Be sure to document the time you evaluate the patient, especially in urgent, emergent, or hospital settings.

Identifying Data.   These include age, gender, marital status, and occupation. The *source of history* or *referral* can be the patient, a family member or friend, an officer, a consultant, or the medical record. Designating the *source of referral* helps you to assess the type of information provided and any possible biases.

Reliability.   Document this information if relevant. For example, "The patient is vague when describing symptoms, and details are confusing." This judgment reflects the quality of the information provided by the patient and is usually made at the end of the interview.

Chief Complaint(s).   *Make every attempt to quote the patient's own words.*

For example, "My stomach hurts and I feel awful." Sometimes patients have no specific complaints. Report their goals instead. For example, "I have come for my regular check-up" or "I've been admitted for a thorough evaluation of my heart."

Present Illness.   This section of the history is a complete, clear, and chronologic account of the problems prompting the patient to seek care. The narrative should include the onset of the problem, the setting in which it has developed, its manifestations, and any treatments.

● Each principal symptom should be well-characterized, with descriptions of (1) location; (2) quality; (3) quantity or severity; (4) timing, including onset, duration, and frequency; (5) the setting in which it occurs; (6) factors that have aggravated or relieved the symptom; and (7) associated manifestations. These *seven attributes* are invaluable for understanding all patient symptoms. See Chapter 3, *Interviewing and the Health History,* pp. 55–98. It is also important to include "pertinent positives" and "pertinent negatives" from sections of the *Review of Systems* related to the *Chief Complaint(s)*. These designate the presence or absence of symptoms relevant to the *differential diagnosis,* which refers to the most likely diagnoses explaining the patient's condition.

● Other information is frequently relevant, such as risk factors for coronary artery disease in patients with chest pain, or current medications in patients with syncope.

● The *Present Illness* should reveal the patient's responses to his or her symptoms and what effect the illness has had on the patient's life. Always remember, *the data flow spontaneously from the patient, but the task of oral and written organization is yours.*

● Patients often have more than one symptom or concern. Each *symptom* merits its own paragraph and a full description.

● *Medications* should be noted, including name, dose, route, and frequency of use. Also list home remedies, nonprescription drugs, vitamins, mineral or herbal supplements, oral contraceptives, and medicines borrowed from family members or friends. Ask patients to bring in all their medications so you can see exactly what they take.

● *Allergies,* including *specific reactions* to each medication, such as rash or nausea, must be recorded, as well as allergies to foods, insects, or environmental factors.

● Note *tobacco use,* including the type. Cigarettes are often reported in pack-years (a person who has smoked 1½ packs a day for 12 years has an 18-pack-year history). If someone has quit, note for how long.

● *Alcohol and drug* use should always be investigated. See Chapter 3, *Interviewing and the Health History,* for suggested questions (pp. 84–85). (Avoid restricting the *Personal and Social History* to these topics if you place them there.)

Past History

● *Childhood illnesses,* such as measles, rubella, mumps, whooping cough, chickenpox, rheumatic fever, scarlet fever, and polio, are included in the *Past History.* Also included are any chronic childhood illnesses.

● Provide information relative to *Adult Illnesses* in each of four areas:

  ● *Medical:* Illnesses such as diabetes, hypertension, hepatitis, asthma, and HIV; hospitalizations; number and gender of sexual partners; and risky sexual practices

  ● *Surgical:* Dates, indications, and types of operations

  ● *Obstetric/Gynecologic:* Obstetric history, menstrual history, methods of contraception, and sexual function

  ● *Psychiatric:* Illness and time frame, diagnoses, hospitalizations, and treatments

● Also cover selected aspects of *Health Maintenance,* especially immunizations and screening tests. For *immunizations,* find out whether the patient has received vaccines for tetanus, pertussis, diphtheria, polio, measles, rubella, mumps, influenza, varicella, hepatitis B, *Haemophilus influenzae* type B, and pneumococci. For *screening tests,* review tuberculin tests, Pap smears, mammograms, stool tests for occult blood, and cholesterol tests, together with results and when they were last performed. If the patient does not know this information, written permission may be needed to obtain old medical records.

Family History.   Under *Family History,* outline or diagram the age and health, or age and cause of death, of each immediate relative, including parents, grandparents, siblings, children, and grandchildren. *Review each of the following conditions and record whether they are present or absent in the family:* hypertension, coronary artery disease, elevated cholesterol levels, stroke, diabetes, thyroid or renal disease, arthritis, tuberculosis, asthma or lung disease, headache, seizure disorder, mental illness, suicide, substance abuse, and allergies, as well as symptoms reported by the patient. Ask about any history of breast, ovarian, colon, or prostate cancer. Ask about any genetically transmitted diseases.

Personal and Social History.   The *Personal and Social History* captures the patient's personality and interests, sources of support, coping style, strengths, and fears. It should include occupation and the last year of schooling; home situation and significant others; sources of stress, both recent and long-term; important life experiences, such as military service, job history, financial situation, and retirement; leisure activities; religious affiliation and spiritual beliefs; and activities of daily living (ADLs). Baseline level of function is particularly important in older or disabled patients (see p. 906 for the ADLs frequently assessed in older patients). The *Personal and Social History* also conveys lifestyle habits that promote health or create risk such as *exercise and diet,* including frequency of exercise; usual daily food intake; dietary supplements or restrictions; use of coffee, tea, and other caffeinated beverages; and *safety measures,* including use of seat belts, bicycle helmets, sunblock, smoke detectors, and other devices related to specific hazards. You may want to include any *alternative health care* practices.

You will come to thread personal and social questions throughout the interview to make the patient feel more at ease.

Review of Systems.   Understanding and using *Review of Systems* questions are often challenging for beginning students. Think about asking a series of questions going from "head to toe." It is helpful to prepare the patient for the questions to come by saying, "The next part of the history may feel like a hundred questions, but they are important and I want to be thorough." Most *Review of Systems* questions pertain to *symptoms,* but on occasion some clinicians also include diseases like pneumonia or tuberculosis.

Start with a fairly general question as you address each of the different systems. This focuses the patient's attention and allows you to shift to more specific questions about systems that may be of concern. Examples of starting questions are "How are your ears and hearing?" "How about your lungs and breathing?" "Any trouble with your heart?" "How is your digestion?" "How about your bowels?" Note that you will vary the need for additional questions depending on the patient's age, complaints, and general state of health and your clinical judgment.

The *Review of Systems* questions may uncover problems that the patient has overlooked, particularly in areas unrelated to the *present illness.* Significant health events, such as a major prior illness or a parent's death, require full exploration. Remember that *major health events should be moved to the Present Illness or Past History in your write-up.* Keep your technique flexible.

Interviewing the patient yields various findings that you organize into formal written format only after the interview and examination are completed.

Some clinicians do the *Review of Systems* during the physical examination, asking about the ears, for example, as they examine them. If the patient has only a few symptoms, this combination can be efficient. If there are multiple symptoms, however, the flow of both the history and the examination can be disrupted, and necessary note-taking becomes awkward.

Listed below is a standard series of review-of-system questions. As you gain experience, the "yes or no" questions, placed at the end of the interview, will take no more than several minutes.

General: Usual weight, recent weight change, any clothes that fit more tightly or loosely than before. Weakness, fatigue, or fever.

Skin: Rashes, lumps, sores, itching, dryness, changes in color; changes in hair or nails; changes in size or color of moles.

Head, Eyes, Ears, Nose, Throat (HEENT): *Head:* Headache, head injury, dizziness, lightheadedness. *Eyes:* Vision, glasses or contact lenses, last examination, pain, redness, excessive tearing, double or blurred vision, spots, specks, flashing lights, glaucoma, cataracts. *Ears:* Hearing, tinnitus, vertigo, earaches, infection, discharge. If hearing is decreased, use or nonuse of hearing aids. *Nose and sinuses:* Frequent colds; nasal stuffiness, discharge, or itching; hay fever; nosebleeds; sinus trouble. *Throat (or mouth and pharynx):* Condition of teeth and gums; bleeding gums; dentures, if any, and how they fit; last dental examination; sore tongue; dry mouth; frequent sore throats; hoarseness.

Neck: "Swollen glands"; goiter; lumps, pain, or stiffness in the neck.

Breasts: Lumps, pain, or discomfort; nipple discharge; self-examination practices.

Respiratory: Cough, sputum (color, quantity), hemoptysis, dyspnea, wheezing, pleurisy, last chest x-ray. You may wish to include asthma, bronchitis, emphysema, pneumonia, and tuberculosis.

Cardiovascular: Heart trouble, high blood pressure, rheumatic fever, heart murmurs; chest pain or discomfort; palpitations, dyspnea, orthopnea, paroxysmal nocturnal dyspnea, edema; results of past electrocardiograms or other cardiovascular tests.

Gastrointestinal: Trouble swallowing, heartburn, appetite, nausea. Bowel movements, stool color and size, change in bowel habits, pain with defecation, rectal bleeding or black or tarry stools, hemorrhoids, constipation, diarrhea. Abdominal pain, food intolerance, excessive belching or passing of gas. Jaundice, liver, or gallbladder trouble; hepatitis.

Peripheral vascular: Intermittent claudication; leg cramps; varicose veins; past clots in the veins; swelling in calves, legs, or feet; color change in fingertips or toes during cold weather; swelling with redness or tenderness.

Urinary: Frequency of urination, polyuria, nocturia, urgency, burning or pain during urination, hematuria, urinary infections, kidney or flank pain, kidney stones, ureteral colic, suprapubic pain, incontinence; in males, reduced caliber or force of the urinary stream, hesitancy, dribbling.

Genital: *Male:* Hernias, discharge from or sores on the penis, testicular pain or masses, scrotal pain or swelling, history of sexually transmitted diseases and their treatments. Sexual habits, interest, function, satisfaction, birth control methods, condom use, and problems. Concerns about HIV infection. *Female:* Age at menarche; regularity, frequency, and duration of periods; amount of bleeding; bleeding between periods or after intercourse; last menstrual period; dysmenorrhea; premenstrual tension. Age at menopause, menopausal symptoms, postmenopausal bleeding. If the patient was born before 1971, exposure to diethylstilbestrol (DES) from maternal use during pregnancy (linked to cervical carcinoma). Vaginal discharge, itching, sores, lumps, sexually transmitted diseases and treatments. Number of pregnancies, number and type of deliveries, number of abortions (spontaneous and induced), complications of pregnancy, birth-control methods. Sexual preference, interest, function, satisfaction, any problems, including dyspareunia. Concerns about HIV infection.

Musculoskeletal: Muscle or joint pain, stiffness, arthritis, gout, backache. If present, describe location of affected joints or muscles, any swelling, redness, pain, tenderness, stiffness, weakness, or limitation of motion or activity; include timing of symptoms (e.g., morning or evening), duration, and any history of trauma. Neck or low back pain. Joint pain with systemic features such as fever, chills, rash, anorexia, weight loss, or weakness.

Psychiatric: Nervousness; tension; mood, including depression, memory change, suicide attempts, if relevant.

Neurologic: Changes in mood, attention, or speech; changes in orientation, memory, insight, or judgment; headache, dizziness, vertigo; fainting, blackouts, seizures, weakness, paralysis, numbness or loss of sensation, tingling or "pins and needles," tremors or other involuntary movements; seizures.

Hematologic: Anemia, easy bruising or bleeding, past transfusions, transfusion reactions.

Endocrine: Thyroid trouble, heat or cold intolerance, excessive sweating, excessive thirst or hunger, polyuria, change in glove or shoe size.

THE COMPREHENSIVE ADULT PHYSICAL EXAMINATION

Beginning the Examination: Setting the Stage

Before you begin the physical examination, take time to prepare for the tasks ahead. Think through your approach to the patient, your professional demeanor, and how to make the patient feel comfortable and relaxed. Review the measures that promote the patient's physical comfort and make any adjustments needed in the lighting and surrounding environment.

See Chapter 18, Assessing Children: Infancy Through Adolescence, for the comprehensive examination of infants, children, and adolescents.

Preparing for the Physical Examination

- Reflect on your approach to the patient.
- Adjust the lighting and the environment.
- Make the patient comfortable.
- Check your equipment.
- Choose the sequence of examination.

Reflect on Your Approach to the Patient. When first examining patients, feelings of insecurity are inevitable, but these will soon diminish with experience. Be straightforward. Identify yourself as a student. Try to appear calm, organized, and competent, even when you feel differently. Forgetting part of the examination is common, especially at first! Simply examine that area out of sequence, but smoothly. It is not unusual to go back to the bedside and ask to check one or two items that you might have overlooked.

Beginners will need to spend more time than experienced clinicians on selected portions of the examination, such as the ophthalmoscopic examination or cardiac auscultation. To avoid alarming the patient, warn the patient ahead of time by saying, for example, "I would like to spend extra time listening to your heart and the heart sounds, but this doesn't mean I hear anything wrong."

Most patients view the physical examination with some anxiety. They feel vulnerable, physically exposed, apprehensive about possible pain, and uneasy about what the clinician may find. At the same time, they appreciate your concern about their problems and respond to your attentiveness. With these considerations in mind, the skillful clinician is thorough without wasting time, systematic without being rigid, gentle yet not afraid to cause discomfort should this be required. The skillful clinician examines each region of the body, and at the same time senses the whole patient, notes the wince or worried glance, and shares information that calms, explains, and reassures.

Over time, you will begin sharing your findings with the patient. As a beginner, *avoid interpreting your findings*. You are not the patient's primary caregiver, and your views may be conflicting or wrong. As you grow in experience and responsibility, sharing findings will become more appropriate. If the patient has specific concerns, discuss them with your teachers before providing reassurance. At times, you may discover abnormalities such as an ominous mass or a deep oozing ulcer. Always avoid showing distaste, alarm, or other negative reactions.

Adjust the Lighting and the Environment. Surprisingly, several environmental factors affect the calibre and reliability of your physical findings. To achieve superior techniques of examination, it is important to "set the stage" so that both you and the patient are comfortable. You will find that awkward positions impair the quality of your examination. Take the time to adjust the bed to a convenient height (but be sure to lower it when finished!), and ask the patient to move toward you if this makes it easier to examine a region of the body more carefully.

Good lighting and a quiet environment make important contributions to what you see and hear but may be hard to arrange. Do the best you can. If a television interferes with listening to heart sounds, politely ask the nearby patient to lower the volume. Most people cooperate readily. Be courteous and remember to thank the patient as you leave.

Tangential lighting is optimal for inspecting structures such as the jugular venous pulse, the thyroid gland, and the apical impulse of the heart. It casts light across body surfaces that throws contours, elevations, and depressions, whether moving or stationary, into sharper relief.

When light is perpendicular to the surface or diffuse, shadows are reduced and subtle undulations across the surface are lost. Experiment with focused, tangential lighting across the tendons on the back of your hand; try to see the pulsations of the radial artery at your wrist.

Check Your Equipment. Equipment necessary for the physical examination includes the following:

TANGENTIAL LIGHTING

PERPENDICULAR LIGHTING

EQUIPMENT FOR THE PHYSICAL EXAMINATION

- An ophthalmoscope and an otoscope. If the otoscope is to be used to examine children, it should allow for pneumatic otoscopy.
- A flashlight or penlight
- Tongue depressors
- A ruler and flexible tape measure, preferably marked in centimeters
- Often a thermometer
- A watch with a second hand
- A sphygmomanometer
- A stethoscope with the following characteristics:

(continued)

EQUIPMENT FOR THE PHYSICAL EXAMINATION (CONTINUED)

- Ear tips that fit snugly and painlessly. To get this fit, choose ear tips of the proper size, align the ear pieces with the angle of your ear canals, and adjust the spring of the connecting metal band to a comfortable tightness.
  - Thick-walled tubing as short as feasible to maximize the transmission of sound: approximately 30 cm (12 inches), if possible, and no longer than 38 cm (15 inches)
  - A bell and a diaphragm with a good changeover mechanism
- Gloves and lubricant for oral, vaginal, and rectal examinations
- Vaginal specula and equipment for cytological and perhaps bacteriological study
- A reflex hammer
- Tuning forks, ideally one of 128 Hz and one of 512 Hz
- Q-tips, safety pins, or other disposable objects for testing two-point discrimination
- Cotton for testing the sense of light touch
- Two test tubes (optional) for testing temperature sensation
- Paper and pen or pencil

Make the Patient Comfortable. Your access to the patient's body is a unique and time-honored privilege of your role as a clinician. Showing concern for privacy and patient modesty must be ingrained in your professional behavior. These attributes help the patient feel respected and at ease. Be sure to close nearby doors and draw the curtains in the hospital or examining room before the examination begins.

You will acquire the art of *draping the patient* with the gown or draw sheet as you learn each segment of the examination in the chapters ahead. *Your goal is to visualize one area of the body at a time.* This preserves the patient's modesty but also helps you to focus on the area being examined. With the patient sitting, for example, untie the gown in back to better listen to the lungs. For the breast examination, uncover the right breast but keep the left chest draped. Redrape the right chest, then uncover the left chest and proceed to examine the left breast and heart. For the abdominal examination, only the abdomen should be exposed. Adjust the gown to cover the chest and place the sheet or drape at the inguinal area.

To help the patient prepare for potentially awkward segments, it is considerate to briefly describe your plans before starting. As you proceed with the examination, keep the patient informed, especially when you anticipate embarrassment or discomfort, as when checking for the femoral pulse. Also try to gauge how much the patient wants to know. Is the patient curious about the lung findings or your method for assessing the liver or spleen?

Make sure your instructions to the patient at each step in the examination are courteous and clear. For example, "I would like to examine your heart now, so please lie down."

As in the interview, be sensitive to the patient's feelings and physical comfort. Watching the patient's facial expressions and even asking "Is it okay?" as you move through the examination often reveals unexpressed worries or sources of pain. To ease discomfort, it may help to adjust the slant of the patient's bed or examining table. Rearranging the pillows or adding blankets for warmth shows your attentiveness to the patient's well-being.

When you have completed the examination, tell the patient your general impressions and what to expect next. For hospitalized patients, make sure the patient is comfortable and rearrange the immediate environment to his or her satisfaction. Be sure to lower the bed to avoid risk for falls and raise the bedrails if needed. As you leave, wash your hands, clean your equipment, and dispose of any waste materials.

Choose the Sequence of the Examination.   It is important to recognize that *the key to a thorough and accurate physical examination is developing a systematic sequence of examination.* Organize your comprehensive or focused examination around three general goals:

● Maximize the patient's comfort.

● Avoid unnecessary changes in position.

● Enhance clinical efficiency.

In general, move from "head to toe." Avoid examining the patient's feet, for example, before checking the face or mouth. You will quickly see that some segments of the examination are best obtained while the patient is sitting, such as examination of the head and neck and of the thorax and lungs, whereas others are best obtained with the patient supine, such as the cardiovascular and abdominal examinations.

Often you will need to examine a patient *at bed rest,* especially in the hospital, where patients frequently cannot sit up in bed or stand. This often dictates changes in your sequence of examination. You can examine the head, neck, and anterior chest with the patient lying supine. Then roll the patient onto each side to listen to the lungs, examine the back, and inspect the skin. Roll the patient back and finish the rest of the examination with the patient again supine.

With practice, you will develop your own sequence of examination, keeping the need for thoroughness and patient comfort in mind. At first, you may need notes to remind you what to look for as you examine each region of the body, but with a few months of practice, you will acquire a routine sequence of your own. This sequence will become habit and remind you to return to a segment of the examination you may have skipped, helping you to be thorough.

For an overview of the physical examination sequence, study the outline on the next page.

THE PHYSICAL EXAMINATION: SUMMARY OF SUGGESTED SEQUENCE

- General survey
- Vital signs
- Skin: upper torso, anterior and posterior
- Head and neck, including thyroid and lymph nodes
- *Optional:* nervous system (mental status, cranial nerves, upper extremity motor strength, bulk, tone; cerebellar function)
- Thorax and lungs
- Breasts
- Musculoskeletal as indicated: upper extremities

- Cardiovascular, including JVP, carotid upstrokes and bruits, PMI, etc.

- Cardiovascular, for S_3 and murmur of mitral stenosis

- Cardiovascular, for murmur of aortic insufficiency
- *Optional:* thorax and lungs—anterior
- Breasts and axillae
- Abdomen
- Peripheral vascular; *Optional:* skin— lower torso and extremities

- Nervous system: lower extremity motor strength, bulk, tone, sensation; reflexes; Babinskis
- Musculoskeletal, as indicated
- *Optional:* skin, anterior and posterior
- *Optional:* nervous system, including gait
- *Optional:* musculoskeletal, comprehensive
- *Women:* pelvic and rectal examination
- *Men:* prostate and rectal examination

Key to the Symbols for the Patient's Position

Sitting

Lying supine, with head of bed raised 30 degrees

Same, turned partly to left side

Sitting, leaning forward

Lying supine

Standing

Lying supine, with hips flexed, abducted, and externally rotated, and knees flexed (lithotomy position)

Lying on the left side (left lateral decubitus)

Each symbol pertains until a new one appears. Two symbols separated by a slash indicate either or both positions.

Techniques of Examination

Now focus on the more detailed description of the physical examination in the section below. Review the cardinal techniques of examination, sequencing and positioning for the examination, and the need for universal precautions.

Cardinal Techniques of Examination. Note that the physical examination relies on four classic techniques: inspection, palpation, percussion, and auscultation. You will see in later chapters that several maneuvers are also used to amplify physical findings, such as having the patient lean forward to better detect the murmur of aortic regurgitation or balloting the patella to check for joint effusion.

● Cardinal Techniques of Examination

- Inspection   Close observation of the details of the patient's appearance, behavior, and movement such as facial expression, mood, body habitus and conditioning, skin conditions such as petechiae or ecchymoses, eye movements, pharyngeal color, symmetry of thorax, height of jugular venous pulsations, abdominal contour, lower extremity edema, and gait.

- Palpation   Tactile pressure from the palmar fingers or fingerpads to assess areas of skin elevation, depression, warmth, or tenderness; lymph nodes; pulses; contours and sizes of organs and masses; and crepitus in the joints.

- Percussion   Use of the striking or *plexor finger*, usually the third, to deliver a rapid tap or blow against the distal *pleximeter finger*, usually the distal third finger of the left hand laid against the surface of the chest or abdomen, to evoke a sound wave such as resonance or dullness from the underlying tissue or organs. This sound wave also generates a tactile vibration against the pleximeter finger.

- Auscultation   Use of the diaphragm and bell of the stethoscope to detect the characteristics of heart, lung, and bowel sounds, including location, timing, duration, pitch, and intensity. For the heart this involves sounds from closing of the four valves and flow into the ventricles as well as murmurs. Auscultation also permits detection of bruits or turbulence over arterial vessels.

Standard and Universal Precautions.   The Centers for Disease Control and Prevention (CDC) have issued several guidelines to protect patients and examiners from the spread of infectious disease. All clinicians examining patients are well advised to study and observe these precautions at the CDC Web sites. Advisories for standard and methicillin-resistant *Staphylococcus aureus* (*MRSA*) precautions and for universal precautions are briefly summarized next.[10–12]

- *Standard and MRSA precautions:* Standard precautions are based on the principle that all blood, body fluids, secretions, excretions except sweat, nonintact skin, and mucous membranes may contain transmissible infectious agents. These practices apply to all patients in any setting. They include hand hygiene; when to use gloves, gowns, and mouth, nose, and eye protection; respiratory hygiene and cough etiquette; patient isolation criteria; precautions relating to equipment, toys, and solid surfaces, and handling of laundry; and safe needle-injection practices.

Be sure to wash your hands before and after examining the patient. This will show your concern for the patient's welfare and display your awareness of a critical component of patient safety. Antimicrobial fast-drying soaps are often within easy reach. *Change your white coat frequently,* because cuffs can become damp and smudged.

● *Universal precautions:* Universal precautions are a set of guidelines designed to prevent transmission of human immunodeficiency virus (HIV), hepatitis B virus (HBV), and other blood-borne pathogens when providing first aid or health care. The following fluids are considered potentially infectious: all blood and other body fluids containing visible blood, semen, and vaginal secretions; and cerebrospinal, synovial, pleural, peritoneal, pericardial, and amniotic fluids. Protective barriers include gloves, gowns, aprons, masks, and protective eyewear. All health care workers should *observe the important precautions for safe injections and prevention of injury from needlesticks, scalpels, and other sharp instruments and devices.* Report to your health service immediately if such injury occurs.

Scope and Positioning for the Examination. As you review the Techniques of Examination summarized on pp. 19–23, note that clinicians vary in where they place different segments of the examination, especially the examinations of the musculoskeletal system and the nervous system. Some of these options are indicated in red in the right-hand column.

As you develop your own sequence of examination, *an important goal is to minimize how often you ask the patient to change position* from supine to sitting, or from standing to lying supine. Some suggestions for patient positioning during the different segments of the examination are also indicated in the right-hand column in *red.*

*This book recommends examining the patient from the patient's **right side**,* moving to the opposite side or foot of the bed or examining table as necessary. This is the standard position for the physical examination and has several advantages compared with the left side: it is more reliable to estimate jugular venous pressure from the right, the palpating hand rests more comfortably on the apical impulse, the right kidney is more frequently palpable than the left, and examining tables are frequently positioned to accommodate a right-handed approach.

Left-handed students are encouraged to adopt right-sided positioning, even though at first it may seem awkward. It still may be easier to use the left hand for percussing or for holding instruments such as the otoscope or reflex hammer.

Overview—The Physical Examination

Read carefully this "head-to-toe" sequence, the techniques for examining each region of the body, and how to optimize patient comfort and minimize changes in the patient position.

General Survey. Observe the patient's general state of health, height, build, and sexual development. Obtain the patient's weight. Note posture, motor activity, and gait; dress, grooming, and personal hygiene; and any odors of the body or breath. Watch the patient's facial expressions and note manner, affect, and reactions to people and things in the environment. Listen to the patient's manner of speaking and note the state of awareness or level of consciousness.

The survey continues throughout the history and examination.

Vital Signs. Measure the blood pressure. Count the pulse and respiratory rate. If indicated, measure the body temperature.

The **patient is sitting** on the edge of the bed or examining table. Stand in front of the patient, moving to either side as needed.

Skin. Observe the skin of the face and its characteristics. Assess skin moisture or dryness and temperature. Identify any lesions, noting their location, distribution, arrangement, type, and color. Inspect and palpate the hair and nails. Study the patient's hands. Continue your assessment of the skin as you examine the other body regions.

Head, Eyes, Ears, Nose, Throat (HEENT). *Head:* Examine the hair, scalp, skull, and face. *Eyes:* Check visual acuity and screen the visual fields. Note the position and alignment of the eyes. Observe the eyelids and inspect the sclera and conjunctiva of each eye. With oblique lighting, inspect each cornea, iris, and lens. Compare the pupils, and test their reactions to light. Assess the extraocular movements. With an ophthalmoscope, inspect the ocular fundi. *Ears:* Inspect the auricles, canals, and drums. Check auditory acuity. If acuity is diminished, check lateralization (Weber test) and compare air and bone conduction (Rinne test). *Nose and sinuses:* Examine the external nose; using a light and a nasal speculum, inspect the nasal mucosa, septum, and turbinates. Palpate for tenderness of the frontal and maxillary sinuses. *Throat (or mouth and pharynx):* Inspect the lips, oral mucosa, gums, teeth, tongue, palate, tonsils, and pharynx. *(You may wish to assess the cranial nerves during this portion of the examination.)*

The room should be darkened for the ophthalmoscopic examination. This promotes pupillary dilation and visibility of the fundi.

Neck. Inspect and palpate the cervical lymph nodes. Note any masses or unusual pulsations in the neck. Feel for any deviation of the trachea. Observe the sound and effort of the patient's breathing. Inspect and palpate the thyroid gland.

Move behind the sitting patient to feel the thyroid gland and to examine the back, posterior thorax, and lungs.

Back. Inspect and palpate the spine and muscles of the back. Observe shoulder height for symmetry.

Posterior Thorax and Lungs. Inspect and palpate the spine and muscles of the *upper* back. Inspect, palpate, and percuss the chest. Identify the level of diaphragmatic dullness on each side. Listen to the breath sounds; identify any adventitious (or added) sounds, and, if indicated, listen to the transmitted voice sounds (see p. 304).

Breasts, Axillae, and Epitrochlear Nodes. In a woman, inspect the breasts with her arms relaxed, then elevated, and then with her hands pressed on her hips. In either sex, inspect the axillae and feel for the axillary nodes. Feel for the epitrochlear nodes.

The patient is **still sitting**. Move to the front again.

A Note on the Musculoskeletal System: By this time, you have made some preliminary observations of the musculoskeletal system. You have inspected the hands, surveyed the upper back, and at least in women, made a fair estimate of the shoulders' range of motion. Use these and subsequent observations to decide whether a full musculoskeletal examination is warranted. If indicated, *with the patient still sitting,* examine the hands, arms, shoulders, neck, and temporomandibular joints. Inspect and palpate the joints and check their range of motion. *(You may choose to examine upper extremity muscle bulk, tone, strength, and reflexes at this time, or you may decide to wait until later.)*

Palpate the breasts, while at the same time continuing your inspection.

The patient position is supine. Ask the patient to lie down. You should stand at the *right side* of the patient's bed.

Anterior Thorax and Lungs.
Inspect, palpate, and percuss the chest. Listen to the breath sounds, any adventitious sounds, and, if indicated, transmitted voice sounds.

Cardiovascular System.
Observe the jugular venous pulsations and measure the jugular venous pressure in relation to the sternal angle. Inspect and palpate the carotid pulsations. Listen for carotid bruits.

Elevate the head of the bed to approximately 30° for the cardiovascular examination, adjusting as necessary to see the jugular venous pulsations.

Inspect and palpate the precordium. Note the location, diameter, amplitude, and duration of the apical impulse. Listen at each auscultatory area with the diaphragm of the stethoscope. Listen at the apex and the lower sternal border with the bell. Listen at each auscultatory area with the diaphragm of a stethoscope. Listen at the apex and the lower sternal border with the bell. Listen for the first and second heart sounds and for physiologic splitting of the second heart sound. Listen for any abnormal heart sounds or murmurs.

Ask the patient to roll partly onto the left side while you listen at the apex for S_3 or mitral stenosis. The patient should sit, lean forward, and exhale while you listen for the murmur of *aortic regurgitation.*

Abdomen.
Inspect, auscultate, and percuss the abdomen. Palpate lightly, then deeply. Assess the liver and spleen by percussion and then palpation. Try to feel the kidneys, and palpate the aorta and its pulsations. If you suspect kidney infection, percuss posteriorly over the costovertebral angles.

Lower the head of the bed to the flat position. **The patient should be supine.**

Lower Extremities.
Examine the legs, assessing three systems while the patient is still supine. Each of these three systems can be further assessed when the patient stands.

The patient is **supine.**

With the Patient Supine

- *Peripheral Vascular System.* Palpate the femoral pulses and, if indicated, the popliteal pulses. Palpate the inguinal lymph nodes. Inspect for lower extremity edema, discoloration, or ulcers. Palpate for pitting edema.

- *Musculoskeletal System.* Note any deformities or enlarged joints. If indicated, palpate the joints, check their range of motion, and perform any necessary maneuvers.

- *Nervous System.* Assess lower extremity muscle bulk, tone, and strength; also assess sensation and reflexes. Observe any abnormal movements.

With the Patient Standing

● *Peripheral Vascular System.* Inspect for varicose veins.

● *Musculoskeletal System.* Examine the alignment of the spine and its range of motion, the alignment of the legs, and the feet.

● *Genitalia and Hernias in Men.* Examine the penis and scrotal contents and check for hernias.

● *Nervous System.* Observe the patient's gait and ability to walk heel-to-toe, walk on the toes, walk on the heels, hop in place, and do shallow knee bends. Do a Romberg test and check for pronator drift.

The patient is **standing**. You should sit on a chair or stool.

Nervous System. The complete examination of the nervous system can also be done at the end of the examination. It consists of the five segments described below: *mental status, cranial nerves* (including funduscopic examination), *motor system, sensory system,* and *reflexes.*

The patient is **sitting or supine**.

Mental Status.   If indicated and not done during the interview, assess the patient's orientation, mood, thought process, thought content, abnormal perceptions, insight and judgment, memory and attention, information and vocabulary, calculating abilities, abstract thinking, and constructional ability.

Cranial Nerves.   If not already examined, check sense of smell, strength of the temporal and masseter muscles, corneal reflexes, facial movements, gag reflex, and strength of the trapezia and sternomastoid muscles.

Motor System.   Muscle bulk, tone, and strength of major muscle groups. *Cerebellar function:* rapid alternating movements (RAMs), point-to-point movements, such as finger-to-nose (F → N) and heel-to-shin (H → S); gait.

Sensory System.   Pain, temperature, light touch, vibration, and discrimination. Compare right with left sides and distal with proximal areas on the limbs.

Reflexes.   Including biceps, triceps, brachioradialis, patellar, Achilles deep tendon reflexes; also plantar reflexes or Babinski reflex (see pp. 696–702).

Additional Examinations.   The *rectal* and *genital* examinations are often performed at the end of the physical examination. Patient positioning is as indicated.

Rectal Examination in Men.   Inspect the sacrococcygeal and perianal areas. Palpate the anal canal, rectum, and prostate. If the patient cannot stand, examine the genitalia before doing the rectal examination.

The patient is **lying on his left side** for the rectal examination (or standing and bending forward).

Genital and Rectal Examinations in Women. Examine the external genitalia, vagina, and cervix. Obtain a Pap smear. Palpate the uterus and adnexa bimanually.

The patient is **supine in the lithotomy position**. You should be seated during examination with the speculum, then standing during bimanual examination of the uterus, adnexa (and rectum as indicated).

B I B L I O G R A P H Y

CITATIONS

1. U.S. Preventive Services Task Force. The guide to clinical preventive services 2007: recommendations of the U.S. Preventive Services Task Force. Washington DC: U.S. Department of Health and Human Services, Agency for Healthcare Research and Quality, September 2007. Available at: http://www.ahrq.gov/clinic/pocketgd07/pocketgd07.pdf. Accessed February 9, 2008.
2. Boulware LE, Marinopoulos S, Phillips KA, et al. Systematic review: the value of the periodic health evaluation. Ann Intern Med 146(4):289–300, 2007.
3. Oboler SK, Prochazka AV, Gonzales R, et al. Public expectations and attitudes for annual physical examinations and testing. Ann Intern Med 136(9):652–659, 2002.
4. Laine C. The annual physical examination: needless ritual or necessary routine? Ann Intern Med 136(9):701–702, 2002.
5. Culica D, Rohrer J, Ward M, et al. Medical check-ups: who does not get them? Am J Public Health 92(1):88–91, 2002.
6. Hesrud DD. Clinical preventive medicine in primary care: background and practice. Rational and current preventive practice. Mayo Clin Proc 75(4):1165–1172, 2000.
7. Simel DL, Rennie D. The clinical examination: an agenda to make it more rational. JAMA 277(7):572–574, 1997.
8. Sackett DL. A primer on the precision and accuracy of the clinical examination. JAMA 267(19):2638–2644, 1992.
9. Evidence-Based Working Group. Evidence-based medicine: a new approach to teaching the practice of medicine. JAMA 268(17):2420–2425, 1992.
10. Centers for Disease Control and Prevention (CDC). Standard precautions. Excerpt from the guidelines for isolation precautions: preventing transmission of infectious agents in healthcare settings 2007. Available at: http://www.cdc.gov/ncidod/dhqp/gl_isolation_standard.html. Accessed February 7, 2008.
11. Centers for Disease Control and Prevention. Information about MRSA for healthcare personnel. Available at: http://www.cdc.gov/ncidod/dhqp/ar_mrsa_healthcareFS.html#. Accessed February 7, 2008.
12. Centers for Disease Control and Prevention. Universal precautions for the prevention for transmission of HIV and other bloodborne infections. Updated 1996. At http://www.cdc.gov/ncidod/dhqp/bp_universal_precautions.html#. Accessed February 7, 2008.

ADDITIONAL REFERENCES

Anatomy and Physiology

Agur AMR, Dalley AF, Grant JC, et al. Grant's Atlas of Anatomy, 11th ed. Philadelphia: Lippincott Williams & Wilkins, 2005.

Berne RM, Koeppen BM. Physiology, 6th ed. Philadelphia: Mosby–Elsevier, 2008.

Buja LM, Krueger GRF, Netter FH. Netter's Illustrated Human Pathology. Teterboro, NJ: Icon Learning Systems, 2005.

Gray H, Standring S, Ellis H, et al. Gray's Anatomy: The Anatomical Basis of Clinical Practice, 39th ed. New York: Elsevier–Churchill Livingstone, 2005.

Guyton AC, Hall JE. Textbook of Medical Physiology, 11th ed. Philadelphia: WB Saunders, 2005.

Moore KL, Dalley AF, Agur AMR. Clinically Oriented Anatomy, 5th ed. Baltimore: Lippincott Williams & Wilkins, 2006.

Medicine, Surgery, and Geriatrics

Barker LR, Burton JR, Zeive PD. Barker, Burton, and Zeive's Principles of Ambulatory Medicine, 7th ed. Philadelphia: Lippincott Williams & Wilkins, 2007.

Brunicardi FC, Schwartz SI, eds. Schwartz's Principles of Surgery, 8th ed. New York: McGraw-Hill Medical, 2006.

Cassel C, Leipzig RM, Cohen HJ, et al. Geriatric Medicine: An Evidence-based Approach, 4th ed. New York: Springer, 2003.

Cecil RL, Goldman L, Ausiello DA. Cecil Textbook of Medicine, 23rd ed. Philadelphia: WB Saunders–Elsevier, 2008.

Hazzard WR. Principles of Geriatric Medicine and Gerontology, 5th ed. New York: McGraw-Hill Professional, 2003.

Kasper DL, Harrison TR, eds. Harrison's Principles of Internal Medicine, 16th ed. New York: McGraw-Hill, 2005.

Mandell GL. Essential Atlas of Infectious Diseases, 3rd ed. Philadelphia: Current Medicine, 2004.

Mandell GL, Gordon R, Bennett JE, et al., eds. Mandell, Douglas, and Bennett's Principles and Practice of Infectious Diseases, 6th ed. Philadelphia: Elsevier–Churchill Livingstone, 2005.

Mandell GL, Mildvan D. Atlas of AIDS, 3rd ed. Philadelphia: Current Medicine, 2001.

Sabiston DC, Townsend CM, eds. Sabiston Textbook of Surgery: The Biological Basis of Modern Surgical Practice, 18th ed. Philadelphia: WB Saunders–Elsevier, 2008.

Youngkin EQ, Davis MS. Women's Health: A Primary Care Clinical Guide, 3rd ed. Upper Saddle River, NJ: Pearson–Prentice Hall, 2004.

Health Promotion and Counseling

American Public Health Association. Public Health Links (for public health professionals). Available at: http://www.apha.org/about/Public+Health+Links. Accessed June 7, 2008.

Centers for Disease Control and Prevention. Vaccines and immunizations. Available at: http://www.cdc.gov/vaccines/. Accessed June 7, 2008.

Hesrud DD. Clinical preventive medicine in primary care: background and practice. Rational and current preventive practice. Mayo Clin Proc 75(4):1165–1172, 2000.

National Quality Measures Clearinghouse. Agency for Healthcare Research and Quality (AHRQ). Available at: http://www.qualitymeasures.ahrq.gov. Accessed June 7, 2008.

National Guideline Clearinghouse. Agency for Healthcare Research and Quality (AHRQ). Available at: http://www.ahrq.gov/clinic/cps3dix.htm. Accessed June 7, 2008.

> **The Bates' suite offers these additional resources to enhance learning and facilitate understanding of this chapter:**
>
> - Bates' *Pocket Guide to Physical Examination and History Taking*, 6th edition
> - Bates' *Nursing Online*
> - Bates' *Visual Guide to Physical Examination*, 4th edition
> - thePoint online resources, http://thepoint.lww.com
> - Student CD-ROM included with the book

Clinical Reasoning, Assessment, and Recording Your Findings

Once you have gained your patient's trust, gathered a detailed history, and completed the requisite portions of the physical examination, you have reached the critical step of formulating your *Assessment* and *Plan*. You must now analyze your findings and identify the patient's problems. You must share your impressions with the patient, eliciting any concerns and making sure that he or she understands and agrees to the steps ahead. Finally, you must document your findings in the patient's record in a succinct and legible format that communicates the patient's story and your clinical reasoning and plan to other members of the health care team.

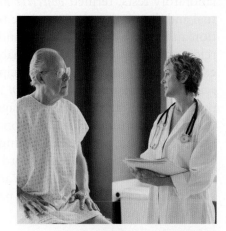

This chapter follows a step-wise approach designed to help you acquire the important skills of clinical reasoning, assessment, and recording your findings after the patient visit. As you listen to patients and examine them, you begin to cluster information into patterns that fall into a list of problems, termed *Assessment* or *Impression*. In a well-constructed record, each problem is listed in order of priority, clarified by an explanation of supporting findings and a differential diagnosis, and followed by a *Plan* for addressing that problem. Plans are often wide-ranging, from tests needed to patient education, a change in medication, referral to another clinician, or a return visit for counseling and support.

Clinical Reasoning, Assessment, and Recording Your Findings—Chapter Overview

- Assessment and Plan: The process of clinical reasoning
- Recording your findings: The record of Mrs. N and the challenges of clinical data
- Recording your findings: Checklist for a clear and accurate record
- Evaluating clinical evidence
- Lifelong learning: Integrating clinical reasoning, assessment, and analysis of clinical evidence

Your clinical reasoning process is pivotal to determining how you interpret the patient's history and physical examination, single out the problems listed in your Assessment, and move from each problem to its action plan. With experience, lifelong learning and pursuit of the clinical literature, and collaboration with colleagues, your clinical reasoning will expand and grow throughout your clinical career. The patient's record serves a dual purpose—it reflects your analysis of the patient's health status, and it documents the unique features of the patient's history, examination, laboratory and test results, assessment, and plan in a formal written format.

The comprehensive health history and physical examination build the foundation of your clinical assessment. As you have seen in Chapter 1, through skilled interviewing you gather the history from the patient or the family, termed *subjective data*, and conduct the physical examination and laboratory tests, termed *objective data*. This information is primarily factual and descriptive. As you move to Assessment, you go beyond description and observation to analysis and interpretation. You select and cluster relevant pieces of information, analyze their possible meanings, and try to explain them logically using principles of biopsychosocial and biomedical science. The *Assessment* and *Plan* include the patient's responses to the problems identified and to your diagnostic and therapeutic plans. A successful *Plan* requires good interpersonal skills and sensitivity to the patient's goals, economic means, competing responsibilities, and family structure and dynamics. Your patient record facilitates clinical thinking, promotes communication and coordination among the many professionals caring for your patient, and documents the patient's problems and management for medicolegal purposes.

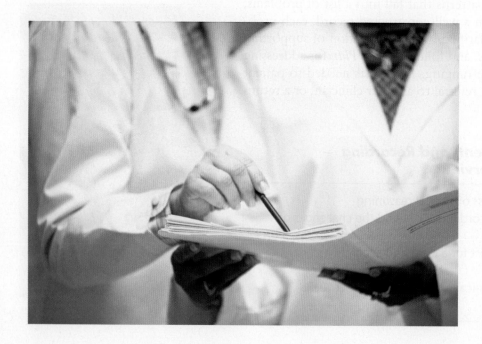

ASSESSMENT AND PLAN: THE PROCESS OF CLINICAL REASONING

Because assessment takes place in the clinician's mind, the process of clinical reasoning may seem inaccessible and even mysterious to beginning students. Experienced clinicians often think quickly, with little overt or conscious effort. They differ widely in personal style, communication skills, clinical training, experience, and interests. Some clinicians may find it difficult to explain the logic behind their clinical thinking. As an active learner, it is expected that you will ask teachers and clinicians to elaborate on the fine points of their clinical reasoning and decision making.[1,2]

Cognitive psychologists have shown that clinicians use three types of reasoning for clinical problem solving: pattern recognition, development of schemas, and application of relevant basic and clinical science.[3–6] As you gain experience, your clinical reasoning will begin at the outset of the patient encounter, not at the end. Study the steps described below, then apply them to the *Case of Mrs. N* that follows. Think about these steps as you see your first patients. As with all patients, focus on determining "What explains this patient's concerns?" and "What are the problems and diagnoses?"[7,8]

Identifying Problems and Making Diagnoses: Steps in Clinical Reasoning

- Identify abnormal findings.
- Localize findings anatomically.
- Interpret findings in terms of probable process.
- Make hypotheses about the nature of the patient's problem.
- Test the hypotheses and establish a working diagnosis.
- Develop a plan agreeable to the patient.

- **Identify abnormal findings.** Make a list of the patient's *symptoms,* the *signs* you observed during the physical examination, and any laboratory reports available to you.

- **Localize these findings anatomically.** This step may be easy. The symptom of scratchy throat and the sign of an erythematous inflamed pharynx, for example, clearly localize the problem to the pharynx. A complaint of headache leads you quickly to the structures of the skull and brain. Other symptoms, however, may present greater difficulty. Chest pain, for example, can originate in the coronary arteries, the stomach and esophagus, or the muscles and bones of the chest. If the pain is exertional and relieved by rest, either the heart or the musculoskeletal components of the chest wall may be involved. If the patient notes pain only when carrying groceries with the left arm, the musculoskeletal system becomes the likely culprit.

When localizing findings, be as specific as your data allow, but bear in mind that you may have to settle for a body region, such as the chest, or a body system, such as the musculoskeletal system. On the other hand, you may be able to define the exact structure involved, such as the left pectoral muscle. Some symptoms and signs cannot be localized, such as fatigue or fever, but are useful in the next set of steps.

● **Interpret the findings in terms of the probable process.** Patient problems often stem from a *pathologic process* involving diseases of a body structure. There are several such processes, variably classified, including congenital, inflammatory or infectious, immunologic, neoplastic, metabolic, nutritional, degenerative, vascular, traumatic, and toxic. Possible pathologic causes of headache, for example, include concussion from trauma, subarachnoid hemorrhage, or even compression from a brain tumor. Fever and stiff neck, or nuchal rigidity, are two of the classic signs of headache from meningitis. Even without other signs, such as rash or papilledema, they strongly suggest an infectious process.

Other problems are *pathophysiologic,* reflecting derangements of biologic functions, such as congestive heart failure or migraine headache. Still other problems are *psychopathologic,* such as disorders of mood like depression or headache as an expression of a somatization disorder.

● **Make hypotheses about the nature of the patient's problem.** Here you draw on all the knowledge and experience you can muster, and it is here that reading is most useful for learning about patterns of abnormalities and diseases that help you cluster your patient's findings.

By consulting the clinical literature, you embark on the lifelong goal of **evidence-based decision-making.**[9,10]

Until you gain broader knowledge and experience, you may not be able to develop highly specific hypotheses, but proceed as far as you can with the data and knowledge you have. The following steps should help:

CLINICAL REASONING: DEVELOPING HYPOTHESES ABOUT PATIENT PROBLEMS

1. *Select the most specific and critical findings to support your hypothesis.* If the patient reports "the worst headache of her life," nausea, and vomiting, for example, and you find a change in mental status, papilledema, and meningismus, build your hypothesis around elevated intracranial pressure rather than gastrointestinal disorders. Although other symptoms are useful diagnostically, they are much less specific.

2. Using your inferences about the structures and processes involved, *match your findings against all the conditions you know that can produce them.* For example, you can match your patient's papilledema with a list of conditions affecting intracranial pressure. Or you can compare the symptoms and signs associated with the patient's headache with

(continued)

CLINICAL REASONING: DEVELOPING HYPOTHESES ABOUT PATIENT PROBLEMS (CONTINUED)

the various infectious, vascular, metabolic, or neoplastic conditions that might produce this clinical picture.

3. *Eliminate the diagnostic possibilities that fail to explain the findings.* You might consider cluster headache as a cause of Mrs. N's headaches (see The Case of Mrs. N, pp. 31–35), but eliminate this hypothesis because it fails to explain the patient's throbbing bifrontal localization with intermittent nausea and vomiting. Also, the pain pattern is atypical for cluster headache—it is not unilateral, boring, or occurring repetitively at the same time over a period of days, nor is it associated with lacrimation or rhinorrhea.

4. *Weigh the competing possibilities and select the most likely diagnosis* from among the conditions that might be responsible for the patient's findings. You are looking for a close match between the patient's clinical presentation and a typical case of a given condition. Other clues help in this selection, too. The *statistical probability* of a given disease in a patient of this age, sex, ethnic group, habits, lifestyle, and locality should greatly influence your selection. You should consider the possibilities of osteoarthritis and metastatic prostate cancer in a 70-year-old man with back pain, for example, but not in a 25-year-old woman with the same complaint. The *timing of the patient's illness* also makes a difference. Headache in the setting of fever, rash, and stiff neck that develops suddenly over 24 hours suggests quite a different problem than recurrent headache over a period of years associated with stress, visual scotoma, and nausea and vomiting relieved by rest.

5. Finally, as you develop possible explanations for the patient's problem, *give special attention to potentially life-threatening and treatable conditions* such as meningococcal meningitis, bacterial endocarditis, pulmonary embolus, or subdural hematoma. Here you make every effort to minimize the risk for missing conditions that may occur less frequently or be less probable but that, if present, would be particularly ominous. *One rule of thumb is always to include "the worst case scenario" in your list of differential diagnoses* and make sure you have ruled out that possibility based on your findings and patient assessment.

See section on Evaluating Clinical Evidence, pp. 43–49.

- **Test your hypotheses.** Now that you have made a hypothesis about the patient's problem, you are ready to *test your hypothesis.* You are likely to need further history, additional maneuvers on physical examination, or laboratory studies or x-rays to confirm or rule out your tentative diagnosis or to clarify which of two or three possible diagnoses are most likely. When the diagnosis seems clear-cut—a simple upper respiratory infection or a case of hives, for example—these steps may not be necessary.

- **Establish a working diagnosis.** You can now establish a working definition of the problem. Make this at the highest level of explicitness and certainty that the data allow. You may be limited to a symptom, such as "tension headache, cause unknown." At other times, you can define a problem explicitly in terms of its structure, process, and cause. Examples include "bacterial meningitis, pneumococcal," "subarachnoid hemor-rhage, left temporoparietal lobe," or "hypertensive cardiovascular disease with left ventricular dilatation and congestive heart failure."

Although diagnoses are based primarily on identifying abnormal struc-tures, altered processes, and specific causes, you will frequently see patients whose complaints do not fall neatly into these categories. Some symp-toms defy analysis and are medically unexplained. You may never be able to move beyond simple descriptive categories such as "fatigue" or "anorexia." Other problems relate to stressful events in the patient's life. Events such as losing a job or loved one may increase the risk for subsequent illness. Identifying these events and helping the patient develop coping strategies are just as important as managing a headache or a duodenal ulcer.

See Chapter 5, Behavior and Mental Status, section on "Medically Unexplained Symptoms," pp. 136–137.

Another increasingly prominent category on problem lists is *Health Main-tenance*. Routinely listing Health Maintenance helps you track several important health concerns more effectively: immunizations, screening measures (e.g., mammograms, prostate examinations), instructions regard-ing nutrition and breast or testicular self-examinations, recommendations about exercise or use of seat belts, and responses to important life events.

● **Develop a plan agreeable to the patient.** Identify and record a *Plan* for each patient problem. Your *Plan* flows logically from the problems or diagnoses you have identified. Specify which steps are needed next. These steps range from tests to confirm or further evaluate a diagnosis; to con-sultations for subspecialty evaluation; to additions, deletions, or changes in medication; to arranging a family meeting. You will find that you will follow many of the same diagnoses over time; however, your *Plan* is often more fluid, encompassing changes and modifications that emerge from each patient visit. The *Plan* should make reference to diagnosis, therapy, and patient education.

Before finalizing your *Plan*, it is important to share your assessment and clinical thinking with the patient and seek out his or her opinions, concerns, and willingness to proceed with any further testing or evaluation. Remem-ber that patients may need to hear the same information multiple times and ways before they comprehend it. The patient should always be an active participant in the plan of care.

RECORDING YOUR FINDINGS: THE CASE OF MRS. N AND THE CHALLENGES OF CLINICAL DATA

Now turn to the case of Mrs. N and scrutinize the history, physical exami-nation, assessment, and plan. Apply your own clinical reasoning to the findings presented and begin to analyze her concerns. See if you agree with the Assessment and Plan and the priority of the problems listed.

THE CASE OF MRS. N

8/25/08 11:00 AM
Mrs. N is a pleasant, 54-year-old widowed saleswoman residing in Amarillo, Texas.
Referral. None
Source and Reliability. Self-referred; seems reliable.

Chief Complaint: "My head aches."

Present Illness: For about 3 months, Mrs. N has had increasing problems with frontal headaches. These are usually bifrontal, throbbing, and mild to moderately severe. She has missed work on several occasions because of associated nausea and vomiting. Headaches now average once a week, usually related to stress, and last 4 to 6 hours. They are relieved by sleep and putting a damp towel over the forehead. There is little relief from aspirin. No associated visual changes, motor-sensory deficits, or paresthesias.

"Sick headaches" with nausea and vomiting began at age 15, recurred throughout her mid-20s, then decreased to one every 2 or 3 months and almost disappeared.

The patient reports increased pressure at work from a new and demanding boss; she is also worried about her daughter (see *Personal and Social History*). She thinks her headaches may be like those in the past, but wants to be sure because her mother died following a stroke. She is concerned that they interfere with her work and make her irritable with her family. She eats three meals a day and drinks three cups of coffee per day; cola at night.

    Medications. Aspirin, 1 to 2 tablets every 4 to 6 hours as needed. "Water pill" in the past for ankle swelling, none recently.
    *Allergies. Ampicillin causes rash.
    Tobacco. About 1 pack of cigarettes per day since age 18 (36 pack-years).
    Alcohol/drugs. Wine on rare occasions. No illicit drugs.

Past History

Childhood Illnesses.   Measles, chickenpox. No scarlet fever or rheumatic fever.

Adult Illnesses.   **Medical:** Pyelonephritis, 1998, with fever and right flank pain; treated with ampicillin; developed generalized rash with itching several days later. Reports kidney x-rays were normal; no recurrence of infection. **Surgical:** Tonsillectomy, age 6; appendectomy, age 13. Sutures for laceration, 2001, after stepping on glass. **Ob/Gyn:** 3-3-0-3, with normal vaginal deliveries. 3 living children. Menarche age 12. Last menses 6 months ago. Little interest in sex, and not sexually active. No concerns about HIV infection. **Psychiatric:** None.

Health Maintenance.   **Immunizations:** Oral polio vaccine, year uncertain; tetanus shots × 2, 1991, followed with booster 1 year later; flu vaccine, 2000, no reaction. **Screening tests:** Last Pap smear, 2004, normal. No mammograms to date.

*You may wish to add an asterisk or underline important points.

(continued)

Gravida (G)-Parity, or # deliveries (P)-Miscarriages (M)-Living (L), or G-P-M-L 3-3-0-3

THE CASE OF MRS. N (CONTINUED)

Family History

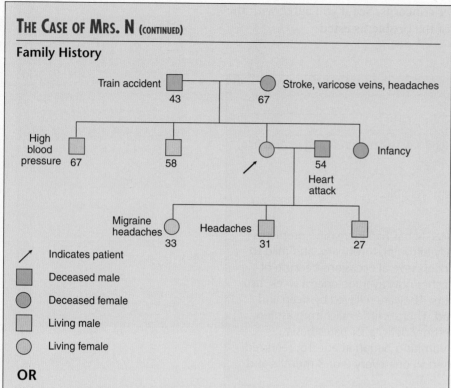

Train accident 43 — 67 Stroke, varicose veins, headaches

High blood pressure 67

58

54 Heart attack

Infancy

Migraine headaches 33

Headaches 31

27

Indicates patient

Deceased male

Deceased female

Living male

Living female

OR

Father died at age 43 in train accident. Mother died at age 67 from stroke; had varicose veins, headaches

One brother, 61, with hypertension, otherwise well; one brother, 58, well except for mild arthritis; one sister, died in infancy of unknown cause

Husband died at age 54 of heart attack

Daughter, 33, with migraine headaches, otherwise well; son, 31, with headaches; son, 27, well

No family history of diabetes, tuberculosis, heart or kidney disease, cancer, anemia, epilepsy, or mental illness.

Personal and Social History: Born and raised in Lake City, finished high school, married at age 19. Worked as sales clerk for 2 years, then moved with husband to Amarillo, had 3 children. Returned to work 15 years ago because of financial pressures. Children all married. Four years ago Mr. N died suddenly of a heart attack, leaving little savings. Mrs. N has moved to a small apartment to be near daughter, Dorothy. Dorothy's husband, Arthur, has an alcohol problem. Mrs. N's apartment now a haven for Dorothy and her 2 children, Kevin, 6 years, and Linda, 3 years. Mrs. N feels responsible for helping them; feels tense and nervous but denies depression. She has friends but rarely discusses family problems: "I'd rather keep them to myself. I don't like gossip." No church or other organizational support. She is typically up at 7:00 A.M., works 9:00 to 5:30, eats dinner alone.

Exercise and diet. Gets little exercise. Diet high in carbohydrates.
Safety measures. Uses seat belt regularly. Uses sunblock. Medications kept in an unlocked medicine cabinet. Cleaning solutions in unlocked cabinet below sink. Mr. N's shotgun and box of shells in unlocked closet upstairs.

(continued)

The Family History can be recorded as a diagram or a narrative. The diagram is more helpful than the narrative for tracing genetic disorders. The negatives from the family history should follow either format.

THE CASE OF MRS. N (CONTINUED)

Review of Systems

General. *Has *gained* about 10 lbs in the past 4 years.

Skin. No rashes or other changes.

Head, Eyes, Ears, Nose, Throat (HEENT). See *Present Illness.* No history of head injury. *Eyes:* Reading glasses for 5 years, last checked 1 year ago. No symptoms. *Ears:* Hearing good. No tinnitus, vertigo, infections. *Nose, sinuses:* Occasional mild cold. No hay fever, sinus trouble. **Throat (or mouth and pharynx):* Some bleeding of gums recently. Last dental visit 2 years ago. Occasional canker sore.

Neck. No lumps, goiter, pain. No swollen glands.

Breasts. No lumps, pain, discharge. Does breast self-examination sporadically.

Respiratory. No cough, wheezing, shortness of breath. Last chest x-ray, 1986, St. Mary's Hospital; unremarkable.

Cardiovascular. No known heart disease or high blood pressure; last blood pressure taken in 2003. No dyspnea, orthopnea, chest pain, palpitations. Has never had an electrocardiogram (ECG).

Gastrointestinal. Appetite good; no nausea, vomiting, indigestion. Bowel movement about once daily, *though sometimes has hard stools for 2 to 3 days when especially tense; no diarrhea or bleeding. No pain, jaundice, gallbladder or liver problems.

Urinary. No frequency, dysuria, hematuria, or recent flank pain; nocturia × 1, large volume. *Occasionally loses some urine when coughs hard.

Genital. No vaginal or pelvic infections. No dyspareunia.

Peripheral Vascular. Varicose veins appeared in both legs during first pregnancy. For 10 years, has had swollen ankles after prolonged standing; wears light elastic pantyhose; tried "water pill" 5 months ago, but it didn't help much; no history of phlebitis or leg pain.

Musculoskeletal. Mild, aching, low-back pain, often after a long day's work; no radiation down the legs; used to do back exercises but not now. No other joint pain.

Psychiatric. No history of depression or treatment for psychiatric disorders. See also *Present Illness* and *Personal and Social History*.

Neurologic. No fainting, seizures, motor or sensory loss. Memory good.

Hematologic. Except for bleeding gums, no easy bleeding. No anemia.

Endocrine. No known thyroid trouble, temperature intolerance. Sweating average. No symptoms or history of diabetes.

Physical Examination

Mrs. N is a short, overweight, middle-aged woman, who is animated and responds quickly to questions. She is somewhat tense, with moist, cold hands. Her hair is fixed neatly and her clothes are immaculate. Her color is good, and she lies flat without discomfort.

(continued)

THE CASE OF MRS. N (CONTINUED)

Vital Signs. Ht (without shoes) 157 cm (5'2"). Wt (dressed) 65 kg (143 lb). BMI 26. BP 164/98 right arm, supine; 160/96 left arm, supine; 152/88 right arm, supine with wide cuff. Heart rate (HR) 88 and regular. Respiratory rate (RR) 18. Temperature (oral) 98.6°F.

Skin. Palms cold and moist, but color good. Scattered cherry angiomas over upper trunk. Nails without clubbing, cyanosis.

Head, Eyes, Ears, Nose, Throat (HEENT). *Head:* Hair of average texture. Scalp without lesions, normocephalic/atraumatic (NC/AT). *Eyes:* Vision 20/30 in each eye. Visual fields full by confrontation. Conjunctiva pink; sclera white. Pupils 4 mm constricting to 2 mm, round, regular, equally reactive to light. Extraocular movements intact. Disc margins sharp, without hemorrhages, exudates. No arteriolar narrowing or A-V nicking. *Ears:* Wax partially obscures right tympanic membrane (TM); left canal clear, TM with good cone of light. Acuity good to whispered voice. Weber midline. AC > BC. *Nose:* Mucosa pink, septum midline. No sinus tenderness. *Mouth:* Oral mucosa pink. Several interdental papillae red, slightly swollen. Dentition good. Tongue midline, with 3 × 4 mm shallow white ulcer on red base on undersurface near tip; tender but not indurated. Tonsils absent. Pharynx without exudates.

Neck. Neck supple. Trachea midline. Thyroid isthmus barely palpable, lobes not felt.

Lymph Nodes. Small (<1 cm), soft, nontender, and mobile tonsillar and posterior cervical nodes bilaterally. No axillary or epitrochlear nodes. Several small inguinal nodes bilaterally, soft and nontender.

Thorax and Lungs. Thorax symmetric with good excursion. Lungs resonant. Breath sounds vesicular with no added sounds. Diaphragms descend 4 cm bilaterally.

Cardiovascular. Jugular venous pressure 1 cm above the sternal angle, with head of examining table raised to 30°. Carotid upstrokes brisk, without bruits. Apical impulse discrete and tapping, barely palpable in the 5th left interspace, 8 cm lateral to the midsternal line. Good S_1, S_2; no S_3 or S_4. A II/VI medium-pitched midsystolic murmur at the 2nd right interspace; does not radiate to the neck. No diastolic murmurs.

Breasts. Pendulous, symmetric. No masses; nipples without discharge.

Abdomen. Protuberant. Well-healed scar, right lower quadrant. Bowel sounds active. No tenderness or masses. Liver span 7 cm in right midclavicular line; edge smooth, palpable 1 cm below right costal margin (RCM). Spleen and kidneys not felt. No costovertebral angle tenderness (CVAT).

Genitalia. External genitalia without lesions. Mild cystocele at introitus on straining. Vaginal mucosa pink. Cervix pink, parous, and without discharge. Uterus anterior, midline, smooth, not enlarged. Adnexa not palpated due to obesity and poor relaxation. No cervical or adnexal tenderness. Pap smear taken. Rectovaginal wall intact.

Rectal. Rectal vault without masses. Stool brown, negative for occult blood.

Extremities. Warm and without edema. Calves supple, nontender.

(continued)

THE CASE OF MRS. N (CONTINUED)

Peripheral Vascular. Trace edema at both ankles. Moderate varicosities of saphenous veins both in lower extremities. No stasis pigmentation or ulcers. Pulses (2 + = brisk, or normal):

	Radial	Femoral	Popliteal	Dorsalis Pedis	Posterior Tibial
RT	2+	2+	2+	2+	2+
LT	2+	2+	2+	Absent	2+

Musculoskeletal. No joint deformities. Good range of motion in hands, wrists, elbows, shoulders, spine, hips, knees, ankles.

Neurologic. *Mental Status:* Tense but alert and cooperative. Thought coherent. Oriented to person, place, and time. *Cranial Nerves:* II–XII intact. *Motor:* Good muscle bulk and tone. Strength 5/5 throughout. *Cerebellar:* Rapid alternating movements (RAMs), point-to-point movements intact. Gait stable, fluid. *Sensory:* Pinprick, light touch, position sense, vibration, and stereognosis intact. Romberg negative. *Reflexes:*

	Biceps	Triceps	Brachio-radialis	Patellar	Achilles	Plantar
RT	2+	2+	2+	2+	1+	↓
LT	2+	2+	2+	2+/2+	1+	↓

OR

Laboratory Data

None currently. See Plan.

See Muscle Strength Grading, p. 680.

Two methods for recording reflexes may be used: a tabular form or a stick picture diagram; 2+ = brisk, or normal. See p. 696 for grading system.

ASSESSMENT AND PLAN

1. **Migraine headaches.** A 54-year-old woman with migraine headaches since childhood, with a throbbing vascular pattern and frequent nausea and vomiting. Headaches are associated with stress and relieved by sleep and cold compresses. There is no papilledema, and there are no motor or sensory deficits on the neurologic examination. The differential diagnosis includes tension headache, also associated with stress, but there is no relief with massage, and the pain is more throbbing than aching. There are no fever, stiff neck, or focal findings to suggest meningitis, and the lifelong recurrent pattern makes subarachnoid hemorrhage unlikely (usually described as "the worst headache of my life").

(continued)

ASSESSMENT AND PLAN (CONTINUED)

Plan:

- Discuss features of migraine vs. tension headaches.
- Discuss biofeedback and stress management.
- Advise patient to avoid caffeine, including coffee, colas, and other carbonated beverages.
- Start NSAIDs for headache, as needed.
- If needed next visit, begin prophylactic medication because patient is having more than three migraines per month.

2. **Elevated blood pressure.** Systolic hypertension with wide cuff is present. May be related to obesity, also to anxiety from first visit. No evidence of end-organ damage to retina or heart.

Plan:

- Discuss standards for assessing blood pressure.
- Recheck blood pressure in 1 month, using wide cuff.
- Check basic metabolic panel; review urinalysis.
- Introduce weight reduction, exercise programs, or both (see #4).
- Reduce salt intake.

3. **Cystocele with occasional stress incontinence.** Cystocele on pelvic examination, probably related to bladder relaxation. Patient is perimenopausal. Incontinence reported with coughing, suggesting alteration in bladder neck anatomy. No dysuria, fever, flank pain. Not taking any contributing medications. Usually involves small amounts of urine, no dribbling, so doubt urge or overflow incontinence.

Plan:

- Explain cause of stress incontinence.
- Review urinalysis.
- Recommend Kegel's exercises.
- Consider topical estrogen cream to vagina next visit if no improvement.

4. **Overweight.** Patient 5'2", weighs 143 lbs. BMI is ~26.

Plan:

- Explore diet history, ask patient to keep food intake diary.
- Explore motivation to lose weight, set target for weight loss by next visit.
- Schedule visit with dietitian.
- Discuss exercise program, specifically, walking 30 minutes most days a week.

5. **Family stress.** Son-in-law with alcohol problem; daughter and grandchildren seeking refuge in patient's apartment, leading to tensions in these relationships. Patient also has financial constraints. Stress currently situational. No current evidence of major depression.

Plan:

- Explore patient's views on strategies to cope with stress.
- Explore sources of support, including Al-Anon for daughter and financial counseling for patient.
- Continue to monitor for depression.

6. **Occasional musculoskeletal low back pain.** Usually with prolonged standing. No history of trauma or motor vehicle accident. Pain does not

(continued)

ASSESSMENT AND PLAN (CONTINUED)

radiate; no tenderness or motor-sensory deficits on examination. Doubt disc or nerve root compression, trochanteric bursitis, sacroiliitis.

Plan:

- Review benefits of weight loss and exercises to strengthen low back muscles.

7. **Tobacco abuse.** 1 pack per day for 36 years.

   Plan:

   - Check peak flow or FEV_1/FVC on office spirometry.
   - Give strong warning to stop smoking.
   - Offer referral to tobacco cessation program.
   - Offer patch, current treatment to enhance abstinence.

8. **Varicose veins, lower extremities.** No complaints currently.

9. **History of right pyelonephritis, 1998.**

10. **Ampicillin allergy.** Developed rash but no other allergic reaction.

11. **Health maintenance.** Last Pap smear 2004; has never had a mammogram.

    Plan:

    - Teach patient breast self-examination; schedule mammogram.
    - Pap smear sent today.
    - Provide three stool guaiac cards; next visit discuss screening colonoscopy.
    - Suggest dental care for mild gingivitis.
    - Advise patient to move medications and caustic cleaning agents to locked cabinet, if possible, above shoulder height.

Generating the Problem List. Now that you have completed your assessment and written record, you will find it helpful to generate a *Problem List* that summarizes the patient's problems for the front of the office or hospital chart. *List the most active and serious problems first, and record their date of onset.* Some clinicians make separate lists for active or inactive problems; others make one list in order of priority. On follow-up visits the *Problem List* helps you remember to check the status of problems the patient may not mention. The *Problem List* also allows other members of the health care team to review the patient's health status at a glance.

A sample *Problem List* for Mrs. N is provided on the following page. You may wish to give each problem a number and use the number when referring to specific problems in subsequent notes.

Clinicians organize problem lists differently, even for the same patient. Problems can be symptoms, signs, past health events such as a hospital admission or surgery, or diagnoses. You might choose different entries from those above. Good lists vary in emphasis, length, and detail, depending on the clinician's philosophy, specialty, and role as a provider. Some clinicians would find this

PROBLEM LIST: THE CASE OF MRS. N

Date Entered	Problem No.	Problem
8/30/08	1	Migraine headaches
	2	Elevated blood pressure
	3	Cystocele with occasional stress incontinence
	4	Overweight
	5	Family stress
	6	Low back pain
	7	Tobacco abuse since age 18
	8	Varicose veins
	9	History of right pyelonephritis 1998
	10	Allergy to ampicillin
	11	Health maintenance

list too long. Others would be more explicit about "family stress" or "varicose veins."

The list illustrated here includes problems that need attention now, like Mrs. N's headaches, as well as problems that need future observation and attention, such as her blood pressure and cystocele. Listing the allergy to ampicillin warns you not to prescribe medications in the penicillin family. Some symptoms such as canker sores and hard stools do not appear on this list because they are minor concerns and do not require attention during this visit. Problem lists with too many relatively insignificant items diminish in value. If these symptoms increase in importance, they can always be added at a later visit.

The Challenges of Clinical Data. As you can see from the case of Mrs. N, organizing the patient's clinical data poses several challenges. The beginning student must decide whether to cluster the patient's symptoms and signs into one problem or into several problems. The amount of data may appear unmanageable. The quality of the data may be prone to error. Guidelines to help you address these challenges are provided in the following paragraphs.

● **Clustering data into single versus multiple problems.** One of the greatest difficulties facing students is how to cluster clinical data. Do selected data fit into one problem or several problems? The patient's *age* may help—young people are more likely to have a single disease, whereas older people tend to have multiple diseases. The *timing* of symptoms is often useful. For example, an episode of pharyngitis 6 weeks ago is probably unrelated to fever, chills, pleuritic chest pain, and cough that prompt an office visit today. To use timing effectively, you need to know the natural history of various diseases and conditions. A yellow penile discharge followed 3 weeks later by a painless penile ulcer suggests two problems: gonorrhea and primary syphilis. In contrast, a penile ulcer followed in 6 weeks by a maculopapular skin rash and generalized lymphadenopathy suggest two stages of the same problem: primary and secondary syphilis.

Involvement of *different body systems* may help you to cluster the clinical data. If symptoms and signs occur in a single system, one disease may explain them. Problems in different, apparently unrelated systems often require more than one explanation. Again, knowledge of disease patterns is necessary. You might decide, for example, to group a patient's high blood pressure and sustained apical impulse together with flame-shaped retinal hemorrhages, place them in the cardiovascular system, and label the constellation "hypertensive cardiovascular disease with hypertensive retinopathy." You would develop another explanation for the patient's mild fever, left lower quadrant tenderness, and diarrhea.

Some diseases involve more than one body system. As you gain knowledge and experience, you will become increasingly adept at recognizing *multisystem conditions* and building plausible explanations that link together their seemingly unrelated manifestations. To explain cough, hemoptysis, and weight loss in a 60-year-old plumber who has smoked cigarettes for 40 years, you probably even now would rank lung cancer high in your differential diagnosis. You might support your diagnosis with your observation of the patient's cyanotic fingernails. With experience and continued reading, you will recognize that his other symptoms and signs can be linked to the same diagnosis. Dysphagia would reflect extension of the cancer to the esophagus, pupillary asymmetry would suggest pressure on the cervical sympathetic chain, and jaundice could result from metastases to the liver.

In another case of multisystem disease, a young man who presents with odynophagia, fever, weight loss, purplish skin lesions, leukoplakia, generalized lymphadenopathy, and chronic diarrhea is likely to have AIDS. Related risk factors should be explored promptly.

- **Sifting through an extensive array of data.** It is common to confront a relatively long list of symptoms and signs, and an equally long list of potential explanations. One approach is to *tease out separate clusters of observations and analyze one cluster at a time,* as just described. You can also *ask a series of key questions* that may steer your thinking in one direction and allow you to temporarily ignore the others. For example, you may ask what produces and relieves the patient's chest pain. If the answer is exercise and rest, you can focus on the cardiovascular and musculoskeletal systems and set the gastrointestinal system aside. If the pain is substernal, burning, and occurs only after meals, you can logically focus on the gastrointestinal tract. A series of discriminating questions helps you form a decision tree or algorithm that is helpful in collecting and analyzing clinical data and reaching logical conclusions and explanations.

- **Assessing the quality of the data.** Almost all clinical information is subject to error. Patients forget to mention symptoms, confuse the events of their illness, avoid recounting embarrassing facts, and often slant their stories to what the clinician wants to hear. Clinicians misinterpret patient statements, overlook information, fail to ask "the one key question," jump prematurely to conclusions and diagnoses, or forget an important part of the examination, such as the funduscopic examination in a woman with headache. You can avoid some of these errors by acquiring the habits of skilled clinicians, summarized below.

TIPS FOR ENSURING THE QUALITY OF PATIENT DATA

- Ask open-ended questions and listen carefully and patiently to the patient's story.
- Craft a thorough and systematic sequence to history taking and physical examination.
- Keep an open mind toward both the patient and the data.
- Always include "the worst-case scenario" in your list of possible explanations of the patient's problem, and make sure it can be safely eliminated.
- Analyze any mistakes in data collection or interpretation.
- Confer with colleagues and review the pertinent medical literature to clarify uncertainties.
- Apply principles of data analysis to patient information and testing.

Compose the record as soon after seeing the patient as possible, before your findings fade from memory. At first you may take notes, but work toward recording each segment of the health history during the interview, leaving spaces for filling in details later. Jot down blood pressure, heart rate, and key abnormal findings to prompt your recall when you complete the record later.

See Table 2-1, p. 53, for a Sample Progress Note for the follow-up visit of Mrs. N.

RECORDING YOUR FINDINGS: CHECKLIST FOR A CLEAR AND ACCURATE RECORD

A clear, well-organized clinical record is one of the most important adjuncts to patient care. Your skill in recording your patient's history and physical examination should evolve in parallel with your growing skills in clinical reasoning and your ability to formulate the patient's *Assessment* and *Plan*. Your goal should be a clear, concise, but comprehensive report that documents the key findings of your patient assessment and communicates the patient's problems in a succinct and *legible* format to other providers and members of the health care team. Even though your institution or agency may have printed or electronic forms for recording patient information, you should always be able to generate your own record.

Regardless of your experience, certain principles will help you to organize a good record. Think especially about the *order and readability* of the record and the *amount of detail* needed. How much detail to include often poses a vexing problem. As a student, you may wish (or be required) to be quite detailed. This helps to build your descriptive skills, vocabulary, and speed—admittedly a time-consuming process. Ultimately, however, the pressures of workload and time management will force some compromises. Nonetheless, a good record always provides the supporting evidence from the history, physical examination, and laboratory findings for all the problems or diagnoses identified.

CHECKLIST FOR A CLEAR AND ACCURATE RECORD

Is the Order Clear?

Order is imperative. Make sure that future readers, including yourself, can easily find specific points of information. Keep the *subjective* items of the history, for example, in the history; do not let them stray into the physical examination. Did you . . .

- Make the headings clear?
- Accent your organization with indentations and spacing?
- Arrange the *Present Illness* in chronologic order, starting with the current episode, then filling in relevant background information?

Do the Data Included Contribute Directly to the Assessment?

You should spell out the supporting evidence—both positive and negative—for every problem or diagnosis that you identify. Be sure there is sufficient detail to support your Assessment and Plan.

Are Pertinent Negatives Specifically Described?

Often portions of the history or examination suggest that an abnormality might exist or develop in that area.

For the patient with notable bruises, record the "pertinent negatives," such as the absence of injury or violence, familial bleeding disorders, or medications or nutritional deficits that might lead to bruising.

For the patient who is depressed but not suicidal, record both facts. In the patient with a transient mood swing, on the other hand, a comment on suicide is unnecessary.

Are There Overgeneralizations or Omissions of Important Data?

Remember that data not recorded are data lost. No matter how vividly you can recall selected details today, you will probably not remember them in a few months. The phrase "neurologic exam negative," even in your own handwriting, may leave you wondering in a few months' time, "Did I really do the sensory exam?"

Is There Too Much Detail?

Is there excess repetition of information or redundancy?

Is important information buried in a mass of detail, to be discovered by only the most persistent reader? *Omit most of your negative findings* unless they relate directly to the patient's complaints or to specific exclusions in

(continued)

CHECKLIST FOR A CLEAR AND ACCURATE RECORD (CONTINUED)

your diagnostic assessment. *Do not list abnormalities that you did not observe. Instead, concentrate on a few major ones, such as* "no heart murmurs," and try to describe structures in a concise, positive way. You can omit certain body structures even though you examined them, such as normal eyebrows and eyelashes.

"Cervix pink and smooth" indicates you saw no redness, ulcers, nodules, masses, cysts, or other suspicious lesions, but this description is shorter and readable.

Are Phrases and Short Words Used Appropriately?
Is There Unnecessary Repetition of Data?

Omit unnecessary words, such as those in parentheses in the examples. This saves valuable time and space.

"Cervix is pink (in color)." "Lungs are resonant (to percussion)." "Liver is tender (to palpation)." "Both (right and left) ears with cerumen." "II/IV systolic ejection murmur (audible)." "Thorax symmetric (bilaterally)."

Omit repetitive introductory phrases such as "The patient reports no . . . , " because readers assume the patient is the source of the history unless otherwise specified.

Use short words instead of longer, fancier ones when they mean the same thing, such as "felt" for "palpated" or "heard" for "auscultated."

Describe what you observed, not what you did. "Optic discs seen" is less informative than "disc margins sharp," even if it marks your first glimpse as an examiner!

Is the Written Style Succinct? Are There Excessive Abbreviations?

Records are scientific and legal documents, so they should be clear and understandable.

Using words and brief phrases instead of whole sentences is common, but abbreviations and symbols should be used only if they are readily understood.

Likewise, an overly elegant style is less appealing than a concise summary.

Be sure your record is legible; otherwise, all that you have recorded is worthless to your readers.

Are Diagrams and Precise Measurements Included Where Appropriate?

Diagrams add greatly to the clarity of the record.

1 x 1 cm mobile elastic nodules

1 x 1.5 cm hard central node

2 x 2 cm hard mass with dimpling of skin

liver 6 cm below RCM

spleen 4 cm below LCM on inspiration

(continued)

CHECKLIST FOR A CLEAR AND ACCURATE RECORD (CONTINUED)

To ensure accurate evaluations and future comparisons, make measurements in centimeters, not in fruits, nuts, or vegetables.

"1 × 1 cm lymph node" versus a "pea-sized lymph node . . ." Or "2 × 2 cm mass on the left lobe of the prostate" versus a "walnut-sized prostate mass."

Is the Tone of the Write-Up Neutral and Professional?

It is important to be objective. Hostile, moralizing, or disapproving comments have no place in the patient's record. Never use inflammatory or demeaning words, penmanship, or punctuation.

Comments such as "Patient DRUNK and LATE TO CLINIC AGAIN!!" are unprofessional and set a bad example for other providers reading the chart. They also might prove difficult to defend in a legal setting.

EVALUATING CLINICAL EVIDENCE

Symptoms, physical findings, tests, and x-rays should help reduce uncertainty about whether a patient does or does not have a given condition. Clinical data, including laboratory work, however, are inherently imperfect. Learn to apply the principles of *reliability, validity, sensitivity, specificity,* and *predictive value* to your clinical findings and the tests you order. These test characteristics will help you decide how confident you can be in your findings and test results as you assess the presence or absence of a disease or problem. You should also understand and apply two additional concepts: the *kappa (κ) measurement of agreement* and *likelihood ratios (LRs)*. These seven statistical tools are common measures for assessing evidence that you will find in the clinical literature. Take the time to work through these measures with your teachers, and practice using them. They will enhance lifelong learning, strengthen your clinical reasoning, and enrich decision making in your clinical practice.

Displaying Clinical Data. To use these principles, it is important to display the data in the 2 × 2 format diagrammed on the following page. Always using this format will ensure the accuracy of your calculations of sensitivity, specificity, and predictive value. Note that the presence or absence of disease implies use of a *gold standard* to establish whether the disease is truly present or absent. This is usually the best test available, such as a coronary angiogram for assessing coronary artery disease or a tissue biopsy for malignancy.

PRINCIPLES OF TEST SELECTION AND USE

Reliability. Indicates how well repeated measurements of the same relatively stable phenomenon will give the same result, also known as precision. Reliability may be measured for one observer or for more than one observer.

Example: If on several occasions one clinician consistently percusses the same span of a patient's liver dullness, *intraobserver reliability* is good. If, on the other hand, several observers find quite different spans of liver dullness on the same patient, *interobserver reliability* is poor.

Validity. Indicates how closely a given observation agrees with "the true state of affairs," or the best possible measure of reality.

Example: Blood pressure measurements by mercury-based sphygmomanometers are less valid than intra-arterial pressure tracings.

Sensitivity. Identifies the proportion of people who test positive in a group of people known to have the disease or condition, or the proportion of people who are *true positives* compared with the total number of people who actually have the disease. When the observation or test is negative in people with the disease, the result is termed *false negative. Good observations or tests have a sensitivity of more than 90%, and help rule out disease because there are few false negatives. Such observations or tests are especially useful for screening.*

Example: The sensitivity of Homan's sign in the diagnosis of deep venous thrombosis (DVT) of the calf is 50%. In other words, compared with a group of patients with deep vein thrombosis confirmed by phlebogram, a much better test, only 50% will have a positive Homan's sign, so this sign, if absent, is not helpful because 50% of patients may have a DVT.

To help remember this, experts state "when the *Se*nsitivity of a symptom or sign is high, a *N*egative response rules *out* the target disorder, and the acronym for this property is "*SnNout.*"[11]

Specificity. Identifies the proportion of people who test negative in a group of people known to be *without* a given disease or condition, or the proportion of people who are "true negatives" compared with the total number of people without the disease. When the observation or test is positive in people without the disease, the result is termed *false positive.* Good observations or tests have a specificity of more than 90% and help "rule in" disease because the test is rarely positive when disease is absent, and there are few false positives.

Example: The specificity of serum amylase in patients with possible acute pancreatitis is 70%. In other words, of 100 patients without pancreatitis, 70% will have a normal serum amylase; in 30%, the serum amylase will be falsely elevated.

Likewise, when the *Sp*ecificity is high, a *P*ositive test result rules *in* the target disorder. The acronym is "*SpPin.*"[11]

(continued)

PRINCIPLES OF TEST SELECTION AND USE (CONTINUED)

Predictive Value. Indicates how well a given symptom, sign, or test result—either positive or negative—predicts the presence or absence of disease.

Positive predictive value is the probability of disease in a patient with a positive (abnormal) test, or the proportion of "true positives" out of the total population tested.

Example: In a group of women with palpable breast nodules in a cancer screening program, the proportion with confirmed breast cancer would constitute the *positive predictive value* of palpable breast nodules for diagnosing breast cancer.

Negative predictive value is the probability of not having the condition or disease when the test is negative, or normal, or the proportion of "true negatives" out of the total population tested.

Example: In a group of women without palpable breast nodules in a cancer screening program, the proportion without confirmed breast cancer constitutes the *negative predictive value* of absence of breast nodules.

Note that the numbers related to presence or absence of disease, as determined by the gold standard, are always displayed **down the table** in the left and right columns (*present = a + c; absent = b + d*). Numbers related to the observation or test are always displayed **across the table** in the upper and lower rows (*test positive = a + b; test negative = c + d*).

Now you are ready to make your calculations:

$$\text{Sensitivity} = \frac{a}{a+c} = \frac{\text{true positive observations (95)}}{\text{total persons with disease (95 + 5)}} \times 100 = 95\%$$

$$\text{Specificity} = \frac{d}{b+d} = \frac{\text{true negative observations (90)}}{\text{total persons with disease (90 + 10)}} \times 100 = 90\%$$

$$\text{Positive predictive value} = \frac{a}{a+b} = \frac{\text{true positive observations (95)}}{\text{total positive observations (95 + 10)}} \times 100 = 90.5\%$$

$$\text{Negative predictive value} = \frac{d}{c+d} = \frac{\text{true negative observations (90)}}{\text{total negative observations (90 + 5)}} \times 100 = 94.7\%$$

Now return to the table on the previous page. *The **vertical red bars** designate sensitivity (a/a + c) and specificity (d/b + d), and the **horizontal red bars** designate positive predictive value (a/a + b) and negative predictive value (d/c + d).* The data displayed indicate that the hypothetical test has excellent test characteristics. The sensitivity and specificity of the test are both more than 90%, as are the positive and negative predictive values. Such a test would be clinically useful for assessing a disease or condition in your patient.

Note that the predictive value of a test or observation depends heavily on the *prevalence* of the condition within the population studied. Prevalence is the proportion of people in a defined population at any given point in time who have the condition in question. When the prevalence of a condition is *low,* the positive predictive value of the test will fall. When the prevalence is *high,* the sensitivity, specificity, and positive predictive value are high, and the negative predictive value approaches zero. To work further on these relationships, turn to the following boxes on Prevalence and Predictive Value, and practice making the calculations described.

PREVALENCE AND PREDICTIVE VALUE

Two examples further illustrate these principles and show *how predictive values vary with prevalence.* Consider first (*Example 1*) an imaginary population *A* with 1,000 people. The prevalence of disease *X* in this population is high—40%. You can quickly calculate that 400 of these people have *X.* You then set out to detect these cases with an observation or test that is 90% sensitive and 80% specific. Of the 400 people with *X,* the observation reveals .90 × 400, or 360 (the true positives). It misses the other 40 (400 − 360, the false negatives). Out of the 600 people without *X,* the observation or test proves negative in .80 × 600, or 480. These people are truly free of *X,* as the observation suggests (the true negatives). But the observation misleads you in the remaining 120 (600 − 480). These people are

(continued)

PREVALENCE AND PREDICTIVE VALUE (CONTINUED)

falsely labeled as having X when they are really free of it (the false positives). These figures are summarized below:

Example 1. Prevalence of Disease X = 40%

As a clinician who does not have perfect knowledge of who really does or does not have disease X, you are faced with a total of 480 people with positive observations. You must try to distinguish between the true and the false positives and will undoubtedly use additional kinds of data to help you in this task. Given only the sensitivity and specificity of your observation, however, you can determine the probability that a positive observation is a true positive, and you may wish to explain it to the concerned patient. This probability is calculated as follows:

$$\textit{Positive predictive value} = \frac{a}{a+b} = \frac{\text{true positives (360)}}{\text{total positives (360 + 120)}} \times 100 = 75\%$$

Thus, 3 out of 4 of the people with positive observations really have the disease, and 1 out of 4 does not.

By a similar calculation, you can determine the probability that a negative observation is a true negative. The results here are reasonably reassuring to the involved patient:

$$\textit{Negative predictive value} = \frac{d}{c+d} = \frac{\text{true negatives (480)}}{\text{total negatives (40 + 480)}} \times 100 = 92\%$$

As *prevalence* of the disease in a population diminishes, however, the predictive value of a positive observation diminishes remarkably, while the predictive value of a negative observation rises further. In *Example 2,* in a second population, *B,* of 1,000 people, only 1% have disease X. Now there are only 10 cases of X and 990 people without X. If this population is

(continued)

PREVALENCE AND PREDICTIVE VALUE (CONTINUED)

screened with the same observation, which has a 90% sensitivity and an 80% specificity, here are the results:

Example 2. Prevalence of Disease X = 1%

You are now confronted with possibly upsetting 207 people (all those with positive observations) to detect 9 out of the 10 real cases. The predictive value of a positive observation is only 4%. Improving the specificity of your observation without diminishing its sensitivity would be very helpful, if it were possible. For example, if you could increase the specificity of the observation from 80% to 98% (given the same prevalence of 1% and sensitivity of 90%), the positive predictive value of the observation would improve from 4% to 31%—scarcely ideal but certainly better. Good observations or tests have a sensitivity and specificity of 90% or greater.

Because prevalence strongly affects the predictive value of an observation, prevalence too influences the assessment process. Because coronary artery disease is much more common in middle-aged men than in young women, you should pursue angina as a cause of chest pain more actively in the former group. The effect of prevalence on predictive value explains why your odds of making a correct assessment are better when you hypothesize a common condition rather than a rare one. The combination of fever, headache, myalgias, and cough probably has the same sensitivity and specificity for influenza throughout the year, but your chance of making this diagnosis correctly by using this cluster of symptoms is much greater during a winter flu epidemic than it is during a quiet August.

Prevalence varies importantly with clinical setting as well as with season. Chronic bronchitis is probably the most common cause of hemoptysis among patients seen in a general medical clinic. In the oncology clinic of a tertiary medical center, however, lung cancer might head the list, while in a group of postoperative patients on a general surgical service, irritation from an endotracheal tube or pulmonary infarction might be most likely. In certain parts of Asia, in contrast, one should think first of a worm called a lung fluke. When you hear hoofbeats in the distance, according to the familiar saying, bet on horses, not on zebras, unless, of course, you're visiting the zoo.

Two other statistics are also clinically useful: the κ statistic for measuring degree of observer agreement, and *likelihood ratios*. Students are encouraged to pursue these concepts through further reading.[12–14]

Likelihood ratio (LR). Conveys the odds that a finding occurs in a patient with the condition compared to a patient without the condition. When the LR is greater than 1.0, the probability of the condition goes up; when the LR is less than 1.0, the probability of the condition goes down.

- A positive LR = $\dfrac{\text{sensitivity}}{(1 - \text{specificity})}$

- A negative LR = $\dfrac{\text{specificity}}{(1 - \text{sensitivity})}$

Kappa (κ) measurement of inter-observer agreement. Measures the degree of observer agreement, or precision, of a clinical finding compared to agreement by chance alone, similar to a correlation coefficient.

Conventional levels of κ are slight agreement = 0.0–0.2; fair = 0.2–0.4; moderate = 0.4–0.6; substantial = 0.8–1.0.[11]

Example. The LR of subarachnoid hemorrhage is 10 if neck stiffness is present, and 0.4 if neck stiffness is absent. Subarachnoid hemorrhage is 10 times more likely when neck stiffness is present than absent. A negative history of neck stiffness is 0.4 times as likely in a patient with, as opposed to a patient without, subarachnoid hemorrhage.

Example. Two clinicians agree 89% of the time that a patient has a migraine headache. Calculations show that their expected agreement is 59% based on chance alone. Their remaining potential agreement beyond chance (100%–59%) is 41%, and their actual agreement beyond chance is 30% (89%–59%). The κ measure of their agreement is 30%/41%, or 0.73. The chance of two clinicians agreeing that migraine is present is moderately high.

LIFELONG LEARNING: INTEGRATING CLINICAL REASONING, ASSESSMENT, AND ANALYSIS OF CLINICAL EVIDENCE

The concepts of sensitivity and specificity help in both the collection and the analysis of data. They even underlie some of the basic strategies of interviewing. Questions with high sensitivity, if answered in the affirmative, may be particularly useful for screening and for gathering evidence to support a hypothesis. For example, "Have you had any discomfort or pain in your chest?" is a highly sensitive question for diagnosing angina pectoris. For patients with this condition, there would be few false-negative responses. Thus, it is a good first screening question. However, because there are many other causes of chest discomfort, it is not highly specific. Pain that is retrosternal, pressing, and less than 10 minutes in duration—each a reasonably sensitive attribute of angina—would add importantly to your growing evidence for the diagnosis. To confirm your hypothesis, a more specific question, if answered in the affirmative, is needed, such as "Is the pain precipitated by exertion?" or "Is the pain relieved by rest?"

Data for testing hypotheses also come from the physical examination. Heart murmurs are good examples of findings with varying sensitivity and specificity. The vast majority of patients with significant valvular *aortic stenosis* have systolic ejection murmurs audible in the aortic area. Presence of a systolic murmur has a high sensitivity for aortic stenosis. This finding is present in most cases. The false-negative rate is low. On the other hand, many other conditions produce systolic murmurs, such as increased blood flow across a normal valve, or the sclerotic changes associated with aging, termed aortic sclerosis, so the finding of a systolic murmur is not very specific. Using such a murmur as your only criterion for diagnosing aortic stenosis would lead to many false positives.

In contrast, a high-pitched, soft blowing decrescendo diastolic murmur best heard along the left sternal border is quite specific for *aortic regurgitation*. Such a murmur is almost never heard in normal people, and it is present in very few other conditions, so there are few false positives.

Combining data from the history and physical examination allows you to test your hypotheses, screen for selected conditions, build your case, and clinch a diagnosis even before obtaining further diagnostic tests. Consider the following list of evidence: cough, fever, a shaking chill, left-sided pleuritic chest pain, dullness throughout the left lower posterior lung field with crackles, bronchial breathing, and egophony. Cough and fever are good screening items for pneumonia, the next items support the hypothesis, and bronchial breathing with egophony in this distribution is very specific for lobar pneumonia. A chest x-ray would confirm the diagnosis.

Absence of selected symptoms and signs is also diagnostically useful, especially when they are usually present in a given condition (i.e., their sensitivity is high). For example, if a patient with cough and left-sided pleuritic chest pain does not have fever, bacterial pneumonia becomes much less likely (except possibly in infancy and old age). Likewise, in a patient with severe dyspnea, the absence of orthopnea makes left ventricular failure less probable as an explanation for shortness of breath.

Skilled clinicians use this kind of logic even if they are unaware of its statistical underpinnings. They start to generate tentative hypotheses as soon as the patient describes the *Chief Complaint*, then build evidence for one or more of these hypotheses and discard others as they continue with the history and examination. In developing a *Present Illness,* they borrow items from other parts of the history, such as the *Past Medical History,* the *Family History,* and the *Review of Systems.* In a 55-year-old man with chest pain, the skilled clinician does not stop with the attributes of pain, but moves on to probe risk factors from coronary artery disease such as family history, hypertension, diabetes, lipid abnormalities, and smoking. In both the history and physical examination, the clinician searches explicitly for other possible manifestations of cardiovascular disease such as congestive heart failure or the claudication or diminished lower extremity pulses of atherosclerotic peripheral vascular disease. By generating hypotheses early and testing them sequentially, experienced clinicians improve their efficiency and enhance the relevance and value of the data they collect. They dig and collect less ore but find more gold.

This sequence of collecting data and testing hypotheses is diagrammed below.

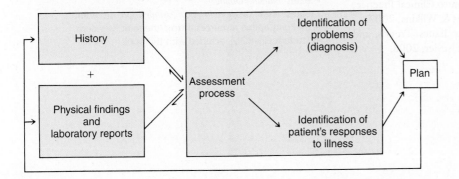

After the plan has been implemented, the process recycles. The clinician gathers more data, assesses the patient's progress, modifies the problem list if indicated, and adjusts the plan accordingly. As you gain experience, the interplay of assessment, data collection, and knowledge from the clinical literature will become increasingly familiar. You will come to value the challenges and rewards of clinical reasoning and assessment that make patient care so meaningful.

BIBLIOGRAPHY

CITATIONS

1. Peterson MC, Holbrook JH, Von Hales DE, et al. Contributions of the history, physical examination, and laboratory investigation in making medical diagnoses. West J Med 156(2): 163–165, 1992.
2. Hampton JR, Harrison MJ, Mitchell JRA, et al. Relative contributions of history-taking, physical examination, and laboratory investigation to diagnosis and management of medical outpatients. Brit Med J 2(5969):486–489, 1975.
3. Bowen J. Educational strategies to promote clinical diagnostic reasoning. New Engl J Med 355(21): 2217–2225, 2006.
4. Coderre S, Mandin H, Harasym P, et al. Diagnostic reasoning strategies and diagnostic success. Med Educ 37(8):695–703, 2003.
5. Elstein A, Schwarz A. Clinical problem solving and diagnosis decision making: selective review of the cognitive literature. Brit Med J 324(7339):729–732, 2002.
6. Norman, G. Research in clinical reasoning: past history and current trends. Med Educ 39(4):418–427, 2005.
7. Schneiderman H. Bedside Diagnosis. An Annotated Bibliography of Literature on Physical Examination and Interviewing, 3rd ed. Philadelphia: American College of Physicians, 1997.
8. McGee S. Evidence Based Physical Diagnosis, 2nd ed. St. Louis: Saunders/Elsevier, 2007.
9. Evidence-Based Medicine Working Group. Evidence-based medicine: a new approach to teaching the practice of medicine. JAMA 268(17):2420–2425, 1992.

10. Guyatt G. Users' Guide to the Medical Literature: A Manual for Evidence-Based Clinical Practice. New York: McGraw-Hill Medical, 2008.

11. Sackett D. A primer on the precision and accuracy of the clinical examination. JAMA 267(19):2638–2644, 1992.

12. Fletcher RH, Fletcher SW. Clinical Epidemiology: The Essentials, 4th ed. Philadelphia: Lippincott Williams & Wilkins, 2005.

13. Black E (ed). Diagnostic Strategies in Common Medical Problems, 2nd ed. Philadelphia: American College of Physicians, 1999.

14. Sackett DL. Evidence-Based Medicine: How to Practice and Teach EBM, 2nd ed. New York: Churchill Livingstone, 2000.

ADDITIONAL REFERENCES

Alfaro-LeFevre R. Critical Thinking and Clinical Judgment: A Practical Approach to Outcome-Focused Thinking, 4th ed. St. Louis: WB Saunders–Elsevier, 2009.

Carpenito LJ. Nursing Diagnosis: Application to Clinical Practice, 12th ed. Philadelphia: Lippincott Williams & Wilkins, 2007.

Cherry B, Jacob SR. Contemporary Nursing: Issues, Trends, and Management, 4th ed. St. Louis: Mosby–Elsevier, 2008.

Fletcher RH, Fletcher SW. Clinical Epidemiology: The Essentials, 4th ed. Philadelphia: Lippincott Williams & Wilkins, 2005.

Innui TS. Establishing the doctor–patient relationship: science, art, or competence? Schweiz Med Wochenschr 128:225, 1998.

Laditka JN, Laditka SB, Mastanduno MP. Hospital utilization for ambulatory care sensitive conditions: health outcome disparities associated with race and ethnicity. Soc Sci Med 57(8):1429–1441, 2003.

Nettina SM. The Lippincott Manual of Nursing Practice Handbook, 3rd ed. Ambler, PA: Lippincott Williams & Wilkins, 2006.

Sackett DL. Evidence-based Medicine: How to Practice and Teach EBM, 2nd ed. New York: Churchill Livingstone, 2000.

The Bates' suite offers these additional resources to enhance learning and facilitate understanding of this chapter:

- Bates' *Pocket Guide to Physical Examination and History Taking*, 6th edition
- Bates' *Nursing Online*
- Bates' *Visual Guide to Physical Examination*, 4th edition
- thePoint online resources, http://thepoint.lww.com
- Student CD-ROM included with the book

TABLE
2-1

Sample Progress Note

A month later, Mrs. N returns for a follow-up visit. The format of the office progress note is quite variable, but it should meet the same standards as the initial assessment. The note should be clear, sufficiently detailed, and easy to follow. It should reflect your clinical reasoning and delineate your assessment and plan. Be sure to learn the documentation standards for billing in your institution, because this can affect the detail and type of information needed in your progress notes.

The note below follows the SOAP format: **S**ubjective, **O**bjective, **A**ssessment, and **P**lan. You will see many other styles, some focused on the "patient-centered" record. The terms for SOAP are often not listed, but implied. Frequently clinicians record the history and physical examination, then document the plan with the listing of each problem and its assessment.

9/25/08

Mrs. N returns to the clinic for follow-up of her migraine headaches. She states that she has fewer headaches since avoiding caffeinated beverages. She is now drinking decaffeinated coffee and has stopped drinking colas. She has joined a support group and started exercising to reduce stress. She is still having one to two headaches a month with some nausea, but they are less severe and generally relieved with NSAIDs. She denies any fever, stiff neck, associated visual changes, motor-sensory deficits, or paresthesias.

She has been checking her blood pressure at home. It is running about 150/90. She is walking 30 minutes three times a week in her neighborhood and has reduced her total daily calorie intake. She has been unable to stop smoking She has been doing the Kegel's exercises but still has some leakage with coughing or laughing.

Medications: Motrin 400 mg up to
three times daily as needed for headache
Allergies: Ampicillin causes rash
Tobacco: 1 pack per day since age 18

Physical Examination: Pleasant, overweight, middle-aged woman, who is animated and somewhat tense. Ht 157 cm (5' 2"). Wt 63 kg (140 lbs). BMI 26. BP 150/90. HR 86 and regular. RR 16. Afebrile.
Skin: No suspicious nevi. *HEENT*: Normocephalic, atraumatic. Pharynx without exudates. *Neck*: Supple, without thyromegaly. *Lymph nodes*: No lymphadenopathy. *Lungs*: Resonant and clear. *CV*: JVP 6 cm above the right atrium; carotid upstrokes brisk, no bruits. Good S_1, S_2. No murmurs heard today. No S_3, S_4. *Abdomen*: Active bowel sounds. Soft, nontender, no hepatosplenomegaly. *Extremities*: Without edema.

Labs: Basic metabolic panel and urinalysis from 8/25/08 unremarkable. Pap smear normal.

Impression and Plan

1. Migraine headaches—now down to one to two per month due to reductions in caffeinated beverages and stress. Headaches are responding to NSAIDs.
   • Will defer daily prophylactic medication for now because patient is having less than three headaches per month and feels better
   • Affirm need to stop smoking and to continue exercise program
   • Affirm patient's participation in support group to reduce stress

2. Elevated blood pressure—BP remains elevated at 150/90.
   • Will initiate therapy with a diuretic
   • Patient to take blood pressure three times a week and bring recordings to next office visit
   • Affirm need to exercise, lose weight, and stop smoking

3. Cystocele with occasional stress incontinence—stress incontinence improved with Kegel's exercises but still with some urine leakage. Urinalysis from last visit—no infection
   • Initiate vaginal estrogen cream
   • Continue Kegel's exercises

4. Overweight—has lost ~ 4 lbs.
   • Continue exercise
   • Review diet history; affirm weight reduction.

5. Family stress—patient handling this better. See Plans above.

6. Occasional low back pain—no complaints today

7. Tobacco abuse—see Plans above

8. Health maintenance—Pap smear sent last visit. Mammogram scheduled. Colonoscopy recommended.

Interviewing and the Health History

The health history interview is a conversation with a purpose. As you learn to elicit the patient's history, you will draw on many of the interpersonal skills that you use every day, but with unique and important differences. Unlike social conversation, in which you can freely express your own needs and interests and are responsible only for yourself, the primary goal of the clinician–patient interview is to improve the well-being of the patient. At its most basic level, the purpose of conversation with a patient is three-fold: to establish a trusting and supportive relationship, to gather information, and to offer information.[1–3]

Relating effectively with patients is among the most valued skills of clinical care. As a beginning clinician, you will focus your energies on gathering information. At the same time, by using techniques that promote trust and convey respect, you will allow the patient's story to unfold in its most full and detailed form. Establishing a supportive interaction helps the patient feel more at ease when sharing information and itself becomes the foundation for therapeutic clinician–patient relationships.[4] Because illness can make patients feel discouraged and isolated, "A feeling of connectedness with the doctor, of being deeply heard and understood, reduces this feeling of isolation and despair. This feeling is the very heart of healing."[5]

This chapter introduces you to the essentials of interviewing. It emphasizes the approach to gathering the health history, but covers all the fundamental habits that you will continually use and refine in your conversations with patients. You will learn the guiding principles for skilled interviewing and how to forge trusting patient relationships. You will read about preparing for the interview, the sequence of the interviewing process, important interviewing techniques, and strategies for addressing various challenges that may arise in patient encounters. To help you navigate this journey, look over the Interviewing Milestones at the end of this section that mark the complex tasks of a skilled interview.

As a clinician facilitating the patient's story, you will generate a series of hypotheses about the nature of the patient's concerns. You will then test these various hypotheses by asking for more detailed information. You will also explore the patient's feelings and beliefs about his or her problem. Eventually, as your clinical experience grows, you will respond with your understanding of the patient's concerns. If you discover that the patient's greatest need is for support and empathy, encouraging the patient to discuss the *experience of*

illness is itself therapeutic, as shown by the words below from a patient with long-standing and severe arthritis:

> The patient had never talked about what the symptoms meant to her. She had never said: "This means that I can't go to the bathroom by myself, put my clothes on, even get out of bed without calling for help."
>
> When we finished the physical examination I said something like: "Rheumatoid arthritis really has not been nice to you." She burst into tears, and her daughter did also, and I sat there, very close to losing it myself.
>
> She said: "You know, no one has ever talked about it as a personal thing before. No one's ever talked to me as if this were a thing that mattered, a personal event."
>
> That was the significant thing about the encounter. I didn't really have much else to offer. . . . But something really significant had happened between us, something that she valued and would carry away with her.[6]

As you can see from this story, the *process* of interviewing patients requires a highly refined sensitivity to the patient's feelings and behavioral cues and is much more than just asking a series of questions. This process differs significantly from the *format* for the health history presented in Chapter 1. Both are fundamental to your work with patients but serve different purposes:

- The *health history format* is a structured framework for organizing patient information in *written or verbal form* for other health care providers; it focuses the clinician's attention on specific kinds of information that must be obtained from the patient.

- The *interviewing process* that actually generates these pieces of information is much more fluid and demands effective communication and relational skills. It requires not only knowledge of the data that you need to obtain but also the ability to elicit accurate information and the interpersonal skills that allow you to respond to the patient's feelings and concerns.

Underlying the new interviewing skills that you will learn is a mindset that allows you to collaborate with the patient and build a healing relationship.

Different Kinds of Health Histories.
As you learned in Chapter 1, the kinds of information you seek vary according to several factors. The scope and degree of detail depend on the patient's needs and concerns, the clinician's goals for the encounter, and the clinical setting (e.g., inpatient or outpatient, amount of time available, primary care or subspecialty).

- For new patients, in most settings, you will do a *comprehensive health history*.

- For patients who seek care for specific complaints, for example, cough or painful urination, a more limited interview tailored to that specific problem may be indicated; this is sometimes known as a *problem-oriented history*.

See Chapter 1, Overview: Physical Examination and History Taking, pp. 3–24.

● For patients who seek care for ongoing or chronic problems, an interview focusing on the patient's self-management, status of the problem(s), and functional capacity including quality of life, is most appropriate.[7]

In a primary care setting, clinicians frequently choose to address issues of health promotion, such as tobacco cessation or reduction of high-risk sexual behaviors. A subspecialist may do an in-depth history to evaluate one problem that incorporates a wide range of areas of inquiry. Knowing the content and relevance of all the components of a comprehensive health history enables you to select the kinds of information most helpful for meeting both clinician and patient goals. Be assured that you will fully gain the knowledge of what types of information to pursue, and when to pursue them, as you deepen your clinical experience.

Interviewing Milestones

Getting Ready: The Approach to the Interview

Taking time for self-reflection. Reviewing the medical record. Reviewing your clinical behavior and appearance. Adjusting the environment. Taking notes.

Learning About the Patient: The Sequence of the Interview

Greeting the patient and establishing rapport. Inviting the patient's story. Setting the agenda for the interview. Expanding and clarifying the patient's story. Creating a shared understanding of the patient's concerns. Negotiating a plan. Following up and closing the interview.

Building the Relationship: The Techniques of Skilled Interviewing

Active listening. Guided questioning. Nonverbal communication. Empathic responses. Validation. Reassurance. Partnering. Summarization. Transitions. Empowering the patient.

Adapting Your Interview to Specific Situations

The silent patient. The confusing patient. The patient with impaired capacity. The talkative patient. The angry or disruptive patient. Interviewing across a language barrier. The patient with low literacy. The deaf or hard-of-hearing patient. The blind patient. The patient with limited intelligence. The patient seeking personal advice.

Sensitive Topics that Call for Special Skills

The sexual history. Mental health. Alcohol and drug use. Family violence. Death and dying.

Societal Aspects of Interviewing

Demonstrating cultural humility. Sexuality in the clinician–patient relationship. Ethics and professionalism.

GETTING READY: THE APPROACH TO THE INTERVIEW

Interviewing patients requires planning. You are undoubtedly eager to begin your relationship with the patient, but first consider several steps that are crucial to success: taking time for self-reflection, reviewing the medical record, setting goals for the interview, reviewing your behavior and appearance, adjusting the environment, and being ready to take brief notes.

Taking Time for Self-Reflection.   As clinicians, we encounter a wide variety of patients, each one unique. Establishing relationships with people from a broad spectrum of ages, social classes, races, ethnicities, and states of *health or illness* is an uncommon opportunity and privilege. Being consistently respectful and open to individual differences is one of the clinician's challenges. Because we bring our own values, assumptions, and biases to every encounter, we must look inward to clarify how our own expectations and reactions may affect what we hear and how we behave. *Self-reflection is a continual part of professional development in clinical work. It brings a deepening personal awareness to our work with patients, which is one of the most rewarding aspects of patient care.*[8]

Reviewing the Medical Record.   Before seeing the patient, review the medical record. This helps you gather information and plan what areas you need to explore with the patient. Look closely at identifying data such as age, gender, address, and health insurance, and peruse the problem list, the medication list, and details such as the documentation of allergies. The chart often provides valuable information about past diagnoses and treat-

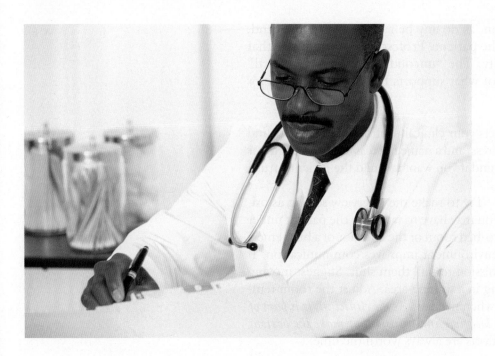

ments, but do not let previous documentation prevent you from developing new approaches or ideas. Remember that information in the medical record comes from different observers and that standardized forms reflect different institutional norms. Moreover, the medical record is not designed to capture the essence of the unique person you are about to meet. Data may be incomplete or even disagree with what you learn from the patient—understanding such discrepancies may prove helpful to the patient's care.

Setting Goals for the Interview.   Before you begin talking with the patient, it is important to clarify your goals for the interview. As a student, your goal may be to obtain a comprehensive health history so that you can submit a write-up to your teacher. As a clinician, your goals range from completing forms for standard health care institutions, to following up on health care issues, to testing hypotheses generated by your review of the chart. *A clinician must balance these provider-centered goals with patient-centered goals.* There can be tension between the needs of the provider, the institution, and the patient and family. Part of the clinician's task is to consider these multiple agendas. By taking a few minutes to think through your goals ahead of time, you will find it easier to strike a healthy balance among the various purposes of the interview to come.

Reviewing Your Clinical Behavior and Appearance.   Just as you carefully observe the patient throughout the interview, the patient will be watching you. Consciously or not, you send messages through both your words and your behavior. Be sensitive to those messages and manage them as well as you can. Posture, gestures, eye contact, and tone of voice all convey the extent of your interest, attention, acceptance, and understanding. The skilled interviewer seems calm and unhurried, even when time is limited. Reactions that betray disapproval, embarrassment, impatience, or boredom block communication, as do any behaviors that condescend, stereotype, criticize, or belittle the patient. Professionalism requires that the physician maintain equanimity. The "unconditional positive regard" espoused by Carl Rogers is part of what supports healing in relationships with patients.[9]

Your personal appearance also affects your clinical relationships. Patients find cleanliness, neatness, conservative dress, and a name tag reassuring. Remember to keep *the patient's perspective* in mind if you want to build the patient's trust.

Adjusting the Environment.

Try to make the interview setting as private and comfortable as possible. You may have to talk with the patient under difficult circumstances, such as a two-bed room or the corridor of a busy emergency department, but a proper environment improves communication. If there are privacy curtains, ask permission to pull them shut. Suggest moving to an empty room instead of talking in a waiting area. Adjust the room temperature for the patient's comfort when needed. *As the clinician, it is part of your job to make adjustments to the location and seating that make the patient and you more comfortable.* These efforts are always worth the time.

Taking Notes.

As a novice, you may need to write down much of what you learn during the interview. Even though experienced clinicians recall much of the interview without taking notes, no one can remember all the details of a comprehensive history. Jot down short phrases, specific dates, or words rather than trying to put them into a final format, but do not let note-taking or written or electronic forms distract you from the patient. Maintain good eye contact, and whenever the patient is talking about sensitive or disturbing material, put down your pen or move away from the keyboard. Most patients are accustomed to note-taking, but for those who find it uncomfortable, explore their concerns and explain your need to make an accurate record. When using an electronic health record, review the patient's record before entering the room; elicit the patient's story while directly facing the patient, maintaining eye contact, and observing all nonverbal behavior; and address the viewing screen only after the establishment of the relationship and with the patient included in the process.[10]

LEARNING ABOUT THE PATIENT: THE SEQUENCE OF THE INTERVIEW

Once you have devoted time and thought to preparing for the interview, you are fully ready to listen to the patient, elicit the patient's concerns, and learn about the patient's health. In general, an interview moves through several stages. *Throughout this sequence you, as the clinician, must always be attuned to the patient's feelings, help the patient express them, respond to their content, and validate their significance.* A typical sequence follows.

Learning About the Patient: The Sequence of the Interview

- Greeting the patient and establishing rapport
- Establishing the agenda for the interview
- Inviting the patient's story
- Identifying and responding to emotional cues
- Expanding and clarifying the patient's story
- Generating and testing diagnostic hypotheses
- Creating a shared understanding of the problem
- Negotiating a plan, including further evaluation, treatment, patient education and self-management support, and prevention
- Planning for follow-up and closing

As a student, you will concentrate primarily on gathering the patient's story and creating a shared understanding of the problem. As you become a practicing clinician, reaching agreement on a plan for further evaluation and treatment becomes more important. Whether the interview is comprehensive or focused, you should move through this sequence with close attention to the patient's feelings and affect, always working on strengthening the relationship. Attention to the patient's perspective when gathering data and forming hypotheses, including the patient's feelings, ideas, expectations, and their effects on daily function, facilitates a broader range of therapeutic interventions.

Greeting the Patient and Establishing Rapport.

The initial moments of your encounter with the patient lay the foundation for your ongoing relationship. How you greet the patient and other visitors in the room, provide for the patient's comfort, and arrange the physical setting all shape the patient's first impressions.

As you begin, *greet the patient* by name and introduce yourself, giving your own name. If possible, shake hands with the patient. If this is the first contact, explain your role, including your status as a student and how you will be involved in the patient's care. Repeat this part of the introduction on subsequent meetings until you are confident that the patient knows who you are: "Good Morning, Mr. Peters. I am Susannah Martinez, a third-year medical student. You may remember me. I was here yesterday talking with you about your heart problems. I am part of the medical team taking care of you."

Using a formal title to address the patient—Mr. O'Neil or Ms. Washington for example—is always best.[11,12] Except with children or adolescents, avoid first names unless you have specific permission from the patient or family. Addressing an unfamiliar adult as "granny" or "dear" can depersonalize and demean. If you are unsure how to pronounce the patient's name, don't be afraid to ask. You can say: "I am afraid of mispronouncing your name. Could you say it for me?" Then repeat it to make sure that you heard it correctly.

When visitors are in the room, be sure to acknowledge and greet each one in turn, inquiring about each person's name and relationship to the patient.

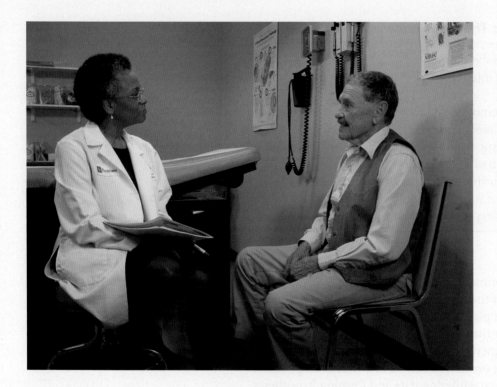

Whenever visitors are present, *you are obligated to maintain the patient's confidentiality.* Let the patient decide if visitors or family members should remain in the room, and ask for the patient's permission before conducting the interview in front of them. For example, "I am comfortable with having your sister stay for the interview, Mrs. Jones, but I want to make sure that this is also what you want" or "Would you prefer if I spoke to you alone or with your sister present?"

Always be attuned to the patient's comfort. In the office or clinic, help the patient find a suitable place for coats and belongings. In the hospital, after greeting the patient, ask how the patient is feeling and if you are coming at a convenient time. Arranging the bed to make the patient more comfortable or allowing a few minutes for the patient to say goodbye to visitors or finish using the bedpan demonstrates your awareness of the patient's needs. In any setting, look for signs of discomfort, such as shifting position or facial expressions showing pain or anxiety. You must attend to pain or anxiety first, both to encourage the patient's trust and to allow enough ease for the interview to proceed.

Consider the best way to *arrange the room* and how far you should be from the patient. Remember that cultural background and individual taste influence preferences about interpersonal space. Choose a distance that facilitates conversation and allows good eye contact. You should probably be within several feet, close enough to be intimate but not intrusive. Pull up a chair and, if possible, sit at eye level with the patient. Move any physical barriers, like desks or bedside tables, out of the way. In an outpatient setting, sitting on a rolling stool, for example, allows you to change distances in response to patient cues. Avoid arrangements that convey disrespect or inequality of power, such as interviewing a woman already positioned for a pelvic examination. Such arrangements are unacceptable. Lighting also makes a difference. If you sit between a patient and a bright light or window, although your view might be good, the patient may have to squint uncomfortably to see you, making the interaction more like an interrogation than a supportive interview.

As you begin the interview, give the patient your undivided attention. Spend enough time on small talk to put the patient at ease, and avoid looking down to take notes, read the chart, or scan a computer screen. In a first meeting, demonstrate interest in the patient as a person. In a non-acute situation, for example, you can begin by asking, "So that I can get to know you, tell me about yourself."[13]

Establishing the Agenda.   Now that you have established rapport, you are ready to pursue the patient's reason for seeking health care. This reason is traditionally designated the *chief complaint,* but in the ambulatory setting, where there are often three or four reasons for the visit, the phrase *presenting problem(s)* may be preferable.[14,15] An additional benefit to this phrase is that it does not characterize the patient as a complainer. Begin with ***open-ended questions*** that allow full freedom of response: "What concerns bring you here today?" or "How can I help you?" Helpful open-ended questions are "Are there specific concerns that prompted you to schedule this appointment?" and "What made you decide to come in to see us today?" Note that these questions encourage the patient to express any possible concerns and do not restrict the patient to a medical problem *per se*. Sometimes patients do not give a specific problem; they ask for "just a check-up." They may even give one reason to the nurse, and another to the doctor. An important fact to remember is that the first problem the patient brings up is not necessarily the most important one. In fact, when the chief reason for coming is psychosocial, it is usually *not* the first reason the patient mentions. The order in which problems are related is not connected to their clinical importance.[16]

Identifying all the concerns at the beginning of the interview allows the patient and the clinician to negotiate which concerns are most pressing for the visit, and which can be postponed to a follow-up appointment. Questions such as "Is there anything else?" or "Have we got everything?" help elicit the patient's complete list of reasons for coming to the office. The clinician may also have concerns such as elevated blood pressure or discussing an abnormal laboratory result. Identifying the full agenda or even the "real reason" for the visit at the outset makes use of the time available more meaningful, facilitates time management, and reduces the short shrift given to late-emerging concerns, although negotiating the agenda at the outset still does not always avert the "hand on the doorknob syndrome."[17]

Inviting the Patient's Story.   Once you have elicited, negotiated, and prioritized the agenda, invite the patient's story by asking about the foremost concern and saying, "Tell me more about . . ." Continue to encourage the patient to tell his or her story in his or her own words, using *a nonfocusing approach*.[18] Avoid biasing the patient's story—*inject no new information* and *do not interrupt*. Instead use active listening skills: lean forward as you listen; add continuers such as nodding your head and phrases like "uh huh," "go on," or "I see." Train yourself to *follow the patient's leads*. If you intervene too early or ask specific questions prematurely, you risk trampling on the very information you are seeking.[14] Studies show that clinicians interrupt patients during office visits after only 18 seconds.[16] Once interrupted, patients usually do not return to telling their stories. After the patient's initial description of each issue, use a *focusing approach to explore the patient's story in more depth*. Ask *"How would you describe the pain?" "What happened next?" "What else did you notice?"* Using additional guided questioning helps you avoid missing any of the patient's concerns.

See p. 71 for discussions of *continuers*.

Identifying and Responding to the Patient's Emotional Cues.

Emotional distress is frequently associated with illness; 30% to 40% of patients show significant levels of anxiety and depression in primary care practices.[19] Patient visits tend to be longer when clinicians miss opportunities to acknowledge emotional clues.[17] Patients may withhold their true concerns in up to 75% of acute care visits[15] but offer various clues to their concerns that may be direct or indirect, verbal or nonverbal, and expressed as ideas or emotions.[20] Acknowledging and responding to these clues help build rapport, expand the clinician's understanding of the illness, and improve patient satisfaction.

See pp. 69–72 for discussions of *guided questioning*.

If the patient does not mention the impact of the illness, probe the broader personal context of the illness by asking "How has this affected you?" or "What do you make of this?" Seek the patient's related emotions directly or indirectly by stating "How did you feel about that?" or "Many people would be frustrated by something like this." In addition, explore the patient's ideas about the effect of the illness on his or her life.[18] See the box below for a taxonomy of the clues about the patient's perspective on illness.

CLUES TO THE PATIENT'S PERSPECTIVE ON ILLNESS[20]

- Direct statement(s) by the patient of explanations, emotions, expectations, and effects of the illness[9]
- Expression of feelings about the illness
- Attempts to explain or understand symptoms
- Speech clues (e.g., repetition,[21] prolonged reflective pauses[22])
- Sharing a personal story
- Behavior clues indicative of unidentified concerns, dissatisfaction, or unmet needs such as reluctance to accept recommendations, seeking a second opinion, or early return appointment

---

Learn to respond immediately when you hear an emotional cue. Appropriate response techniques include reflection, synonyms, and feedback indicating support and partnership. A mnemonic for responding to emotional cues is *NURS: N*aming—"That sounds like a scary experience"; *U*nderstanding or legitimization—"It's understandable that you feel that way"; and *R*especting—"You've done better than most people would with this."

Expanding and Clarifying the Patient's Story. After eliciting the patient's story as fully as possible in a nondirective manner and exploring the patient's lived experience of the illness, guide the patient to elaborating on the areas of the health history that seem most significant. As a clinician, you must clarify the attributes of each symptom, including context, associations, and chronology. For pain and many other symptoms, understanding these essential characteristics, summarized below as the seven key attributes of a symptom, is critical.

To pursue the seven attributes, two mnemonics may help:

● **OLD CARTS,** or **O**nset, **L**ocation, **D**uration, **C**haracter, **A**ggravating/ **A**lleviating Factors, **R**adiation, and **T**iming, and

● **OPQRST,** or **O**nset, **P**alliating/**P**rovoking Factors, **Q**uality, **R**adiation, **S**ite, and **T**iming

---

THE SEVEN ATTRIBUTES OF A SYMPTOM

1. *Location.* Where is it? Does it radiate?
2. *Quality.* What is it like?
3. *Quantity or severity.* How bad is it? (For pain, ask for a rating on a scale of 1 to 10.)
4. *Timing.* When did (does) it start? How long does it last? How often does it come?
5. *Setting in which it occurs.* Include environmental factors, personal activities, emotional reactions, or other circumstances that may have contributed to the illness.
6. *Remitting or exacerbating factors.* Is there anything that makes it better or worse?
7. *Associated manifestations.* Have you noticed anything else that accompanies it?

Whenever possible, *use the patient's words,* making sure you clarify their meaning. Although using medical jargon is highly seductive, it confuses and frustrates patients. Be aware of how quickly jargon like "take a history" and "work you up" can creep into your discussions. Choose instead plain English words such as "I'd like to learn more about your illness" or "Doing these tests can help us understand what's causing your illness."

It is important to establish *the sequence and time course* of each of the patient's symptoms if you are to arrive at accurate assessments. Encourage a chronologic account by asking such questions as "What then?" or "What happened next?" or "Please start at the beginning, or the last time you felt well, and go step by step." To fill in specific details, guide the patient's story by employing different types of questions and the techniques of skilled interviewing. Use focused questions to elicit information that the patient has not already offered. *In general, an interview moves back and forth from open-ended questions to*

See the Techniques of Skilled Interviewing and discussion of focused questions, pp. 69–72.

increasingly focused questions and then on to another open-ended question, returning the lead in the interview to the patient.

Generating and Testing Diagnostic Hypotheses.

Over time, as you gain experience listening to patient concerns, you will develop the skills of clinical reasoning. You will *generate and test diagnostic hypotheses* about what disease process might be present. Identifying the various attributes of each of the patient's symptoms and pursuing related details are fundamental to recognizing patterns of disease and to generating the *differential diagnosis*. As you learn more about diagnostic patterns and epidemiology, knowing what data you are listening for and asking for further information become more automatic.

Some students visualize the process of evoking a full description of the symptom as "the cone":

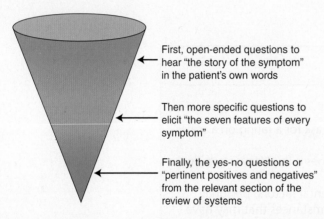

First, open-ended questions to hear "the story of the symptom" in the patient's own words

Then more specific questions to elicit "the seven features of every symptom"

Finally, the yes-no questions or "pertinent positives and negatives" from the relevant section of the review of systems

Each symptom has its own "cone," which becomes a paragraph in the History of Present Illness in the written record.

Appropriate questions about symptoms are also suggested in each of the chapters on the regional physical examinations. This is one way that you build evidence for and against various diagnostic possibilities. The challenge is to not let this kind of inquiry dominate the interview and displace learning about the patient's perspective, conveying concern for the patient's well-being, and building the relationship.[5]

For example, in a patient with a cough, these questions would come from the Respiratory section of the Review of Systems, on pp. 20–21.

See also Chapter 2, Clinical Reasoning, Assessment, and Recording Your Findings, pp. 25–53.

Creating a Shared Understanding of the Problem.

Recent literature makes it clear that delivering effective health care requires exploring the deeper meanings patients attach to their symptoms. Although the "seven attributes of a symptom" add important details to the patient's history, the **disease/illness distinction model** helps you understand the full range of what every good interview needs to cover.[23] This model acknowledges the very different yet complementary perspectives of the clinician and the patient. *Disease* is the explanation that the *clinician* brings to the symptoms. It is the way that the clinician organizes what he or she learns from the patient that leads to a clinical diagnosis. *Illness* can be defined as how the *patient* experiences all aspects of the disease, including its effects on relationships, function, and sense of well-being. Many factors may shape this experience, including prior personal or family health, the effect of symptoms on everyday life, individual outlook and style of coping, and expectations about medical care. The melding of these perspectives forms the basis for planning evaluation and treatment. *The clinical interview needs to incorporate both these views of reality.*

Even a chief complaint as straightforward as sore throat can illustrate these divergent views. The patient may be most concerned about pain and difficulty swallowing, missing time from work, or a cousin who was hospitalized with tonsillitis. The clinician, however, may focus on specific points in the history that differentiate streptococcal pharyngitis from other etiologies, or on a questionable history of allergy to penicillin. To understand the patient's expectations, the clinician needs to go beyond just the attributes of a symptom. Learning about the patient's perception of illness means asking patient-centered questions in the four domains listed below. This information is crucial to patient satisfaction, effective health care, and patient follow-through.[18,24]

EXPLORING THE PATIENT'S PERSPECTIVE

- The patient's **F**eelings, including fears or concerns, about the problem
- The patient's **I**deas about the nature and the cause of the problem
- The effect of the problem on the patient's life and **F**unction
- The patient's **E**xpectations of the disease, of the clinician, or of health care, often based on prior personal or family experiences

---

Exploring the patient's perspective encompasses different types of questions. To uncover the patient's feelings the clinician might ask, "What concerns you most about the pain?" or "How has this been for you?" To explore the patient's thoughts about the cause of the problem you could say "Why do you think you have this stomachache?" or "What have you tried?" because therapeutic attempts suggest explanatory models. A patient may worry that the pain is a symptom of serious disease and want reassurance. Alternatively, the patient may be less concerned about the cause of the pain and just want relief. To determine the effect of the illness on the patient's lifestyle and function, particularly for patients with chronic illness, ask, "What can't you do now that you could do before? How has your backache (shortness of breath, etc.) affected your ability to work? Your life at home? Your social activities? Your role as a parent? Your function in intimate relationships? The way you feel about yourself as a person?" You need to find out what the patient expects from you, the clinician, or from health care in general . . . "I am glad that the pain is almost gone, how specifically can I help you now?" Even if the stomach pain is almost gone, the patient may need a work excuse to take to an employer. A mnemonic for the patient's perspective on the illness is *FIFE—Feelings, Ideas, effect on Function, and Expectations.*

Negotiating a Plan. Learning about the disease and conceptualizing the illness give you and the patient the opportunity to create a complete and congruent picture of the problem. This multifaceted picture then forms the basis for planning further evaluation (e.g., physical examination, laboratory tests, consultations) and negotiating a treatment plan. It also plays an important role in building rapport with your patient. Advanced skills, such as motivational interviewing and the therapeutic use of the clinician–patient relationship, are beyond the scope of this book.

See also Chapter 2, Clinical Reasoning, Assessment, and Recording Your Findings, for more specific techniques for negotiating a plan.

Planning for Follow-Up and Closing.   You may find that ending the interview is difficult. Patients often have many questions, and if you have done your job well, they are engaged and affirmed as they talk with you. Let the patient know that the end of the interview is approaching to allow time for the patient to ask any final questions. Make sure the patient understands the mutual plans you have developed. For example, before gathering your papers or standing to leave the room, you can say, "We need to stop now. Do you have any questions about what we've covered?" As you close, reviewing future evaluation, treatments, and follow-up is helpful. "So, you will take the medicine as we discussed, get the blood test before you leave today, and make a follow-up appointment for 4 weeks. Do you have any questions about this?" Address any related concerns or questions that the patient raises.

The patient should have a chance to ask any final questions; however, the last few minutes are not the time to bring up new topics. If that happens and the concern is not life-threatening, simply assure the patient of your interest and make plans to address the problem at a future time. "That knee pain sounds concerning. Why don't you make an appointment for next week so we can discuss it?" Reaffirming your continued commitment to improving the patient's health is always appreciated.

BUILDING A THERAPEUTIC RELATIONSHIP: THE TECHNIQUES OF SKILLED INTERVIEWING

Building the Relationship.   You probably had many reasons to become a health care professional, but one of them was undoubtedly the desire to serve others. To succeed in fulfilling this laudable goal, you must sustain this motivation throughout your rigorous training and transform this goal into a set of behavioral approaches to your patients.

The paradigm that embeds your relationship with the patient into the therapeutic process itself now has many names and models, such as the biopsychosocial model and patient-centered care, among others.[5,18,26,27] Comparing these various models reveals common elements that include interest in the patient as a whole person, an empowering approach to the patient role, and involvement of the clinician's self on an emotional and reflective level.[28] There is now robust literature demonstrating that an approach to patient care anchored in these principles is not only more satisfying for the patient and the clinician but also more effective in achieving good health care outcomes.[8,29]

This section describes the skills that form the basic tools of interviewing. Some of these habits are purely techniques that you can readily put into practice. Some are constructs that will inform your interviewing behaviors. You will employ these interviewing skills to achieve the tasks described earlier in the Sequence of the Interview (see p. 61) more effectively. You need to practice using these tools and find ways to be observed or recorded so that you can receive feedback on your progress. Several of these fundamental skills are listed below and then described in more detail. Pick one or two of them to incorporate into your next patient interview. Then refer back to this chapter to build your repertoire of skills.

The Techniques of Skilled Interviewing

- Active listening
- Guided questioning
- Nonverbal communication
- Empathic responses
- Validation
- Reassurance
- Partnering
- Summarization
- Transitions
- Empowering the patient

Active Listening. Underlying all the various techniques is the habit of *active listening*. Active listening is the process of closely attending to what the patient is communicating, being aware of the patient's emotional state, and using verbal and nonverbal skills to encourage the speaker to continue and expand. This allows you to understand precisely at multiple levels of the patient's experience.[30] This takes practice. It is easy to drift into thinking about your next question or the differential diagnosis when you and the patient are best served by your concentration on listening.

Guided Questioning: Options for Expanding and Clarifying the Patient's Story.
There are several ways you can ask for more information from the patient without interfering with the flow of the patient's story. Your goal is to facilitate the patient's fullest communica-

- Moving from open-ended to focused questions
- Using questioning that elicits a graded response
- Asking a series of questions, one at a time
- Offering multiple choices for answers
- Clarifying what the patient means
- Encouraging with continuers
- Using echoing

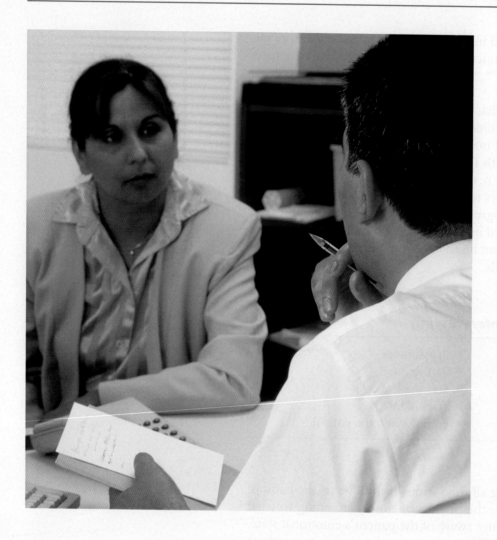

tion. Learning the following specific techniques allows you to encourage patient disclosures, while minimizing the risk for distorting their ideas or missing significant details. This is how you avoid asking a series of specific questions, which takes more time and makes the patient feel more passive.

Moving from Open-Ended to Focused Questions.   Your questioning should proceed from general to specific. Think once again about the "cone," open at the top then tapering to a focal point. Start with the most general questions like "How can I help?" to still open but focused ones like "Tell me more about your experience with the medicine." Then pose closed questions like "Did the new medicine cause any problems?" Begin with a truly open-ended question that does not inadvertently include an answer. A possible sequence might be

"Tell me about your chest pain." (Pause)

"What else?" (Pause)

"Where did you feel it?" (Pause) "Show me."

"Anywhere else?" (Pause) "Did it travel anywhere?" (Pause) "To which arm?"

You should avoid *leading questions* that include the answer in the question or suggest your desired response: "Has your pain been improving?" or "You don't have any blood in your stools, do you?" If you ask "Is your pain like a pressure?" and the patient answers yes, your words may turn into the patient's words. Adopt the more neutral "Please describe your pain."

Questioning that Elicits a Graded Response. If necessary, ask questions that require *a graded response* rather than a single answer. "How many steps can you climb before you get short of breath?" is better than "Do you get short of breath climbing stairs?"

Asking a Series of Questions, One at a Time. Be sure to *ask one question at a time.* "Any tuberculosis, pleurisy, asthma, bronchitis, pneumonia?" may lead to a negative answer out of sheer confusion. Try "Do you have any of the following problems?" Be sure to pause and establish eye contact as you list each problem.

Offering Multiple Choices for Answers. Sometimes patients seem quite unable to describe their symptoms without help. To minimize bias, *offer multiple-choice answers:* "Which of the following words best describes your pain: aching, sharp, pressing, burning, shooting, or something else?" Almost any specific question can provide at least two possible answers. "Do you bring up any phlegm with your cough, or is it dry?"

Clarifying What the Patient Means. At times, patients use words that are ambiguous or have unclear associations. To understand their meaning, you need to *request clarification,* as in "Tell me exactly what you meant by 'the flu'" or "You said you were behaving just like your mother. What did you mean?"

Encouraging With Continuers. Without specifying content, you can use posture, gestures, or words to encourage the patient to say more. Pausing with a nod of the head or remaining silent, yet attentive and relaxed, is a *cue for the patient to continue.* Leaning forward, making eye contact, and using phrases like "Mm-hmm," or "Go on," or "I'm listening" all maintain the flow of the patient's story.

Echoing. A simple repetition of the patient's last words, or *echoing,* encourages the patient to express both factual details and feelings, as in the following example:

Patient: "The pain got worse and began to spread." (Pause)

Response: "Spread?" (Pause)

Patient: "Yes, it went to my shoulder and down my left arm to the fingers. It was so bad that I thought I was going to die." (Pause)

Response: "Going to die?"

Patient: "Yes, it was just like the pain my father had when he had his heart attack, and I was afraid the same thing was happening to me."

This reflective technique has helped to reveal not only the location and severity of the pain but also its meaning to the patient. It did not bias the story or interrupt the patient's train of thought.

Nonverbal Communication.   Communication that does not involve speech occurs continuously and provides important clues to feelings and emotions. Becoming more sensitive to nonverbal messages allows you to both "read the patient" more effectively and send messages of your own. Pay close attention to eye contact, facial expression, posture, head position and movement such as shaking or nodding, interpersonal distance, and placement of the arms or legs—crossed, neutral, or open. Be aware that some nonverbal language is universal and some is culturally bound.

Just as mirroring your position can signify the patient's increasing sense of connectedness, matching your position to the patient's can signify increased rapport. You can also mirror the patient's *paralanguage,* or qualities of speech, such as pacing, tone, and volume, to increase rapport. Moving closer or physical contact like placing your hand on the patient's arm can convey empathy or help the patient gain control of difficult feelings. Bringing nonverbal communication to the conscious level is the first step to using this crucial form of patient interaction.

Empathic Responses.   Conveying empathy greatly strengthens patient rapport. As patients talk with you they may express—with or without words—feelings they may or may not have consciously acknowledged. These feelings are crucial to understanding their illnesses and to establishing a trusting relationship. *To provide empathy, you must first identify the patient's feelings.* This requires a willingness and interest on your part in hearing about and eliciting emotional content. At first, this may seem unfamiliar or uncomfortable. When you sense important but unexpressed feelings from the patient's face, voice, words, or behavior, inquire about them rather than assuming that you know how the patient feels. You may simply ask, "How did you feel about that?" Unless you let patients know that you are interested in feelings as well as facts, you may miss important insights.

Once you have identified the feelings, respond with understanding and acceptance. Responses may be as simple as "I understand," "That sounds upsetting," or "You seem sad." Empathy may also be nonverbal—for example, offering a tissue to a crying patient or gently placing your hand on the patient's arm. For a response to be empathic, it must reflect a precise understanding of what the patient is feeling. If your response acknowledges how upset a patient must have been at the death of a parent, when in fact the death relieved the patient of a long-standing financial and emotional burden, you have misunderstood the situation. Instead of making assumptions, you can ask directly about the patient's emotional response. "I am sorry about the death of your father. What has that been like for you?"

Validation.   Another important way to make a patient feel affirmed is to validate or acknowledge the legitimacy of his or her emotional experience. A patient who has been in a car accident but has no physical injury may still be experiencing significant distress. Stating something like, "Being in that accident must have been very scary. Car accidents are always unsettling because they remind us of our vulnerability and mortality. That could explain why you still feel upset," reassures the patient. It helps the patient feel that such emotions are legitimate and understandable.

Reassurance.   When you are talking with patients who are anxious or upset, it is tempting to try to reassure them. You may find yourself saying, "Don't worry. Everything is going to be all right." Although this may be appropriate in nonprofessional relationships, in your role as a clinician, such comments are usually counterproductive. You may fall into reassuring the patient about the wrong thing. Moreover, premature reassurance may block further disclosures, especially if the patient feels that the clinician is uncomfortable with the anxiety or has not appreciated the extent of the patient's distress. Such admissions require encouragement, not a cover-up.

The first step to effective reassurance is simply identifying and acknowledging the patient's feelings. This promotes a feeling of connection. The actual reassurance comes much later after you have completed the interview, the physical examination, and perhaps some laboratory studies. At that point, you can interpret for the patient what you think is happening and deal openly with expressed concerns. The reassurance comes from conveying information in a competent manner, making the patient feel confident that problems have been fully understood and will be addressed.

Partnering.   When building your relationships with patients, make explicit your desire to work with them in an ongoing way. When you discuss a diagnosis or express uncertainty about how to explain their symptoms, it is reassuring to state that regardless of what happens with their disease, you are committed to a continuing partnership. Even in your role as student, especially in a hospital setting, this support can make a big difference.

Summarization.   Giving a capsule summary of the patient's story during the course of the interview serves several different functions. It communicates to the patient that you have been listening carefully. It identifies what you know and what you don't know. "Now, let me make sure that I have the full story. You said you've had a cough for 3 days, that it's especially bad at night, and that you have started to bring up yellow phlegm. You have not had a fever or felt short of breath, but you do feel congested, with difficulty breathing through your nose." Following with an attentive pause or asking "Anything else?" lets the patient add other information and corrects any misunderstanding.

You can use summarization at different points in the interview to structure the visit, especially at times of transition (see below). This technique also allows you, the clinician, to organize your clinical reasoning and to convey your thinking to the patient, making the relationship more collaborative. *It is also a useful technique for learners when they draw a blank on what to ask the patient next.*

Transitions. Patients have many reasons to feel vulnerable during a health care visit. To put them more at ease, tell them when you are changing directions during the interview. Just as clear signs along the highway give a sense of confidence, this "signposting" gives patients a greater sense of control. As you move from one part of the history to the next and on to the physical examination, orient the patient with brief transitional phrases like "Now I'd like to ask some questions about your past health." Make clear what the patient should expect or do next. "Before we move on to reviewing all your medications, was there anything else about past health problems?" "Now I would like to examine you. I will step out for a few minutes. Please undress and put on this gown." Specifying that the gown should close in the back protects the patient's modesty and can make examiners more comfortable.

Empowering the Patient. The clinician–patient relationship is inherently unequal. Your feelings of inexperience as a student predictably transition over time to confidence in your knowledge, skills, and authority in your role as clinician. But patients have many reasons to feel vulnerable. They may be in pain or worried about a symptom. They may be unfamiliar or overwhelmed with accessing the health care system and processes that you take for granted. Differences of gender, ethnicity, race, or class may also contribute to power differentials. However, ultimately, patients are responsible for their own care.[31] Patients who are self-confident and understand your recommendations are most likely to adopt your advice, make lifestyle changes, or take medications as prescribed.

Listed next are principles that help you share power with your patients. Although many of them have been discussed in other sections of this chapter, the need to reinforce patients' primary responsibility for their health is so fundamental that it is worth summarizing them here.

EMPOWERING THE PATIENT: PRINCIPLES OF SHARING POWER

- Evoke the patient's perspective.
- Convey interest in the person, not just the problem.
- Follow the patient's leads.
- Elicit and validate emotional content.
- Share information with the patient, especially at transition points during the visit.
- Make your clinical reasoning transparent to the patient.
- Reveal the limits of your knowledge.

ADAPTING YOUR INTERVIEW TO SPECIFIC SITUATIONS

Interviewing patients may precipitate several behaviors and situations that seem perplexing or even vexing. Your ability to handle these situations will evolve throughout your career. *Always remember the importance of listening to the patient and clarifying the patient's concerns.*

The Silent Patient.   Novice interviewers are often uncomfortable with periods of silence and feel obligated to keep the conversation going. Silence has many meanings and many purposes. Patients frequently fall silent for short periods to collect thoughts, remember details, or decide whether you can be trusted with certain information. The period of silence usually feels much longer to the clinician than it does to the patient. The clinician should appear attentive and give brief encouragement to continue when appropriate. During periods of silence, watch the patient closely for nonverbal cues, such as difficulty controlling emotions.

Patients with depression or dementia may lose their usual spontaneity of expression, give short answers to questions, and then fall silent. If you have already tried guiding them through recent events or a typical day, try shifting your inquiry to the symptoms of depression or begin an exploratory mental status examination.

See Chapter 5, Behavior and Mental Status, pp. 135–162.

At times, silence may be the patient's response to how you are asking questions. Are you asking too many short-answer questions in rapid succession? Have you offended the patient in any way by signs of disapproval or criticism? Have you failed to recognize an overwhelming symptom such as pain, nausea, or dyspnea? If so, you may need to ask the patient directly, "You seem very quiet. Have I done something to upset you?"

The Confusing Patient.   Some patients present a confusing array of *multiple symptoms*. They seem to have every symptom that you ask about, or "a positive review of systems." With these patients, focus on the meaning or function of the symptom, emphasizing the patient's perspective (see p. 67), and guide the interview into a psychosocial assessment. There is little profit to exploring each symptom in detail. Although the patient may have several illnesses, a somatization disorder may be in play.

See Chapter 5, Behavior and Mental Status, Medically Unexplained Symptoms, pp. 136–137, and Table 5-1, Somatoform Disorders: Types and Approach, pp. 158–159.

At other times, you may feel baffled, frustrated, and confused because you cannot make sense out of the patient's story. The history is vague and difficult to understand, ideas are poorly connected, and language is hard to follow. Even though you word your questions carefully, you cannot seem to get clear answers. The patient's manner of relating to you may also seem peculiar, distant, aloof, or inappropriate. Symptoms may be described in bizarre terms: "My fingernails feel too heavy" or "My stomach knots up like a snake." Perhaps there is a mental status change like psychosis or delirium, a mental illness such as schizophrenia, or a neurologic disorder. Consider delirium in acutely ill or intoxicated patients and dementia in the elderly. Such patients give histories that are inconsistent and cannot provide a clear chronology about what has happened. Some may even confabulate to fill in the gaps in their memories.

See Table 20-2, Delirium and Dementia, p. 931.

When you suspect a psychiatric or neurologic disorder, do not spend too much time gathering a detailed history. You will only tire and frustrate both the patient and yourself. Shift to the mental status examination, focusing on level of consciousness, orientation, memory, and capacity to understand. You can work in the initial questions smoothly by asking, "When was your last appointment at the clinic? Let's see . . . that was about how long ago?" "Your address now is. . . ? . . . and your phone number?" You can check these responses against the chart or seek permission to speak with family members or friends and then obtain their perspectives.

See Chapter 5, Behavior and Mental Status, The Mental Status Examination, pp. 145–154.

The Patient With Altered Capacity.

Some patients cannot provide their own histories because of delirium from illness, dementia, or other health or mental health conditions. Others are unable to relate certain parts of the history, such as events related to a febrile illness or a seizure. Under these circumstances, you need to determine whether the patient has "*decision-making capacity*," or the ability to understand information related to health, to make medical choices based on reason and a consistent set of values, and to declare preferences about treatments. The term *capacity* is preferable to the term "*competence*," which is a legal term. You do not need to consult psychiatry to assess capacity unless mental illness impairs decision making. For many patients with psychiatric conditions or even cognitive impairments, their ability to make decisions remains intact.

For patients with capacity, obtain their consent before talking about their health with others. Even if patients communicate only with facial expressions or gestures, you must maintain confidentiality and elicit their input. Assure patients that any shared history will be kept confidential, and clarify what you can discuss with others. Your knowledge about the patient can be quite comprehensive, yet others may offer surprising and important information. A spouse, for example, may report significant family strains, depressive symptoms, or drinking habits that the patient has denied. Consider dividing the interview into two segments—one with the patient and the other with both the patient and a second informant. Each interview has its own value. Information from other sources often gives you helpful ideas for planning the patient's care, but remains confidential. Also learn the tenets of the *Health Insurance Portability and Accountability Act (HIPAA)* passed by Congress in 1996, which sets strict standards for disclosure for both institutions and providers when sharing patient information. [32]

For patients with impaired capacity, you will often need to find a *surrogate informant or decision maker* to assist with the history. Check whether the patient has a *durable power of attorney for health care* or a *health care proxy*. If not, in many cases, a spouse or family member who can represent the patient's wishes can fill this role.

Apply the basic principles of interviewing to your conversations with patients' relatives or friends. Find a private place to talk. Introduce yourself, state your purpose, inquire how they are feeling under the circumstances, and recognize and acknowledge their concerns. As you listen to their versions of the history, assess the quality of their relationship with the patient because it may color their credibility. Establish how they know the patient. For example, when a child is brought in for health care, the accompanying adult may not be the primary or even frequent caregiver, just the most available ride. Always seek the best-informed source. Occasionally, a relative or friend insists on being with the patient during your evaluation. Try to find out why, and assess the patient's wishes.

The Talkative Patient.

The garrulous, rambling patient may be just as difficult as the silent or confused patient. Faced with limited time and the need to "get the whole story," you may grow impatient, even exasperated. Although this problem has no perfect solution, several techniques are helpful. Give the patient free rein for the first 5 or 10 minutes, listening closely to the conversation. Perhaps the patient simply needs a good listener and is expressing pent-up concerns, or the patient's style is to tell stories. Does the patient seem obsessively detailed? Is the patient unduly anxious or apprehensive? Is there flight of ideas or a disorganized thought process that suggests a thought disorder? What about confabulation?

Focus on what seems most important to the patient. Show your interest by asking questions in those areas. Interrupt only if necessary, but be courteous. Learn how to set limits when needed. Remember that part of your task is structuring the interview to gain important information about the patient's health. A brief summary may help you change the subject yet validate any concerns. "Let me make sure that I understand. You have described many concerns. In particular I heard about two different kinds of pain, one on your left side that goes into your groin and is fairly new, and one in your upper abdomen after you eat that you have had for months. Let's focus just on the side pain first. Can you tell me what it feels like?"

See Summarization, p. 73.

Finally, do not show your impatience. If time runs out, explain the need for a second meeting. Setting a time limit for the next appointment may be helpful. "I know we have much more to talk about. Can you come again next week? We will have a full hour then."

The Crying Patient.

Crying signals strong emotions, ranging from sadness to anger or frustration. If the patient is on the verge of tears, pausing, gentle probing, or responding with empathy gives the patient permission to cry. Usually crying is therapeutic, as is your quiet acceptance of the patient's distress or pain. Offer a tissue and wait for the patient to recover. Make a supportive remark like "I am glad you were able to express your feelings." Most patients will soon compose themselves and resume their story. Aside from an acute grief or loss, it is unusual for crying to escalate and become uncontrollable.

Crying makes many people uncomfortable. If this is true for you, you need to learn how to accept displays of emotion so that as a clinician you can support patients at these moving and significant times.

The Angry or Disruptive Patient. Many patients have reasons to be angry: they are ill, they have suffered a loss, they lack their accustomed control over their own lives, and they feel relatively powerless in the health care system.[33] They may direct this anger toward you. It is possible that this hostility toward you is justified . . . were you late for your appointment, inconsiderate, insensitive, or angry yourself? If so, acknowledge the fact and try to make amends. More often, however, patients displace their anger onto the clinician as a reflection of their frustration or pain.

Accept angry feelings from patients. Allow them to express such emotions without getting angry in return. Avoid joining such patients in their hostility toward another provider, the clinic, or the hospital, even when privately you may feel sympathetic. You can validate their feelings without agreeing with their reasons. "I understand that you felt very frustrated by the long wait and answering the same questions over and over. Our complex health care system can seem very unsupportive when you are not feeling well." After the patient has calmed down, help find steps that will avert such situations in the future. Rational solutions to emotional problems are not always possible, however, and people need time to express and work through their angry feelings.

Some angry patients become overtly disruptive. Few people can disturb the clinic or emergency department more quickly than patients who are angry, belligerent, or out of control. Before approaching such patients, alert the security staff—as a clinician, maintaining a safe environment is one of your responsibilities. Stay calm, appear accepting, and avoid being confrontational in return. Keep your posture relaxed and nonthreatening and your hands loosely open. At first do not try to make disruptive patients lower their voices or stop if they are haranguing you or the staff. Listen carefully. Try to understand what they are saying. Once you have established rapport, gently suggest moving to a different location that is more private and will cause less disruption.

The Interview Across a Language Barrier. Nothing will convince you more of the importance of the history than not being able to talk with the patient, an increasingly common experience. More than 46 million people in the United States do not speak English as their primary language, and the command of English for approximately 21 million is less than fluent.[34] Such people are less likely to have regular primary or preventive care and more likely to report problems with care or even experience medical errors. Learning to work with qualified interpreters is not only cost-effective but important for optimal care.[34–36]

If your patient speaks a different language, make every effort to find an interpreter. A few broken words and gestures are no substitutes for the full story. The ideal interpreter is a neutral person who is familiar with both languages and cultures. Recruiting family members or friends to serve as interpreters can be hazardous—confidentiality may be violated, meanings may be distorted, and transmitted information may be incomplete. Untrained interpreters may try to speed up the interview by telescoping lengthy replies into a few words, losing much of what may be significant detail.

As you begin working with the interpreter, establish rapport and review what information would be most useful. Explain that you need the interpreter to translate everything, not to condense or summarize. *Make your questions clear, short, and simple.* You can also help the interpreter by outlining your goals for each segment of the history. After going over your plans, arrange the room so that you have easy eye contact and nonverbal communication with the patient. Then speak directly to the patient . . . "How long have you been sick?" rather than "How long has the patient been sick?" Having the interpreter close by the patient, or even behind you, keeps you from moving your head back and forth as though you were watching a tennis match.

When available, bilingual written questionnaires are invaluable, especially for the review of systems. First, however, be sure that patients can read in their language; otherwise, ask for help from the interpreter. In some clinical settings, there are speakerphone translators; use them if there are no better options.

GUIDELINES FOR WORKING WITH AN INTERPRETER

- Choose a trained interpreter in preference to a hospital worker, volunteer, or family member.
- Use the interpreter as a resource for cultural information.
- Orient the interpreter to the components you plan to cover in the interview; include reminders to translate everything the patient says.
- Arrange the room so that you and the patient have eye contact and can read each other's nonverbal cues. Seat the interpreter next to the patient.
- Allow the interpreter and the patient to establish rapport.
- Address the patient directly. Reinforce your questions with nonverbal behaviors.
- Keep sentences *short* and *simple*. Focus on the most important concepts to communicate.
- Verify mutual understanding by asking the patient to repeat back what he or she has heard.
- Be patient. The interview will take more time and may provide less information.

The Patient With Low Literacy. Before giving written instructions, assess the patient's ability to read. Literacy levels are highly variable, and marginal reading skills are more prevalent than commonly believed. Explore the many reasons people do not read: language barriers, learning disorders, poor vision, or lack of education. Some patients feel uncomfortable about disclosing their problems with reading. Asking about educational level may be helpful, but practical approaches are more fruitful. Ask, "How comfortable are you with filling out medical forms?" or ask the patient to read whatever instructions you have written. (This will also address any difficulty with your handwriting.) Another rapid screen is to hand the patient a written text upside down—most patients who read will turn the page around immediately. Lack of reading skill may explain why the patient has not taken medications as prescribed or adhered to recommended treatments. Respond sensitively, and do not confuse the degree of literacy with level of intelligence.

The Patient With Impaired Hearing. Communicating with the deaf presents many of the same challenges as communicating with patients who speak a different language. Even people with partial hearing may define themselves as deaf, a distinct cultural group. Find out the patient's preferred method of communicating. Patients may use American Sign Language, a unique language with its own syntax, or various other combinations of signs and speech. Thus, communication is often truly cross-cultural. Ask when hearing loss occurred relative to the development of speech and other language skills. Query the kinds of schools the patient has attended. These questions help you determine whether the patient identifies with the deaf culture or the hearing culture. Written questionnaires are also useful. If the patient prefers sign language, find an interpreter and use the principles identified earlier. Time-consuming handwritten questions and answers may be the only solution, although literacy skills may also be an issue.

Hearing deficits vary. If the patient has a hearing aid, find out if the patient is using it. Make sure it is working. For patients with unilateral hearing loss, sit on the hearing side. A person who is *hard of hearing* may not be aware of the problem, a situation you will have to tactfully address. Eliminate background noise such as television or hallway conversation as much as possible. For patients who have partial hearing or can read lips, face them directly, in good light. Patients should wear their glasses to better pick up visual cues that help them understand you.

Speak at a normal volume and rate and do not let your voice trail off at the ends of sentences. Avoid covering your mouth or looking down at papers while speaking. Remember that even the best lip readers comprehend only a percentage of what is said, so having patients repeat what you have said is important. When closing, write out any oral instructions.

The Patient With Impaired Vision. When meeting with a blind patient, shake hands to establish contact and explain who you are and why you are there. If the room is unfamiliar, orient the patient to the surroundings and report if anyone else is present. It still may be helpful to adjust the light. Encourage visually impaired patients to wear glasses whenever possible. Remember to use words because postures and gestures are unseen.

The Patient With Limited Intelligence. Patients of moderately limited intelligence can usually give adequate histories. In fact, you may even be able to omit their disability from their evaluations. If you suspect problems, however, pay special attention to the patient's schooling and ability to function independently. How far have such patients gone in school? If they didn't finish, why not? What kinds of courses have they taken? How did they do? Have they had any testing done? Are they living alone? Do they need assistance with activities such as transportation or shopping? The sexual history is equally important and often overlooked. Find out if the patient is sexually active and provide information that may be needed about pregnancy or sexually transmitted diseases.

If you are unsure about the patient's level of intelligence, make a smooth transition to the mental status examination and assess simple calculations, vocabulary, memory, and abstract thinking.

See Chapter 5, Behavior and Mental Status, pp. 135–162.

For patients with severe mental retardation, you will have to turn to the family or caregivers to elicit the history. Identify the person who accompanies the patient, but always show interest in the patient first. Establish rapport, make eye contact, and engage in simple conversation. As with children, avoid "talking down" or using affectations of speech or condescending behavior. The patient, family members, caregivers, or friends will notice and appreciate your respect.

The Patient With Personal Problems.   Patients may ask you for advice about personal problems that fall outside the range of your clinical expertise. Should the patient quit a stressful job, for example, or move out of state? Instead of responding, ask about the different approaches the patient has considered and related pros and cons, others who have provided advice, and what supports are available for different choices. Letting the patient talk through the problem with you is more valuable and therapeutic than any answer you could give.

SENSITIVE TOPICS THAT CALL FOR SPECIFIC APPROACHES

Clinicians talk with patients about many subjects that are emotionally charged. These discussions can be particularly awkward when clinicians are inexperienced or assessing patients they do not know well. Even seasoned clinicians are affected by societal taboos enveloping certain subjects: abuse of alcohol or drugs, sexual practices, death and dying, financial concerns, racial and ethnic bias, family interactions, domestic violence, psychiatric illnesses, physical deformities, bowel function, and others. Many of these topics trigger strong personal responses related to family, cultural, and societal value systems. Mental illness, drug use during pregnancy, and same-sex practices are three obvious examples of issues that evoke biases that can affect the patient interview. This section explores challenges to the clinician in several of these sensitive areas.

Several basic principles can help guide your response to sensitive topics:

GUIDELINES FOR BROACHING SENSITIVE TOPICS

- *The single most important rule is to be nonjudgmental.* The clinician's role is to learn about the patient and help the patient achieve better health. Disapproval of behaviors or elements in the health history will only interfere with this goal.

(continued)

> ### GUIDELINES FOR BROACHING SENSITIVE TOPICS (CONTINUED)
>
> - *Explain why you need to know certain information.* This makes patients less apprehensive. For example, say to patients, "Because sexual practices put people at risk for certain diseases, I ask all of my patients the following questions."
> - Find opening questions for sensitive topics and learn the specific kinds of information needed for your assessments.
> - Finally, consciously acknowledge whatever discomfort you are feeling. Denying your discomfort may lead you to avoid the topic altogether.

Look into other strategies for becoming more comfortable with sensitive areas. Examples include general reading about these topics in medical and lay literature; talking to selected colleagues and teachers openly about your concerns; taking special courses that help you explore your own feelings and reactions; and ultimately, reflecting on your own life experience. Take advantage of all these resources. Whenever possible, listen to experienced clinicians, then practice similar discussions with your own patients. The range of topics that you can explore with comfort will widen progressively.

The Sexual History. Asking questions about sexual behavior can be life-saving. Sexual behaviors determine risks for pregnancy, sexually transmitted diseases (STDs), and AIDS—good interviewing helps prevent or reduce these risks. Sexual practices may be directly related to the patient's symptoms and integral to both diagnosis and treatment. Many patients have questions or concerns about sexuality that they would discuss more freely if you ask about sexual health. Finally, sexual dysfunction may result from use of medication or from misinformation that, if recognized, can be readily addressed.

You can introduce questions about sexual behavior at multiple points in an interview. If the chief complaint involves genitourinary symptoms, include questions about sexual health as part of "expanding and clarifying" the patient's story. For women, you can ask these questions as part of the Obstetric/Gynecologic section of the Past Medical History. You can bring them into discussions about Health Maintenance, along with diet, exercise, and screening tests, or as part of the lifestyle issues or important relationships covered in the Personal and Social History. Or, in a comprehensive history, you can ask about sexual practices during the Review of Systems. Do not forget this area of inquiry just because the patient is elderly or has a disability or chronic illness.

An orienting sentence or two is often helpful. "To assess your risk for various diseases, I need to ask you some questions about your sexual health and practices" or "I routinely ask all patients about their sexual function." For more specific complaints you might state, "To figure out why you have this discharge and what we should do about it, I need to ask some questions about your sexual activity." Try to be matter-of-fact in your style; the patient will be likely to follow your lead. *Use specific language.* Refer to genitalia with explicit words such as penis or vagina and avoid phrases like "private parts." Choose words that the patient understands or explain what you mean. "By intercourse, I mean when a man inserts his penis into a woman's vagina."

In general, ask about both specific sexual behaviors and satisfaction with sexual function. Here are examples of questions that help patients reveal their concerns:

See specific questions in Chapter 13, Male Genitalia and Hernias, pp. 504–505, and Chapter 14, Female Genitalia, pp. 527–528.

● "When was the last time you had intimate physical contact with someone?" Did that contact include sexual intercourse?" Using the term "sexually active" can be ambiguous. Patients have been known to reply, "No, I just lie there."

● "Do you have sex with men, women, or both?" Individuals may have sex with persons of the same gender, yet not consider themselves gay, lesbian, or bisexual. Some gay and lesbian patients have had sex with the opposite gender. Your questions should always be about the behaviors.

● "How many sexual partners have you had in the last 6 months? In the last 5 years? In your lifetime?" Again, these questions give the patient an easy opportunity to acknowledge multiple partners. Ask also about routine use of condoms. "Do you *always* use condoms?"

● It is important to ask all patients, "Do you have any concerns about HIV infection or AIDS?" even if no explicit risk factors are evident.

Note that these questions make no assumptions about marital status, sexual preference, or attitudes toward pregnancy or contraception. Listen to each of the patient's responses, and ask additional questions as indicated. To elicit information about sexual behaviors, you will need to ask more specific and focused questions than in other parts of the interview.

The Mental Health History. Cultural constructs of mental and physical illness vary widely, causing marked differences in acceptance and attitudes. Think how easy it is for patients to talk about diabetes and taking insulin compared with discussing schizophrenia and using psychotropic medications. Ask open-ended questions initially. "Have you ever had any problem with emotional or mental illnesses?" Then move to more specific questions such as "Have you ever visited a counselor or psychotherapist?" "Have you ever been prescribed medication for emotional issues?" "Have you or has anyone in your family ever been hospitalized for an emotional or mental health problem?"

For patients with depression or thought disorders such as schizophrenia, a careful history of their illness is in order. Depression is common worldwide but still remains underdiagnosed and undertreated. Be sensitive to reports of mood changes or symptoms such as fatigue, unusual tearfulness, appetite or weight changes, insomnia, and vague somatic complaints. Two opening screening questions are: "Over the past 2 weeks, have you felt down, depressed, or hopeless?" and "Over the past 2 weeks, have you felt little interest or pleasure in doing things?"[37] If the patient seems depressed, also ask about thoughts of suicide: "Have you ever thought about hurting your-self or ending your life?" As with chest pain, you must evaluate severity—both depression and angina are potentially lethal.

Many patients with schizophrenia or other psychotic disorders can function in the community and tell you about their diagnoses, symptoms, hospital-izations, and current medications. You should investigate their symptoms and assess any effects on mood or daily activities.

For further approaches, turn to Chapter 5, Behavior and Mental Status, p. 143.

Alcohol and Illicit Drugs.
Many clinicians hesitate to ask patients about use of alcohol and drugs, whether prescribed or illegal. Misuse of alcohol or drugs often directly contributes to symptoms and the need for care and treat-ment. Despite the high lifetime prevalence of substance abuse disorders—more than 13% for alcohol and 4% for illegal drugs in the United States—they remain underdiagnosed.[38]

Avoid letting personal feelings interfere with your role as a clinician. It is your job to gather data, assess the effects on the patient's health, and plan a therapeutic response. Clinicians should routinely ask about current and past use of alcohol or drugs, patterns of use, and family history. Make sure to include adolescents and older adults in your questioning.[39,40]

Alcohol.   Questions about alcohol and other drugs follow naturally after questions about caffeine and cigarettes. "What do you like to drink?" or "Tell me about your use of alcohol" are good opening questions that avoid the easy yes or no response. Remember to assess what the patient considers alcohol—some patients do not use this term for wine or beer. To detect problem drink-ing, use several well-validated short screening tools that do not take much time. Two additional questions: "Have you ever had a drinking problem?" and "When was your last drink?" along with a drink within 24 hours are suspicious for problem drinking.[41] The most widely used screening questions are the **CAGE** questions about **C**utting down, **A**nnoyance if criticized, **G**uilty feel-ings, and **E**ye-openers.

THE CAGE QUESTIONNAIRE

Have you ever felt the need to **Cut down** on drinking?
Have you ever felt **Annoyed** by criticism of your drinking?
Have you ever felt **Guilty** about drinking?
Have you ever taken a drink first thing in the morning (**Eye-opener**) to steady your nerves or get rid of a hangover?

(Adapted from Mayfield D, McCleod G, Hall P. The CAGE questionnaire: validation of a new alcoholism screening instrument. Am J Psychiatry 131:1121–1123, 1974.)

Two or more affirmative answers to the CAGE Questionnaire suggest alco-hol misuse and have a sensitivity that ranges from 43% to 94% and specificity that ranges from 70% to 96%.[37,42] If you detect misuse, you need to ask about blackouts (loss of memory about events during drinking), seizures, accidents or injuries while drinking, job problems, conflict in personal relationships, or legal problems. Also ask specifically about drinking while driving or operating machinery.[43,44]

Illicit Drugs.   As with alcohol, your questions about drugs should be more focused if you are to get answers that help you distinguish use from misuse. A good opening question is, "Have you ever used any drugs other than those required for medical reasons?"[45] From there, you can ask specifically about either patterns of use (last use, how often, substances used, amount) or inquire about modes of consumption. "Have you ever injected a drug?" "Have you ever smoked or inhaled a drug?" "Have you ever taken a pill for nonmedical reasons?" As fashions in drugs of abuse change, it is important to stay up to date about the most current hazards and risks from overdose.

Another approach is to adapt the CAGE questions to screening for substance abuse by adding "or drugs" to each question. Once you identify substance abuse, continue further with questions like "Are you always able to control your use of drugs?" "Have you had any bad reactions?" "What happened . . . Any drug-related accidents, injuries, or arrests? Job or family problems?" . . . "Have you ever tried to quit? Tell me about it."

Family Violence.   Because of the high prevalence of physical, sexual, and emotional abuse, many authorities recommend the routine screening of all female patients for domestic violence. Other patients at increased risk are children and the elderly.[46,47] As with other sensitive topics, start this part of the interview with general "normalizing" questions: "Because abuse is common in many women's lives, I've begun to ask about it routinely." "Are there times in your relationships that you feel unsafe or afraid?" "Many women tell me that someone at home is hurting them in some way. Is this true for you?" "Within the last year, have you been hit, kicked, punched, or otherwise hurt by someone you know? If so, by whom?" As with other segments of the history, use a pattern that goes from general to specific, less difficult to more difficult.

Physical abuse—often not mentioned by either victim or perpetrator—should be considered in the following settings:

CLUES TO POSSIBLE PHYSICAL ABUSE

- If injuries are unexplained, seem inconsistent with the patient's story, are concealed by the patient, or cause embarrassment
- If the patient has delayed getting treatment for trauma
- If there is a past history of repeated injuries or "accidents"
- If the patient or person close to the patient has a history of alcohol or drug abuse
- If the partner tries to dominate the interview, will not leave the room, or seems unusually anxious or solicitous

---

When you suspect abuse, it is important to spend part of the encounter alone with the patient. You can use the transition to the physical examination as a reason to ask the other person to leave the room. If the patient is also resistant, you should not force the situation, potentially placing the victim in jeopardy. Be attuned to diagnoses that have a higher association with abuse, such as pregnancy and somatization disorder.

Child abuse is unfortunately also common. Asking parents about their approach to discipline is a routine part of well-child care. You can also ask parents how they cope with a baby who will not stop crying or a child who misbehaves: "Most parents get very upset when their baby cries (or their child has been naughty). How do you feel when your baby cries?" "What do you do when your baby won't stop crying?" "Do you have any fears that you might hurt your child?" Find out how other caregivers or companions handle these situations as well.

See Chapter 18, Assessing Children: Infancy Through Adolescence, p. 751.

Death and the Dying Patient.
There is a growing and important emphasis in health care education on improving clinician training related to death and dying. Many clinicians avoid talking about death because of their own discomfort and anxiety. Work through your own feelings with the help of reading and discussion. Basic concepts of care are appropriate even for beginning students because you will come into contact with patients of all ages near the end of their lives.

For a discussion of end-of-life decision making, grief and bereavement, and advance directives, turn to Chapter 20, The Older Adult, p. 909.

Kubler-Ross has described five stages in a person's response to loss or the anticipatory grief of impending death: denial and isolation, anger, bargaining, depression or sadness, and acceptance.[48] These stages may occur sequentially or overlap in any order or combination. At each stage, follow the same approach. Be sensitive to the patient's feelings about dying; watch for cues that the patient is open to talking about them. Make openings for patients to ask questions: "I wonder if you have any concerns about the procedure? . . . your illness? . . . what it will be like when you go home?" Explore these concerns and provide whatever information the patient requests. Avoid unwarranted reassurance. If you explore and accept patients' feelings, answer their questions, and demonstrate your commitment to staying with them throughout their illness, reassurance will grow where it really matters—within the patients themselves.

Dying patients rarely want to talk about their illnesses at each encounter, nor do they wish to confide in everyone they meet. Give them opportunities to talk, and listen receptively, but if they stay at a social level, respect their preferences. Remember that illness—even a terminal one—is only a part of the total person. A smile, a touch, an inquiry about a family member, a comment on the day's events, or even some gentle humor affirms and sustains the unique individual you are caring for. Communicating effectively means getting to know the whole patient; that is part of the helping process.

Understanding the patient's wishes about treatment at the end of life is an important clinician responsibility. Failing to establish communication about end-of-life decisions is widely viewed as a flaw in clinical care. Even if discussions of death and dying are difficult for you, you must learn to ask specific questions. The condition of the patient and the health care setting often determine what needs to be discussed. For patients who are acutely ill and in the hospital, discussions about what the patient wants to have done in the event of a cardiac or respiratory arrest are usually mandatory. Asking about *Do Not Resuscitate (DNR) status* is often difficult when you have no previous relationship with the patient or lack knowledge of the patient's values and life experience. Find out about the patient's frame of reference because the media give many patients an unrealistic view of the effectiveness of resuscitation. "What experiences have you had with the death of a close friend or relative?" "What do you know about cardiopulmonary resuscitation (CPR)?" Educate patients about the likely success of CPR, especially if they are chronically ill or advanced in age. Assure them that relieving pain and taking care of their other spiritual and physical needs will be a priority.

In general, it is important to encourage any adult, but especially the elderly or chronically ill, to establish a *health proxy* who can act as the patient's health decision maker. This part of the interview can be a "values history" that identifies what is important to the patient and makes life worth living, and the point when living would no longer be worthwhile. Ask how patients spend their time every day, what brings them joy, and what they look forward to. Make sure to clarify the meaning of statements like, "You said that you don't want to be a burden to your family. What exactly do you mean by that?" Explore the patient's religious or spiritual frame of reference so that you and the patient can make the most appropriate decisions about health care.

See discussion of the Patient With Altered Capacity, pp. 76–77.

SOCIETAL ASPECTS OF INTERVIEWING

Demonstrating Cultural Humility—A Changing Paradigm.
Communicating effectively with patients from every background has always been an important professional skill. Nonetheless, the disparities in risks of disease, morbidity, and mortality are marked and broadly documented across different population groups, reflecting inequities in health care access, income level, type of insurance, educational level, language proficiency, and provider decision making.[49,50] To level these disparities, clinicians are increasingly urged to focus on their own attributes and responsiveness as they experience diversity in their clinical practices.

See Chapters 4–20, sections on Health Promotion and Counseling and selected notations in the Examples of Abnormalities columns.

Cultural competence has been commonly viewed as "the capacity to function effectively as an individual and an organization within the context of the cultural beliefs, behaviors, and needs" presented by patients and their communities.[51,52] Nevertheless, experts caution that too often cultural competence is reduced to a static and decontextualized set of traits and beliefs for particular ethnic groups.[53] This can inadvertently objectify such patients as "other," implicitly reinforcing the perspectives of the dominant (often Western) culture.[54] Instead, "culture is ever-changing and always being revised within the dynamic context of its enactment."[53] However, "this dynamic is often compromised by various sociocultural mismatches between patients and providers."[55] Such mismatches arise from providers' lack of knowledge about patient beliefs and lived experiences as well as the unintentional and intentional enactment of stereotypes and bias during patient encounters.

Instead, move toward the precepts of *cultural humility*. Cultural humility is defined as a "process that requires humility as individuals continually engage in self-reflection and self-critique as lifelong learners and reflective practitioners."[55] It is a process that includes "the difficult work of examining cultural beliefs and cultural systems of both patients and providers to locate the points of cultural dissonance or synergy that contribute to patients' health outcomes."[56] It calls for clinicians to "bring into check the power imbalances that exist in the dynamics of (clinician)–patient communication" and maintain mutually respectful and dynamic partnerships with patients and communities. To attain these attributes, seek out the more effective training models that continue to emerge.[57-62]

Begin your commitment to self-reflective practice by studying the vignettes that follow. These examples illustrate how cultural differences and unconscious bias can unwittingly lead to poor communication and disrupt the quality and outcomes of patient care.

CULTURAL HUMILITY: SCENARIO 1

A 28-year-old taxi driver from Ghana who had recently moved to the United States complained to a friend about U.S. medical care. He had gone to the clinic because of fever and fatigue. He described being weighed, having his temperature taken, and having a cloth wrapped tightly, to the point of pain, around his arm. The clinician, a 36-year-old woman from Washington, D.C., had asked the patient many questions, examined him, and wanted to take blood, which the patient had refused. The patient's final comment was ". . . and she didn't even give me chloroquine!"—his primary reason for seeking care. The man from Ghana was expecting few questions, no examination, and treatment for malaria, which is what fever usually means in Ghana.

In this example, cross-cultural miscommunication is understandable and thus less threatening to explore. Unconscious bias leading to miscommunication, however, occurs in many clinical interactions. Consider the scenario below that is closer to daily practice.

CULTURAL HUMILITY: SCENARIO 2

A 16-year-old high school student came to the local teen health center because of painful menstrual cramps that were interfering with concentrating at school. She was dressed in a tight top and short skirt and had multiple piercings, including in her eyebrow. The 30-year-old male clinician asked the following questions: "Are you passing all of your classes?

(continued)

CULTURAL HUMILITY: SCENARIO 2 (CONTINUED)

What kind of job do you want after high school? What kind of birth control do you want?" The teenager felt pressured into accepting birth control pills, even though she had clearly stated that she had never had intercourse and planned to postpone it until she got married. She was an honor student and planning to go to college, but the clinician did not elicit these goals. The clinician glossed over her cramps by saying, "Oh, you can just take some ibuprofen. Cramps usually get better as you get older." The patient will not take the birth control pills that were prescribed, nor will she seek health care soon again. She experienced the encounter as an interrogation, so failed to gain trust in her clinician. In addition, the clinician's questions made assumptions about her life and did not show respect for her health concerns. Even though the provider pursued important psychosocial domains, she received ineffective health care because of conflicting cultural values and unreflected clinician bias.

In both of these cases, the failure stems from mistaken assumptions or biases. In the first case, the clinician did not consider the many variables affecting patient beliefs about health and expectations for care. In the second case, the clinician allowed stereotypes to dictate the agenda instead of listening to the patient and respecting her as an individual. Each of us has our own cultural background and our own biases. These do not simply fade away as we become clinicians.

As you provide care for an ever-expanding and diverse group of patients, you must recognize how culture shapes not just the patient's beliefs, but also your own. *Culture* is the system of shared ideas, rules, and meanings that influences how we view the world, experience it emotionally, and behave in relation to other people. It can be understood as the "lens" through which we perceive and make sense out of the world we inhabit. The meaning of culture is much broader than the term "ethnicity." Cultural influences are not limited to minority groups; they are relevant to everyone.

Avoid allowing knowledge about specific cultural groups to turn into stereotyping rather than understanding. For example, you may have learned that Hispanic patients convey their pain in a more dramatic fashion. Recognize that this is a stereotype. You must evaluate each patient with pain as an individual, not decreasing the amount of analgesic you would typically use, but being aware of your reactions to the patient's style. Work on an appropriate and informed clinical approach to all patients by becoming aware of your own values and biases, developing communication skills that transcend cultural differences, and building therapeutic partnerships based on respect for each patient's life experience. This type of framework, described in the next section, will allow you to approach each patient as a unique individual.

> ## THE THREE DIMENSIONS OF CULTURAL HUMILITY
>
> - *Self-awareness.* Learn about your own biases . . . we all have them.
> - *Respectful communication.* Work to eliminate assumptions about what is "normal." Learn directly from your patients—they are the experts on their culture and illness.
> - *Collaborative partnerships.* Build your patient relationships on respect and mutually acceptable plans.

Self-Awareness.   Start by exploring your own cultural identity. How do you describe yourself in terms of ethnicity, class, region or country of origin, religion, and political affiliation? Don't forget the characteristics that we often take for granted—gender, life roles, sexual orientation, physical ability, and race—especially if we are in majority groups. What aspects of your family of origin do you identify with, and how are you different from your family of origin? How do these identities influence your beliefs and behaviors?

A more challenging task in learning about ourselves is to bring our own values and biases to a conscious level. *Values* are the standards we use to measure our own and others' beliefs and behaviors. These may appear to be absolutes. *Biases* are the attitudes or feelings that we attach to perceived differences. Being attuned to difference is normal; in fact, in the distant past, detecting differences may have preserved life. Intuitively knowing members of one's own group is a survival skill that we may have outgrown as a society but that is still actively at work.

Feeling guilty about our biases makes it hard to recognize and acknowledge them. Start with less threatening constructs, like the way an individual relates to time, a culturally determined phenomenon. Are you always on time—a positive value in the dominant Western culture? Or do you tend to run a little late? How do you feel about people whose habits are opposite to yours? Next time you attend a meeting or class, notice who is early, on time, or late. Is it predictable? Think about the role of physical appearance. Do you consider yourself thin, mid-size, or heavy? How do you feel about your weight? What does prevailing U.S. culture teach us to value in physique? How do you feel about people who have different weights?

Respectful Communication.   Given the complexity of culture, no one can possibly know the health beliefs and practices of every culture and subculture. Let your patients be the experts on their own unique cultural perspectives. Even if patients have trouble describing their values or beliefs in the abstract, they should be able to respond to specific questions. Find out about the patient's cultural background. Use some of the same questions discussed earlier in the section, Creating a Shared Understanding of the Problem (see pp. 66–67). Maintain an open, respectful, and inquiring attitude. "What did you hope to get from this visit?" If you have established rapport and trust, patients will be willing to teach you. Be aware of questions that contain assumptions. And always be ready to acknowledge your areas of ignorance or bias. "I know very little about Ghana. What would have happened at a clinic there if you had these concerns?" Or, with the second patient and with much more difficulty,

"I mistakenly made assumptions about you that are not right. I apologize. Would you be willing to tell me more about yourself and your future goals?"

Learning about specific cultures is valuable because it broadens what you, as a clinician, identify as areas you need to explore. Do some reading about the life experiences of individuals in ethnic or racial groups that live in your area. There may be reasons for loss of trust in clinicians and health care delivery.[63] Go to movies that are filmed in different countries or explicitly present the perspective of different cultures. Learn about the concerns of different consumer groups with visible health agendas. Get to know healers of different disciplines and learn about their practices. Most importantly, be open to learning from your patients. Do not assume that what you have learned about a cultural group applies to the individual before you.

Collaborative Partnerships.   Through continual work on self-awareness and seeing through the "lens" of others, the clinician lays the foundation for the collaborative relationship that best supports the patient's health. Communication based on trust, respect, and a willingness to reexamine assumptions allows patients to express concerns that may run counter to the dominant culture. These concerns may be associated with strong feelings such as anger or shame. You, the clinician, must be willing to listen to and validate these feelings, and not let your own feelings prevent you from exploring painful areas. You must also be willing to reexamine your beliefs about what is the "right approach" to clinical care in a given situation. Make every effort to be flexible and creative in your plans and respectful of patients' knowledge about their own best interests. By consciously distinguishing what is truly important to the patient's health from what is just the standard advice, you and your patients can construct the unique approach to their health care that is in concert with their beliefs and effective clinical care. Remember that if the patient stops listening, fails to follow your advice, or does not return, your health care has not been successful.

Sexuality in the Clinician–Patient Relationship.   Clinicians of both genders occasionally find themselves physically attracted to their patients. Similarly, patients may make sexual overtures or exhibit flirtatious behavior toward clinicians. The emotional and physical intimacy of the clinician–patient relationship may lend itself to these sexual feelings.

If you become aware of such feelings in yourself, accept them as a normal human response, and bring them to conscious level so they will not affect your behavior. Denying these feelings makes it more likely for you to act inappropriately. *Any* sexual contact or romantic relationship with patients is *unethical;* keep your relationship with the patient within professional bounds, and seek help if you need it.[64–66]

Sometimes clinicians meet patients who are frankly seductive or make sexual advances. You may be tempted to ignore this behavior because you are not sure that it really happened, or you are just hoping it will go away. Calmly but firmly, make it clear that your relationship is professional, not personal. If unwelcome overtures continue, leave the room and find a chaperone to continue the interview. You should also reflect on your image. Has your clothing or demeanor been unconsciously seductive? Have you been overly warm with the patient? Although it is your responsibility to avoid contributing to these problems, usually you are not at fault. Often these problems reflect the patient's discomfort with feeling less powerful.

Ethics and Professionalism.   You may wonder why an introductory chapter on interviewing contains a section on clinical ethics. The potential power of clinician–patient communication calls for guidance beyond our innate sense of morality.[67] *Ethics* are a set of principles crafted through reflection and discussion to define right and wrong. *Medical ethics,* which guide our professional behavior, are neither static nor simple, but several principles have guided clinicians throughout the ages. Although in most situations your gut sense of right and wrong will be all that you need, even as students, you will face decisions that call for the application of ethical principles.

Some of the traditional and still fundamental maxims embedded in the healing professions are listed below. This body of ethics has been termed *"principalism."* As the field of clinical ethics expands, other ethical systems come into play: *utilitarianism*, or providing the greatest good for the greatest number, building on the work of John Stuart Mill; *feminist ethics*, which invoke problems of marginalization of social groups; *casuistry*, or the analysis of paradigmatic prior cases as relevant; and *communitarianism*, which emphasizes the interests of communities and societies over individuals and social responsibilities bearing on the need to maintain the institutions of civil society.[68]

BUILDING BLOCKS OF PROFESSIONAL ETHICS IN PATIENT CARE

- *Nonmaleficence or primum non nocere* is commonly stated as, "First, do no harm." In the context of an interview, giving information that is incorrect or not really related to the patient's problem can do harm. Avoiding relevant topics or creating barriers to open communication can also do harm.
- *Beneficence* is the dictum that the clinician needs to "do good" for the patient. As clinicians, your actions need to be motivated by what is in the patient's best interest.
- *Autonomy* reminds us that patients have the right to determine what is in their own best interest. This principle has become increasingly important over time and is consistent with collaborative rather than paternalistic clinician–patient relationships.
- *Confidentiality* can be one of the most challenging principles. As a clinician, you are obligated not to repeat what you learn from or know about a patient. This privacy is fundamental to our professional relationships with patients. In the daily flurry of activity in a hospital, it is all too easy to let something slip. You must be on your guard.

As students, you are exposed to some of the ethical challenges that you will confront later as practicing clinicians. However, there are dilemmas unique to students that you will face from the time that you begin taking care of patients. The following vignettes capture some of the most common experiences. They raise a variety of ethical and practical issues that are overlapping.

ETHICS AND PROFESSIONALISM: SCENARIO 1

You are a third-year medical student on your first clinical rotation in the hospital. It is late in the evening when you are finally assigned to the patient you are to "work up" and present the next day at preceptor rounds. You go to the patient's room and find the patient exhausted from the day's events and clearly ready to settle down for the night. You know that your intern and attending physician have already done their evaluations. Do you proceed with a history and physical that is likely to take 1 to 2 hours? Is this process only for your education? Do you ask permission before you start? What do you include?

Here you are confronted with the tension between *the need to learn by doing* and *doing no harm to patients.* There is a utilitarian ethical principle that reminds us that if clinicians-in-training do not learn, there will be no future caregivers. Yet the dictums to do no harm and prioritize what is in the patient's best interests are clearly in conflict with that future need. As a student, this dilemma will arise often.

Obtaining *informed consent* is the means to address this ethical dilemma. Making sure the patient realizes that you are in training and new at patient evaluation is always important. It is impressive how often patients willingly let students be involved in their care. It is an opportunity for patients to give back to their caregivers. Even when clinical activities appear to be purely for educational purposes, there may be a benefit to the patient. Multiple caregivers provide multiple perspectives, and the experience of being heard can be therapeutic.

ETHICS AND PROFESSIONALISM: SCENARIO 2

It is after 10 PM, and you and your resident are on the way to complete the required advance directives form with a frail, elderly patient who was admitted earlier that day with bilateral pneumonia. The form, which includes a discussion of Do Not Resuscitate orders, must be completed before the team can sign out and leave for the day. Just then, your resident is paged to an emergency and asks you to go ahead and meet with the patient to complete the form; the resident will cosign it later. You had a lecture on advance directives and end-of-life discussions in your first year of medical school but have never seen a clinician discuss this with a patient. You have not yet met the patient, nor have you had a chance to really look at the form. What should you do? Do you inform the resident that you have never done this before nor even seen it done? Do you need to inform the patient that this is totally new for you? Who should decide whether you are competent to do this independently?

In this situation, you are being asked to take responsibility for clinical care that exceeds your level of comfort and perhaps your competence. This can happen in a number of situations, such as being asked to evaluate a clinical situation without proper back-up or to draw blood or start an IV before practicing under supervision. For the patient in the second scenario, you may have many of the following thoughts: "the patient needs to have this completed before going to sleep and so will benefit"; "the risk to the patient from discussing advance directives is minimal"; "you are pretty good with elderly patients and think that you might be able to do this"; "what if the patient actually arrests that night and you are responsible for what happens?"; and finally, "if you bother the resident now he or she will be angry and that may affect your evaluation." There is educational value in being pushed to the limits of your knowledge to solve problems and to gain confidence in functioning independently. But what is the right thing to do in this situation?

The principles listed above only partially help you sort this out because only part of your quandary relates to your relationship with the patient. Much of the tension in this scenario has to do with the dynamics of a health care team and your role on that team. You are there to help with the work of the team, but you are primarily there to learn. Current formulations of medical ethics address those issues and others. One such formulation is the Tavistock Principles.[69] These principles construct a framework for analyzing health care situations that extends beyond our direct care of individual patients to complicated choices about the interactions of health care teams and the distribution of resources for the well-being of society. A broadly representative group that initially met in Tavistock Square in London in 1998 has continued to elaborate an evolving document of ethical principles for guiding health care behavior for both individuals and institutions across the health care spectrum. A current iteration of the Tavistock Principles follows.

THE TAVISTOCK PRINCIPLES

Rights: People have a right to health and health care.

Balance: Care of the individual patient is central, but the health of populations is also our concern.

Comprehensiveness: In addition to treating illness, we have an obligation to ease suffering, minimize disability, prevent disease, and promote health.

Cooperation: Health care succeeds only if we cooperate with those we serve, each other, and those in other sectors.

Improvement: Improving health care is a serious and continuing responsibility.

Safety: Do no harm.

Openness: Being open, honest, and trustworthy is vital in health care.

In the second scenario, think about the Tavistock Principles of *openness and cooperation*, in addition to the balance between *do no harm* and *beneficence*. You need to work with your team in a way that is honest and reliable to do the best for the patient. You can also see that there are no clear or easy answers in such situations. What responses are available to you to address these and other quandaries?

You need to reflect on your beliefs and assess your level of comfort with a given situation. Sometimes there may be alternative solutions. For example, in Scenario 1, the patient may really be willing to have the history and physical examination done at that late hour, or perhaps you can negotiate a time for the next morning. In Scenario 2, you might find another person who is more qualified to complete the form or to supervise when you do it. Alternatively, you may choose to go ahead and complete the form, alerting the patient to your inexperience and obtaining the patient's consent. You will need to choose which situations warrant voicing your concerns, even at the risk of a bad evaluation.

Seek coaching on how to express your reservations in a way that ensures that they will be heard. As a clinical student, you will need settings for discussing these immediately relevant ethical dilemmas with other students and with more senior trainees and faculty. Small groups that are structured to address these kinds of issues are particularly useful in providing validation and support. Take advantage of such opportunities whenever possible.

ETHICS AND PROFESSIONALISM: SCENARIO 3

You are the student on the clinical team that has been taking care of Ms. Robbins, a 64-year-old woman admitted for an evaluation of weight loss and weakness. During the hospitalization, she had a biopsy of a mass in her chest in addition to many other tests. You have gotten to know her well, spending a lot of time with her to answer questions, explain procedures, and learn about her and her family. You have discussed her fears about what "they" will find and know that she likes to know everything possible about her health and medical care. You have even heard her express frustrations with her attending physician at not always being given the "straight story." It is late Friday afternoon, but you promised Ms. Robbins that you would come by one more time before the weekend and let her know if the results of the biopsy were back yet. Just before you go to her room, the resident tells you that the pathology is back from her biopsy and shows metastatic cancer, but the attending physician does not want the team to say anything until he comes in on Monday.

What are you going to do? You feel that it is wrong to avoid the situation by not going to her room. You also believe that the patient's preference and anxiety are best served by finding out then and not waiting for 3 days. You do not want to go against the attending physician's clear instructions, however, both because you respect the fact that it is his patient and because that feels dishonest.

In this situation, telling the patient about her biopsy results is dictated by several ethical principles: the patient's best interests, autonomy, and your integrity. The other part of the ethical dilemma concerns communicating your plan to the attending. Sometimes the most challenging part of such dilemmas tests your will to follow through with the right course of action. Although it may appear to be a lose-lose situation, a respectful and honest discussion with the attending, respectfully articulating what is in the patient's best interest, will usually be heard. Enlist the support of your resident or other helpful attendings if that is possible. Learning how to navigate difficult discussions will be a useful professional skill.

B I B L I O G R A P H Y

CITATIONS

1. Cohen-Cole SA. The Medical Interview: The Three Function Approach. St. Louis: MosbyYear Book, 1991.

2. Bird J, Cohen-Cole SA. The three function model of the medical interview. Adv Psychosom Med 20:65–88, 1990.

3. Lazare A, Putnam SM, Lipkin M Jr. Three functions of the medical interview. In: Lipkin M Jr, Putnam SM, Lazare A, et al, eds. The Medical Interview: Clinical Care, Education, and Research. New York: Springer-Verlag, 1995.

4. Novack DH. Therapeutic aspects of the clinical encounter. In Lipkin M Jr, Putnam SM, et al, eds. The Medical Interview: Clinical Care, Education, and Research. New York: Springer-Verlag:32, 1995.

5. Suchman AL, Matthews DA. What makes the patient-doctor relationship therapeutic? Exploring the connectional dimension of medical care. Ann Intern Med 108(1):25–130, 1988.

6. Hastings C. The lived experiences of the illness: making contact with the patient. In: Benne P, Wrubel J, eds. The Primacy of Caring: Stress and Coping in Health and Illness. Menlo Park CA: Addison-Wesley, 1989.

7. Wagner EH, Austin BT, Korff MV. Organizing care for patients with chronic illness. Milbank Q 74(4):511–544, 1996.

8. Epstein RM. Mindful practice. JAMA 282(9):833–839, 1999.

9. Balint M. The Doctor, His Patient and the Illness. 2nd ed. New York: International Universities Press, 1964.

10. Ventres W, Kooienga S, Vuvkovic N, et al. Physicians, patients and the electronic health record: an ethnographic analysis. Ann Fam Med 4(2):124–131, 2006.

11. Conant EB. Addressing patients by their first names. N Engl J Med 308(4):226, 1998.

12. Heller ME. Addressing patients by their first names. N Engl J Med 308(18):1107, 1987.

13. Platt FW, Gaspar DL, Coulehan JL, et al. "Tell me about yourself": the patient-centered interview. Ann Int Med 134(11):1079–1085, 2001.

14. Baron RJ. An introduction to medical phenomenology: I can't hear you while I'm listening. Ann Intern Med 103(4):606–611, 1985.

15. Bass LW, Cohen RL. Ostensible versus actual reasons for seeking pediatric attention: another look at the parental ticket of admission. Pediatrics 70(6):870–874, 1982.

16. Beckman HB, Frankel RM. The effect of physician behavior on the collection of data. Ann Intern Med 101(4):692–696, 1984.

17. White J, Levinson W, Roter D. "Oh, by the way…:" the closing moments of the medical visit. J Gen Intern Med 9(1):24–28, 1994.

18. Smith RC. Patient-Centered Interviewing: An Evidence-Based Method. Philadelphia: Lippincott Williams & Wilkins, 2002.

19. Von Korff M, Shapiro S, Burke JD, et al. Anxiety and depression in a primary care clinic. Arch Gen Psychiatry 44(2):152–156, 1987.

20. Lang F, Floyd MR, Beine KL. Clues to patients' explanations and concerns about their illnesses: a call for active listening. Arch Fam Med 9(3):222–227, 2000.

21. Brown JB, Weston W, Stewart M. Patient-centered interviewing part II: finding common ground. Can Fam Physician 35:153–157, 1989.

22. Neighbour R. The Inner Consultation: How to Develop an Effective and Intuitive Consulting Style. Lancaster, England: MTP Press Ltd.:164–178, 1987.

23. Kleinman A, Eisenberg L, Good B. Culture, illness, and care: clinical lessons from anthropological and cross-cultural research. Ann Intern Med 88(2):251–258, 1978.

24. Smith RC, Lyles JS, Mettler J, et al. The effectiveness of an intensive teaching experience for residents in interviewing: a randomized controlled study. Ann Intern Med 128(2):118–126, 1998.

25. Miller WM, Rollnick S. Motivational Interviewing–Preparing People for Change. 2nd ed. New York: Guilford Press, 2002.

26. Engel GL. The need for a new medical model: a challenge for biomedicine. Science 196(4286):126–129, 1977.

27. Engel GL, Morgan WL Jr. Interviewing the Patient. Philadelphia: WB Saunders, 1973.

28. Bayer–Fetzer Conference on physician–patient communication in medical education. Essential elements of communication in medical encounters: the Kalamazoo Consensus Statement. Acad Med 76(4):390–393, 2001.

29. Stewart M. Questions about patient-centered care: answers from quantitative research. In: Stewart M, et al, eds. Patient-Centered Medicine: Transforming the Clinical Method. Abington, UK: Radcliffe Medical Press: 263–268, 2003.

30. Coulehan JL, Block MR. The Medical Interview: Mastering Skills for Clinical Practice, 4th ed. Philadelphia: FA Davis Company, 2001.

31. Lipkin M Jr, Putnam SM, Lazare A, et al (eds). The Medical Interview: Clinical Care, Education, and Research. New York: Springer-Verlag, 1995.

32. Office for Civil Rights–HIPAA, U.S. Department of Health and Human Services. Available at: http://www.hhs.gov/ocr/hipaa/. Accessed February 17, 2008.

33. Platt FW. Field Guide to the Difficult Patient Interview. Philadelphia: Lippincott Williams and Wilkins, 1999.

34. Jacobs EA, Shephard DS, Suya JA, et al. Overcoming language barriers in health care: costs and benefits in interpreter services. Am J Public Health 94(5):866–869, 2004.

35. Jacobs EA, Sadowski LS, Rathous PJ. The impact of enhanced interpreter service intervention on hospital costs and patient satisfaction. J Gen Intern Med 22(suppl 2):306–311, 2007.

36. Hardt E, Jacobs EA, Chen A. Insights into the problems that language barriers may pose for the medical interview. J Gen Intern Med 21(12):1357–1358, 2006.

37. U.S. Preventive Services Task Force. Screening and behavioral counseling interventions in primary care to reduce alcohol misuse: recommendation statement. Rockville, MD, Agency for Healthcare Research and Quality, April 2004. Available at: http://www.ahrq.gov/clinic/3rduspstf/alcohol/alcomisrs.htm. Accessed February 18, 2008.

38. Regier DA, Farmer ME, Rae DS, et al. Comorbidity of mental disorders with alcohol and other drug abuse. Results from the Epidemiologic Catchment Area (ECA) study. JAMA 264(19):2511–2518, 1990.

39. Saitz R. Unhealthy alcohol use. N Engl J Med 352(67):596–607, 2005.

40. Carni J, Farre M. Drug addiction. N Engl J Med 349(10): 975–986, 2003.

41. Cyr MG, Wartman SA. The effectiveness of routine screening questions in the detection of alcoholism. JAMA 259(1):51–54, 1988.

42. Ewing JA. Detecting alcoholism: the CAGE questionnaire. JAMA 252(14):1905–1907, 1984.

43. National Institute on Alcohol Abuse and Alcoholism. Helping patients who drink too much. A clinician's guide. Available at: http://pubs.niaaa.nih.gov/publications/Practitioner/Clinicians Guide2005/clinicians_guide.htm. Accessed February 18, 2008.

44. National Institute on Alcohol Abuse and Alcoholism. Alcohol Alert No. 62. Alcohol–an important issue in women's health. July 2004. Available at: http://pubs.niaaa.nih.gov/publications/aa62/aa62.htm. Accessed February 18, 2008.

45. Cocco KM, Carey KB. Psychometric properties of the drug abuse screening test in psychiatric outpatients. Psychol Assessment 10(4):408–414, 1998.

46. U.S. Preventive Services Task Force. Screening for family and intimate partner violence: recommendation statement. Rockville MD, Agency for Healthcare Research and Quality, March 2004. Available at: http://www.ahrq.gov/clinic/3rduspstf/famviolence/famviolrs.htm. Accessed February 18, 2008.

47. Rhodes KV, Frankel RM, Levinthal N, et al. "You're not the victim of domestic violence, are you?" Provider-patient communication about domestic violence. Ann Intern Med 147(9): 620–627, 2007.

48. Kübler-Ross E. On Death and Dying. New York: Macmillan, 1997.

49. Smedley BA, Stith AY, Nelson AR (eds). Committee on Understanding and Eliminating Racial and Ethnic Disparities in Health Care. Unequal Treatment: Confronting Racial and Ethnic Disparities in Health Care. Washington DC: Institute of Medicine, 2003.

50. Agency for Healthcare Quality and Research. National Health Care Disparities Report 2006–Highlights. Available at: http://www.ahrq.gov/qual/nhdr06/nhdr06high.pdf. Accessed February 17, 2008.

51. Office of Minority Health, U.S. Department of Health and Human Services. National standards on culturally and linguistically appropriate services (CLAS). Available at: http://www.omhrc.gov/templates/browse.aspx?lvl=2&lvlID=15. Accessed February 16, 2008.

52. Office of Minority Health, U.S. Department of Health and Human Services. National standards on culturally and linguistically appropriate health care. Executive summary. Available at: http://www.omhrc.gov/assets/pdf/checked/executive.pdf. Accessed February 16, 2008.

53. Hunt LM. Beyond cultural competence. Park Ridge Bulletin 24:3–4, 2001. Available at: http://www.parkridgecenter.org/Page1882.html. Accessed February 16, 2008.

54. Kumas-Tan Z, Beagan B, Loppie C, et al. Measures of cultural competence: examining hidden assumptions. Acad Med 82(6): 548–557, 2007.

55. Tervalon M, Murray-Garcia J. Cultural humility versus cultural competence: a critical distinction in defining physician training outcomes in multicultural education. J Health Care Poor Underserved 9(2):117–125, 1998.

56. Tervalon M. Components of culture in health for medical students' education. Acad Med 78(6):570–576, 2003.

57. Smith WR, Betancourt JR, Wynia MK, et al. Recommendations for teaching about racial and ethnic disparities in health and health care. Ann Intern Med 147(9):654–665, 2007.

58. National Center for Cultural Competence. Georgetown University Center for Child and Human Development. Available at: http://www11.georgetown.edu/research/gucchd/nccc/index.html. Accessed February 16, 2008. See also: Tools and Processes for Self Assessment. Available at: http://www11.georgetown.edu/research/gucchd/nccc/foundations/assessment.html. Accessed February 16, 2008

59. Jacobs EA, Kohrman C, Lemon M, et al. Teaching physicians-in-training to address racial disparities in health: a community-hospital partnership. Public Health Rep 18(4):349–356, 2003.

60. Juarez JA, Marvel K, Brezinski KL, et al. Bridging the gap: a curriculum to teach residents cultural humility. Fam Med 38(2):97–102, 2006.

61. Office of Minority Health, U.S. Department of Health and Human Services. Think cultural health: bridging the health care gap through cultural competency continuing education programs. Available at: http://www.thinkculturalhealth.org/. Accessed February 16, 2008.

62. National Consortium for Multicultural Education for Health Professionals. Available at: http://culturalmeded.stanford.edu/. Accessed February 17, 2008.

63. Jacobs EA, Rolle I, Ferrans CE, et al. Understanding African Americans' views of the trustworthiness of physicians. J Gen Intern Med 21(6):642–647, 2006.

64. Committee on Ethics, American College of Obstetricians and Gynecologists. ACOG Committee Opinion No. 373. Sexual misconduct. Obstet Gynecol 110(2 Pt 1):441–444, 2007.

65. Gabbard GO, Nadelson C. Professional boundaries in the physician-patient relationship. JAMA 273(18):1445–1449, 1995.

66. Council on Ethical and Judicial Affairs. American Medical Association: sexual misconduct in the practice of medicine. JAMA 266(19):2741–2745, 1991.

67. ABIM Foundation, American Board of Internal Medicine, ACP-ASIM Foundation, American College of Physicians-American Society of Internal Medicine, European Federation of Internal Medicine. Medical professionalism in the new millennium: a physician charter. Ann Intern Med 136(3): 243–246, 2002.

68. Giordano J. The ethics of interventional pain management: basic concepts and theories: problems and practice. Presentation at: Texas Tech University Health Sciences Center, February 15, 2008, Lubbock, TX.

69. Berwick D, Davidoff F, Hiatt H, et al. Refining and implementing the Tavistock principles for everybody in health care. Brit Med J 323(7313):616–619, 2001.

ADDITIONAL REFERENCES

Building a Therapeutic Relationship: The Techniques of Skilled Interviewing

Billings JA, Stoeckle JD. The Clinical Encounter: A Guide to the Medical Interview and Case Presentation, 2nd ed. St. Louis: Mosby, 1999.

Côté L, Leclère H. How clinical teachers perceive the doctor-patient relationship and themselves as role models. Acad Med 75(11):1117–1124, 2000.

Delbanco TL. Enriching the doctor-patient relationship by inviting the patient's perspective. Ann Intern Med 116(5):414–418, 1993.

Frankel RM, Quill TE, McDanial SH. The biopsychosocial approach: past, present, and future. Rochester, NY: University of Rochester Press, 2003.

Kurtz SM, Silverman J, Draper J. Teaching and learning communication skills in medicine, 2nd ed. Oxford, San Francisco: Radcliffe Publishers, 2005.

McAulay V. The changing doctor–patient relationship: diagnoses are made from careful history and examination. BMJ 320 (7238):873–874, 2000.

Adapting Interviewing Techniques to Specific Situations

Agency for Healthcare Research and Quality. Evidence Report/Technology Assessment No. 87. Literacy and Health Outcomes. January 2004. Available at: http://www.ahrq.gov/downloads/pub/evidence/pdf/literacy/literacy.pdf. Accessed June 8, 2008.

Americans with Disabilities Act Home Page, U.S. Department of Justice. Available at http://www.ada.gov/#Anchor-47857. Accessed June 7, 2008.

Barnett S. Cross-cultural communication with patients who use American sign language. Fam Med 34(5):376–382, 2002.

Grantmakers in Health: In the right words: addressing language and culture in providing health care. Issues in Brief 18:1–54, 2003.

Iezzoni LI, O'Day BL, Killeen M, et al. Communicating about health care: observations from persons who are deaf or hard of hearing. Ann Intern Med 140(5):356–362, 2004.

Marcus EN. The silent epidemic—the health effects of illiteracy. N Engl J Med 355(4):339–341, 2006.

McDaniel SH, Campbell TL, Hepworth J, et al. Family-Oriented Primary Care, 2nd ed. New York: Springer, 2005.

Putsch RW. Cross-cultural communication: the special case of interpreters in health care. JAMA 254(23):3344–3348, 1985.

Rivadeneyra R, Elderkin-Thompson V, Silver RC, et al. Patient centeredness in medical encounters requiring an interpreter. Am J Med 108(6):470–474, 2000.

Schwartzberg JG, Cowett A, VanGeest J, et al. Communication techniques for patients with low health literacy: a survey of physicians, nurses, and pharmacists. Am J Health Behav 31(Suppl. 1):S96–104, 2007.

Sensitive Topics That Call for Specific Approaches

Cochran SD, Mays VM. Physical health complaints among lesbians, gay men, and bisexual and homosexually experienced heterosexual individuals: results from the California Quality of Life Survey. Am J Public Health 97(11):2048–2055, 2007.

End of Life/Palliative Education Resource Center. Available at: http://www.eperc.mcw.edu/index.htm. Accessed June 8, 2008.

Fiellin DA, Reid MC, O'Connor PG. Screening for alcohol problems in primary care: a systematic review. Arch Intern Med 160(13):1977–1989, 2000.

Lee R. Health care problems of lesbian, gay, bisexual, and transgender patients. West J Med 172(6):403–408, 2000.

Marlatt GA, Donovan DM. Relapse Prevention: Maintenance Strategies in the Treatment of Addictive Behaviors, 2nd ed. New York: Guilford Press, 2005.

Miller WR, Rollnick S. Motivational Interviewing, 2nd ed. New York: Guilford Press, 2002.

Rastegar DA, Fingerhood MI. Addiction Medicine: An Evidence-based Handbook. Philadelphia: Lippincott Williams & Wilkins, 2005.

Vandemark LM, Mueller M. Mental health after sexual violence: the role of behavioral and demographic risk factors. Nurs Res 57(3):175–181, 2008.

Societal Aspects of Interviewing

Carrillo JE, Green AR, Betancourt JR. Cross-cultural primary care: a patient-based approach. Ann Intern Med 130:829–834, 1999.

Council on Ethical and Judicial Affairs, American Medical Association. Sexual misconduct in the practice of medicine. JAMA 266(19):2741–2745, 1991.

Doyal L. Closing the gap between professional teaching and practice. BMJ 322(7288):685–686, 2001.

Enbom JA, Parshley P, Kollath J. A follow-up evaluation of sexual misconduct complaints: the Oregon Board of Medical Examiners, 1998 through 2002. Am J Obstet Gynecol 190(6): 1642–1650; discussion, 1650–1653; 6A, 2004.

Fadiman A. The Spirit Catches You and You All Fall Down. New York: Farrar, Straus and Giroux, 1997.

Gabbard GO, Nadelson C. Professional boundaries in the physician–patient relationship. JAMA 273(18):1445–1449, 1995.

Medical professionalism in the new millennium: a physician charter. Ann Intern Med 136(3):243–246, 2002.

Lo B. Resolving Ethical Dilemmas: A Guide for Clinicians, 3rd ed. Philadelphia: Lippincott Williams & Wilkins, 2005.

Makoul G. Essential elements of communication in medical encounters: the Kalamazoo consensus statement. Acad Med 76(4):390–393, 2001.

Robinson GE, Stewart DE. A curriculum on physician–patient sexual misconduct and teacher–learner mistreatment. Part 1: Content. Can Med Assoc J 154(1):643–649, 1996.

The Bates' suite offers these additional resources to enhance learning and facilitate understanding of this chapter:

- *Bates' Pocket Guide to Physical Examination and History Taking,* 6th edition
- *Bates' Nursing Online*
- *Bates' Visual Guide to Physical Examination,* 4th edition
- thePoint online resources, http://thepoint.lww.com
- Student CD-ROM included with the book

Regional Examinations

2

Beginning the Physical Examination: General Survey, Vital Signs, and Pain

Once you understand the patient's concerns and have elicited a careful history, you are ready to begin the physical examination. At first you may feel unsure of how the patient will relate to you. With practice, your skills in physical examination will grow, and you will gain confidence. Through study and repetition, the examination will flow more smoothly, and you will soon shift your attention from technique and how to handle instruments to what you hear, see, and feel. Touching the patient's body will seem more natural, and you will learn to minimize any discomfort to the patient. Before long, as you gain proficiency, what once took between 1 and 2 hours will take considerably less time.

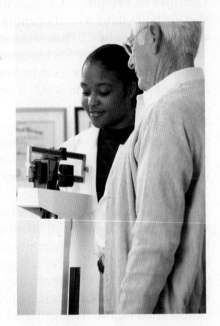

This chapter, reorganized for this edition, addresses *Common or Concerning Symptoms* that relate to general health. *Health Promotion and Counseling* focuses on important habits for a healthy lifestyle—optimal weight and nutrition, exercise, and blood pressure and diet. This section provides information that will be useful as you counsel patients about their Body Mass Index (BMI), particularly because being overweight or obese poses a growing health threat to all age groups in our population. The remaining sections of the chapter follow the sequence of the patient visit.

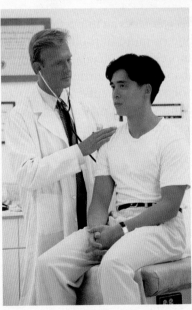

- *General Survey*—The General Survey begins with the first moments of the patient encounter. How do you perceive the patient's apparent state of health, demeanor and facial affect or expression, grooming, posture, and gait? Height and weight, usually recorded before the patient enters the examining room, add important detail to the General Survey.

- *Vital Signs*—These include blood pressure, heart rate, respiratory rate, and temperature and their ranges of normal.

- *Pain, the Fifth Vital Sign*—This edition brings new information on how to assess pain, commonly underdiagnosed and a major focus of caring for patients in all health professions.

THE HEALTH HISTORY

Common or Concerning Symptoms

- Changes in weight
- Fatigue and weakness
- Fever, chills, night sweats
- Pain

Changes in Weight.   Changes in weight result from changes in body tissues or body fluid. Good opening questions include "How often do you check your weight?" "How is it compared to a year ago?" For changes, ask, "Why do you think it has changed?" "What would you like to weigh?" If weight gain or loss appears to be a problem, ask about the amount of change, its timing, the setting in which it occurred, and any associated symptoms.

Weight gain occurs when caloric intake exceeds caloric expenditure over time and typically appears as increased body fat. Weight gain may also reflect abnormal accumulation of body fluids. When the retention of fluid is relatively mild, it may not be visible, but several pounds of fluid usually appear as *edema*.

In the overweight patient, for example, when did the weight gain begin? Was the patient heavy as an infant or a child? Using milestones appropriate to the patient's age, inquire about weight at the following times: birth, kindergarten, high school or college graduation, discharge from military service, marriage, after each pregnancy, menopause, and retirement. What were the patient's life circumstances during the periods of weight gain? Has the patient tried to lose weight? How? With what results?

Weight loss is an important symptom with many causes. Mechanisms include one or more of the following: decreased intake of food for reasons such as anorexia, dysphagia, vomiting, and insufficient supplies of food; defective absorption of nutrients through the gastrointestinal tract; increased metabolic requirements; and loss of nutrients through the urine, feces, or injured skin. A person may also lose weight when a fluid-retaining state improves or responds to treatment.

Try to determine whether the drop in weight is proportional to any change in food intake, or whether it has remained normal or even increased.

Rapid changes in weight, over a few days, suggest changes in body fluids, not tissues.

↑ wgt
- fat vs. edema

Causes of weight loss include *gastrointestinal diseases; endocrine disorders* (diabetes mellitus, hyperthyroidism, adrenal insufficiency); *chronic infections; malignancy; chronic cardiac, pulmonary, or renal failure; depression;* and *anorexia nervosa or bulimia* (see Table 4-1, Eating Disorders and Excessively Low BMI, p. 128).

Weight loss with relatively high food intake suggests *diabetes mellitus, hyperthyroidism,* or *malabsorption.* Consider also binge eating (bulimia) with clandestine vomiting.

Symptoms associated with weight loss often suggest a cause, as does a thorough psychosocial history. Who cooks and shops for the patient? Where does the patient eat? With whom? Are there any problems with obtaining, storing, preparing, or chewing food? Does the patient avoid or restrict certain foods for medical, religious, or other reasons?

Poverty, old age, social isolation, physical disability, emotional or mental impairment, lack of teeth, ill-fitting dentures, alcoholism, and drug abuse increase the likelihood of malnutrition.

Throughout the history, be alert for signs of malnutrition. Symptoms may be subtle and nonspecific, such as weakness, easy fatigability, cold intolerance, flaky dermatitis, and ankle swelling. Securing a good history of eating patterns and quantities is essential. Ask general questions about intake at different times throughout the day, such as "Tell me what you typically eat for lunch." "What do you eat for a snack?" "When?"

See Table 4-2, Nutrition Screening, p. 129.

Fatigue and Weakness.   Like weight loss, *fatigue* is a nonspecific symptom with many causes. It refers to a sense of weariness or loss of energy that patients describe in various ways. "I don't feel like getting up in the morning" . . . "I don't have any energy" . . . "I just feel blah". . . "I'm all done in" . . . "I can hardly get through the day" . . . "By the time I get to the office I feel as if I've done a day's work." Because fatigue is a normal response to hard work, sustained stress, or grief, try to elicit the life circumstances in which it occurs. Fatigue unrelated to such situations requires further investigation.

Fatigue is a common symptom of depression and anxiety states, but also consider *infections* (such as hepatitis, infectious mononucleosis, and tuberculosis); *endocrine disorders* (hypothyroidism, adrenal insufficiency, diabetes mellitus, panhypopituitarism); *heart failure; chronic disease of the lungs, kidneys, or liver; electrolyte imbalance; moderate to severe anemia; malignancies; nutritional deficits;* and *medications.*

Use open-ended questions to explore the attributes of the patient's fatigue, and encourage the patient to fully describe what he or she is experiencing. Important clues about etiology often emerge from a good psychosocial history, exploration of sleep patterns, and a thorough review of systems.

Weakness is different from fatigue. It denotes a demonstrable loss of muscle power and will be discussed later with other neurologic symptoms (see pp. 665).

Weakness, especially if localized in a neuroanatomical pattern, suggests possible *neuropathy* or *myopathy.*

Fever, Chills, and Night Sweats.   *Fever* refers to an abnormal elevation in body temperature (see p. 120 for definitions of normal). Ask about fever if patients have an acute or chronic illness. Find out whether the patient has used a thermometer to measure the temperature. Bear in mind that errors in technique can lead to unreliable information. Has the patient felt feverish or unusually hot, noted excessive sweating, or felt chilly and cold? Try to distinguish between subjective *chilliness,* and a *shaking chill* with shivering throughout the body and chattering of teeth.

Recurrent shaking chills suggest more extreme swings in temperature and systemic *bacteremia.*

Feeling cold, goosebumps, and shivering accompany a rising temperature, while feeling hot and sweating accompany a falling temperature. Normally the body temperature rises during the day and falls during the night. When fever exaggerates this swing, *night sweats* occur. Malaise, headache, and pain in the muscles and joints often accompany fever.

Feelings of heat and sweating also accompany menopause. Night sweats occur in *tuberculosis* and *malignancy.*

Fever has many causes. Focus your questions on the timing of the illness and its associated symptoms. Become familiar with patterns of infectious diseases that may affect your patient. Inquire about travel, contact with sick people, or other unusual exposures. Be sure to inquire about medications because they may cause fever. In contrast, recent ingestion of aspirin, acetaminophen, corticosteroids, and nonsteroidal anti-inflammatory drugs may mask fever and affect the temperature recorded at the time of the physical examination.

Pain.   Pain is one of the most common symptoms prompting office care. Each year, approximately 70 million Americans report persistent or intermittent pain, often underassessed and undertreated.[1-3] Adopt a comprehensive approach to guide your subsequent physical examination and management. Because of its importance in patient well-being, turn to the new section later in this chapter to guide your approach to patients with pain.

See Acute and Chronic Pain, pp. 121–124 later in this chapter for discussion of etiologies of pain and strategies for assessment.

HEALTH PROMOTION AND COUNSELING

Important Topics for Health Promotion and Counseling

- Optimal weight, nutrition, and diet
- Exercise

Optimal Weight, Nutrition, and Diet.   Fewer than half of U.S. adults maintain a healthy weight, with a BMI of 19 or above but less than 25. Obesity has increased in every segment of the U.S. population, regardless of age, gender, ethnicity, or socioeconomic status. Review the alarming statistics about the rising prevalence of obesity nationally and worldwide in the table below.

See Table 4-3, Obesity-Related Risk Factors and Diseases, p. 130.

● Obesity At a Glance

- More than 60% of U.S. adults are overweight or obese (BMI >25).
- More than 14% of U.S. children and adolescents are overweight.
- Health Disparities: the prevalence of being overweight or obese is higher in selected ethnic and income groups:
  - Women: black women—69%; white women—47%
  - Women: women with an income <130% of the poverty threshold are 50% more likely to be obese than those at higher income levels
  - Men: black men—58%; white men—62%
  - Adolescents: highest prevalence in Mexican-American boys, black girls, white boys from lower-income families
- Overweight and obesity increase risk of heart disease, numerous types of cancers, type 2 diabetes, stroke, arthritis, sleep apnea, and depression.

(continued)

● Obesity At a Glance (continued)

- More than 50% of people with non-insulin-dependent diabetes and 20% of people with hypertension or elevated cholesterol are overweight or obese.
- Obesity is increasing worldwide: although being poor in the world's poorest countries is associated with underweight and malnutrition, being poor in a middle-income country adopting a Western lifestyle is associated with increased risk of obesity.
- Only 42% of obese U.S. adults report that health care professionals have advised them to lose weight.

(Sources: Surgeon General, U.S. Department of Health and Human Services. Surgeon General's Call to Action to Prevent and Decrease Overweight and Obesity. Overweight and Obesity: At a Glance. Available at: http://www.surgeongeneral.gov/topics/obesity/calltoaction/fact_glance.htm. Accessed January 19, 2008; McTigue KM, Harris R, Hemphill B, et al. Screening and interventions for obesity in adults: summary of the evidence for the U.S. Preventive Services Task Force. Ann Intern Med 139(11):933–949, 2003; Hossain P, Kawar B, El Hahas M. Obesity and diabetes in the developing world: a growing challenge. N Engl J Med 356(3):213–215, 2007.)

To promote optimal patient weight and nutrition, adopt the four-pronged approach outlined below. Even reducing weight by 5% to 10% can improve blood pressure, lipid levels, and glucose tolerance and reduce the risk of diabetes or hypertension.

TIPS FOR PROMOTING OPTIMAL WEIGHT AND NUTRITION

- Measure BMI and waist circumference; identify risk of overweight and obesity.
- Establish additional risk factors for heart disease and obesity-related diseases.
- Assess dietary intake.
- Assess the patient's motivation to change; provide counseling about nutrition and exercise.

See Table 4-4, Obesity: Stages of Change Model and Assessing Readiness, p. 131.

Take advantage of the excellent resources available for patient assessment and counseling summarized in the following sections. Review the role of weight in the growing prevalence of *metabolic syndrome* (see p. 344).

See Table 4-3, Obesity-Related Risk Factors and Diseases, p. 130.

Responding to the BMI.   Classify the BMI according to the national guidelines in the following table. If the BMI is *above 25*, assess the patient for *additional risk factors* for heart disease and other obesity-related diseases: hypertension, high LDL cholesterol, low HDL cholesterol, high triglycerides, high blood glucose, family history of premature heart disease, physical inactivity, and cigarette smoking. Patients with a BMI over 25 and two or more risk factors should pursue weight loss, especially if the waist circumference is elevated.

● Classification of Overweight and Obesity by BMI

	Obesity Class	BMI (kg/m²)
Underweight		<18.5
Normal		18.5–24.9
Overweight		25.0–29.9
Obesity	I	30.0–34.9
	II	35.0–39.9
Extreme obesity	III	≥40

(Source: National Institutes of Health and National Heart, Lung, and Blood Institute: Clinical Guidelines on the Identification, Evaluation, and Treatment of Overweight and Obesity in Adults: The Evidence Report. NIH Publication 98-4083. June 1998.)

Assessing Dietary Intake.   Advising patients about diet and weight loss is important, especially in light of the many, often contradictory dieting options in the popular press. Review three excellent guidelines for counseling your patients:

See Table 4-5, Healthy Eating: U.S.D.A. Food Pyramid, p. 132.

● National Institutes of Health and National Heart, Lung, and Blood Institute. Clinical Guidelines on the Identification, Evaluation, and Treatment of Overweight and Obesity in Adults. Available at: http://www.nhlbi.nih.gov/guidelines/obesity/ob_home.htm. Accessed January 19, 2008.[7]

● U.S. Preventive Services Task Force. Screening for Obesity in Adults: recommendations and rationale. Rockville MD. Agency for Healthcare Research and Quality, November 2003. Available at: http://www.ahrq.gov/clinic/3rduspstf/obesity/obesrr.htm. Accessed January 19, 2008.[8]

● U.S. Department of Health and Human Services and U.S. Department of Agriculture. Dietary Guidelines for Americans 2005. Available at: http://www.health.gov/dietaryguidelines/dga2005/document/pdf/DGA2005.pdf. Accessed January 19, 2008.[9]

Diet recommendations hinge on assessment of the patient's motivation and readiness to lose weight and individual risk factors. The *Clinical Guidelines on the Identification, Evaluation, and Treatment of Overweight and Obesity in Adults*[7] recommend the following general guidelines:

● A 10% weight reduction over 6 months, or a decrease of 300 to 500 kcal/day, for people with BMIs between 27 and 35

● A weight loss goal of ½ to 1 pound per week because more rapid weight loss does not lead to better results at 1 year.[8]

These guidelines recommend low-calorie diets of 800 to 1500 kcal per day. Interventions that combine nutrition education, diet, and moderate exercise with behavioral strategies are most likely to succeed (see p. 108). The *Clinical Guidelines* cite evidence supporting the role of moderate physical activity in weight loss and weight loss maintenance programs: it enhances and may assist with maintenance of weight; it increases cardiorespiratory fitness; and it may decrease abdominal fat.

If the BMI falls *below 18.5*, be concerned about possible anorexia nervosa, bulimia, or other medical conditions. These conditions are summarized in Table 4-1, Eating Disorders and Excessively Low BMI, p. 128. (See also pp. 104–106 for health promotion and counseling for overweight or underweight patients.)

Once you have assessed food intake, nutritional status, and motivation to adopt healthy eating behaviors or lose weight, give patients the "nine major messages" of the Dietary Guidelines for Americans 2005, as summarized and adapted below.

See Table 4-5, Healthy Eating: U.S.D.A. Food Pyramid, p. 132.

PROMOTING PATIENT HEALTH: NINE KEY MESSAGES[9]

- Consume a variety of foods within and among the basic food groups while staying within energy needs.
- Control calorie intake and portion size to manage body weight.
- Maintain moderate physical activity for at least 30 minutes each day, for example, walking 3 to 4 miles per hour.
- Increase daily intake of fruits and vegetables, whole grains, and nonfat or low-fat milk and milk products.
- Choose fats wisely, keeping intake of saturated fat, *trans* fat found in partially hydrogenated vegetable oils, and cholesterol low.
- Choose carbohydrates—sugars, starches, and fibers—wisely for good health.
- Choose and prepare foods with little salt.
- If you drink alcoholic beverages, do so in moderation.
- Keep food safe to eat.

Be prepared to help adolescent females and women of childbearing age increase intake of iron and folic acid. Assist adults older than 50 years to identify foods rich in vitamin B_{12} and calcium. Advise older adults and those with dark skin or low exposure to sunlight to increase intake of vitamin D.

See Table 4-6, Nutrition Counseling: Sources of Nutrients, p. 133.

Blood Pressure and Diet.   With respect to blood pressure, there is reliable evidence that regular and frequent exercise, decreased sodium intake and increased potassium intake, and maintenance of a healthy weight reduce the risk for developing hypertension as well as lower blood pressure in adults who are already hypertensive. Explain to patients that most dietary sodium comes from salt (sodium chloride). The recommended daily allowance (RDA)

See Table 4-7, Patients With Hypertension: Recommended Changes in Diet, p. 133.

of sodium is less than 2400 mg, or 1 teaspoon, per day. Patients need to read food labels closely, especially the Nutrition Facts panel. Low-sodium foods are those with sodium listed at less than 5% of the RDA of 2400 mg or less. For nutritional interventions to reduce the risk for cardiac disease, turn to p. 347.

Exercise.   Fitness is a key component of both weight control and weight loss. Currently, 30 minutes of moderate activity, defined as walking 2 miles in 30 minutes on most days of the week or its equivalent, is recommended. Patients can increase exercise by such simple measures as parking farther away from their place of work or using stairs instead of elevators. A safe goal for weight loss is ½ to 2 pounds per week.

● Moderate and Vigorous Exercise

A 154-pound man (5'10") will use up about the number of calories listed doing each activity below. **Those who weigh more will use more calories, and those who weigh less will use fewer.** The calorie values listed include both calories used by the activity and calories used for normal body functioning.

	Approximate Calories Used by a 154-pound Man	
	In 1 hour	In 30 minutes
Moderate Physical Activities:		
Hiking	370	185
Light gardening/yard work	330	165
Dancing	330	165
Golf (walking and carrying clubs)	330	165
Bicycling (less than 10 miles per hour)	290	145
Walking (3 ½ miles per hour)	280	140
Weight training (general light workout)	220	110
Stretching	180	90
Vigorous Physical Activities:		
Running/jogging (5 miles per hour)	590	295
Bicycling (more than 10 miles per hour)	590	295
Swimming (slow freestyle laps)	510	255
Aerobics	480	240
Walking (4 ½ miles per hour)	460	230
Heavy yard work (chopping wood)	440	220
Weight lifting (vigorous effort)	440	220
Basketball (vigorous)	440	220

(Source: U.S. Department of Agriculture: Inside the Pyramid—Calories used. Available at http://www.mypyramid.gov/pyramid/calories_used_table.html. Accessed January 23, 2008.)

THE GENERAL SURVEY

The *General Survey* of the patient's appearance, height, and weight begins with the opening moments of the patient encounter, but you will find that your observations of the patient's appearance crystallize as you start the physical examination. The best clinicians continually sharpen their powers of observation and description, like naturalists identifying birds from silhouettes backlit against the sky. It is important to heighten the acuity of your clinical perceptions of the patient's mood, build, and behavior. These details enrich and deepen your emerging clinical impression. A skilled observer can depict distinguishing features of the patient's general appearance so well in words that a colleague could spot the patient in a crowd of strangers.

Many factors contribute to the patient's body habitus—socioeconomic status, nutrition, genetic makeup, degree of fitness, mood state, early illnesses, gender, geographic location, and age cohort. Recall that the patient's nutritional status affects many of the characteristics you scrutinize during the *General Survey:* height and weight, blood pressure, posture, mood and alertness, facial coloration, dentition and condition of the tongue and gingiva, color of the nail beds, and muscle bulk, to name a few. Be sure to make the assessment of height, weight, BMI, and risk for obesity a routine part of your clinical practice.

You should now recapture the observations you have been making since the first moments of your interaction and refine them throughout your assessment. Does the patient hear you when greeted in the waiting room or examination room? Rise with ease? Walk easily or stiffly? If hospitalized when you first meet, what is the patient doing—sitting up and enjoying television? . . . or lying in bed? . . . What occupies the bedside table—a magazine? . . . a flock of "get well" cards? . . . a Bible or a rosary? . . . an emesis basin? . . . or nothing at all? Each of these observations should raise one or more tentative hypotheses about the patient for you to consider during future assessments.

 GENERAL APPEARANCE

Apparent State of Health. Try to make a general judgment based on observations throughout the encounter. Support it with the significant details.

Acutely or chronically ill, frail, or fit and robust.

Level of Consciousness. Is the patient awake, alert, and responsive to you and others in the environment? If not, promptly assess the level of consciousness.

See Chapter 17, The Nervous System, Level of Consciousness, p. 706.

Signs of Distress.   For example, does the patient show evidence of these problems?

● Cardiac or respiratory distress

Clutching the chest, pallor, diaphoresis; labored breathing, wheezing, cough

● Pain

Wincing, sweating, protectiveness of painful area; facial grimacing; unusual posture favoring one limb or body area

● Anxiety or depression

Anxious face, fidgety movements, cold and moist palms; inexpressive or flat affect, poor eye contact, psychomotor slowing. See Chapter 5, Behavior and Mental Status, p. 147.

Skin Color and Obvious Lesions.   See Chapter 6, The Skin, Hair, and Nails, for details.

Pallor, cyanosis, jaundice, rashes, bruises

Dress, Grooming, and Personal Hygiene.   How is the patient dressed? Is clothing appropriate to the temperature and weather? Is it clean, properly buttoned, and zipped? How does it compare with clothing worn by people of comparable age and social group?

Excess clothing may reflect the cold intolerance of *hypothyroidism,* hide skin rash or needle marks, or signal personal lifestyle preferences.

Glance at the patient's shoes. Have holes been cut in them? Are the laces tied? Or is the patient wearing slippers?

Cut-out holes or slippers may indicate gout, bunions, or other painful foot conditions. Untied laces or slippers also suggest edema.

Is the patient wearing any unusual jewelry? Where? Is there any body piercing?

Copper bracelets are sometimes worn for *arthritis*. Piercing may appear on any part of the body.

Note the patient's hair, fingernails, and use of cosmetics. They may be clues to the patient's personality, mood, or lifestyle. Nail polish and hair coloring that have "grown out" may signify decreased interest in personal appearance.

"Grown-out" hair and nail polish can help you estimate the length of an illness if the patient cannot give a history. Fingernails chewed to the quick may reflect stress.

Do personal hygiene and grooming seem appropriate to the patient's age, lifestyle, occupation, and socioeconomic group? These are norms that vary widely, of course.

Unkempt appearance may be seen in *depression* and *dementia,* but this appearance must be compared with the patient's probable norm.

Facial Expression. Observe the facial expression at rest, during conversation about specific topics, during the physical examination, and in interaction with others. Watch for eye contact. Is it natural? Sustained and unblinking? Averted quickly? Absent?	The stare of *hyperthyroidism;* the immobile face of *parkinsonism;* the flat or sad affect of *depression.* Decreased eye contact may be cultural, or may suggest anxiety, fear, or sadness.
Odors of the Body and Breath. Odors can be important diagnostic clues, such as the fruity odor of diabetes or the scent of alcohol. (For the scent of alcohol, the CAGE questions, p. 84, will help you determine possible misuse.)	Breath odors of alcohol, acetone (diabetes), pulmonary infections, uremia, or liver failure
Never assume that alcohol on a patient's breath explains changes in mental status or neurologic findings.	People with alcoholism may have other serious and potentially correctable problems such as hypoglycemia, subdural hematoma, or postictal state
Posture, Gait, and Motor Activity. What is the patient's preferred posture?	Preference for sitting up in *left-sided heart failure,* and for leaning forward with arms braced in *chronic obstructive pulmonary disease*
Is the patient restless or quiet? How often does the patient change position? How fast are the movements?	Fast, frequent movements of *hyperthyroidism;* slowed activity of *hypothyroidism*
Is there any apparent involuntary motor activity? Are some body parts immobile? Which ones?	Tremors or other involuntary movements; paralyses. See Table 17-4, Tremors and Involuntary Movements (pp. 720–721).
Does the patient walk smoothly, with comfort, self-confidence, and balance, or is there a limp or discomfort, fear of falling, loss of balance, or any movement disorder?	See Table 17-10, Abnormalities of Gait and Posture (p. 730).
Height. If possible, measure the patient's height in stocking feet. Is the patient unusually short or tall? Is the build slender and lanky, muscular, or stocky? Is the body symmetric? Note the general body proportions and look for any deformities.	Very short stature in *Turner's syndrome,* childhood renal failure, and *achondroplastic* and *hypopituitary dwarfism;* long limbs in proportion to the trunk in hypogonadism and *Marfan's syndrome;* height loss in *osteoporosis* and vertebral compression fractures.
Weight. Is the patient emaciated, slender, plump, obese, or somewhere in between? If the patient is obese, is the fat distributed evenly or concentrated over the trunk, the upper torso, or around the hips?	Generalized fat in simple obesity; truncal fat with relatively thin limbs in *Cushing's syndrome* and *metabolic syndrome*

Whenever possible, weigh the patient with shoes off. Weight provides one index of caloric intake, and changes over time yield other valuable diagnostic data. Remember that changes in weight can occur with changes in body fluid status, as well as in fat or muscle mass.

Calculating the BMI. Use your measurements of height and weight to calculate the *Body Mass Index,* or *BMI.* Body fat consists primarily of adipose in the form of triglycerides and is stored in subcutaneous, inter-abdominal, and intramuscular fat deposits that are difficult to measure directly. The BMI incorporates estimated but more accurate measures of body fat than weight alone. Note that BMI criteria for overweight and obesity are not rigid cut-points but guidelines for estimating increasing risks to patient health and well-being from both excess and low weight. For older adults, there is a disproportionate risk for undernutrition.

BMI standards are derived from two surveys: the National Health Examination Survey, consisting of three survey cycles between 1960 and 1970, and the National Health and Nutrition Examination Survey, conducted over three cycles between the 1970s and the 1990s.

There are several ways to calculate the BMI, as shown in the accompanying table. Choose the method most suited to your practice. The National Institutes of Health and the National Heart, Lung, and Blood Institute caution that people who are very muscular may have a high BMI but still be healthy.[7] Likewise, the BMI for people with low muscle mass and reduced nutrition may appear inappropriately "normal."

If the BMI is 35 or higher, measure the patient's *waist circumference.* With the patient standing, measure the waist just above the hip bones. The patient may have excess body fat if the waist measures:

- ≥35 inches for women

- ≥40 inches for men

Methods to Calculate Body Mass Index (BMI)

$$\left(\frac{110 \times 700}{62}\right) \div 62 = 20.03$$

Unit of Measure	Method of Calculation
Weight *in pounds*, height *in inches*	(1) Body Mass Index Chart (see table below)
	(2) $\left(\dfrac{\text{Weight (lbs)} \times 700^*}{\text{Height (inches)}}\right) \div \text{Height (inches)}$
Weight *in kilograms*, height *in meters squared*	(3) $\dfrac{\text{Weight (kg)}}{\text{Height (m}^2)}$
Either	(4) "BMI Calculator" at Web site www.nhlbisupport.com/bmi/bmicalc.htm

*Several organizations use 704.5, but the variation in BMI is negligible. Conversion formulas: 2.2 lbs = 1 kg; 1.0 inch = 2.54 cm; 100 cm = 1 meter.

(Source: National Institutes of Health and National Heart, Lung, and Blood Institute: Body Mass Index Calculator. Available at: http://www.nhlbisupport.com/bmi/bmicalc.htm. Accessed January 22, 2008.)

Body Mass Index Table

	Normal						Overweight					Obese									
BMI	19	20	21	22	23	24	25	26	27	28	29	30	31	32	33	34	35	36	37	38	39
Height (inches)									Body Weight (pounds)												
58	91	96	100	105	110	115	119	124	129	134	138	143	148	153	158	162	167	172	177	181	186
59	94	99	104	109	114	119	124	128	133	138	143	148	153	158	163	168	173	178	183	188	193
60	97	102	107	112	118	123	128	133	138	143	148	153	158	163	168	174	179	184	189	194	199
61	100	106	111	116	122	127	132	137	143	148	153	158	164	169	174	180	185	190	195	201	206
62	104	109	115	120	126	131	136	142	147	153	158	164	169	175	180	186	191	196	202	207	213
63	107	113	118	124	130	135	141	146	152	158	163	169	175	180	186	191	197	203	208	214	220
64	110	116	122	128	134	140	145	151	157	163	169	174	180	186	192	197	204	209	215	221	227
65	114	120	126	132	138	144	150	156	162	168	174	180	186	192	198	204	210	216	222	228	234
66	118	124	130	136	142	148	155	161	167	173	179	186	192	198	204	210	216	223	229	235	241
67	121	127	134	140	146	153	159	166	172	178	185	191	198	204	211	217	223	230	236	242	249
68	125	131	138	144	151	158	164	171	177	184	190	197	203	210	216	223	230	236	243	249	256
69	128	135	142	149	155	162	169	176	182	189	196	203	209	216	223	230	236	243	250	257	263
70	132	139	146	153	160	167	174	181	188	195	202	209	216	222	229	236	243	250	257	264	271
71	136	143	150	157	165	172	179	186	193	200	208	215	222	229	236	243	250	257	265	272	279
72	140	147	154	162	169	177	184	191	199	206	213	221	228	235	242	250	258	265	272	279	287
73	144	151	159	166	174	182	189	197	204	212	219	227	235	242	250	257	265	272	280	288	295
74	148	155	163	171	179	186	194	202	210	218	225	233	241	249	256	264	272	280	287	295	303
75	152	160	168	176	184	192	200	208	216	224	232	240	248	256	264	272	279	287	295	303	311
76	156	164	172	180	189	197	205	213	221	230	238	246	254	263	271	279	287	295	304	312	320

(Source: Adapted from National Institutes of Health and National Heart, Lung, and Blood Institute: Clinical Guidelines on the Identification, Evaluation and Treatment of Overweight and Obesity in Adults: The Evidence Report. June 1998. Available at: www.nhlbi.nih.gov/guidelines/obesity/bmi_tbl.pdf. Accessed January 22, 2008.)

Height and Weight Across the Lifespan. Height and weight in childhood and adolescence reflect the many behavioral, cognitive, and physiologic changes of growth and development. Developmental milestones, markers for growth spurts, and sexual maturity ratings can be found in Chapter 18, Assessing Children: Infancy Through Adolescence. With aging, some of these changes reverse, as described in Chapter 20, The Older Adult. Height may decrease, posture may become more stooping from kyphosis of the thoracic spine, and extension of the knees and hips may diminish. The abdominal muscles may relax, changing the abdominal contour, and fat may accumulate at the hips and lower abdomen. Be alert to these changes as you assess older patients.

THE VITAL SIGNS

Now you are ready to measure the *Vital Signs*—the blood pressure, heart rate, respiratory rate, and temperature. You may find that the vital signs are already taken and recorded in the chart; if abnormal, you will often wish to repeat them yourself. You can also make these important measurements later as you start the cardiovascular and thorax and lung examinations, but frequently they provide important initial information that influences the direction of your evaluation.

Check either the blood pressure or the pulse first. If the blood pressure is high, measure it again later in the examination. Count the radial pulse with your fingers, or the apical pulse with your stethoscope at the cardiac apex. Continue either of these techniques and count the respiratory rate without alerting the patient—breathing patterns may change if the patient knows breaths are being counted. The temperature is taken with tympanic thermometers or digital electronic probes. Further details on techniques for ensuring accuracy of the vital signs are provided in the following pages.

See Table 9-3, Abnormalities of the Arterial Pulse and Pressure Waves (p. 377). See Table 4-8, Abnormalities in Rate and Rhythm of Breathing (p. 134).

BLOOD PRESSURE

Choice of Blood Pressure Cuff (Sphygmomanometer). More than 72 million Americans have elevated blood pressure.[10] To detect blood pressure elevations, an accurate instrument is essential. Blood pressure devices may be mercury, aneroid, or electronic, and there are international protocols for evaluating their accuracy.[11–13]

Self-monitoring of blood pressure by well-instructed patients using approved devices improves blood pressure control, especially when it is done two times daily at the upper arm with automatic readouts.[14–16]

Take the time to choose a cuff of appropriate size for your patient's arm. Follow the guidelines on the next page, and advise your patients about how to choose the best cuff for home use. Urge them to have their home devices recalibrated routinely.

SELECTING THE CORRECT BLOOD PRESSURE CUFF

- Width of the inflatable bladder of the cuff should be about 40% of upper arm circumference (about 12–14 cm in the average adult).
- Length of the inflatable bladder should be about 80% of upper arm circumference (almost long enough to encircle the arm).
- The standard cuff is 12 × 23 cm, appropriate for arm circumferences up to 28 cm.

If the cuff is too *small* (narrow), the blood pressure will read *high;* if the cuff is too *large* (wide), the blood pressure will read *low* on a small arm and *high* on a large arm.

Technique for Measuring Blood Pressure.[17]   Before assessing the blood pressure, take several steps to make sure your measurement will be accurate. Proper technique is important and reduces the inherent variability arising from the patient or examiner, the equipment, and the procedure itself.

STEPS TO ENSURE ACCURATE BLOOD PRESSURE MEASUREMENT

- Ideally, instruct the patient to avoid smoking or drinking caffeinated beverages for 30 minutes before the blood pressure is measured.
- Check to make sure the examining room is quiet and comfortably warm.
- Ask the patient to sit quietly for at least 5 minutes in a chair, rather than on the examining table, with feet on the floor. The arm should be supported at heart level.
- Make sure the arm selected is *free of clothing*. There should be no arterio-venous fistulas for dialysis, scarring from prior brachial artery cutdowns, or signs of lymphedema (seen after axillary node dissection or radiation therapy).
- Palpate the brachial artery to confirm that it has a viable pulse.
- Position the arm so that the brachial artery, at the antecubital crease, is *at heart level*—roughly level with the 4th interspace at its junction with the sternum.
- If the patient is seated, rest the arm on a table a little above the patient's waist; if standing, try to support the patient's arm at the midchest level.

If the brachial artery is 7 to 8 cm *below* heart level, the blood pressure will read approximately 6 cm higher; if the brachial artery is 6 to 7 cm *higher,* the blood pressure will read 5 cm lower.[18,19]

Now you are ready to measure the blood pressure.

● Center the inflatable bladder over the brachial artery. The lower border of the cuff should be about 2.5 cm above the antecubital crease. Secure the cuff snugly. Position the patient's arm so that it is slightly flexed at the elbow.

A loose cuff or a bladder that balloons outside the cuff leads to falsely high readings.

● To determine how high to raise the cuff pressure, first estimate the systolic pressure by palpation. As you feel the radial artery with the fingers of one hand, rapidly inflate the cuff until the radial pulse disappears. Read this pressure on the manometer and add 30 mm Hg to it. Use of this sum as the target for subsequent inflations prevents discomfort from unnecessarily high cuff pressures. It also avoids the occasional error caused by an *auscultatory gap*—a silent interval that may be present between the systolic and the diastolic pressures.

An unrecognized auscultatory gap may lead to serious under-estimation of systolic pressure (150/98 in the example below) or overestimation of diastolic pressure.

● Deflate the cuff promptly and completely and wait 15 to 30 seconds.

● Now place the bell of a stethoscope lightly over the brachial artery, taking care to make an air seal with its full rim. Because the sounds to be heard, the *Korotkoff sounds,* are relatively low in pitch, they are generally heard better with the bell.

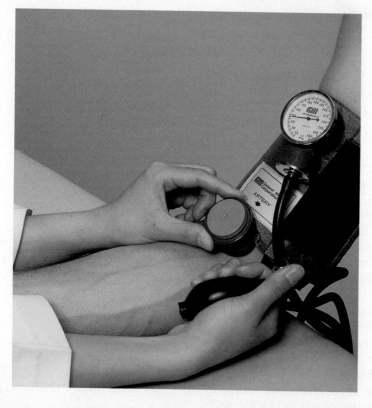

200 — Systolic pressure

160 — } Auscultatory gap

mm Hg

120 — Diastolic pressure

80 —

40 —

0 —

If you find an auscultatory gap, record your findings completely (e.g., 200/98 with an auscultatory gap from 170–150).

An auscultatory gap is associated with arterial stiffness and athero-sclerotic disease.[20]

● Inflate the cuff rapidly again to the level just determined, and then deflate it slowly at a rate of about 2 to 3 mm Hg per second. Note the level at which you hear the sounds of at least two consecutive beats. This is the systolic pressure.

mm Hg

160

120

80

40

Artery occluded; no flow — **Silence**

Systolic pressure

Artery compressed; blood flow audible — **Sounds of turbulent flow**

Diastolic pressure

Artery not compressed; flow free and audible — **Silence**

Arterial pulse tracing

Effect of cuff on arterial blood flow

Auscultatory findings

● Continue to lower the pressure slowly until the sounds become muffled and then disappear. To confirm the disappearance of sounds, listen as the pressure falls another 10 to 20 mm Hg. Then deflate the cuff rapidly to zero. The disappearance point, which is usually only a few mm Hg below the muffling point, provides the best estimate of true diastolic pressure in adults.

In some people, the muffling point and the disappearance point are farther apart. Occasionally, as in aortic regurgitation, the sounds never disappear. If the difference is ≥10 mm Hg, record both figures (e.g., 154/80/68).

● Read both the systolic and the diastolic levels to the nearest 2 mm Hg. Wait 2 or more minutes and repeat. Average your readings. If the first two readings differ by more than 5 mm Hg, take additional readings.

● When using a mercury sphygmomanometer, keep the manometer vertical (unless you are using a tilted floor model) and make all readings at eye level with the meniscus. When using an aneroid instrument, hold the dial so that it faces you directly. Avoid slow or repetitive inflations of the cuff, because the resulting venous congestion can cause false readings.

By making the sounds less audible, venous congestion may produce artificially low systolic and high diastolic pressures.

● Blood pressure should be taken in both arms at least once. Normally, there may be a difference in pressure of 5 mm Hg and sometimes up to 10 mm Hg. Subsequent readings should be made on the arm with the higher pressure.

Pressure difference of more than 10–15 mm Hg in *subclavian steal syndrome, aortic dissection*

Classification of Normal and Abnormal Blood Pressure.

In its seventh report in 2003, the Joint National Committee on Prevention, Detection, Evaluation, and Treatment of High Blood Pressure recommended using the mean of two or more properly measured seated blood pressure readings, taken on two or more office visits, for diagnosis of hypertension.[17] Blood pressure measurement should be verified in the contralateral arm.

The Joint National Committee has identified four levels of systolic and diastolic hypertension. Note that either component may be high.

Assessment of hypertension also includes its effects on target "end organs"—the eyes, heart, brain, and kidneys. Look for hypertensive retinopathy, left ventricular hypertrophy, and neurologic deficits suggesting stroke. Renal assessment requires urinalysis and blood tests of renal function.

● JNCVII Blood Pressure Classification—Adults Older Than 18 Years

Category	Systolic (mm Hg)	Diastolic (mm Hg)
Normal	<120	<80
Prehypertension	120–139	80–89
Hypertension		
Stage 1	140–159	90–99
Stage 2	≥160	≥100

Note that the blood pressure goal for patients with hypertension, diabetes, or renal disease is <130/80.

When the systolic and diastolic levels fall in different categories, use the higher category. For example, 170/92 mm Hg is Stage 2 hypertension; 135/100 mm Hg is Stage 1 hypertension. In *isolated systolic hypertension,* systolic blood pressure is ≥140 mm Hg, and diastolic blood pressure is <90 mm Hg.

Treatment of *isolated systolic hypertension* in patients 60 years or older reduces total mortality and both mortality and complications from cardiovascular disease.[21,22]

The Hypertensive Patient with Unequal Blood Pressures in the Arms and Legs. To detect coarctation of the aorta, make two further blood pressure measurements at least once in every hypertensive patient:

- Compare blood pressures in the arms and legs.

- Compare the volume and timing of the radial and femoral pulses. Normally, volume is equal and the pulses occur simultaneously.

Coarctation of the aorta arises from narrowing of the thoracic aorta, usually proximal but sometimes distal to the left subclavian artery.

Coarctation of the aorta and *occlusive aortic disease* are distinguished by hypertension in the upper extremities and low blood pressure in the legs and by diminished or delayed femoral pulses.[23]

To determine blood pressure in the leg, use a wide, long thigh cuff that has a bladder size of 18 × 42 cm, and apply it to the midthigh. Center the bladder over the posterior surface, wrap it securely, and listen over the popliteal artery. If possible, the patient should be prone. Alternatively, ask the supine patient to flex one leg slightly, with the heel resting on the bed. When cuffs of the proper size are used for both the leg and the arm, blood pressures should be equal in the two areas. (The usual arm cuff, improperly used on the leg, gives a falsely high reading.)

HEART RATE AND RHYTHM

Examine the arterial pulses, the heart rate and rhythm, and the amplitude and contour of the pulse wave.

Heart Rate. The radial pulse is commonly used to assess the heart rate. With the pads of your index and middle fingers, compress the radial artery until a maximal pulsation is detected. If the rhythm is regular and the rate seems normal, count the rate for 30 seconds and multiply by 2. If the rate is unusually fast or slow, however, count it for 60 seconds. The range of normal is 50–90 beats per minute.[24]

Rhythm. To begin your assessment of rhythm, feel the radial pulse. If there are any irregularities, check the rhythm again by listening with your stethoscope at the cardiac apex. Beats that occur earlier than others may not be detected peripherally, and the heart rate can be seriously underestimated. Is the rhythm regular or irregular? If irregular, try to identify a pattern: (1) Do early beats appear in a basically regular rhythm? (2) Does the irregularity vary consistently with respiration? (3) Is the rhythm totally irregular?

See Table 9-1, Selected Heart Rates and Rhythms (p. 375), and Table 9-2, Selected Irregular Rhythms (p. 376).

Relatively low levels of blood pressure should always be interpreted in the light of past readings and the patient's present clinical state.

A pressure of 110/70 mm Hg would usually be normal, but could also indicate significant hypotension if past pressures have been high.

If indicated, assess *orthostatic, or postural, blood pressure* (see Chapter 20, the Older Adult, p. 916). Measure blood pressure and heart rate in two positions—*supine* after the patient is resting up to 10 minutes, then within 3 minutes after the patient *stands up*. Normally, as the patient rises from the horizontal to the standing position, systolic pressure drops slightly or remains unchanged, while diastolic pressure rises slightly. Orthostatic hypotension is a drop in systolic blood pressure of ≥20 mm Hg or in diastolic blood pressure of ≥10 mm Hg within 3 minutes of standing.[25,26]

A fall in systolic pressure of 20 mm Hg or more, especially when accompanied by symptoms and tachycardia, indicates *orthostatic (postural) hypotension*. Causes include drugs, moderate or severe blood loss, prolonged bed rest, and diseases of the autonomic nervous system.

RESPIRATORY RATE AND RHYTHM

Observe the *rate, rhythm, depth,* and *effort of breathing.* Count the number of respirations in 1 minute either by visual inspection or by subtly listening over the patient's trachea with your stethoscope during your examination of the head and neck or chest. Normally, adults take ~20 breaths per minute in a quiet, regular pattern. An occasional sigh is normal. Check to see if expiration is prolonged.

See Table 4-8, Abnormalities in Rate and Rhythm of Breathing (p. 134).

Prolonged expiration in COPD.

TEMPERATURE

The average *oral temperature,* usually quoted at 37°C (98.6°F), fluctuates considerably. In the early morning hours, it may fall as low as 35.8°C (96.4°F), and in the late afternoon or evening, it may rise as high as 37.3°C (99.1°F). *Rectal temperatures* are *higher* than oral temperatures by an average of 0.4 to 0.5°C (0.7 to 0.9°F), but this difference is also quite variable. In contrast, *axillary temperatures* are *lower* than oral temperatures by approximately 1°, but take 5 to 10 minutes to register and are generally considered less accurate than other measurements.

Most patients prefer oral to rectal temperature measurements. However, taking oral temperatures is not recommended when patients are unconscious, restless, or unable to close their mouths. Temperature readings may be inaccurate and thermometers broken by unexpected movements of the patient's jaws.

Oral Temperatures.   For *oral temperatures,* choose a glass or an electronic thermometer. When using a *glass thermometer,* shake the thermometer down to 35°C (96°F) or below, insert it under the tongue, instruct the patient to close both lips, and wait 3 to 5 minutes. Then read the thermometer, reinsert it for a minute, and read it again. If the temperature is still rising, repeat this procedure until the reading remains stable. Note that hot or cold liquids, and even smoking, can alter the temperature reading. In these situations, it is best to delay measuring the temperature for 10 to 15 minutes. Due to breakage and mercury exposure, glass thermometers are giving way to electronic thermometers.

Electronic Thermometers.   If using an electronic thermometer, carefully place the disposable cover over the probe and insert the thermometer under the tongue. Ask the patient to close both lips, and then watch closely for the digital readout. An accurate temperature recording usually takes about 10 seconds.

Rectal Temperatures.   For a *rectal temperature,* ask the patient to lie on one side with the hip flexed. Select a rectal thermometer with a stubby tip, lubricate it, and insert it about 3 cm to 4 cm (1½ inches) into the anal canal, in a direction pointing to the umbilicus. Remove it after 3 minutes, then read. Alternatively, use an electronic thermometer after lubricating the probe cover. Wait about 10 seconds for the digital temperature recording to appear.

Tympanic Membrane Temperatures.   Taking the *tympanic membrane temperature* is an increasingly common practice and is quick, safe, and reliable if performed properly. Make sure the external auditory canal is free of cerumen, which lowers temperature readings. Position the probe in the canal so that the infrared beam is aimed at the tympanic membrane (otherwise the measurement will be invalid). Wait 2 to 3 seconds until the digital temperature reading appears. This method measures core body temperature, which is higher than the normal oral temperature by approximately 0.8°C (1.4°F).

Fever or pyrexia refers to an elevated body temperature. *Hyperpyrexia* refers to extreme elevation in temperature, above 41.1°C (106°F), while *hypothermia* refers to an abnormally low temperature, below 35°C (95°F) rectally.

Rapid respiratory rates tend to increase the discrepancy between oral and rectal temperatures. In these situations, rectal temperatures are more reliable.

Causes of *fever* include infection, trauma such as surgery or crush injuries, malignancy, blood disorders such as acute hemolytic anemia, drug reactions, and immune disorders such as collagen vascular disease.

The chief cause of *hypothermia* is exposure to cold. Other predisposing causes include reduced movement as in paralysis, interference with vasoconstriction as from sepsis or excess alcohol, starvation, hypothyroidism, and hypoglycemia. Elderly people are especially susceptible to hypothermia and also less likely to develop fever.

Tympanic measurements are more variable than oral or rectal measurements, including right and left comparisons in the same person.[27]

SPECIAL SITUATIONS

Weak or Inaudible Korotkoff Sounds.   Consider technical problems such as erroneous placement of your stethoscope, failure to make full skin contact with the bell, and venous engorgement of the patient's arm from repeated inflations of the cuff. Consider also the possibility of shock.

When you cannot hear Korotkoff sounds at all, you may be able to estimate the systolic pressure by palpation. Alternative methods such as Doppler techniques or direct arterial pressure tracings may be necessary.

To intensify Korotkoff sounds, one of the following methods may be helpful:

- Raise the patient's arm before and while you inflate the cuff. Then lower the arm and determine the blood pressure.

- Inflate the cuff. Ask the patient to make a fist several times, and then determine the blood pressure.

Arrhythmias.   Irregular rhythms produce variations in pressure and therefore unreliable measurements. Ignore the effects of an occasional premature contraction. With frequent premature contractions or atrial fibrillation, determine the average of several observations and note that your measurements are approximate. Verify your findings with an electrocardiogram.

Palpation of an irregularly irregular rhythm reliably indicates *atrial fibrillation.* For all other irregular patterns, an ECG is needed to identify the type of rhythm.

White Coat Hypertension.   "White coat hypertension" describes hypertension in people whose blood pressure measurements are higher in the office than at home or in more relaxed settings, usually >140/90. This phenomenon occurs in 10% to 25% of patients, especially women and anxious individuals, and may last for several visits. Try to relax the patient and remeasure the blood pressure later in the encounter.

Home or ambulatory hypertension, unlike "white coat" or isolated office hypertension, signals increased risk of cardiovascular disease.[28–31]

The Obese or Very Thin Patient.   For the obese arm, it is important to use a wide cuff of 15 cm. If the arm circumference exceeds 41 cm, use a thigh cuff of 18 cm. For the very thin arm, a pediatric cuff may be indicated.

Using a small cuff overestimates systolic blood pressure in obese patients.[32]

ACUTE AND CHRONIC PAIN

Understanding Acute and Chronic Pain.   The International Association for the Study of Pain defines *pain* as "an unpleasant sensory and emotional experience" associated with tissue damage, described in terms of such damage, or both. The experience of pain is complex and multifactorial. Pain involves sensory, emotional, and cognitive processing but may lack a specific physical etiology.[1]

Chronic pain may be a spectrum disorder related to mental health and somatic conditions. See Chapter 5, Behavior and Mental Status, "Symptoms and Behavior," pp. 136–140.

Chronic pain is defined in several ways: pain not associated with cancer or other medical conditions that persists for more than 3 to 6 months; pain lasting more than 1 month beyond the course of an acute illness or injury; or pain recurring at intervals of months or years.[33] Chronic noncancer pain affects 5% to 33% of patients in primary care settings. More than 40% of patients report that their pain is poorly controlled.[34]

Assessing the Patient's History. Adopt a comprehensive approach to understanding the patient's pain, carefully listening to the patient's description of the many features of pain and contributing factors. Accept the patient's self-report, which experts state is the most reliable indicator of pain.[1]

Location. Ask the patient to point to the pain, because lay terms may not be specific enough to localize the site of origin.

Severity. Assessing the severity of the pain is especially important. Use a consistent method to determine severity. Three scales are common: the Visual Analog Scale and two scales using ratings from 1 to 10—the Numeric Rating Scale and the Faces Pain Scale. Multidimensional tools like the Brief Pain Inventory are also available; these take longer to administer but address the effects of pain on the patient's activity level.[35] The Faces Pain Scale is reproduced below, because it can be used by children as well as patients with language barriers or cognitive impairment.[36]

1. Explain to the child that each face is for a person who feels happy because he or she has no pain (hurt, or whatever word the child uses) or feels sad because he or she has some or a lot of pain.
2. Point to the appropriate face and state, "This face . . .":
   0—"is very happy because he [or she] doesn't hurt at all."
   1—"hurts just a little bit."
   2—"hurts a little more."
3—"hurts even more."
4—"hurts a whole lot."
5—"hurts as much as you can imagine although you don't have to be crying to feel this bad."
3. Ask the child to choose the face that best describes how he or she feels. Be specific about which pain (e.g., "shot" or incision) and what time (e.g., Now? Earlier before lunch?)

(Adapted with permission from Wong DL, Hockenberry-Eaton M, Wilson D, Winkelstein ML, Schwartz P. Wong's Essentials of Pediatric Nursing, 6th ed. St. Louis, 2001: 1301. Copyrighted by Mosby, Inc.)

Associated Features. Ask the patient to describe the pain and how the pain started. Is it related to a site of injury, movement, or time of day? What is the quality of the pain—sharp, dull, burning? Ask if the pain radiates or follows a particular pattern. What makes the pain better or worse? Pursue the seven features of pain, as you would with any symptom.

See Chapter 3, The Seven Attributes of a Symptom, p. 165.

Attempted Treatments, Medications, Related Illnesses, and Impact on Daily Activities. Be sure to ask about any treatments that the patient has tried, including medications, physical therapy, and alternative medicines. A comprehensive medication history helps you to identify drugs that interact with analgesics and reduce their efficacy.

Identify any comorbid conditions such as arthritis, diabetes, HIV/AIDS, substance abuse, sickle cell disease, or psychiatric disorders. These can have significant effects on the patient's experience of pain.

Chronic pain is the leading cause of disability and impaired performance at work. Inquire about the effects of pain on the patient's daily activities, mood, sleep, work, and sexual activity.

Health Disparities.   Be aware of the well-documented health disparities in pain treatment and delivery of care, which range from lower use of analgesics in emergency rooms for African-American and Hispanic patients to disparities in use of analgesics for cancer, postoperative, and low back pain.[33] Studies show that clinician stereotypes, language barriers, and unconscious clinician biases in decision making all contribute to these disparities. Critique your own communication style, seek information and best practice standards, and improve your techniques of patient education and empowerment as first steps in ensuring uniform and effective pain management.

See Institute of Medicine report, *Unequal Treatment: Confronting Racial and Ethnic Disparities in Health Care*, 2002.[37]

Types of Pain.   Be familiar with recent advances in the scientific understanding of pain processes, helpfully described in several excellent modules for clinicians available online.[1,33,38] Review the summary of types of pain in the following box to aid in your diagnosis and management.

TYPES OF PAIN[1,33,39]	
Nociceptive or somatic pain	Pain related to tissue damage is termed *nociceptive*, or *somatic*. Nociceptive pain can be either acute and remitting or chronic and persistent. This form of pain is mediated by the afferent A-delta and C-fibers of the sensory system that respond to noxious stimuli and is modulated by both neurotransmitters and psychological processes. Modulating neurotransmitters include endorphins, histamines, acetylcholine, and monoamines like serotonin, norepinephrine, and dopamine. These afferent nociceptors can be sensitized by inflammatory mediators.

(continued)

TYPES OF PAIN[1,33,39] (CONTINUED)

Neuropathic pain   Pain resulting from direct injury to the peripheral or central nervous system is termed *neuropathic*. Over time, neuropathic pain may become independent of the inciting injury, becoming burning, lancinating, or shock-like in quality and persisting beyond healing from the initial injury. Mechanisms postulated to evoke neuropathic pain include central nervous system brain or spinal cord injury from stroke or trauma; peripheral nervous system disorders causing entrapment or pressure on spinal nerves, plexuses, or peripheral nerves; and referred pain syndromes with increased or prolonged pain responses to inciting stimuli. These triggers appear to induce changes in pain signal processing through "neuronal plasticity" leading to pain that persists beyond healing from the initial injury.[33]

Psychogenic and   *Psychogenic pain* relates to the many factors that
idiopathic pain   influence the patient's report of pain—psychiatric conditions like anxiety or depression, personality and coping style, cultural norms, and social support systems. *Idiopathic pain* is pain without an identifiable etiology.

Pain Management.   Treatment of pain requires sophisticated knowledge of nonopioid, opioid, and adjuvant analgesics and modalities of behavioral and physical therapy, which are beyond the scope of this book. Seek training in pain therapeutics, and turn to the medical literature for helpful reviews on the challenges and advances in pain management.[3,34,40] Clinicians are often reluctant to administer narcotics because of fear of inducing addiction. Make use of the following definitions, and take advantage of validated screening tools for opioid assessment in patients with pain.[41,42]

Focus on the *Four A's* to monitor patient outcomes:

● *A*nalgesia

● *A*ctivities of daily living

● *A*dverse effects

● *A*berrant drug-related behaviors

ADDICTION, PHYSICAL DEPENDENCE, AND TOLERANCE[43]

Tolerance: A state of adaptation in which exposure to a drug induces changes that result in a diminution of one or more of the drug's effects over time.

Physical Dependence: A state of adaptation that is manifested by a drug class-specific withdrawal syndrome that can be produced by abrupt cessation, rapid dose reduction, decreasing blood level of the drug, and/or administration of an antagonist.

Addiction: A primary, chronic, neurobiologic disease, with genetic, psychosocial, and environmental factors influencing its development and manifestations. It is characterized by behaviors that include one or more of the following: impaired control over drug use, compulsive use, continued use despite harm, and craving.

RECORDING YOUR FINDINGS

Your write-up of the physical examination begins with a general description of the patient's appearance, based on the General Survey. Note that initially you may use sentences to describe your findings; later you will use phrases. The style below contains phrases appropriate for most write-ups.

Recording the Physical Examination— The General Survey and Vital Signs

Choose vivid and graphic adjectives, as if you are painting a picture in words. Avoid clichés such as "well-developed" or "well-nourished" or "in no acute distress," because they could apply to any patient and do not convey the special features of the patient before you.

Record the vital signs taken at the time of your examination. They are preferable to those taken earlier in the day by other providers. (Common abbreviations for blood pressure, heart rate, and respiratory rate are self-explanatory.)

"Mrs. Scott is a young, healthy-appearing woman, well-groomed, fit, and cheerful. Height is 5'4", weight 135 lbs, BMI 24, BP 120/80, right and left arms, HR 72 and regular, RR 16, temperature 37.5°C."

OR

"Mr. Jones is an elderly male who looks pale and chronically ill. He is alert, with good eye contact but unable to speak more than two or three words at a time due to shortness of breath. He has intercostal muscle retraction when breathing and sits upright in bed. He is thin, with diffuse muscle wasting. Height is 6'2", weight 175 lbs, BP 160/95, right arm, HR 108 and irregular, RR 32 and labored, temperature 101.2°F."

Suggests exacerbation of chronic obstructive pulmonary disease

BIBLIOGRAPHY

CITATIONS

1. American Medical Association. Pain Management: The Online Series. Module 1.Pathophysiology of Pain and Pain Assessment. September 2007. Available at: http://www.ama-cmeonline.com/pain_mgmt/. Accessed January 19, 2008.
2. Upshur CC, Luckmann RS, Savageau JA. Primary care provider concerns about management of chronic pain in community clinic populations. J Gen Int Med 21(6):652–655, 2006.
3. Sinatra R. Opioid analgesics in primary care: challenges and new advances in the management of noncancer pain. J Am Board Fam Med 19(2):165–167, 2006.
4. Surgeon General, U.S. Department of Health and Human Services. Surgeon General's Call to Action to Prevent and Decrease Overweight and Obesity. Overweight and Obesity: At a Glance. Available at: http://www.surgeongeneral.gov/topics/obesity/calltoaction/fact_glance.htm. Accessed January 19, 2008.
5. McTigue KM, Harris R, Hemphill B, et al. Screening and interventions for obesity in adults: summary of the evidence for the U.S. Preventive Services Task Force. Ann Intern Med 139(11): 933–949, 2003.
6. Hossain P, Kawar B, El Hahas M. Obesity and diabetes in the developing world: a growing challenge. N Engl J Med 356(3): 213–215, 2007.
7. National Institutes of Health and National Heart, Lung, and Blood Institute. Clinical Guidelines on the Identification,

Evaluation, and Treatment of Overweight and Obesity in Adults. Available at: http://www.nhlbi.nih.gov/guidelines/obesity/ob_home.htm. Accessed January 19, 2008.

8. U.S. Preventive Services Task Force. Screening for Obesity in Adults: Recommendations and Rationale. Rockville, MD, Agency for Healthcare Research and Quality, November 2003. Available at: http://www.ahrq.gov/clinic/3rduspstf/obesity/obesrr.htm. Accessed January 19, 2008.

9. U.S. Department of Health and Human Services and U.S. Department of Agriculture. Dietary Guidelines for Americans 2005. Available at: http://www.health.gov/dietaryguidelines/dga2005/document/pdf/DGA2005.pdf. Accessed January 19, 2008.

10. American Heart Association. Heart Disease and Stroke Statistics, 2007 Update. Available at: http://www.americanheart.org/downloadable/heart/1166712318459HS_StatsInsideText.pdf) and Cardiovascular Disease Statistics. Available at: http://www.americanheart.org/presenter.jhtml?identifier=4478). See also: National Center for Health Statistics. Fast Stats A to Z. Available at: http://www.cdc.gov/nchs/fastats/heart.htm. Accessed December 2, 2007.

11. O'Brien E, Asmar R, Beilin L, et al. European Society of Hypertension recommendations for conventional, ambulatory, and more blood pressure measurement. J Hypertens 21(5):821–848, 2005.

12. O'Brien E, Pickering T, Asmar R, et al. International protocol for validation of blood pressure measuring devices in adults. Blood Press Monit 7(1):3–17, 2002.

13. O'Brien E, Waider B, Parati G, et al. Blood pressure measuring devices: recommendations of the European Society of Hypertension. BMJ 322(7285):531–536, 2001.

14. Verberk WJ, Kroon AA, Kessles AGH, et al. Home blood pressure measurement: a systematic review. J Am Coll Cardiol 46(5):743–751, 2005.

15. McManus RJ, Mant J, Roalfe A, et al. Targets and self monitoring in hypertension: randomized controlled trial and cost effectiveness analysis. BMJ 331(7515):493, epub 2005.

16. Bakx JC, van der Wel MC, van Weel. Self monitoring of high blood pressure. BMJ 331(7515):466–467, 2005.

17. Chobanian AV, Bakris GL, Black HR, et al. The Seventh Report of the Joint National Committee on Prevention, Detection, Evaluation, and Treatment of High Blood Pressure—The JNC 7 Report. JAMA 289(19):2560–2572, 2003. Available at: http://www.nhlbi.nih.gov/guidelines/hypertension/jnc7full.pdf. Accessed January 20, 2008.

18. McGee S. Blood pressure. In: Evidence-Based Physical Diagnosis, 2nd ed. St. Louis: Saunders, 2007:153–173.

19. Mitchell PL, Parlin RW, Blackburn H. Effect of vertical displacement of the arm on indirect blood-pressure measurements. N Engl J Med 271:72–74, 1064.

20. Cavallini MC, Roman MJ, Blank SG, et al. Association of the auscultatory gap with vascular disease in hypertensive patients. Ann Intern Med 124(10):877–883, 1996.

21. Chaudhry SI, Krumholz HM, Foody JM. Systolic hypertension in older persons. JAMA 292(9):1074–1080, 2004.

22. Chobanian A. Isolated systolic hypertension in the elderly. N Engl J Med 357(8):789–796, 2007.

23. Brickner ME, Hillis LD, Lange RA. Congenital heart disease in adults: first of two parts. N Engl J Med 342(2):256–263, 2000.

24. Spodick DH. Normal sinus heart rate: appropriate rate thresholds for sinus tachycardia and bradycardia. South Med J 89(7):666–667, 1996.

25. Carslon JE. Assessment of orthostatic blood pressure: measurement technique and clinical applications. South Med J 92(2):167–173, 1999.

26. Consensus Committee of the American Autonomic Society and the American Academy of Neurology. Consensus statement on the definition of orthostatic hypotension, pure autonomic failure, and multiple system atrophy. Neurology 46(5):1470, 1996.

27. McGee S. Chapter 16, Temperature. In Evidence-Based Physical Diagnosis, 2nd ed. St. Louis: Saunders, 2007:174–186.

28. Bobrie G, Genes N, Vaur L, et al. Is "isolated home" hypertension as opposed to "isolated office" hypertension a sign of greater cardiovascular risk? Arch Int Med 161(18):2205–2211, 2001.

29. Clement DL, De Buysere ML, DeBacquer DA, et al. Prognostic value of ambulatory blood-pressure recordings in patients with treated hypertension. N Engl J Med 348(24):2407–2415, 2003.

30. Rickerby J. The role of home blood pressure measurement in managing hypertension: an evidence-based review. J Hum Hypertens 16(7):469–472, 2002.

31. Pickering TG, Shimbo D, Hass D. Ambulatory blood pressure monitoring. N Engl J Med 354(22):2368–2374, 2006.

32. Fonseca-Reyes S, de Alba-García JG, Parra-Carrillo JZ, et al. Effect of standard cuff on blood pressure readings in patients with obese arms: how frequent are arms of a 'large circumference'? Blood Press Monit 8(3):101–106, 2003.

33. American Medical Association. Pain Management: The Online Series. Pathophysiology of pain and pain assessment. Module 7—Assessing and Treating Persistent Nonmalignant Pain: an overview. September 2007. Available at: http://www.ama-cmeonline.com/pain_mgmt/. Accessed January 19, 2008.

34. Nicholson B, Passik SD. Management of chronic noncancer pain in the primary care setting. South Med J 100(10):1028–1036, 2007.

35. Daut RL, Cleeland CS, Flanery RC. Development of the Wisconsin Brief Pain Questionnaire to assess pain in cancer and other diseases. Pain 17(2):197–210, 1983.

36. Bieri D, Reeve R, Champion GD, et al. The Faces Pain Scale for the self-assessment of the severity of pain experienced by children: development, initial validation and preliminary investigation for ratio scale properties. Pain 41(2):139–150, 1990.

37. Smedley BR, Stith AY, Nelson AR (eds). Committee on Understanding and Eliminating Racial and Ethnic Disparities in Health Care. Unequal Treatment: Confronting Racial and Ethnic Disparities in Health Care. Washington, DC: National Academies Press, 2002.

38. American Medical Association. Pain Management: The Online Series. Pathophysiology of pain and pain assessment. Module 3. Pain management: Barriers to Pain Management & Pain in Special Populations. September 2007. Available at: http://www.ama-cmeonline.com/pain_mgmt/. Accessed January 19, 2008.

39. Foley K. Opioids and chronic neuropathic pain. N Engl J Med 348(13):1279–1280, 2003.

40. Gilron I, Watson PN, Cahill CM, et al. Neuropathic pain: a practical guide for the clinician. CMAJ 175(3):256–275, 2006.

41. Butler SF, Budman SH, Fernandez K, et al. Validations of a screener and opioid assessment measure for patients with chronic pain. Pain 112(1–2):65–75, 2004.

42. Webster LR, Webster RM. Predicting aberrant behaviors in opioid-treated patients: preliminary validation of the Opioid Risk Tool. Pain Med 6(6):432–442, 2005.

43. American Pain Society. Definitions Related to the Use of Opioids for the Treatment of Pain. A consensus statement from the American Academy of Pain Medicine, the American Pain Society, and the American Society of Addiction Medicine, 2001. Available at: http://www.ampainsoc.org/advocacy/opioids2.htm. Accessed January 20, 2008.

ADDITIONAL REFERENCES

Weight and Nutrition

American Academy of Family Physicians. Nutrition Screening Initiative. Available at: http://www.aafp.org/afp/980301ap/edits.html. Accessed June 8, 2008.

Ashar BH, Rowland Seymour A. Advising patients who use dietary supplements. Am J Med 121(12):91–97, 2008.

Ashen MD, Blumenthal RS. Low HDL cholesterol levels. N Engl J Med 353(12):1252–1260, 2005.

Ford ES, Wayne G, Dietz WH, et al. Prevalence of the metabolic syndrome among U.S. adults: findings from the Third National Health and Nutrition Examination Survey. JAMA 287(3):356–359, 2002.

Huang HY, Caballero B, Change S, et al. The efficacy and safety of multivitamins and mineral supplement use to prevent cancer and chronic disease in adults: a systematic review for a National Institutes of Health State-of-the-Science Conference. Ann Intern Med 145(5):372–385, 2006.

Lien LF, Brown AJ, Ard JD, et al. Effects of PREMIER lifestyle modifications on participants with and without the metabolic syndrome. Hypertension 50(4):609–616, 2007.

Mehler PS. Bulimia nervosa. N Engl J Med 349(9):875–880, 2003.

National Institute of Diabetes & Digestive & Kidney Diseases. National Diabetes Statistics. Available at: http://diabetes.niddk.nih.gov/dm/pubs/statistics/index.htm. Accessed January 15, 2008.

Pearson TA, Blair SN, Daniels SR, et al. AHA guidelines for primary prevention of cardiovascular disease and stroke: 2002 update. Circulation 106:388–391, 2002.

Sacks FM, Svetkey LP, Vollmer WM, et al. Effects on blood pressure of reduced dietary sodium and the dietary approaches to stop hypertension (DASH) diet. N Engl J Med 344(1):3–10, 2001.

Samaha FF, Iqbal N, Seshadri P, et al. A low-carbohydrate as compared with a low-fat diet in severe obesity. N Engl J Med 34(21):2074–2081, 2003.

Stevens VJ, Obarzanek E, Cook NR, et al. Long-term weight loss and changes in blood pressure: results of the trials of hypertension prevention, Phase II. Ann Intern Med 134(1):1–11, 2001.

Blood Pressure

Beevers G, Lip GY, O'Brien E. ABC of hypertension. Blood pressure measurement. Part I. Sphygmomanometry: factors common in all techniques. BMJ 322(7292):981–985, 2001.

Beevers G, Lip GY, O'Brien E. ABC of hypertension. Blood pressure measurement. Part II. Conventional sphygmomanometry: technique of auscultatory blood pressure measurement. BMJ 322(7293):1043–1047, 2001.

Bobrie G, Genes N, Vaur L, et al. Is "isolated home" hypertension as opposed to "isolated office" hypertension a sign of greater cardiovascular risk? Arch Intern Med 161(18):2205–2211, 2001.

McAlister FA, Straus SE. Evidence-based treatment of hypertension. Measurement of blood pressure: an evidence based review. BMJ 322:908–911, 2001.

Perry HM, Davis BR, Price TR, et al, for the Systolic Hypertension in the Elderly Program Cooperative Research Group. Effect of treating isolated systolic hypertension on the risk of developing various types and subtypes of stroke: the Systolic Hypertension in the Elderly Program (SHEP). JAMA 284(4):465–471, 2000.

Tholl U, Forstner K, Anlauf M. Measuring blood pressure: pitfalls and recommendations. Nephrol Dial Transplant 19:766, 2004.

U.S. Preventive Services Task Force. Screening for High Blood Pressure: U.S. Preventive Services Task Force Reaffirmation Recommendation Statement. AHRQ Publication No. 08-05105-EF-2, December 2007; first published in Ann Intern Med 147:783–786, 2007. Agency for Healthcare Research and Quality, Rockville, MD. Available at: http://www.ahrq.gov/clinic/uspstf07/hbp/hbprr.htm. Accessed June 8, 2008.

Writing Group of the PREMIER Collaborative Research Group. Effects of comprehensive lifestyle modification on blood pressure control: main results of the PREMIER clinical trial. JAMA 289(16):2083–2093, 2003.

Acute and Chronic Pain

Caraceni A, Portenoy RK. An international survey of cancer pain characteristics and syndromes. IASP Task Force on Cancer Pain. International Association for the Study of Pain. Pain 82(3):263–274, 1999.

Charlton JE, ed. Core Curriculum for Professional Education in Pain, 3rd ed. Seattle: International Association for the Study of Pain, 2005. Available at: http://www.iasp-pain.org/AM/Template.cfm?Section=Publications&Template=/CM/HTMLDisplay.cfm&ContentID=2307#TOC. Accessed June 9, 2008.

The Bates' suite offers these additional resources to enhance learning and facilitate understanding of this chapter:

- Bates' Pocket Guide to Physical Examination and History Taking, 6th edition
- Bates' Nursing Online
- Bates' Visual Guide to Physical Examination, 4th edition
- thePoint online resources, http://thepoint.lww.com
- Student CD-ROM included with the book

TABLE
4-1

Eating Disorders and Excessively Low BMI

In the United States an estimated 5 to 10 million women and 1 million men suffer from eating disorders. These severe disturbances of eating behavior are often difficult to detect, especially in teens wearing baggy clothes or in individuals who binge and then induce vomiting or evacuation. Be familiar with the two principal eating disorders, *anorexia nervosa* and *bulimia nervosa*. Both conditions are characterized by distorted perceptions of body image and weight. Early detection is important, because prognosis improves when treatment occurs in the early stages of these disorders.

Clinical Features

Anorexia Nervosa	*Bulimia Nervosa*
• Refusal to maintain minimally normal body weight (or BMI above 17.5 kg/m²)	• Repeated binge eating followed by self-induced vomiting, misuse of laxatives, diuretics or other medications, fasting, or excessive exercise
• Afraid of appearing fat	• Often with normal weight
• Frequently starving but in denial; lacking insight	• Overeating at least twice a week during 3-month period; large amounts of food consumed in short period (~2 hrs)
• Often brought in by family members	
• May present as failure to make expected weight gains in childhood or adolescence, amenorrhea in women, loss of libido or potency in men	• Preoccupation with eating; craving and compulsion to eat; lack of control over eating; alternating with periods of starvation
• Associated with depressive symptoms such as depressed mood, irritability, social withdrawal, insomnia, decreased libido	• Dread of fatness but may be obese
• Additional features supporting diagnosis: self-induced vomiting or purging, excessive exercise, use of appetite suppressants and/or diuretics	• Subtypes of
• Biologic complications	• *Purging:* bulimic episodes accompanied by self-induced vomiting or use of laxatives, diuretics, or enemas
• *Neuroendocrine changes:* amenorrhea, increased corticotropin-releasing factor, cortisol, growth hormone, serotonin; decreased diurnal cortisol fluctuation, luteinizing hormone, follicle-stimulating hormone, thyroid-stimulating hormone	• *Nonpurging:* bulimic episodes accompanied by compensatory behavior such as fasting, exercise, but without purging
• *Cardiovascular disorders:* bradycardia, hypotension, arrhythmias, cardiomyopathy	• Biologic complications
• *Metabolic disorders:* hypokalemia, hypochloremic metabolic alkalosis, increased BUN, edema	See changes listed for anorexia nervosa, especially weakness, fatigue, mild cognitive disorder; also erosion of dental enamel, parotitis, pancreatic inflammation with elevated amylase, mild neuropathies, seizures, hypokalemia, hypochloremic metabolic acidosis, hypomagnesemia
• *Other:* dry skin, dental caries, delayed gastric emptying, constipation, anemia, osteoporosis	

(Sources: World Health Organization: The ICD-10 Classification of Mental and Behavioral Disorders: Diagnostic Criteria for Research. Geneva, World Health Organization, 1993. American Psychiatric Association: DSM-IV-TR: Diagnostic and Statistical Manual of Mental Disorders, 4th ed. Washington, DC, American Psychiatric Association, 1994. Halmi KA: Eating Disorders: In: Kaplan HI, Sadock BJ, eds. Comprehensive Textbook of Psychiatry, 7th ed. Philadelphia, Lippincott Williams & Wilkins, 1663–1676, 2000. Mehler PS. Bulimia nervosa. N Engl J Med 349(9):875–880, 2003.)

TABLE 4-2

Nutrition Screening

Nutrition Screening Checklist

I have an illness or condition that made me change the kind and/or amount of food I eat.	Yes (2 pts)	_____
I eat fewer than 2 meals per day.	Yes (3 pts)	_____
I eat few fruits or vegetables, or milk products.	Yes (2 pts)	_____
I have 3 or more drinks of beer, liquor, or wine almost every day.	Yes (2 pts)	_____
I have tooth or mouth problems that make it hard for me to eat.	Yes (2 pts)	_____
I don't always have enough money to buy the food I need.	Yes (4 pts)	_____
I eat alone most of the time.	Yes (1 pt)	_____
I take 3 or more different prescribed or over-the-counter drugs each day.	Yes (1 pt)	_____
Without wanting to, I have lost or gained 10 pounds in the last 6 months.	Yes (2 pts)	_____
I am not always physically able to shop, cook, and/or feed myself.	Yes (2 pts)	_____
	TOTAL	_____

Instructions. Check "yes" for each condition that applies, then total the nutritional score. For total scores of 3–5 points (moderate risk) or ≥6 points (high risk), further evaluation is needed (especially for the elderly).

Rapid Screen for Dietary Intake

	Portions Consumed by Patient	Recommended
Grains, cereals, bread group	_____	6–11
Fruit group	_____	2–4
Vegetable group	_____	3–5
Meat/meat substitute group	_____	2–3
Dairy group	_____	2–3
Sugars, fats, snack foods	_____	—
Soft drinks	_____	—
Alcoholic beverages	_____	<2

Instructions. Ask the patient for a 24-hour dietary recall (perhaps two of these) before completing the form.

(Sources: *Nutrition Screening*—American Academy of Family Physicians. The Nutrition Screening Initiative. Available at: www.aafp.org/PreBuilt/ NSI_DETERMINE.pdf. Accessed January 23, 2008; *Rapid Screen for Dietary Intake*—Nestle M. Nutrition. In Woolf SH, Jonas S, Lawrence RS, eds. Health Promotion and Disease Prevention in Clinical Practice. Baltimore, Williams & Wilkins, 1996.)

TABLE
4-3

Obesity-Related Risk Factors and Diseases

Cardiovascular
- Hypertension
- Congestive heart failure
- Cor pulmonale
- Varicose veins
- Pulmonary embolism
- Coronary artery disease

Endocrine
- The metabolic syndrome
- Type 2 diabetes
- Dyslipidemia
- Polycystic ovarian syndrome/ androgenicity
- Amenorrhea/infertility/menstrual disorders

Gastrointestinal
- Gastroesophageal reflux disease (GERD)
- Nonalcoholic fatty liver disease (NAFLD)
- Cholelithiasis
- Hernias
- Colon cancer

Genitourinary
- Urinary stress incontinence
- Obesity-related glomerulopathy
- Hypogonadism (male)
- Breast and uterine cancers
- Pregnancy complications

Integument
- Striae distensae (stretch marks)
- Status pigmentation of legs
- Lymphedema
- Cellulitis
- Intertrigo, carbuncles
- Acanthosis nigricans/skin tags

Muscoloskeletal
- Hyperuricemia and gout
- Immobility
- Osteoarthritis (knees, hips)
- Low back pain

Neurologic
- Stroke
- Idiopathic intracranial hypertension
- Meralgia paresthetica

Psychological
- Depression/low self-esteem
- Body image disturbance
- Social stigmatization

Respiratory
- Dyspnea
- Obstructive sleep apnea
- Hypoventilation syndrome
- Pickwickian syndrome
- Asthma

(Source: American Medical Association. Roadmaps for Clinical Practice—Case Studies in Disease Prevention and Health Promotion—Assessment and Management of Adult Obesity: A Primer for Physicians. Available at: http://www.ama-assn.org/ama1/pub/upload/mm/433/healthrisks.pdf. Accessed January 16, 2008.)

TABLE
4-4

Obesity: Stages of Change Model and Assessing Readiness

Stage	Characteristic	Patient Verbal Cue	Appropriate Intervention	Sample Dialogue
Precontemplation	Unaware of problem, no interest in change	"I'm not really interested in weight loss. It's not a problem."	Provide information about health risks and benefits of weight loss	"Would you like to read some information about the health aspects of obesity?"
Contemplation	Aware of problem, beginning to think of changing	"I know I need to lose weight, but with all that's going on in my life right now, I'm not sure I can."	Help resolve ambivalence; discuss barriers	"Let's look at the benefits of weight loss, as well as what you may need to change."
Preparation	Realizes benefits of making changes and thinking about how to change	"I have to lose weight, and I'm planning to do that."	Teach behavior modification; provide education	"Let's take a closer look at how you can reduce some of the calories you eat and how to increase your activity during the day."
Action	Actively taking steps toward change	"I'm doing my best. This is harder than I thought."	Provide support and guidance, with a focus on the long term	"It's terrific that you're working so hard. What problems have you had so far? How have you solved them?"
Maintenance	Initial treatment goals reached	"I've learned a lot through this process."	Relapse control	"What situations continue to tempt you to overeat? What can be helpful for the next time you face such a situation?"

(Sources: American Medical Association. Roadmaps for Clinical Practice—Case Studies in Disease Prevention and Health Promotion—Assessment and Management of Adult Obesity: A Primer for Physicians. Available at: http://www.ama-assn.org/ama1/pub/upload/mm/433/healthrisks.pdf. Accessed January 16, 2008; Adapted from Prochaska JO, DiClemente CC. Toward a comprehensive model of change. In: Miller WR, ed. *Treating Addictive Behaviors*. New York, NY: Plenum, 1986:3–27.)

TABLE
4-5

Healthy Eating: U.S.D.A. Food Pyramid

PHYSICAL ACTIVITY
30 min – most days
60 min – to prevent weight gain
60-90 min – to sustain weight loss

GRAINS	VEGETABLES	FRUITS	MILK	MEAT & BEANS
Make half your grains whole	Vary your veggies	Focus on fruits	Get your calcium-rich foods	Go lean with protein
Eat at least 3 oz. of whole-grain cereals, breads, crackers, rice, or pasta every day	Eat more dark-green veggies like broccoli, spinach, and other dark leafy greens	Eat a variety of fruit	Go low-fat or fat-free when you choose milk, yogurt, and other milk products	Choose low-fat or lean meats and poultry
1 oz. is about 1 slice of bread, about 1 cup of breakfast cereal, or ½ cup of cooked rice, cereal, or pasta	Eat more orange vegetables like carrots and sweet potatoes	Choose fresh, frozen, canned, or dried fruit	If you don't or can't consume milk, choose lactose-free products or other calcium sources such as fortified foods and beverages	Bake it, broil it, or grill it
	Eat more dry beans and peas like pinto beans, kidney beans, and lentils	Go easy on fruit juices		Vary your protein routine — choose more fish, beans, peas, nuts, and seeds

For a 2,000-calorie diet, you need the amounts below from each food group. To find the amounts that are right for you, go to MyPyramid.gov.

Eat 6 oz. every day	Eat 2½ cups every day	Eat 2 cups every day	Get 3 cups every day; for kids aged 2 to 8, it's 2	Eat 5½ oz. every day

Find your balance between food and physical activity
- Be sure to stay within your daily calorie needs.
- Be physically active for at least 30 minutes most days of the week.
- About 60 minutes a day of physical activity may be needed to prevent weight gain.
- For sustaining weight loss, at least 60 to 90 minutes a day of physical activity may be required.
- Children and teenagers should be physically active for 60 minutes every day, or most days.

Know the limits on fats, sugars, and salt (sodium)
- Make most of your fat sources from fish, nuts, and vegetable oils.
- Limit solid fats like butter, margarine, shortening, and lard, as well as foods that contain these.
- Check the Nutrition Facts label to keep saturated fats, *trans* fats, and sodium low.
- Choose food and beverages low in added sugars. Added sugars contribute calories with few, if any, nutrients.

TABLE 4-6 Nutrition Counseling: Sources of Nutrients

Nutrient	Food Source
Calcium	Dairy foods such as yogurt, milk, and natural cheeses Breakfast cereal, fruit juice with calcium supplements Dark green leafy vegetables such as collards, turnip greens
Iron	Shellfish Lean meat, dark turkey meat Cereals with iron supplements Spinach, peas, lentils Enriched and whole-grain bread
Folate	Cooked dried beans and peas Oranges, orange juice Dark-green leafy vegetables
Vitamin D	Milk (fortified) Eggs, butter, margarine Cereals (fortified)

(Source: Adapted from Dietary Guidelines Committee, 2000 Report. Nutrition and Your Health: Dietary Guidelines for Americans. Washington, DC, Agricultural Research Service, U.S. Department of Agriculture, 2000.)

TABLE 4-7 Patients With Hypertension: Recommended Changes in Diet

Dietary Change	Food Source
Increase foods high in potassium	Baked white or sweet potatoes, cooked greens such as spinach Bananas, plantains, many dried fruits, orange juice
Decrease foods high in sodium	Canned foods (soups, tuna fish) Pretzels, potato chips, pickles, olives Many processed foods (frozen dinners, ketchup, mustard) Batter-fried foods Table salt, including for cooking

(Source: Adapted from Dietary Guidelines Committee, 2000 Report. Nutrition and Your Health: Dietary Guidelines for Americans. Washington, DC, Agricultural Research Service, U.S. Department of Agriculture, 2000.)

TABLE
4-8

Abnormalities in Rate and Rhythm of Breathing

When observing respiratory patterns, think in terms of *rate*, *depth*, and *regularity* of the patient's breathing. Describe what you see in these terms. Traditional terms, such as tachypnea, are given below so that you will understand them, but simple descriptions are recommended for use.

Normal

The respiratory rate is about 14–20 per min in normal adults and up to 44 per min in infants.

Slow Breathing (*Bradypnea*)

Slow breathing may be secondary to such causes as diabetic coma, drug-induced respiratory depression, and increased intracranial pressure.

Sighing Respiration

Breathing punctuated by frequent sighs should alert you to the possibility of hyperventilation syndrome—a common cause of dyspnea and dizziness. Occasional sighs are normal.

Rapid Shallow Breathing (*Tachypnea*)

Rapid shallow breathing has a number of causes, including restrictive lung disease, pleuritic chest pain, and an elevated diaphragm.

Cheyne-Stokes Breathing

Periods of deep breathing alternate with periods of apnea (no breathing). Children and aging people normally may show this pattern in sleep. Other causes include heart failure, uremia, drug-induced respiratory depression, and brain damage (typically on both sides of the cerebral hemispheres or diencephalon).

Obstructive Breathing

In obstructive lung disease, expiration is prolonged because narrowed airways increase the resistance to air flow. Causes include asthma, chronic bronchitis, and COPD.

Rapid Deep Breathing (*Hyperpnea, Hyperventilation*)

Rapid deep breathing has several causes, including exercise, anxiety, and metabolic acidosis. In the comatose patient, consider infarction, hypoxia, or hypoglycemia affecting the midbrain or pons. *Kussmaul breathing* is deep breathing due to metabolic acidosis. It may be fast, normal in rate, or slow.

Ataxic Breathing (*Biot's Breathing*)

Ataxic breathing is characterized by unpredictable irregularity. Breaths may be shallow or deep, and stop for short periods. Causes include respiratory depression and brain damage, typically at the medullary level.

Behavior and Mental Status

As clinicians, we are uniquely poised to screen, detect, investigate, and encourage health-promoting behaviors. Empathic listening and close observation open a unique vista on the patient's outlook, concerns, and habits. Nevertheless, clinicians often miss clues of mental illness and harmful dysfunctional behaviors in patients. This chapter introduces common symptoms and behaviors encountered in routine patient interactions, concepts guiding history-taking related to mental health, priorities for mental health promotion and counseling, and the formal elements of the *mental status examination* that should be conducted when behavioral problems are suspicious indicators of mental health disorders.

Health and human behavior are intimately linked, as amply noted in the Health Promotion and Counseling sections throughout this book. Government statistics, advisories of the Surgeon General, reports from the U.S. Preventive Services Task Force and the Centers for Disease Control and Prevention, and position statements from leading professional societies all attest to the importance of maintaining and promoting the mental and physical health of our patients. Despite the prevalence of mental disorders, detection is difficult and recognition and treatment rates are low. The prevalence of mental disorders in the U.S. population is 30%,[1] yet only approximately 20% of affected patients receive treatment. Even for patients who obtain care, evidence suggests that adherence to treatment guidelines in primary care offices is less than 50%.[2]

It is especially important for clinicians to learn the common features of mental and physical illness, given the shortage of psychiatrists and the compelling need for improved care in office settings. Often patients have more than one mental disorder, with symptoms that mirror medical illnesses. It has been noted that "these disorders are associated with substantial psychosocial morbidity and they are all treatable."[3] Clinicians are well-advised, for example, to learn to look for depression or anxiety in patients with substance abuse and to look for substance abuse in patients with depression or anxiety. Further, it is increasingly important for clinicians to recognize that "difficult patients" are frequently those with multiple unexplained symptoms and underlying psychiatric conditions that are amenable to therapy. Without better "dual diagnosis," patient health, function, and quality of life are at risk.

SYMPTOMS AND BEHAVIOR

Patient Symptoms: What Do They Mean? For beginning clinicians, the challenge is to sort out the array of symptoms encountered in office practice. As we have seen, symptoms may be psychological, relating to mood or anxiety, or *physical*, relating to a body sensation such as pain, fatigue, or palpitations. In the mental health literature, such physical symptoms are often termed *somatic*. Studies reveal that physical symptoms prompt more than 50% of U.S. office visits.[4] Approximately 5% of these symptoms are acute, triggering immediate evaluation. Another 70% to 75% are minor or self-limited and resolve in 6 weeks. Nevertheless, approximately 25% of patients have persisting and recurrent symptoms that elude assessment through the history and physical examination and fail to improve. Overall, 30% of symptoms are *medically unexplained*. Some of them involve single complaints that appear to persist longer than others—for example, back pain, headache, or musculoskeletal complaints. Others occur in clusters presenting as *functional syndromes,* such as irritable bowel syndrome, fibromyalgia, chronic fatigue, temporomandibular joint disorder, and multiple chemical sensitivity.

Medically Unexplained Symptoms. Clinicians face the perplexing task of deciding whether to assign a medical or psychiatric label to medically unexplained symptoms and syndromes. As experts have noted, "for patients with mental and psychosomatic disorders, primary care offices are the first port-of-call."[6] Two-thirds of patients with depression, for example, present with physical complaints, and half report multiple unexplained physical or somatic symptoms.[7] Further, the functional syndromes have been shown to "frequently co-occur and share key symptoms and selected objective abnormalities."[8] For example, the rates of co-occurrence of fibromyalgia and chronic fatigue syndrome in an analysis of 53 studies were 34% to 70%. Failure to recognize the admixture of physical symptoms and functional syndromes with common mental health disorders—anxiety, depression, unexplained or somatoform physical symptoms, and substance abuse—adds to loss of the patient's quality of life and impaired treatment outcomes. Often these patients are "high users" of the health care system and have significant disability.

Patients with medically unexplained symptoms and unrecognized psychiatric problems are frequently labeled "difficult patients." Depression and anxiety make physician ratings of difficult encounters three times more likely, and somatization increases this likelihood nine-fold.[9] Patients with medically unexplained symptoms appear to be a heterogeneous group spanning a continuum from impairment to meeting formal DSM-IV-TR criteria for mood and somatization disorders. Authors of the first randomized controlled intervention trial for patients with medically unexplained symptoms advise viewing this symptom cluster as "a general warning signal of underlying psychological distress, of which depression is an advanced manifestation."[10]

See Table 5-1, Somatoform Disorders, p. 159, for types of somatoform disorders and guidelines for clinician management.

A *physical symptom* can be explained physically or medically or can be unexplained; a *somatoform symptom* lacks an adequate medical or physical explanation. A *somatoform disorder* meets DSM-IV-TR diagnostic criteria.[5]

MENTAL HEALTH DISORDERS AND UNEXPLAINED SYMPTOMS IN PRIMARY CARE SETTINGS

Mental Health Disorders in Primary Care

- Approximately 20% of primary care outpatients have mental disorders, but up to 50% to 75% of these disorders are undetected and untreated.[11,12]
- Prevalence of mental disorders in primary care settings is roughly:[5,11,13,14]
  - Anxiety—20%
  - Mood disorders including dysthymia, depressive, and bipolar disorders—25%
  - Depression—10%
  - Somatoform disorders—10% to 15%
  - Alcohol and substance abuse—15% to 20%

Explained and Unexplained Symptoms

- Physical symptoms account for approximately half of office visits.
- Roughly one-third of physical symptoms are unexplained; in 20% to 25% of patients, physical symptoms become chronic or recurring.[4,7]
- In patients with *unexplained symptoms,* the prevalence of depression and anxiety exceeds 50% and increases with the total number of reported physical symptoms,[4,7] making detection and "dual diagnosis" important clinical goals.

Common Functional Syndromes

- Co-occurrence rates for *common functional syndromes* such as irritable bowel syndrome, fibromyalgia, chronic fatigue, temporomandibular joint disorder, and multiple chemical sensitivity reach 30% to 90%, depending on the disorders compared.[8]
- The prevalence of *symptom overlap* in the common functional syndromes is high: namely, complaints of fatigue, sleep disturbance, musculoskeletal pain, headache, and gastrointestinal problems.
- The common functional syndromes also overlap in rates of functional impairment, psychiatric comorbidity, and response to cognitive and antidepressant therapy.

Patient Identifiers for Selective Mental Health Screening. Unexplained conditions lasting beyond 6 weeks are increasingly recognized as common chronic disorders that should prompt screening for depression, anxiety, or both. Because screening all patients is time-consuming and expensive, experts recommend a two-tier approach: brief screening questions with high sensitivity and specificity for patients at risk, followed by more detailed investigation when indicated. Several groups of patients warrant brief screening because of high rates of coexisting depression and anxiety.

Although explanations are still unclear, recent studies have helped elucidate these *overlap symptoms* and *functional syndromes* and provide streamlined practical screening tools for detecting mental disorders, suitable for office care. A well-established instrument to aid in office diagnosis is the

PATIENT IDENTIFIERS FOR MENTAL HEALTH SCREENING[4,7]

- Medically unexplained physical symptoms—more than half have a depressive or anxiety disorder
- Multiple physical or somatic symptoms or "high symptom count"
- High severity of the presenting somatic symptom
- Chronic pain
- Symptoms for more than 6 weeks
- Physician rating as a "difficult encounter"
- Recent stress
- Low self-rating of health
- High use of healthcare services
- Substance abuse

Chronic pain may be a spectrum disorder in patients with anxiety, depression, or somatic symptoms. See Chapter 4, Beginning the Physical Examination: General Survey, Vital Signs, and Pain, pp. 101–134.

PRIME-MD; however, it contains 26 questions and takes up to 10 minutes to complete. Better delineation of the current multi-item diagnostic categories in the DSM-IV-TR is highly likely over the next 5 to 8 years, and new and more effective techniques for office screening and management continue to emerge.[10,14,15]

HIGH-YIELD SCREENING QUESTIONS FOR OFFICE PRACTICE—BUT FOLLOW-UP SYSTEMS FOR DIAGNOSIS AND TREATMENT NEEDED...

Depression[11,16,17]

- Over the past 2 weeks, have you felt down, depressed, or hopeless?
- Over the past 2 weeks, have you felt little interest or pleasure in doing things (anhedonia)?

Anxiety

- Anxiety disorders include generalized anxiety disorder, social phobia, panic disorder, post-traumatic stress disorder, and acute stress disorder.
- Generalized Anxiety Disorder Scale: 2-item or 7-item[18,19]
- Panic Disorder: In the past 4 weeks, have you had an anxiety attack—suddenly feeling fear or panic?[20]

Hypochondriacal Features

- Whiteley Index: 14-item self-rating scale[15,21]

Alcohol and Substance Abuse

- CAGE questions adapted for alcohol and drug abuse—see Chapter 3, Interviewing and the Health History, p. 84.

Multidimensional

- PRIME-MD (Primary Care Evaluation of Mental Disorders)—for the five most common disorders in primary care: depression, anxiety, alcohol, somatoform, and eating disorders; 26-item patient questionnaire followed by clinician evaluation; takes approximately 10 minutes[22]
- PRIME-MD Patient Health Questionnaire—available as patient health questionnaire for self-rating; takes approximately 3 minutes[13]

Character Disorders. Character disorders, also called *personality disorders*, account for another group of "difficult patients" that frequently escape detection in office practices. These patients have dysfunctional interpersonal coping styles that disrupt and destabilize their relationships, including those with health care providers. Often these maladaptive behavioral traits are formed in early childhood. The DSM-IV-TR classifies 10 types of character disorders, summarized in the table below. They must be of early onset, endure over time and across situations, and not be solely a product of a general medical condition, medication, or abused substance.[23] Lifetime prevalence in community studies is approximately 6%.[24,25] Primary care providers fail to identify roughly half of patients with these disorders, which co-occur with alcohol and substance abuse at high frequencies: 28% and 48%, respectively.[26,27]

● Character Disorders

Personality Type	Characteristic Behavior Patterns
Paranoid	Distrust and suspiciousness
Schizoid	Detachment from social relationships, with a restricted range of emotional expression
Schizotypal	Eccentricities in behavior and cognitive distortions; acute discomfort in close relationships
Antisocial	Disregard for rights of others; a defect in the experience of compunction or remorse for harming others
Borderline	Instability in interpersonal relationships, self-image, and affective regulation
Histrionic	Emotional overreactivity, theatrical behavior, and seductiveness
Narcissistic	Persisting grandiosity, need for admiration, and lack of empathy for others
Avoidant	Social inhibition, feelings of inadequacy, and hypersensitivity to negative evaluation
Dependent	Submission and clinging behavior
Obsessive-compulsive	Rigid, detail-oriented behavior, often associated with compulsions to perform tasks repetitively and unnecessarily

(Source: Schiffer RB. Psychiatric disorders in medical practice. In: Goldman L, Ausiello D, eds. Cecil Textbook of Medicine, 22nd ed. Philadelphia: Saunders, 2004:2628–2639.)

Elaborated profiles of the individual character disorders are beyond the scope of this book but well worth study. Interaction with *patients who have borderline personality disorder* is especially challenging. Prevalence in primary care practices is 6%, though the diagnosis often is missed.[25] More than 90% of patients with this disorder also meet criteria for other personality disorders. Because many borderline symptoms are common in other disorders, such as depression, anxiety, substance abuse, and eating disorders, the underlying diagnosis may go undetected. Patients with borderline personality disorder are impulsive—more than 50% attempt suicide and cut or injure themselves.[28] More than half lose their jobs because of interpersonal problems. Roughly one third experience sexual abuse. When these patients rank their outlook and feelings, they are most likely to report feeling unhappy, depressed, or despondent; mood swings and emotions that spiral out of control, leading to extremes of rage, sadness, and anxiety; fear of rejection or abandonment by those they care for (yet an inability to maintain healthy relationships); and inability to soothe or comfort themselves when distressed and dependency on other people for solace, with a sense of emptiness. Clinicians tend to label these patients as demanding, disruptive, and manipulative. Recognizing the features of borderline personalities leads to early referral, better provider relationships, and the potential to relieve the suffering and pain of these patients' daily life experiences.[23]

THE HEALTH HISTORY

Common or Concerning Symptoms

- Changes in attention, mood, or speech
- Changes in insight, orientation, or memory
- Anxiety, panic, ritualistic behavior, and phobias
- Delirium or dementia

Overview. As with the General Survey, your assessment of mental status begins with the patient's first words. As you gather the health history, you will quickly discern the patient's level of *alertness* and *orientation, mood, attention,* and *memory.* As the history unfolds, you will learn about the patient's *insight* and *judgment,* as well as any *recurring or unusual thoughts or perceptions.* For some, you will need to supplement your interview with specific questions and a more formal evaluation of mental status. Just as symptoms, blood pressure, and valvular murmurs help you to distinguish, for example, health from disease in the cardiovascular system, specific components of mental function illuminate specific concerns and conditions.

Many of the terms pertinent to the mental health history and the mental status examination are familiar to you from social conversation. Take the time to learn their precise meanings in the context of formal evaluation of mental status, as detailed in the next table.

Attention, Mood, Speech; Insight, Orientation, Memory. Much of the information about the patient's *mental status* becomes evident during the interview. As you talk with the patient and listen to the patient's story, assess *level of consciousness; general appearance; mood,* including depression or mania; and *ability to pay attention, remember, understand,* and *speak.* By placing the patient's vocabulary and general fund of information in the context of his or her cultural and educational background, you can often make a rough estimate of intelligence. Likewise, the patient's responses to illness and life circumstances often tell you about his or her degree of *insight and judgment.*

See Table 5-2, Disorders of Mood, p. 160, and Table 17-5, Disorders of Speech, p. 722.

TERMINOLOGY: THE MENTAL STATUS EXAMINATION

Level of consciousness	Alertness or state of awareness of the environment
Attention	The ability to focus or concentrate over time on one task or activity—an inattentive or distractible person with impaired consciousness has difficulty giving a history or responding to questions.
Memory	The process of registering or recording information, tested by asking for immediate repetition of material, followed by storage or retention of information. *Recent or short-term memory* covers minutes, hours, or days; *remote or long-term memory* refers to intervals of years.
Orientation	Awareness of personal identity, place, and time; requires both memory and attention
Perceptions	Sensory awareness of objects in the environment and their interrelationships (external stimuli); also refers to internal stimuli such as dreams or hallucinations
Thought processes	The logic, coherence, and relevance of the patient's thought as it leads to selected goals, or *how* people think
Thought content	*What* the patient thinks about, including level of insight and judgment
Insight	Awareness that symptoms or disturbed behaviors are normal or abnormal; for example, distinguishing between daydreams and hallucinations that seem real
Judgment	Process of comparing and evaluating alternatives when deciding on a course of action; reflects values that may or may not be based on reality and social conventions or norms
Affect	An observable, usually episodic, feeling or tone expressed through voice, facial expression, and demeanor
Mood	A more sustained emotion that may color a person's view of the world (mood is to affect as climate is to weather)
Language	A complex symbolic system for expressing, receiving, and comprehending words; as with consciousness, attention, and memory, language is essential for assessing other mental functions
Higher cognitive functions	Assessed by vocabulary, fund of information, abstract thinking, calculations, construction of objects that have two or three dimensions

If you suspect a problem in orientation and memory, you can ask, "Let's see, your last clinic appointment was when . . . ?" "And the date today?" The more you can integrate your exploration of mental status into a sensitive patient history, the less it will seem like an interrogation.

Anxiety, Panic, Ritualistic Behavior, Phobias.   If the patient has unusual thoughts, preoccupations, beliefs, or perceptions, explore them as they arise during the interview. For example, worries persisting over a 6-month period suggest a possible *generalized anxiety disorder*, the most prevalent psychiatric condition in the United States following substance abuse, with a lifetime prevalence of approximately 5%.[29] Over time, you will come to recognize some of its mimics: *panic disorder*, with its recurrent panic attacks followed by a period of anxiety about further attacks; *obsessive-compulsive disorder*, with its intrusive thoughts and ritualistic behaviors; *posttraumatic stress disorder*, characterized by avoidance, numbing, and hyperarousal; and *social phobia*, with its marked anticipatory anxiety in social situations. For such patients, you will need to supplement your interview with questions in specific areas. You may determine the need to go further and pursue a formal mental status examination. The components of the mental status examination are described in the section on Techniques of Examination, pp. 145–155.

See Table 5-3, Anxiety Disorders, p. 161, and Table 5-4, Psychotic Disorders, p. 162.

Delirium or Dementia.   All patients with documented or suspected brain lesions, psychiatric symptoms, or reports from family members of vague or changed behavioral symptoms need further systematic assessment. Patients may have subtle behavioral changes, difficulty taking medications properly, problems attending to household chores or paying bills, or loss of interest in their usual activities. Other patients may behave strangely after surgery or during an acute illness. Each problem should be identified as expeditiously as possible. Mental function influences the ability to hold a job and is often important in evaluating disability.

See Table 20-2, Delirium and Dementia, p. 931.

May be signs of depression or dementia

HEALTH PROMOTION AND COUNSELING

Important Topics for Health Promotion and Counseling

- Screening for depression and suicidality
- Screening for dementia

The burden of suffering that mental disorders impose is great. They affect 26% of Americans 18 years or older, or approximately 58 million people.[30] This number represents roughly one in four adults in a given year. Serious mental illness affects approximately 6% of the population. Most people with one mental illness, or 45%, meet criteria for two or more other mental disorders. Illness severity is strongly linked to comorbidity. For the general population, focus health promotion and counseling on depression, suicide risk, and dementia, three important conditions often overlooked. Also screen routinely for addiction to alcohol or drugs.

Depression. *Major depression* is a common medical illness and frequently coexists with other mental disorders, notably anxiety disorders and substance abuse. Lifetime prevalence is high, 16%, with an annual prevalence of 6.7%, or almost 15 million adults.[1,30] Depression is twice as likely in women as in men; the prevalence of postpartum depression is 10% to 15%. Depression frequently accompanies serious medical illnesses, including diabetes, heart disease, cancer, stroke, and HIV/AIDS; outcomes and costs of care for these illnesses improve when depression is treated. Primary care providers often miss signs of early depression such as low self-esteem, loss of pleasure in daily activities (*anhedonia*), sleep disorders, and difficulty concentrating or making decisions. Watch carefully for depressive symptoms, especially in patients who are young, female, single, divorced or separated, seriously or chronically ill, or bereaved. Those with a prior history or family history of depression are also at risk.

See Chapter 3, Interviewing and the Health History, pp. 83–84.

The U.S. Preventive Services Task Force recommends screening in clinical settings that can provide accurate diagnosis, treatment, and follow-up.[31,32] Screening tools suitable for the office are readily available. All positive screening results warrant more formal diagnostic evaluation. Failure to diagnose depression can have fatal consequences—suicide rates among patients with major depression are eight times higher than in the general population.

See screening questions on p. 84 and review screening tools readily available for office practice.[17,33–35]

Suicide. Preventing suicide is a national public health imperative. Suicide now ranks as the 11th leading cause of death in the United States and the third leading cause of death for people 10 to 24 years.[36,37] The most recent data, from 2004, reveal an overall rate of 10.9 suicide deaths per 100,000 population. There are 8 to 25 attempts for every completed suicide. Suicide rates are four times higher among men, who are more likely to use firearms and less likely to use poison than women. The highest suicide rates are in white men older than 65 years (14.3 deaths per 100,000). For white men 85 years or older, suicide rates climb to 17.8 deaths per 100,000.

Clues to pending suicide are variable and subtle. More than half of patients completing suicide have visited their physicians in the prior month, and 10% to 40% in the prior week.[38] Two-thirds of suicides occur on the first attempt. Powerful risk factors have been identified: more than 90% of people who die by suicide have depression or other mental disorders, or they are substance abusers. Other risk factors are prior suicide attempts; delusional or psychotic thinking; family history of suicide, mental disorders, or substance abuse; family violence, including physical or sexual abuse; firearms in the home; and incarceration. Pursue any clinical suspicion of suicide by asking patients directly about suicidal ideation and plans. Refer at-risk patients immediately for psychiatric care. Currently, given the low incidence of suicide, clinicians are urged to intensify targeted rather than general screening.

See Chapter 20, The Older Adult, pp. 893–933, Table 20-1, Minimum Geriatric Competencies, p. 930, and Table 20-2, Delirium and Dementia, p. 931.

Alcohol and Substance Abuse. As detailed throughout this chapter, the interactions and comorbidity of alcohol and substance abuse with mental

See Chapter 3, Interviewing and the Health History–Alcohol and disorders and suicide are both extensive and profound. Alcohol, tobacco, and illicit drugs account for more illness, deaths, and disabilities than any other preventable condition. Lifetime prevalence of alcohol and illicit drug use in the United States is 13% and 3%. In recent U.S. surveys, 8% of those 12 years or older, or 19 million people, reported use of illicit drugs in the prior 30 days. An estimated 3% are dependent on or abuse illicit drugs; of these cases, 60% involve marijuana.[39] Because screening for alcohol and drug use is part of *every* patient history, information on screening is found in Chapter 3, Interviewing and the Health History.

Illicit Drugs, pp. 83–84. See also Chapter 11, The Abdomen– Screening for Alcohol Abuse, pp. 429–430.

Important Areas of the Mental Status Examination

- Appearance and behavior
- Speech and language
- Mood
- Thoughts and perceptions
- Cognition, including memory, attention, information and vocabulary, calculations, abstract thinking, and constructional ability

The interplay between mental disorders and physical health is challenging and complex. Mental disorders often take the form of somatic complaints, and physical illnesses provoke behavioral and emotional responses. Always look carefully for pathophysiologic or pharmacologic causes as you probe the context and emotional import of changes in mental status. Personality factors, psychodynamics, or the patient's personal experiences can complicate assessments of mental status. You can explore these areas during the interview. By integrating and correlating your observations and findings from the history and examination, selectively amplified by components or all of the formal mental status examination, you will come to understand the patient as a whole, molded by life experiences, family, and culture.

As you will see in Chapter 17, The Nervous System, mental status and brain structure and function are intimately intertwined. Your assessment of mental status is an integral component of your assessment of the nervous system, and the first segment of your nervous system write-up. With dedication and practice, you will learn to describe the patient's mood, speech, behavior, and cognition and relate these findings to your examination of the cranial nerves, motor and sensory systems, and reflexes.

At first, you may feel reluctant to perform mental status examinations, wondering if they will upset patients, invade their privacy, or result in labeling their thoughts or behavior as pathologic. Such concerns are understandable. An insensitive examination may alarm a patient, and even a skillful examination may bring to conscious awareness a deficit that the patient is trying to ignore. You may wish to discuss some of these concerns with your instructor or other experienced clinicians. As with other realms of clinical assessment, your skills and confidence will improve with experience, and rewards will follow. Remember that patients appreciate an understanding listener, and some will owe their health, their safety, or even their lives to your attention.

The mental status examination consists of the following components:

- Appearance and behavior

- Speech and language

- Mood

- Thoughts and perceptions

- Cognitive function, including memory, attention, information and vocabulary, calculations, abstract thinking, and constructional ability.

The format that follows should help to organize your observations, but it is not intended as a step-by-step guide. When a full examination is indicated, you should be flexible in your approach but thorough in what you cover. In some situations, however, sequence is important. If, during your initial interview, the patient's consciousness, attention, comprehension of words, or ability to speak seems impaired, assess this attribute promptly. Such a patient cannot give a reliable history, and you will not be able to test most of the other mental functions.

 APPEARANCE AND BEHAVIOR

Use here all the relevant observations made throughout the course of your history and examination. Include these areas:

Level of Consciousness.   Is the patient awake and alert? Does the patient seem to understand your questions and respond appropriately and reasonably quickly, or is there a tendency to lose track of the topic and fall silent or even asleep?

See the table on Level of Consciousness (Arousal), Chapter 17, The Nervous System, p. 706.

If the patient does not respond to your questions, escalate the stimulus in steps:

- Speak to the patient by name and in a loud voice.

Lethargic patients are drowsy but open their eyes and look at you, respond to questions, and then fall asleep.

- Shake the patient gently, as if awakening a sleeper.

Obtunded patients open their eyes and look at you, but respond slowly and are somewhat confused.

If there is no response to these stimuli, promptly assess the patient for stupor or coma—severe reductions in level of consciousness.

Posture and Motor Behavior.   Does the patient lie in bed, or prefer to walk around? Note body posture and the patient's ability to relax. Observe the pace, range, and character of movements. Do they seem to be under voluntary control? Are certain parts immobile? Do posture and motor activity change with topics under discussion or with activities or people around the patient?

Tense posture, restlessness, and fidgeting of anxiety; crying, pacing, and hand-wringing of *agitated depression;* hopeless, slumped posture and slowed movements of *depression;* singing, dancing, and expansive movements of a *manic episode.*

Dress, Grooming, and Personal Hygiene.   How is the patient dressed? Is clothing clean, pressed, and properly fastened? How does it compare with

Grooming and personal hygiene may deteriorate in *depression, schizophre-*

clothing worn by people of comparable age and social group? Note the patient's hair, nails, teeth, skin, and, if present, beard. How are they groomed? How do the person's grooming and hygiene compare with those of other people of comparable age, lifestyle, and socioeconomic group? Compare one side of the body with the other.

nia, and *dementia*. Excessive fastidiousness may be seen with *obsessive–compulsive disorder*. One-sided neglect may result from a lesion in the opposite parietal cortex, usually the nondominant side.

Facial Expression.   Observe the face, both at rest and when the patient interacts with others. Watch for variations in expression with topics under discussion. Are they appropriate? Or is the face relatively immobile throughout?

Expressions of anxiety, depression, apathy, anger, elation; facial immobility in parkinsonism

Manner, Affect, and Relationship to People and Things.   Using your observations of facial expressions, voice, and body movements, assess the patient's *affect*, or external expression of the inner emotional state. Does it vary appropriately with topics under discussion, or is the affect, labile, blunted, or flat? Does it seem inappropriate or extreme at certain points? If so, how? Note the patient's openness, approachability, and reactions to others and to the surroundings. Does the patient seem to hear or see things that you do not or seem to be conversing with someone who is not there?

Anger, hostility, suspiciousness, or evasiveness of patients with *paranoia*. Elation and euphoria of *mania*. Flat affect and remoteness of *schizophrenia*. Apathy (dulled affect with detachment and indifference) of *dementia*. Anxiety, depression

SPEECH AND LANGUAGE

Throughout the interview, note the characteristics of the patient's speech, including the following:

Quantity.   Is the patient talkative or relatively silent? Are comments spontaneous or only responsive to direct questions?

Rate.   Is speech fast or slow?

Slow speech of *depression*; accelerated rapid, loud speech in *mania*

Loudness.   Is speech loud or soft?

Articulation of Words.   Are the words spoken clearly and distinctly? Is there a nasal quality to the speech?

Dysarthria refers to defective articulation. *Aphasia* refers to a disorder of language. See Table 17-5, Disorders of Speech, p. 722.

Fluency.   This involves the rate, flow, and melody of speech and the content and use of words. Be alert for abnormalities of spontaneous speech such as:

- Hesitancies and gaps in the flow and rhythm of words

These abnormalities suggest *aphasia*. The patient may have so much difficulty in talking or in understanding others that you may not be able to obtain a history. You may also falsely suspect a psychotic disorder.

- Disturbed inflections, such as a monotone

- Circumlocutions, in which phrases or sentences are substituted for a word the person cannot think of, such as "what you write with" for "pen"

- Paraphasias, in which words are malformed ("I write with a den"), wrong ("I write with a bar"), or invented ("I write with a dar").

If the patient's speech lacks meaning or fluency, proceed with further testing as outlined in the following table.

● Testing for Aphasia

Word Comprehension	Ask the patient to follow a one-stage command, such as "Point to your nose." Try a two-stage command: "Point to your mouth, then your knee."
Repetition	Ask the patient to repeat a phrase of one-syllable words (the most difficult repetition task): "No ifs, ands, or buts."
Naming	Ask the patient to name the parts of a watch.
Reading Comprehension	Ask the patient to read a paragraph aloud.
Writing	Ask the patient to write a sentence.

These tests help you determine the kind of aphasia the patient may have. Remember that deficiencies in vision, hearing, intelligence, and education may also affect performance. Two common kinds of aphasia—Wernicke's and Broca's—are compared in Table 17-5, Disorders of Speech, p. 722.

A person who can write a correct sentence does not have aphasia.

MOOD

Assess mood during the interview by exploring the patient's perceptions of his or her mood. Find out about the patient's usual mood level and how it has varied with life events. "How did you feel about that?", for example, or, more generally, "How is your overall mood?" The reports of relatives and friends may be of great value.

Moods include sadness and deep melancholy; contentment, joy, euphoria, and elation; anger and rage; anxiety and worry; and detachment and indifference.

What has the patient's mood been like? How intense has it been? Has it been labile or fairly unchanging? How long has it lasted? Is it appropriate to the patient's circumstances? In case of depression, have there also been episodes of an elevated mood, suggesting a bipolar disorder?

For depressive and bipolar disorders, see Table 5-2, Disorders of Mood, p. 160.

If you suspect depression, assess its depth and any associated risk of suicide. The following series of questions is useful, proceeding as far as the patient's positive answers warrant:

● Do you get pretty discouraged (or depressed or blue)?

● How low do you feel?

● What do you see for yourself in the future?

● Do you ever feel that life isn't worth living? Or that you would just as soon be dead?

● Have you ever thought of doing away with yourself?

● How did (do) you think you would do it?

● What do you think would happen after you were dead?

Asking about suicidal thoughts does not implant the idea in the patient's mind, and it may be the only way to get the information. Although you may feel uneasy about direct questions, most patients discuss their thoughts and feelings freely, sometimes with considerable relief. By open discussion, you demonstrate your interest and concern for a possibly life-threatening problem.

 ## THOUGHT AND PERCEPTIONS

Thought Processes. Assess the logic, relevance, organization, and coherence of the patient's thought processes as revealed in the patient's words and speech throughout the interview. Does speech progress logically toward a goal? Here you use speech as a window into the patient's mind. Listen for patterns of speech that suggest disorders of thought processes, as outlined in the table below.

● Variations and Abnormalities in Thought Processes

Circumstantiality	Speech characterized by indirection and delay in reaching the point because of unnecessary detail, although components of the description have a meaningful connection. Many people without mental disorders speak circumstantially.	Observed in people with obsessions
Derailment (Loosening of Associations)	Speech in which a person shifts from one subject to others that are unrelated or related only obliquely without realizing that the subjects are not meaningfully connected. Ideas slip off the track between clauses, not within them.	Observed in *schizophrenia, manic episodes,* and other *psychotic disorders*
Flight of Ideas	An almost continuous flow of accelerated speech in which a person changes abruptly from topic to topic. Changes are usually based on understandable associations, plays on words, or distracting stimuli, but the ideas do not progress to sensible conversation.	Most frequently noted in *manic episodes*
Neologisms	Invented or distorted words, or words with new and highly idiosyncratic meanings	Observed in *schizophrenia,* other *psychotic disorders,* and *aphasia*
Incoherence	Speech that is largely incomprehensible because of illogic, lack of meaningful connections, abrupt changes in topic, or disordered grammar or word use. Shifts in meaning occur within clauses. Flight of ideas, when severe, may produce incoherence.	Observed in severe psychotic disturbances (usually *schizophrenia*)
Blocking	Sudden interruption of speech in midsentence or before completion of an idea. The person attributes this to losing the thought. Blocking occurs in normal people.	Blocking may be striking in *schizophrenia.*
Confabulation	Fabrication of facts or events in response to questions, to fill in the gaps in an impaired memory	Seen in Korsakoff's syndrome from alcoholism
Perseveration	Persistent repetition of words or ideas	Occurs in *schizophrenia* and other *psychotic disorders*
Echolalia	Repetition of the words and phrases of others	Occurs in manic episodes and *schizophrenia*
Clanging	Speech in which a person chooses a word on the basis of sound rather than meaning, as in rhyming and punning speech. For example, "Look at my eyes and nose, wise eyes and rosy nose. Two to one, the ayes have it!"	Occurs in *schizophrenia* and *manic episodes*

Thought Content.   You should assess information relevant to thought content during the interview. Follow appropriate leads as they occur rather than using stereotyped lists of specific questions. For example, "You mentioned a few minutes ago that a neighbor was responsible for your entire illness. Can you tell me more about that?" Or, in another situation, "What do you think about at times like these?"

You may need to make more specific inquiries. If so, couch them in tactful and accepting terms. "When people are upset like this, sometimes they can't keep certain thoughts out of their minds," or ". . . things seem unreal. Have you experienced anything like this?" In these ways, find out about any of the patterns shown in the following table.

● Abnormalities of Thought Content

Compulsions	Repetitive behaviors or mental acts that a person feels driven to perform in order to produce or prevent some future state of affairs, although expectation of such an effect is unrealistic
Obsessions	Recurrent, uncontrollable thoughts, images, or impulses that a person considers unacceptable and alien
Phobias	Persistent, irrational fears, accompanied by a compelling desire to avoid the stimulus
Anxieties	Apprehensions, fears, tensions, or uneasiness that may be focused (phobia) or free-floating (a general sense of ill-defined dread or impending doom)
Feelings of Unreality	A sense that things in the environment are strange, unreal, or remote
Feelings of Depersonalization	A sense that one's self is different, changed, or unreal, or has lost identity or become detached from one's mind or body
Delusions	False, fixed, personal beliefs that are not shared by other members of the person's culture or subculture. Examples include: • *Delusions of persecution* • *Delusions of grandeur* • *Delusional jealousy* • *Delusions of reference,* in which a person believes that external events, objects, or people have a particular and unusual personal significance (e.g., that the radio or television might be commenting on or giving instructions to the person) • *Delusions of being controlled* by an outside force • *Somatic delusions* of having a disease, disorder, or physical defect • *Systematized delusions,* a single delusion with many elaborations or a cluster of related delusions around a single theme, all systematized into a complex network

Compulsions, obsessions, phobias, and *anxieties* are often associated with neurotic disorders. See Table 5-3, Anxiety Disorders (p. 161).

Delusions and feelings of unreality or depersonalization are more often associated with *psychotic disorders.* See Table 5-4, Psychotic Disorders (p. 162). Delusions may also occur in delirium, severe mood disorders, and dementia.

Perceptions. Inquire about false perceptions in a manner similar to that used for thought content. For example, "When you heard the voice speaking to you, what did it say? How did it make you feel?" Or, "After you've been drinking a lot, do you ever see things that aren't really there?" Or, "Sometimes after major surgery like this, people hear peculiar or frightening things. Have you experienced anything like that?" In these ways, find out about the following abnormal perceptions.

● Abnormalities of Perception

Illusions	Misinterpretations of real external stimuli
Hallucinations	Subjective sensory perceptions in the absence of relevant external stimuli. The person may or may not recognize the experiences as false. Hallucinations may be auditory, visual, olfactory, gustatory, tactile, or somatic. (False perceptions associated with dreaming, falling asleep, and awakening are not classified as hallucinations.)

Illusions may occur in grief reactions, *delirium,* acute and *post-traumatic stress disorders,* and *schizophrenia.*

Hallucinations may occur in *delirium, dementia* (less commonly), *posttraumatic stress disorder, schizophrenia,* and alcoholism.

Insight and Judgment. These attributes are usually best assessed during the interview.

Insight. Some of your very first questions to the patient often yield important information about insight: "What brings you to the hospital?" "What seems to be the trouble?" "What do you think is wrong?" More specifically, note whether the patient is aware that a particular mood, thought, or perception is abnormal or part of an illness.

Patients with psychotic disorders often lack insight into their illness. Denial of impairment may accompany some neurologic disorders.

Judgment. You can usually assess judgment by noting the patient's responses to family situations, jobs, use of money, and interpersonal conflicts. "How do you plan to get the help you'll need after leaving the hospital?" "How are you going to manage if you lose your job?" "If your husband starts to abuse you again, what will you do?" "Who will attend to your financial affairs while you are in the nursing home?"

Judgment may be poor in delirium, dementia, mental retardation, and psychotic states. Anxiety, mood disorders, intelligence, education, income, and cultural values also influence judgment.

Note whether decisions and actions are based on reality or, for example, on impulse, wish fulfillment, or disordered thought content. What values seem to underlie the patient's decisions and behavior? Allowing for cultural variations, how do these compare with mature adult standards? Because judgment reflects maturity, it may be variable and unpredictable during adolescence.

Disorientation occurs especially when memory or attention is impaired, as in delirium.

COGNITIVE FUNCTIONS

Orientation. By skillful questioning, you can often determine the patient's orientation in the context of the interview. For example, you can ask quite naturally for specific dates and times, the patient's address and telephone number, the names of family members, or the route taken to the hospital. At times—when rechecking the status of a patient with delirium, for example—simple, direct questions may be indicated.

"Can you tell me what time it is now . . . and what day it is?" In either of these ways, determine the patient's orientation for the following:

- *Time*—the time of day, day of the week, month, season, date and year, duration of hospitalization

- *Place*—the patient's residence, the names of the hospital, city, and state

- *Person*—the patient's own name, and the names of relatives and professional personnel

Attention.   These tests of attention are commonly used:

Digit Span.   Explain that you would like to test the patient's ability to concentrate, perhaps adding that this can be difficult when people are in pain, or ill, or feverish. Recite a series of digits, starting with two at a time and speaking each number clearly at a rate of about one per second. Ask the patient to repeat the numbers back to you. If this repetition is accurate, try a series of three numbers, then four, and so on as long as the patient responds correctly. Jot down the numbers as you say them to ensure your own accuracy. If the patient makes a mistake, try once more with another series of the same length. Stop after a second failure in a single series.

Causes of poor performance include *delirium, dementia, mental retardation,* and performance anxiety.

In choosing digits you may use street numbers, zip codes, telephone numbers, and other numerical sequences that are familiar to you, but avoid consecutive numbers, easily recognized dates, and sequences that possibly are familiar to the patient.

Now, starting again with a series of two, ask the patient to repeat the numbers to you backward.

Normally, a person should be able to repeat correctly at least five digits forward and four backward.

Serial 7s.   Instruct the patient, "Starting from a hundred, subtract 7, and keep subtracting 7. . . ." Note the effort required and the speed and accuracy of the responses. Writing down the answers helps you keep up with the arithmetic. Normally, a person can complete serial 7s in 1½ minutes, with fewer than four errors. If the patient cannot do serial 7s, try 3s or counting backward.

Poor performance may result from delirium, the late stage of dementia, mental retardation, loss of calculating ability, anxiety, or depression. Also consider the possibility of limited education.

Spelling Backward.   This can substitute for serial 7s. Say a five-letter word, spell it, e.g., W-O-R-L-D, and ask the patient to spell it backward.

Remote Memory.   Inquire about birthdays, anniversaries, social security number, names of schools attended, jobs held, or past historical events such as wars relevant to the patient's past.

Remote memory may be impaired in the late stage of *dementia.*

Recent Memory. This could involve the events of the day. Ask questions with answers you can check against other sources so you can see if the patient is confabulating (making up facts to compensate for a defective memory). These might include the day's weather, today's appointment time, and medications or laboratory tests taken during the day. (Asking what the patient had for breakfast may be a waste of time unless you can check the accuracy of the answer.)

New Learning Ability. Give the patient three or four words such as "83 Water Street and blue," or "table, flower, green, and hamburger." Ask the patient to repeat them so that you know that the information has been heard and registered. This step, like digit span, tests registration and immediate recall. Then proceed to other parts of the examination. After about 3 to 5 minutes, ask the patient to repeat the words. Note the accuracy of the response, awareness of whether it is correct, and any tendency to confabulate. Normally, a person should be able to remember the words.

Recent memory is impaired in *dementia* and *delirium*. *Amnestic disorders* impair memory or new learning ability significantly and reduce a person's social or occupational functioning, but they do not have the global features of delirium or dementia. Anxiety, depression, and mental retardation may also impair recent memory.

 ## HIGHER COGNITIVE FUNCTIONS

Information and Vocabulary. Information and vocabulary, when observed clinically, provide a rough estimate of a person's intelligence. Assess them during the interview. Ask a student, for example, about favorite courses, or inquire about work, hobbies, reading, favorite television programs, or current events. Explore such topics first with simple questions, then with more difficult ones. Note the person's grasp of information, the complexity of the ideas expressed, and the vocabulary used.

More directly, you can ask about specific facts such as:

    The name of the president, vice president, or governor
    The names of the last four or five presidents
    The names of five large cities in the country

If considered in the context of cultural and educational background, information and vocabulary are fairly good indicators of intelligence. They are relatively unaffected by any but the most severe psychiatric disorders, and may be helpful for distinguishing mentally retarded adults (whose information and vocabulary are limited) from those with mild or moderate *dementia* (whose information and vocabulary are fairly well preserved).

Calculating Ability. Test the patient's ability to do arithmetical calculations, starting at the rote level with simple addition ("What is 4 + 3? . . . 8 + 7?") and multiplication ("What is 5 × 6? . . . 9 × 7?"). The task can be made more difficult by using two-digit numbers ("15 + 12" or "25 × 6") or longer, written examples.

Poor performance may be a useful sign of dementia or may accompany *aphasia*, but it must be assessed in terms of the patient's intelligence and education.

Alternatively, pose practical and functionally important questions, such as "If something costs 78 cents and you give the clerk one dollar, how much should you get back?"

Abstract Thinking. Test the capacity to think abstractly in two ways.

    Proverbs. Ask the patient what people mean when they use some of the following proverbs:

    A stitch in time saves nine.
    Don't count your chickens before they're hatched.

Concrete responses are often given by people with mental retardation, *delirium,* or *dementia* but may also be a function of limited education. Patients with *schizophrenia* may respond concretely or with personal, bizarre interpretations.

The proof of the pudding is in the eating.
A rolling stone gathers no moss.
The squeaking wheel gets the grease.

Note the relevance of the answers and their degree of concreteness or abstractness. For example, "You should sew a rip before it gets bigger" is concrete, whereas "Prompt attention to a problem prevents trouble" is abstract. Average patients should give abstract or semiabstract responses.

Similarities.   Ask the patient to tell you how the following are alike:

An orange and an apple   A church and a theater

A cat and a mouse   A piano and a violin

A child and a dwarf   Wood and coal

Note the accuracy and relevance of the answers and their degree of concreteness or abstractness. For example, "A cat and a mouse are both animals" is abstract, "They both have tails" is concrete, and "A cat chases a mouse" is not relevant.

Constructional Ability.   The task here is to copy figures of increasing complexity onto a piece of blank unlined paper. Show each figure one at a time and ask the patient to copy it as well as possible.

The three diamonds below are rated poor, fair, and good (but not excellent).[40]

In another approach, ask the patient to draw a clock face complete with numbers and hands. The example below is rated excellent.

These three clocks are poor, fair, and good.[40]

If vision and motor ability are intact, poor constructional ability suggests dementia or parietal lobe damage. Mental retardation may also impair performance.

SPECIAL TECHNIQUES

Mini-Mental State Examination (MMSE).   This brief test is useful in screening for cognitive dysfunction or dementia and following their course over time. For more detailed information regarding the MMSE, contact the Publisher, Psychological Assessment Resources, Inc., 16204 North Florida Avenue, Lutz, Florida 33549. Below are some sample questions.

MMSE Sample Items

Orientation to Time
  "What is the date?"

Registration
  "Listen carefully; I am going to say three words. You say them back after I stop. Ready? Here they are . . .
  HOUSE (pause), CAR (pause), LAKE (pause). Now repeat those words back to me." [Repeat up to five times, but score only the first trial.]

Naming
  "What is this?" [Point to a pencil or pen.]

Reading
  "Please read this and do what it says." [Show examinee the words on the stimulus form.]
  CLOSE YOUR EYES

(Reproduced by special permission of the Publisher, Psychological Assessment Resources, Inc., 16204 North Florida Avenue, Lutz, Florida 33549, from the Mini Mental State Examination, by Marshal Folstein and Susan Folstein, Copyright 1975, 1998, 2001 by Mini Mental LLC, Inc. Published 2001 by Psychological Assessment Resources, Inc. Further reproduction is prohibited without permission of PAR, Inc.)

RECORDING YOUR FINDINGS

Recording Behavior and Mental Status

"Mental Status: The patient is alert, well-groomed, and cheerful. Speech is fluent and words are clear. Thought processes are coherent, insight is good. The patient is oriented to person, place, and time. Serial 7s accurate; recent and remote memory intact. Calculations intact."

OR

"Mental Status: The patient appears sad and fatigued; clothes are wrinkled. Speech is slow and words are mumbled. Thought processes are coherent but insight into current life reverses is limited. The patient is oriented to person, place, and time. Digit span, serial 7s, and calculations accurate but responses delayed. Clock drawing is good."

Suggests depression

BIBLIOGRAPHY

CITATIONS

1. Kessler RC, Demnler O, Frank RG, et al. Prevalence and treatment of mental disorders, 1990 to 2003. N Engl J Med 352(24): 2515–2523, 2005.

2. Hepner KA, Rowe M, Rost K, et al. The effect of adherence to practice guidelines on depression outcomes. Ann Intern Med 147(5):320–329, 2007.

3. Schiffer RB. Psychiatric disorders in medical practice. In: Goldman L, Ausiello D, eds. Cecil Textbook of Medicine, 22nd ed. Philadelphia: Saunders, 2004: 2628–2639.

4. Kroenke K. Patients presenting with somatic complaints: epidemiology, psychiatric comorbidity, and management. Int J Methods Psychiatr Res 12(1):34–43, 2003.

5. Kroenke K, Spitzer RL, deGruy, et al. A symptom checklist for screen for somatoform disorders in primary care. Psychosomatics 39(3):263–272, 1998.

6. Rief W, Hessel A, Braehler E. Somatization symptoms and hypochondriacal features in the general population. Psychosomatic Medicine 63(4):595–602, 2001.

7. Kroenke K. The interface between physical and psychological symptoms. Primary Care Companion. J Clin Psychiatry 5(Suppl. 7):11–18, 2003.

8. Aaron LA, Buchwald D. A review of the evidence for overlap among unexplained clinical conditions. Ann Intern Med 134(9): 868–881, 2001.

9. Jackson JL, Kronke K. Managing somatization—medically unexplained should not mean medically ignored. J Gen Int Med 21(7):797–799, 2006.

10. Smith RC, Lyles JS, Gardiner JC, et al. Primary care clinicians treat patients with medically unexplained symptoms: a randomized controlled trial. J Gen Int Med 21(7):671–677, 2006.

11. Staab JP, Datto CJ, Weinreig RM, et al. Detection and diagnosis of psychiatric disorders in primary medical care settings. Med Clin N Am 85(3):579–596, 2001.

12. Ansseau, Dierick M, Buntinkxz F, et al. High prevalence of mental disorders in primary care. J Affect Disord 78(1):49–55, 2004.

13. Spitzer RL, Kroenke K, Williams JBW, et al. Validation and utility of a self-report version of PRIME-MD–the PHQ Primary Care Study. JAMA 282(18):1737–1744, 1999.

14. Kroenke K, Sharpe M, Sykes R. Revising the classification of somatoform disorders: key questions and preliminary recommendations. Psychosomatics 48(4):277–285, 2007.

15. Reif W, Martin A, Rauh E, et al. Evaluation of general practitioners' training: how to manage patients with unexplained physical symptoms. Psychosomatics 47(4):304–311, 2006.

16. U.S. Preventive Services Task Force. Screening for depression: recommendations and rationale. Ann Intern Med 136(10): 760–764, 2002.

17. Whooley MA, Avins AL, Miranda J, et al. Case-finding instruments for depression: two questions are as good as many. J Gen Intern Med 12(7):439–445, 1997.

18. Spitzer RL, Kroenke K, Williams JB, et al. A brief measure for assessing generalized anxiety disorder: the GAD 7. Arch Intern Med 166(10):1092–1097, 2006.

19. Kroenke K, Spitzer RL, Williams JBW, et al. Anxiety disorders in primary care: prevalence, impairment, comorbidity, and detection. Ann Intern Med 146(5):317–325, 2007.

20. Lowe B, Grafe K, Zipfel S, et al. Detecting panic disorder in medical and psychosomatic outpatients: comparative validation of the Hospital Anxiety and Depression Scale, the Patient Health Questionnaire, a screening question, and physicians' diagnosis. J Psychosom Res 55(6):515–519, 2003.

21. Pilowsky U. Dimensions of hypochondriasis. Br J Psychiatry 113(494):89–93, 1967.

22. Spitzer RL, Williams JB, Kroenke K, et al. Utility of a new procedure for diagnosing mental disorders in primary care. The PRIME-MD 1000 study. JAMA 272(22):1749–1756, 1994.

23. Oldham JM. A 44-year-old woman with borderline personality disorder. JAMA 287(8):1029–1037, 2002.

24. Paris J. Borderline personality disorder. CMAJ 172(12): 1579–1583, 2005.

25. Gross R, Olfson M, Gameroff M, et al. Borderline personality disorder in primary care. Arch Intern Med 162(1):53–60, 2002.

26. Grant BF, Stinson FS, Dawson DA, et al. Co-occurrence of 12-month alcohol and drug use disorders and personality disorders in the United States: results from the national epidemiologic survey on alcohol and related conditions. Arch Gen Psychiatry 61(8):361–368, 2004.

27. Compton WM, Thomas YF, Stinson FS, et al. Prevalence, correlates, disability, and comorbidity of DSM-IV drug abuse and dependence in the United States: results from the national epidemiologic survey on alcohol and related conditions. Arch Gen Psychiatry 64(5):566–576, 2007.

28. Conklin CZ, Westen D. Borderline personality disorder in clinical practice. Am J Psychiatry 162(5):867–875, 2005.

29. Fricchione G. Generalized anxiety disorder. N Engl J Med 351(7):675–682, 2004.

30. National Institutes of Mental Health. The numbers count: mental disorders in America. Available at: http://www.nimh.nih.gov/health/publications/the-numbers-count-mental-disorders-in-america.shtml. Accessed February 1, 2008.

31. U.S. Preventive Services Task Force. Screening for depression in adults: recommendations and rationale. Ann Intern Med 136(10):760–764, 2002. Available at: http://www.ahrq.gov/clinic/3rduspstf/depression/depressrr.htm. Accessed February 1, 2008.

32. U.S. Preventive Services Task Force. Screening for depression in adults: summary of the evidence. Ann Intern Med 136(10): 765–776, 2002. Available at: http://www.ahrq.gov/clinic/3rduspstf/depression/depsum1.htm. Accessed February 1, 2008.

33. Williams JW, Noel H, Cordes JA, et al. Is this patient clinically depressed? JAMA 287(9):1160–1170, 2002.

34. Beck AT, Steer RA. Internal consistencies of the original and revised Beck Depression Inventory. J Clin Psychol 40(6): 1365–1367, 1984.

35. Zung A. A self-rating depression scale. Arch Gen Psychiatry, 12(1):63–70, 1965. Also available at: http://healthnet.umassmed.edu/mhealth/ZungSelfRatedDepressionScale.pdf. Accessed February 3, 2008.

36. National Institute of Mental Health. Suicide in the U.S.: statistics and prevention. Available at: http://www.nimh.nih.

gov/health/publications/suicide-in-the-us-statistics-and-prevention.shtml. Accessed January 26, 2008.

37. Centers for Disease Control and Prevention. Suicide facts at a glance. Summer 2007. Available at: http://www.cdc.gov/ncipc/dvp/suicide/SuicideDataSheet.pdf. Accessed January 28, 2008.

38. U.S. Preventive Services Task Force. Screening for suicide risk in adults: recommendations and rationale. May 2004. Available at: http://www.ahrq.gov/clinic/3rduspstf/suicide/suiciderr.htm. Accessed January 26, 2008.

39. U.S. Preventive Services Task Force. Screening for illicit drug use: recommendation statement. January 2008. Available at: http://www.ahrq.gov/clinic/uspstf08/druguse/drugrs.htm #clinical. Accessed February 3, 2008.

40. Strub RL, Black FW. The Mental Status Examination in Neurology, 2nd ed. Philadelphia: F.A. Davis, 1985.

ADDITIONAL REFERENCES

American Psychiatric Association. Diagnostic and Statistical Manual of Mental Disorders, 4th ed. Washington, DC: American Psychiatric Association, 2000.

Antai-Otong D. Managing geriatric psychiatric emergencies: delirium and dementia. Nurs Clin North Am 38(1):123–135, 2003.

Coffey CE, Cummings JL. American Psychiatric Press Textbook of Geriatric Neuropsychiatry, 2nd ed. Washington, DC: American Psychiatric Press, 2000.

Cottler LB, Campbell W, Krishna VAS, et al. Predictors of high rates of suicidal ideation among drug users. J Nerv Ment Dis 193(7):431–437, 2005.

Fancher T, Kravitz R. In the clinic: depression. Ann Intern Med 146(9):ITC5-1–ITC5-16, 2007.

Folstein M, Folstein SE, McHugh PR. "Mini-mental state": a practical method for grading the cognitive state of patients for the clinician. J Psych Res 12(3):189–198, 1975.

Haas LJ, Leiser JP, Magill MK. Management of the difficult patient. Am Fam Phys 72(10):2063–2068, 2005.

Hales RE, Yudofsky SC, eds. Essentials of Clinical Psychiatry, 2nd ed. Washington, DC: American Psychiatric Press, 2004.

Hull SK, Broquet K. How to manage difficult patient encounters. Family Practice Management, June 2007. Available at: www.aafp.org/fpm. Accessed January 5, 2008.

Khan AK, Khan A, Harezlak JH, et al. Somatic symptoms in primary care. Psychosomatics 44(6):471–478, 2003.

Luoma JB, Martin CE, Pearson JL. Contact with mental health and primary care providers before suicide: a review of the evidence. Am J Psychiatry 159(6):909–916, 2002.

Manchikanti L, Giordano J, Boswell MV, et al. Psychological factors as predictors of opioid abuse and illicit drug use in chronic pain patients. J Opioid Manag 3(2):89–100, 2007.

National Center for Health Statistics. Fast stats A to Z: self-inflicted injury/suicide. Available at: http://www.cdc.gov/nchs/fastats/suicide.htm. Accessed January 26, 2008.

Sadock BJ, Sadock VA, Kaplan HI, eds. Kaplan & Sadock's Comprehensive Textbook of Psychiatry, 8th ed. Philadelphia: Lippincott Williams & Wilkins, 2005.

Schiffer RB, Rao SM, Fogel BS, eds. Neuropsychiatry. Philadelphia: Lippincott Williams & Wilkins, 2002.

Silber MH. Chronic insomnia. N Engl J Med 353(8):803–810, 2005.

Weisner C, Mertens J, Parthasarathy S, et al. Integrating primary medical care with addiction treatment: a randomized controlled trial. JAMA 286(14):1715–1723, 2001.

The Bates' suite offers these additional resources to enhance learning and facilitate understanding of this chapter:

- Bates' Pocket Guide to Physical Examination and History Taking, 6th edition
- Bates' Nursing Online
- Bates' Visual Guide to Physical Examination, 4th edition
- thePoint online resources, http://thepoint.lww.com
- Student CD-ROM included with the book

Somatoform Disorders: Types and Approach to Symptoms

TYPES OF SOMATOFORM DISORDERS

Somatoform Disorders[a]

Disorder	Features
Somatization disorder	Chronic, multisystem disorder characterized by complaints of pain, gastrointestinal and sexual dysfunction, and pseudoneurologic symptoms. Onset is usually early in life, and psychosocial and vocational achievements are limited.
Conversion disorder	Syndrome of symptoms of deficits mimicking neurologic or medical illness in which psychological factors are judged to be of etiologic importance
Pain disorder	Clinical syndrome characterized predominantly by pain in which psychological factors are judged to be of etiologic importance
Hypochondriasis	Chronic preoccupation with the idea of having a serious disease. The preoccupation is usually poorly amenable to reassurance
Body dysmorphic disorder	Preoccupation with an imagined or exaggerated defect in physical appearance

Other Somatoform-like Disorders

Factitious disorder	Intentional production or feigning of physical or psychological signs when external reinforcers (e.g., avoidance of responsibility, financial gain) are not clearly present
Malingering	Intentional production or feigning of physical or psychological signs when external reinforcers (e.g., avoidance of responsibility, financial gain) are present
Dissociative disorders	Disruptions of consciousness, memory, identity, or perception judged to be due to psychological factors

APPROACH TO SOMATIC AND UNEXPLAINED SYMPTOMS

Stepped Care Approach to Somatic Symptoms in Primary Care[b]

Is the somatic symptom likely to be...	Clinician action might be...
Acutely serious? (<5% of cases)	Expedited diagnostic workup
Minor/self-limited? (70%–75% of cases)	Address patient expectations
	Symptom-specific therapy
	Follow-up in 2–6 weeks
Chronic or recurrent? (20%–25% of cases)	Screen for depression and anxiety

(table continues on page 159)

Caused or aggravated by a depressive or anxiety disorder?	Antidepressant therapy and/or cognitive-behavioral therapy (CBT)
Due to a functional somatic syndrome?	Syndrome-specific therapy
	Antidepressant therapy and/or CBT
Persistent and medically unexplained?	Regular, time-limited clinic visits
	Consider mental health referral
	Symptom management strategies, if evidence-based (e.g., behavioral treatments, pain self-management programs, pain or other specialty clinics, complementary and alternative medicine)
	Rehabilitative rather than disability approach

Management Guidelines for Patients With Medically Unexplained Symptoms[c]

General Aspects	Show empathy and understanding for the complaints and frustrating experiences the patient has had so far (e.g., explain that medically unexplained symptoms are common).
	Develop a good patient–physician relationship; try to be the "coordinator" of diagnostic procedures and care.
Diagnosis	Explore not only the history of complaints and former treatments, but impairment, (health) anxiety, psychosocial issues.
	Use screeners and self-report questionnaires as economic instruments for detection; use symptom diaries to assess course and influencing factors on symptoms.
	When the patient presents with a new symptom, examine the relevant organ system.
	Show the results of investigations to explain the absence of pathology and to give clear reassurance that there is no serious physical disease.
	Avoid unnecessary diagnostic tests or surgical procedures.
Treatment	Provide regularly scheduled visits (e.g., every 4–6 weeks), especially in the case of a history of very frequent healthcare utilization.
	Explain that treatment is coping, not curing (when pathology cannot be found or does not explain degree of complaints).
	Suggest coping strategies like regular physical activity, relaxation, distraction.
Referral	If referral is necessary to start psychotherapy or psychopharmacotherapy, prepare the patient for the treatment and reassure him/her that you will continue to be his/her "doctor."

(Sources: [a]Schiffer RB. Psychiatric disorders in medical practice. In: Goldman L, Ausiello D, eds. Cecil Textbook of Medicine. 22nd ed. Philadelphia: Saunders 2004, pp. 2628–2639; [b]Kroenke K. Patients presenting with somatic complaints: epidemiology, psychiatric comorbidity, and management. Int J Methods Psychiatr Res 12(1):34–43, 2003; [c]Reif W, Martin A, Rauh E, et al. Evaluation of general practitioners' training: how to manage patients with unexplained physical symptoms. Psychosomatics 47(4):304–311, 2006.)

Disorders of Mood

Mood disorders may be either depressive or bipolar. A bipolar disorder can include manic, hypomanic, or depressive features. *Four types of episodes,* described below, are combined in different ways in diagnosis of mood disorders. A major depressive disorder includes only one or more major depressive episodes. A *bipolar I disorder* includes one or more manic or mixed episodes, usually accompanied by major depressive episodes. A *bipolar II disorder* includes one or more major depressive episodes accompanied by at least one hypomanic episode.

Dysthymic and *cyclothymic disorders* are chronic and less severe conditions that do not meet the criteria of the other disorders. Mood disorders due to general medical conditions or substance abuse are classified separately.

Major Depressive Episode

At least five of the symptoms listed below (including one of the first two) must be present during the same 2-week period. They must also represent a change from the person's previous state.

- Depressed mood (may be an irritable mood in children and adolescents) most of the day, nearly every day
- Markedly diminished interest or pleasure in almost all activities most of the day, nearly every day
- Significant weight gain or loss (not dieting) or increased or decreased appetite nearly every day
- Insomnia or hypersomnia nearly every day
- Psychomotor agitation or retardation nearly every day
- Fatigue or loss of energy nearly every day
- Feelings of worthlessness or inappropriate guilt nearly every day
- Inability to think or concentrate or indecisiveness nearly every day
- Recurrent thoughts of death or suicide, or a specific plan for or attempt at suicide

The symptoms cause significant distress or impair social, occupational, or other important functions. In severe cases, hallucinations and delusions may occur.

Mixed Episode

A mixed episode, which must last at least 1 week, meets the criteria for both major and manic depressive episodes.

Dysthymic Disorder

A depressed mood and symptoms for most of the day, for more days than not, over at least 2 years (1 year in children and adolescents). Freedom from symptoms lasts no more than 2 months at a time.

Manic Episode

A distinct period of abnormally and persistently elevated, expansive, or irritable mood must be present for at least a week (any duration if hospitalization is necessary). During this time, at least three of the symptoms listed below have been persistent and significant. (Four of these symptoms are required if the mood is only irritable).

- Inflated self-esteem or grandiosity
- Decreased need for sleep (feels rested after sleeping 3 hours)
- More talkative than usual or pressure to keep talking
- Flight of ideas or racing thoughts
- Distractibility
- Increased goal-directed activity (either socially, at work or school, or sexually) or psychomotor agitation
- Excessive involvement in pleasurable high-risk activities (buying sprees, foolish business ventures, sexual indiscretions)

The disturbance is severe enough to impair social or occupational functions or relationships. It may necessitate hospitalization for the protection of self or others. In severe cases, hallucinations and delusions may occur.

Hypomanic Episode

The mood and symptoms resemble those in a manic episode but are less impairing, do not require hospitalization, do not include hallucinations or delusions, and have a shorter minimum duration—4 days.

Cyclothymic Episode

Numerous periods of hypomanic and depressive symptoms that last for at least 2 years (1 year in children and adolescents). Freedom from symptoms lasts no more than 2 months at a time.

Tables 5-2 to 5-4 are based, with permission, on the *Diagnostic and Statistical Manual of Mental Disorders,* 4th ed., text revision (*DSM IV-TR*). Washington, DC, American Psychiatric Association, 2000. For further details and criteria, the reader should consult this manual, its successor, or comprehensive textbooks of psychiatry.

Anxiety Disorders

Panic Disorder	A *panic disorder* is defined by recurrent, unexpected panic attacks, at least one of which has been followed by a month or more of persistent concern about further attacks, worry over their implications or consequences, or a significant change in behavior in relation to the attacks. A *panic attack* is a discrete period of intense fear or discomfort that develops abruptly and peaks within 10 minutes. It involves at least four of the following symptoms: (1) palpitations, pounding heart, or accelerated heart rate; (2) sweating; (3) trembling or shaking; (4) shortness of breath or a sense of smothering; (5) a feeling of choking; (6) chest pain or discomfort; (7) nausea or abdominal distress; (8) feeling dizzy, unsteady, lightheaded, or faint; (9) feelings of unreality or depersonalization; (10) fear of losing control or going crazy; (11) fear of dying; (12) paresthesias (numbness or tingling); (13) chills or hot flushes. Panic disorder may occur with or without *agoraphobia*.
Agoraphobia	Agoraphobia is an anxiety about being in places or situations where escape may be difficult or embarrassing or help unavailable. Such situations are avoided, require a companion, or cause marked anxiety.
Specific Phobia	A specific phobia is a marked, persistent, and excessive or unreasonable fear that is cued by the presence or anticipation of a specific object or situation, such as dogs, injections, or flying. The person recognizes the fear as excessive or unreasonable, but exposure to the cue provokes immediate anxiety. Avoidance or fear impairs the person's normal routine, occupational or academic functioning, or social activities or relationships.
Social Phobia	A social phobia is a marked, persistent fear of one or more social or performance situations that involve exposure to unfamiliar people or to scrutiny by others. Those afflicted fear that they will act in embarrassing or humiliating ways, as by showing their anxiety. Exposure creates anxiety and possibly a panic attack, and the person avoids precipitating situations. He or she recognizes the fear as excessive or unreasonable. Normal routines, occupational or academic functioning, or social activities or relationships are impaired.
Obsessive-Compulsive Disorder	This disorder involves obsessions or compulsions that cause marked anxiety or distress. Although they are recognized at some point as excessive or unreasonable, they are very time consuming and interfere with the person's normal routine, occupational functioning, or social activities or relationships.
Acute Stress Disorder	The person has been exposed to a traumatic event that involved actual or threatened death or serious injury to self or others and responded with intense fear, helplessness, or horror. During or immediately after this event, the person has at least three of these dissociative symptoms: (1) a subjective sense of numbing, detachment, or absence of emotional responsiveness; (2) a reduced awareness of surroundings, as in a daze; (3) feelings of unreality; (4) feelings of depersonalization; and (5) amnesia for an important part of the event. The event is persistently reexperienced, as in thoughts, images, dreams, illusions, and flashbacks, or distress from reminders of the event. The person is very anxious or shows increased arousal and tries to avoid stimuli that evoke memories of the event. The disturbance causes marked distress or impairs social, occupational, or other important functions. The symptoms occur within 4 weeks of the event and last from 2 days to 4 weeks.
Posttraumatic Stress Disorder	The event, the fearful response, and the persistent reexperiencing of the traumatic event resemble those in acute stress disorder. Hallucinations may occur. The person has increased arousal, tries to avoid stimuli related to the trauma, and has numbing of general responsiveness. The disturbance causes marked distress, impairs social, occupational, or other important functions, and lasts for more than a month.
Generalized Anxiety Disorder	This disorder lacks a specific traumatic event or focus for concern. Excessive anxiety and worry, which the person finds hard to control, are about a number of events or activities. At least three of the following symptoms are associated: (1) feeling restless, keyed up, or on edge; (2) being easily fatigued; (3) difficulty in concentrating or mind going blank; (4) irritability; (5) muscle tension; (6) difficulty in falling or staying asleep, or restless, unsatisfying sleep. The disturbance causes significant distress or impairs social, occupational, or other important functions.

TABLE
5-4

Psychotic Disorders

Psychotic disorders involve grossly impaired reality testing. Specific diagnoses depend on the nature and duration of the symptoms and on a cause when it can be identified. Seven disorders are outlined below.

Schizophrenia

Schizophrenia impairs major functioning, as at work or school or in interpersonal relations or self-care. For this diagnosis, performance of one or more of these functions must have decreased for a significant time to a level markedly below prior achievement. In addition, the person must manifest at least two of the following for a significant part of 1 month: (1) delusions; (2) hallucinations; (3) disorganized speech; (4) grossly disorganized or catatonic behavior;* and (5) negative symptoms such as a flat affect, alogia (lack of content in speech), or avolition (lack of interest, drive, and ability to set and pursue goals). Continuous signs of the disturbance must persist for at least 6 months.

Subtypes of this disorder include paranoid, disorganized, and catatonic schizophrenia.

Schizophreniform Disorder

A schizophreniform disorder has symptoms similar to those of schizophrenia, but they last less than 6 months, and the functional impairment seen in schizophrenia need not be present.

Schizoaffective Disorder

A schizoaffective disorder has features of both a major mood disturbance and schizophrenia. The mood disturbance (depressive, manic, or mixed) is present during most of the illness and must, for a time, be concurrent with symptoms of schizophrenia (listed above). During the same period of time, there must also be delusions or hallucinations for at least 2 weeks without prominent mood symptoms.

Delusional Disorder

A delusional disorder is characterized by nonbizarre delusions that involve situations in real life, such as having a disease or being deceived by a lover. The delusion has persisted for at least a month, but the person's functioning is not markedly impaired, and behavior is not obviously odd or bizarre. The symptoms of schizophrenia, except for tactile and olfactory hallucinations related to the delusion, have not been present.

Brief Psychotic Disorder

In this disorder, at least one of the following psychotic symptoms must be present: delusions, hallucinations, disordered speech such as frequent derailment or incoherence, or grossly disorganized or catatonic behavior. The disturbance lasts at least 1 day but less than 1 month, and the person returns to his or her prior functional level.

Psychotic Disorder Due to a General Medical Condition

Prominent hallucinations or delusions may be experienced during a medical illness. For this diagnosis, they should not occur exclusively during the course of delirium. The medical condition should be documented and judged to be causally related to the symptoms.

Substance-Induced Psychotic Disorder

Prominent hallucinations or delusions may be induced by intoxication or withdrawal from a substance such as alcohol, cocaine, or opioids. For this diagnosis, these symptoms should not occur exclusively during the course of delirium. The substance should be judged to be causally related to the symptoms.

---

*Catatonic behaviors are psychomotor abnormalities that include stupor, mutism, negativistic resistance to instructions or attempts to move the person, rigid or bizarre postures, and excited, apparently purposeless activity.

The Skin, Hair, and Nails

ANATOMY AND PHYSIOLOGY

The major function of the skin is to keep the body in homeostasis despite daily assaults from the environment. The skin provides boundaries for body fluids while protecting underlying tissues from microorganisms, harmful substances, and radiation. It modulates body temperature and synthesizes vitamin D. Hair, nails, and sebaceous and sweat glands are considered appendages of the skin. The skin and its appendages undergo many changes during aging. Turn to Chapter 20, The Older Adult (pp. 895–896), to review normal and abnormal changes of the skin with aging.

Skin. The skin is the heaviest single organ of the body, accounting for approximately 16% of body weight and covering an area of roughly 1.2 to 2.3 meters squared. It contains three layers: the epidermis, the dermis, and the subcutaneous tissues.

The most superficial layer, the *epidermis,* is thin, devoid of blood vessels, and itself divided into two layers: an outer horny layer of dead keratinized cells and an inner cellular layer where both melanin and keratin are formed. Migration from the inner layer to the top layer takes approximately 1 month.

The epidermis depends on the underlying *dermis* for its nutrition. The dermis is well supplied with blood. It contains connective tissue, sebaceous glands, sweat glands, and hair follicles. It merges below with *subcutaneous,* or *adipose, tissue,* also known as fat.

The color of normal skin depends primarily on four pigments: melanin,

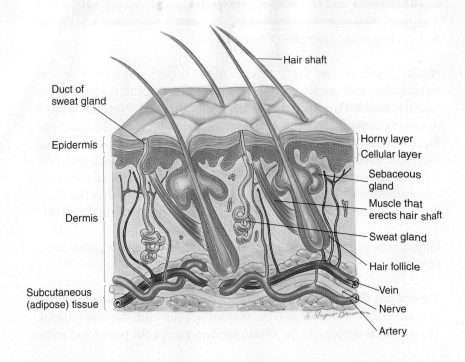

Duct of sweat gland

Epidermis

Dermis

Subcutaneous (adipose) tissue

Hair shaft

Horny layer

Cellular layer

Sebaceous gland

Muscle that erects hair shaft

Sweat gland

Hair follicle

Vein

Nerve

Artery

carotene, oxyhemoglobin, and deoxyhemoglobin. The amount of *melanin*, the brownish pigment of the skin, is genetically determined and is increased by exposure to sunlight. *Carotene* is a golden yellow pigment that exists in subcutaneous fat and in heavily keratinized areas such as the palms and soles.

Hemoglobin, which circulates in the red cells and carries most of the oxygen of the blood, exists in two forms. *Oxyhemoglobin*, a bright red pigment, predominates in the arteries and capillaries. An increase in blood flow through the arteries to the capillaries causes a reddening of the skin, whereas the opposite change usually produces pallor. The skin of light-colored people is normally redder on the palms, soles, face, neck, and upper chest.

- blushing/pale "from shock"

As blood passes through the capillary bed, oxyhemoglobin loses its oxygen to the tissues and changes to *deoxyhemoglobin*—a darker and somewhat bluer pigment. An increased concentration of deoxyhemoglobin in cutaneous blood vessels gives the skin a bluish cast known as *cyanosis*.

Cyanosis is of two kinds, depending on the oxygen level in the arterial blood. If this level is low, cyanosis is *central*. If it is normal, cyanosis is *peripheral*. Peripheral cyanosis occurs when cutaneous blood flow decreases and slows, and tissues extract more oxygen than usual from the blood. Peripheral cyanosis may be a normal response to anxiety or a cold environment.

anxiety/cold

Skin color is also affected by the scattering of light reflected back through the turbid superficial layers of the skin or vessel walls. This scattering makes the color look more blue and less red. The bluish color of a subcutaneous vein results from this effect; it is much bluer than the venous blood obtained on venipuncture.

Hair. Adults have two types of hair: *vellus hair*, which is short, fine, inconspicuous, and relatively unpigmented; and *terminal hair*, which is coarser, thicker, more conspicuous, and usually pigmented. Scalp hair and eyebrows are examples of terminal hair.

Nails. Nails protect the distal ends of the fingers and toes. The firm, rectangular, and usually curving *nail plate* gets its pink color from the vascular *nail bed* to which the plate is firmly attached. Note the whitish moon, or *lunula*, and the free edge of the nail plate. Roughly one fourth of the nail plate (the *nail root*) is covered by the proximal nail fold. The *cuticle* extends from the fold and, functioning as a seal, protects the space between the fold and the plate from external moisture. *Lateral nail folds* cover the sides of the nail plate. Note that the angle between the proximal nail fold and nail plate is normally less than 180°.

Fingernails grow approximately 0.1 mm daily; toenails grow more slowly.

Sebaceous Glands and Sweat Glands. *Sebaceous glands* produce a fatty substance secreted onto the skin surface through the hair follicles. These glands are present on all skin surfaces except the palms and soles.

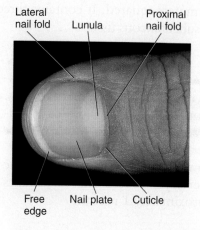

Sweat glands are of two types: eccrine and apocrine. The *eccrine glands* are widely distributed, open directly onto the skin surface, and by their sweat production help to control body temperature. In contrast, the *apocrine glands* are found chiefly in the axillary and genital regions, usually open into hair follicles, and are stimulated by emotional stress. Bacterial decomposition of apocrine sweat is responsible for adult body odor.

THE HEALTH HISTORY

Common or Concerning Symptoms

> - Hair loss
> - Rash
> - Moles

Start your inquiry about the skin with a few open-ended questions: "Have you noticed any changes in your skin?". . . your hair? . . . your nails?. . . "Have you had any rashes? . . . sores? . . . lumps? . . . itching?"

Ask, "Have you noticed any moles you are concerned about? Do you have any moles that have changed in size, shape, color, or sensation? What about any new moles?" If patients have such moles, pursue any personal or family history of melanoma and results of any prior biopsies of the skin.

You may wish to defer further questions about the skin until the physical examination, when you inspect the skin and identify the lesions that the patient is concerned about.

Causes of generalized itching include dry skin, aging, pregnancy, uremia, jaundice, lymphomas and leukemia, drug reaction, and lice.

Approximately half of *melanomas* are initially detected by the patient.[1]

HEALTH PROMOTION AND COUNSELING

Important Topics for Health Promotion and Counseling

> - Risk factors for skin cancers
> - Avoidance of excessive sun exposure

Clinicians play an important role in educating patients about early detection of suspicious moles, protective measures for skin care, and the hazards of excessive sun exposure. Skin cancers are the most common cancers in the United States and usually arise on sun-exposed areas, particularly the head, neck, and hands. Almost all skin cancers are of three types[2,3]:

- *Basal cell carcinoma,* arising in the lowest, or basal, level of the epidermis, accounts for approximately 80% of skin cancers. These cancers arise in sun-exposed areas, usually on the head and neck. They are pearly white and translucent, tend to grow slowly, and rarely metastasize.

● *Squamous cell carcinoma*, in the upper layer of the epidermis, accounts for approximately 16% of skin cancers. These cancers are often crusted and scaly with a red inflamed or ulcerated appearance; they can metastasize.

● *Melanoma*, arising from the pigment-producing melanocytes in the epidermis that give the skin its color, accounts for approximately 4% of skin cancers and is the most lethal type. Although rare, melanomas are the most rapidly increasing U.S. malignancy. Lifetime risk for melanoma in men is 1 in 49, and in women is 1 in 73.[4] Melanomas can spread rapidly to the lymph system and internal organs, and they cause 80% of deaths from skin cancer.[5] Mortality rates are highest in white men, approximately 3.6% per year, possibly because of lower "skin awareness" and lower rates of self-examination.[6]

Risk Factors for Melanoma. Educate your patient about *risk factors for melanoma*. Recently reported analysis of more than 364,000 people screened in the National Melanoma/Skin Cancer Screening Program of the American Academy of Dermatology validates the HARMM model for identifying higher-risk people in the general population during skin cancer screening.[7]

● HARMM Melanoma Risk Model

Risk Factor	Increased Risk of Melanoma
● **H**istory of previous melanoma	3.3
● **A**ge over 50	1.2
● **R**egular dermatologist absent	1.4
● **M**ole changing	2.0
● **M**ale gender	1.4

Number of Risk Factors	Increased Likelihood of Melanoma
● 0–1	1.0
● 2	1.7
● 3	2.5
● 4–5	4.5

(Source: Goldberg MS, Doucette JT, Lim HW, et al. Risk factors for presumptive melanoma in skin cancer screening: American Academy of Dermatology National Melanoma/Skin Cancer Screening Program experience 2001–2005. J Am Acad Dermatology 57(1):60–66, 2007.)

Other risk factors include having 50 or more common moles; one to four atypical or unusual moles, especially if dysplastic[8,9]; red or light hair; actinic lentigenes, or macular brown or tanned spots usually on sun-exposed areas, such as freckles; ultraviolet radiation from heavy sun exposure, sunlamps, or tanning booths; light eye or skin color, especially skin that freckles or burns easily; severe blistering sunburns in childhood; immunosuppression from

HIV or chemotherapy; and family history of melanoma.[6,10] Early detection of melanoma, when 3 mm or less, significantly improves prognosis.

The most commonly recommended screening measure for skin cancer is *total-body skin examination* by a clinician, although data on the utility of this method for nondermatologists are limited. Although the U.S. Preventive Services Task Force has found insufficient evidence to recommend inspection for routine screening, the American Cancer Society recommends skin examination as part of a routine cancer-related check-up every 3 years for people aged 20 to 40 years, and yearly for those older than 40.[11,12] Only a few studies have shown that *skin self-examination* enhances detection,[13–15] but this low-cost method of patient education can promote health awareness in at-risk patients. (See Techniques for Skin Self-Examination on pp. 170–171.)

Detecting Moles.   Patients and clinicians who find moles should apply the *ABCD method* to screen for melanoma. Sensitivity ranges from 50% to 97%, and specificity from 96% to 99%.[1,12,16]

See Table 6-10, Benign and Malignant Nevi, p. 186.

ABCDs of Examining Moles for Possible Melanoma

- **A** for asymmetry of one side of mole compared to the other
- **B** for irregular borders, especially ragged, notched, or blurred
- **C** for variation or change in color, especially blue or black
- **D** for diameter ≥6 mm or different from others, especially if changing, itching, or bleeding

---

Preventing Skin Cancer.   Counsel patients about preventive strategies such as reducing sun exposure and using sunscreens (though these are not conclusively validated as effective).[13] Caution patients to minimize direct sun exposure, especially at midday, when ultraviolet B rays (UV-B), the most common cause of skin cancer, are most intense. Sunscreens fall into two categories: thick, pastelike ointments that block all solar rays, and light-absorbing sunscreens rated by "sun protective factor" (SPF). The SPF is a ratio of the number of minutes for treated versus untreated skin to redden with exposure to UV-B. An SPF of at least 15 is recommended and protects against 93% of UV-B. (There is no scale for UV-A, which causes photoaging, or UV-C, the most carcinogenic ray but blocked in the atmosphere by ozone.) Water-resistant sunscreens that remain on the skin for prolonged periods are preferable. Be aware, however, that use of sunscreens may give patients a false sense of security and increase sun exposure.

TECHNIQUES OF EXAMINATION

Your examination of the skin, hair, and nails begins with the General Survey and continues throughout the physical examination. Take time, however, to ensure that the patient wears a gown and is draped accordingly to facilitate close inspection of the hair, anterior and posterior surfaces of the body, palms and soles, and web spaces between the fingers and toes.

Inspect the entire skin surface in good light, preferably natural light or artificial light that resembles it. Correlate your findings with observations of the mucous membranes, especially when assessing skin color, because diseases may appear in both areas. Techniques for examining these membranes are described in later chapters.

Artificial light often distorts colors and masks jaundice.

To sharpen your observations, you may wish to turn now to the tables at the end of the chapter to better identify skin colors and patterns and types of lesions that you may encounter during the examination.

 SKIN

Inspect and palpate the skin. Note these characteristics:

Color.   Patients may notice a change in their skin color before the clinician does. Ask about it. Look for increased pigmentation (brownness), loss of pigmentation, redness, pallor, cyanosis, and yellowing of the skin.

See Table 6-1, Skin Colors (pp. 174–175).

Assess the red color of oxyhemoglobin and the pallor in its absence where the horny layer of the epidermis is thinnest and causes the least scatter: the fingernails, the lips, and the mucous membranes, particularly those of the mouth and the palpebral conjunctiva. In dark-skinned people, inspecting the palms and soles may also be useful.

Pallor results from decreased redness in *anemia* and decreased blood flow, as occurs in fainting or arterial insufficiency.

Central cyanosis is best identified in the lips, oral mucosa, and tongue. The lips, however, may turn blue in the cold, and melanin in the lips may simulate cyanosis in darker-skinned people.

Causes of *central cyanosis* include advanced lung disease, congenital heart disease, and hemoglobin-opathies.

Cyanosis of the nails, hands, and feet may be central or peripheral in origin. Anxiety or a cold examining room may cause peripheral cyanosis.

Cyanosis in *congestive heart failure* is usually peripheral, reflecting decreased blood flow, but in *pulmonary edema,* it may also be central. *Venous obstruction* may cause peripheral cyanosis.

Look for the yellow color of jaundice in the sclera. Jaundice may also appear in the palpebral conjunctiva, lips, hard palate, undersurface of the tongue, tympanic membrane, and skin. To see jaundice more easily in the lips, blanch out the red color by pressure with a glass slide.

Jaundice suggests liver disease or excessive hemolysis of red blood cells.

For the yellow color that accompanies high levels of carotene, look at the palms, soles, and face.

Carotenemia

Moisture. Examples are dryness, sweating, and oiliness.

Dryness in hypothyroidism; oiliness in acne

Temperature. Use the backs of your fingers to make this assessment. In addition to identifying generalized warmth or coolness of the skin, note the temperature of any red areas.

Generalized warmth in fever, *hyperthyroidism*; coolness in *hypothyroidism*. Local warmth of inflammation or cellulitis (PVD in LE)

Texture. Examples are roughness and smoothness.

Roughness in *hypothyroidism*; velvety texture in *hyperthyroidism*

Mobility and Turgor. Lift a fold of skin and note the ease with which it lifts up (mobility) and the speed with which it returns into place (turgor).

Decreased mobility in edema, *scleroderma*; decreased turgor in dehydration

Lesions. Observe any lesions of the skin, noting their characteristics:

- Their *anatomic location and distribution* over the body. Are they generalized or localized? Do they, for example, involve the exposed surfaces, the intertriginous or skin-fold areas, extensor or flexor areas, or acral (peripheral) areas? Do they involve areas exposed to specific allergens or irritants, such as wrist bands, rings, or industrial chemicals?

Many skin diseases have typical distributions. *Acne* affects the face, upper chest, and back; *psoriasis*, the knees and elbows (among other areas); and *Candida* infections, the intertriginous areas. See patterns in Table 6-2, Skin Lesions—Anatomic Location and Distribution (p. 176).

- Their *patterns and shapes.* For example, are they linear, clustered, annular (in a ring), arciform (in an arc), geographic, or serpiginous (serpent- or worm-like)? Are they dermatomal, covering a skin band that corresponds to a sensory nerve root (see pp. 632–633)

Vesicles in a unilateral dermatomal pattern are typical of herpes zoster.[17] See patterns in Table 6-3, Skin Lesions—Patterns and Shapes (p. 177).

- The *types of skin lesions* (e.g., macules, papules, vesicles, nevi). If possible, find representative and recent lesions that have not been traumatized by scratching or otherwise altered. Inspect them carefully and feel them.

- Their *color*.

See Table 6-4, Primary Skin Lesions (pp. 178–180); Table 6-5, Secondary Skin Lesions (p. 181); Table 6-6, Secondary Skin Lesions—Depressed (p. 182); Table 6-7, Acne Vulgaris—Primary and Secondary Lesions, (p. 183); Table 6-8, Vascular and Purpuric Lesions of the Skin (p. 184); Table 6-9, Skin Tumors (p. 185); and Table 6-10, Benign and Malignant Nevi (p. 186).

SKIN LESIONS IN CONTEXT

tells you to look shit up

After familiarizing yourself with the basic types of lesions, review their appearances in Tables 6-11 and 6-12 and in a well-illustrated textbook of dermatology. Whenever you see a skin lesion, look it up in such a text. The

See Table 6-11, Skin Lesions in Context (pp. 187–188), and Table 6-12, Diseases and type of lesions, their location, and their distribution, together with other information from the history and the examination, should equip you well for this search and, in time, for arriving at specific dermatologic diagnoses.

Evaluating the Bedbound Patient.   People confined to bed, especially when they are emaciated, elderly, or neurologically impaired, are particularly susceptible to skin damage and ulceration. *Pressure sores* result when sustained compression obliterates arteriolar and capillary blood flow to the skin. Sores may also result from the shearing forces created by bodily movements. When a person slides down in bed from a partially sitting position, for example, or is dragged rather than lifted up from a supine position, the movements may distort the soft tissues of the buttocks and close off the arteries and arterioles. Friction and moisture further increase the risk.

Assess every susceptible patient by carefully inspecting the skin that overlies the sacrum, buttocks, greater trochanters, knees, and heels. Roll the patient onto one side to see the sacrum and buttocks. *elbows, occipital, scapula, spine*

Related Skin Conditions (pp. 189–190).

See Table 6-13, Pressure Ulcers (p. 191).

Local redness of the skin warns of impending necrosis, although some deep pressure sores develop without antecedent redness. Ulcers may be seen.

HAIR

Inspect and palpate the hair. Note its quantity, distribution, and texture.

Alopecia refers to hair loss—diffuse, patchy, or total. Sparse hair in *hypothyroidism;* fine, silky hair in *hyperthyroidism*

See Table 6-14, Hair Loss (p. 192).

NAILS

Inspect and palpate the fingernails and toenails. Note their color and shape and any lesions. Longitudinal bands of pigment may be seen in the nails of normal people who have darker skin.

See Table 6-15, Findings in or Near the Nails (pp. 193–194).

SPECIAL TECHNIQUES

Instructions for the Skin Self-Examination.   The American Academy of Dermatology recommends regular self-examination of the skin using the following techniques. The patient will need a full-length mirror, a hand-held mirror, and a well-lit room that provides privacy. Teach the patient the **ABCD** method for assessing moles (see p. 186), and show the patient the photos of benign and malignant nevi in Table 6-10 on p. 186.

PATIENT INSTRUCTIONS FOR THE SKIN SELF-EXAMINATION

Examine your body front and back in the mirror, then right and left sides with arms raised.

Bend elbows and look carefully at forearms, upper underarms, and palms.

Look at the backs of your legs and feet, the spaces between your toes, and the sole.

Examine the back of your neck and scalp with a hand mirror. Part hair for a closer look.

Finally, check your back and buttocks with a hand mirror.

(Source: Adapted from American Academy of Dermatology. SkinCancerNet. Available at: http://www.skincarephysicians.com/skincancernet; and from American Academy of Dermatology. How to perform a self-examination. Available at: http://www.aad.org/public/News/DermInfo/SelfExam.htm. Accessed June 16, 2007.)

RECORDING YOUR FINDINGS

Note that initially you may use sentences to describe your findings; later you will use phrases. The style below contains phrases appropriate for most write-ups.

Recording the Physical Examination—The Skin

"Color pink. Skin warm and moist. Nails without clubbing or cyanosis. No suspicious nevi. No rash, petechiae, or ecchymoses."

OR

"Marked facial pallor, with circumoral cyanosis. Palms cold and moist. Cyanosis in nailbeds of fingers and toes. One raised blue-black nevus, 1 × 2 cm, with irregular border on right forearm. No rash."

Suggests central cyanosis and possible melanoma

OR

"Facial plethora. Skin icteric. Spider angioma over anterior torso. Palmar erythema. Single pearly papule with depressed center and telangiectasias, 1 × 1 cm, on posterior neck above collarline. No suspicious nevi. Nails with clubbing but no cyanosis."

Suggests possible liver disease and basal cell carcinoma

BIBLIOGRAPHY

CITATIONS

1. Whited JD, Grichnik JM. Does this patient have a mole or a melanoma? The rational clinical examination. JAMA 279(9): 696–701, 1998.
2. American Academy of Dermatology. Public Resource Center: 2004 Melanoma fact sheet. Available at: http://www.aad.org/public/News/DermInfo/2004MelanomaFAQ.htm. Accessed June 16, 2007.
3. American Academy of Dermatology. What is skin cancer? Skincare.net. Available at: http://www.skincarephysicians.com/skincancernet/whatis.html. Accessed January 29, 2005.
4. National Cancer Institute. Cancer Topics. Melanoma. Available at: http://www.cancer.gov/cancertopics/types/melanoma/. Accessed June 16, 2007.
5. Miller AJ, Mihm MC. Melanoma. N Engl J Med 355(1): 51–65, 2006.
6. Helfand M, Krages KP. Counseling to Prevent Skin Cancer: A Summary of the Evidence for the U.S. Preventive Services Task Force. Rockville, MD, Agency for Healthcare Research and Quality, October 2003. Available at: http://www.ahrq.gov/clinic/3rduspstf/skcacoun/skcounsum.htm. Accessed June 16, 2007.
7. Goldberg MS, Doucette JT, Lim HW, et al. Risk factors for pre-sumptive melanoma in skin cancer screening: American Academy of Dermatology National Melanoma/Skin Cancer Screening

Program experience 2001–2005. J Am Acad Dermatology 57(1):60–66, 2007.
8. Naeyaert JM, Broches L. Dysplastic nevi. N Engl J Med 349(23):2233–2240, 2003.
9. Tucker MA, Halpern A, Holly EA, et al. Clinically recognized dysplastic nevi: a central risk factor for cutaneous melanoma. JAMA 277(18):1439–1444, 1997.
10. National Cancer Institute. Melanoma: who's at risk? Available at: http://www.cancer.gov/cancertopics/wyntk/melanoma/page7. Accessed June 16, 2007.
11. U.S. Preventive Services Task Force. Screening for Skin Cancer: Recommendations and Rationale. [Article originally published in Am J Prev Med 20(3S):44–46, 2001.] Rockville, MD, Agency for Healthcare Research and Quality. Available at: http://www.ahrq.gov/clinic/ajpmsuppl/skcarr.htm. Accessed June 16, 2007.
12. American Cancer Society. Skin cancer, 2005. Available at: http://www.cancer.org/downloads/PRO/SkinCancer.pdf. Accessed June 16, 2007.
13. U.S. Preventive Services Task Force: Counseling to Prevent Skin Cancer: Recommendations and Rationale. Rockville, MD, Agency for Healthcare Research and Quality, 2003. Available at: http://www.ahrq.gov/clinic/3rduspstf/skcacoun/skcarr.htm. Accessed June 16, 2007.

14. Berwick M, Begg CB, Fine JA, et al. Screening for cutaneous melanoma by skin self-examination. J Natl Cancer Inst 88: 17–23, 1996.

15. Robinson JK, Fisher SG, Turrisi RJ. Predictors of skin self-examination performance. Cancer 95(1):135–146, 2002.

16. American Academy of Dermatology. SkinCancerNet. Skin Examinations. Available at: http://www.skincarephysicians. com/skincancernet/skin_examinations.html#Examination%20 by%20a%20Dermatologist. Accessed June 16, 2007.

17. U.S. Preventive Services Task Force: Screening for Skin Cancer: Summary of the Evidence. [Article originally published in Am J Prev 20(3S):47–58, 2001.] Rockville, MD, Agency for Healthcare Research and Quality, 2001. Available at: http://www.ahrq. gov/clinic/ajpmsuppl/helfand1.htm. Accessed June 16, 2007.

18. Goodheart HP. Goodheart's Photoguide of Common Skin Disorders: Diagnosis and Management, 2nd ed. Philadelphia: Lippincott Williams & Wilkins, 2003.

19. Spicknall KE, Zirwas MJ, English JC 3rd. Clubbing: an update on diagnosis, differential diagnosis, pathophysiology, and clinical relevance. J Am Acad Dermatol 52(6):1020–1028, 2005.

20. Fawcett RS, Hart TM, Lindford S, et al. Nail abnormalities: clues to systemic diseases. Am Fam Phys 69(6):1418–1425, 2004.

21. Hanford RR, Cobb MW, Banner NT. Unilateral Beau's lines associated with a fractured and immobilized wrist. Cutis 56(5): 263–264, 1995.

ADDITIONAL READINGS

Alam M, Ratner D. Cutaneous squamous cell carcinoma. N Engl J Med 344(13):975–983, 2001.

American Academy of Dermatology. Malignant Melanoma. Available at: http://www.aad.org/public/Publications/pamphlets/ MalignantMelanoma.htm. Accessed June 16, 2007.

American Cancer Society. Cancer Statistics Presentation 2007. Available at: http://www.cancer.org/docroot/PRO/content/ PRO_1_1_Cancer_Statistics_2007_Presentation.asp. Accessed June 16, 2007.

Boulton AJM, Kirsner RS, Vileikyte L. Neuropathic diabetic foot ulcers. N Engl J Med 351(1):48–55, 2004.

Fitzpatrick TB, Wolff K, Johnson RA, et al. Fitzpatrick's Color Atlas and Synopsis of Clinical Dermatology, 5th ed. New York: McGraw-Hill, 2005.

Fitzpatrick TB, Wolff K. Fitzpatrick's Dermatology in General Medicine, 7th ed. New York: McGraw-Hill, 2008.

Gnann JW, Whitley RJ. Herpes zoster. N Engl J Med 347(5): 340–346, 2002.

Grimes P. New insights and new therapies in vitiligo. JAMA 293(6):730–735, 2005.

Habif TP. Clinical Dermatology: A Color Guide to Diagnosis and Therapy, 4th ed. New York: Mosby, 2004.

Habif TP. Skin Disease: Diagnosis and Treatment, 2nd ed. Philadelphia: Elsevier–Mosby, 2005.

Hall AH. Chronic arsenic poisoning. Toxicol Lett 128(1–3): 69–72, 2002.

Hall JC. Sauer's Manual of Skin Diseases, 9th ed. Philadelphia: Lippincott Williams & Wilkins, 2006.

Hordinsky M, Sawaya M, Roberts JL. Hirsutism and hair loss in the elderly. Clin Geriatr Med 18(1):121–133, 2002.

Miller AJ, Mihm MC. Melanoma. N Engl J Med 355(1):51–65, 2006.

Lyder CH. Pressure ulcer prevention and management. JAMA 289(2):223–226, 2003.

Myers KA, Farquhar DRE. Does this patient have clubbing? JAMA 286(3):341–347, 2001.

Rubin A, Elbert HC, Ratner D. Basal-cell carcinoma. N Engl J Med 353(21):2262–2269, 2005.

Scanlon E, Stubbs N. Pressure ulcer risk assessment in patients with darkly pigmented skin. Professional Nurse 19(6):339–341, 2004.

Schon MP, Henning-Boehncke W. Psoriasis. N Engl J Med 352(18): 1899–1912, 2005.

Singer AJ, Clark RAF. Cutaneous wound healing. N Engl J Med 341(10):738–746, 1999.

Singh N, Armstrong DG, Lipsky BA. Preventing foot ulcers in patients with diabetes. JAMA 293(2):217–228, 2005.

Swartz MN. Cellulitis. N Engl J Med 350(9):904–912, 2004.

Yancey KB, Egan GA. Pemphigoid: clinical, histologic, immunopathologic, and therapeutic considerations. JAMA 284(3): 350–356, 2000.

The Bates' suite offers these additional resources to enhance learning and facilitate understanding of this chapter:

- Bates' Pocket Guide to Physical Examination and History Taking, 6th edition
- Bates' Nursing Online
- Bates' Visual Guide to Physical Examination, 4th edition
- thePoint online resources, http://thepoint.lww.com
- Student CD-ROM included with the book

TABLE 6-1

Skin Colors

Changes in Pigmentation

A widespread increase in *melanin* may be caused by Addison's disease (hypofunction of the adrenal cortex) or some pituitary tumors. More common are local areas of increased or decreased pigment.

Café-Au-Lait Spot

A slightly but uniformly pigmented macule or patch with a somewhat irregular border, usually 0.5 to 1.5 cm in diameter; benign. Six or more such spots, each with a diameter of >1.5 cm, however, suggest neurofibromatosis (p. 188). (The small, darker macules are unrelated.)

Tinea Versicolor

Common superficial fungal infection of the skin, causing hypopigmented, slightly scaly macules on the trunk, neck, and upper arms (short-sleeved shirt distribution). They are easier to see in darker skin and in some are more obvious after tanning. In lighter skin, macules may look reddish or tan instead of pale.

Vitiligo

In vitiligo, depigmented macules appear on the face, hands, feet, extensor surfaces, and other regions and may coalesce into extensive areas that lack melanin. The brown pigment is normal skin color; the pale areas are vitiligo. The condition may be hereditary. These changes may be distressing to the patient.

?MJ disease?

Cyanosis

Cyanosis is the somewhat bluish color that is visible in these toenails and toes. Compare this color with the normally pink fingernails and fingers of the same patient. Impaired venous return in the leg caused this example of peripheral cyanosis. Cyanosis, especially when slight, may be hard to distinguish from normal skin color.

Jaundice

Jaundice makes the skin diffusely yellow. Contrast this patient's skin color with the examiner's hand. Jaundice is seen most easily and reliably in the sclera, as shown here. It may also be visible in mucous membranes. Causes include *liver disease* and *hemolysis of red blood cells.*

*carotenemia ♀

Carotenemia

The yellowish palm of carotenemia is compared with a normally pink palm, sometimes a subtle finding. Unlike jaundice, carotenemia does not affect the sclera, which remains white. The cause is a diet high in carrots and other yellow vegetables or fruits. Carotenemia is not harmful but indicates the need for assessing dietary intake.

Erythema

Red hue, increased blood flow, seen here as the "slapped cheeks" of *erythema infectiosum* ("fifth disease").

Heliotrope

Violaceous eruption over the eyelids in the collagen vascular disease *dermatomyositis.*

(Sources of photos: *Tinea Versicolor*—Ostler HB, Mailbach HI, Hoke AW, Schwab IR. Diseases of the Eye and Skin: A Color Atlas. Philadelphia, Lippincott Williams & Wilkins, 2004; *Vitiligo, Erythema*—Goodheart HP. Goodheart's Photoguide of Common Skin Disorders: Diagnosis and Management, 2nd ed. Philadelphia, Lippincott Williams & Wilkins, 2003; *Heliotrope*—Hall JC. Sauer's Manual of Skin Diseases, 8th ed. Philadelphia, Lippincott Williams & Wilkins, 2000.)

Skin Lesions—Anatomic Location and Distribution

Herald lesion

Pityriasis Rosea
Reddish oval ringworm-like lesions

Psoriasis
Silvery scaly lesions, mainly on the extensor surfaces

Tinea Versicolor
Tan, flat, scaly lesions

Atopic Eczema
(adult form)
Appears mainly on flexor surfaces

(Source: Hall JC. *Sauer's Manual of Skin Diseases*, 8th ed. Philadelphia, Lippincott Williams & Wilkins, 2000; Photos from: Goodheart HP. Goodheart's Photoguide of Common Skin Disorders: Diagnosis and Management, 2nd ed. Philadelphia, Lippincott Williams & Wilkins, 2003.)

TABLE
6-3

Skin Lesions—Patterns and Shapes

Linear
Example: Linear epidermal nevus

Geographic
Example: Mycosis fungoides

Clustered
Example: Grouped lesions of herpes simplex

Serpiginous
Example: Tinea corporis

serpesant/ worm like

ring-like

Annular, arciform
Example: Annular lesion of tinea faciale (ringworm)

(Sources of photos: *Linear Epidermal Nevus, Herpes Simplex, Tinea Faciale*—Goodheart HP. Goodheart's Photoguide of Common Skin Disorders: Diagnosis and Management, 2nd ed. Philadelphia, Lippincott Williams & Wilkins, 2003; *Mycosis Fungoides, Tinea Corporis*—Hall JC. Sauer's Manual of Skin Diseases, 8th ed. Philadelphia, Lippincott Williams & Wilkins, 2000.)

TABLE
6-4

Primary Skin Lesions (*initial presentation*)

Flat, Nonpalpable Lesions With Changes in Skin Color

Macule—Small flat spot, up to 1.0 cm

HEMANGIOMA

VITILIGO

Patch—Flat spot, 1.0 cm or larger

CAFÉ-AU-LAIT SPOT

Palpable Elevations: Solid Masses

Plaque—Elevated superficial lesion 1.0 cm or larger, often formed by coalescence of papules

PSORIASIS

PSORIASIS

Papule—Up to 1.0 cm

PSORIASIS

Nodule—Marble-like lesion larger than 0.5 cm, often deeper and firmer than a papule

DERMATOFIBROMA

Cyst—Nodule filled with expressible material, either liquid or semisolid

EPIDERMAL INCLUSION CYST

Wheal—A somewhat irregular, relatively transient, superficial area of localized skin edema

URTICARIA

Palpable Elevations With Fluid-Filled Cavities
Vesicle—Up to 1.0 cm; filled with serous fluid

HERPES SIMPLEX

HERPES ZOSTER

(table continues on page 180)

Bulla—1.0 cm or larger; filled with serous fluid

INSECT BITE

INSECT BITE

Pustule—Filled with pus

ACNE

SMALL POX

Burrow (scabies)—A minute, slightly raised tunnel in the epidermis, commonly found on the finger webs and on the sides of the fingers. It looks like a short (5–15 mm), linear or curved gray line and may end in a tiny vesicle. Skin lesions include small papules, pustules, lichenified areas, and excoriations. With a magnifying lens, look for the *burrow* of the mite that causes scabies.

SCABIES

(Sources of photos: *Hemangioma, Café-au-Lait Spot, Psoriasis* [bottom], *Dermatofibroma, Herpes Simplex, Herpes Zoster, Insect Bite* [right]—Hall JC. Sauer's Manual of Skin Diseases, 9th ed. Philadelphia, Lippincott Williams & Wilkins, 2006; *Vitiligo, Psoriasis* [top], *Epidermal Inclusion Cyst, Urticaria, Insect Bite* [left], *Acne, Scabies*—Goodheart HP, Goodheart's Photoguide of Common Skin Disorders: Diagnosis and Management, 2nd ed. Philadelphia, Lippincott Williams & Wilkins, 2003; *Small Pox*—Ostler, HB, Mailbach HI, Hoke AW, Schwab IR. Diseases of the Eye and Skin: A Color Atlas. Philadelphia, Lippincott Williams & Wilkins, 2004.)

Secondary Skin Lesions (*seen in overtreatment, excess scratching, infection of primary lesions*)

Scale—A thin flake of dead exfoliated epidermis.

ICHTHYOSIS VULGARIS

DRY SKIN

Crust—The dried residue of skin exudates such as serum, pus, or blood

Lichenification—Visible and palpable thickening of the epidermis and roughening of the skin with increased visibility of the normal skin furrows (often from chronic rubbing)

IMPETIGO

NEURODERMATITIS

Scars—Connective tissue that arises from injury or disease

80% elasticity/turgor return

Keloids—Hypertrophic scarring that extends beyond the borders of the initiating injury

HYPERTROPHIC SCAR FROM STEROID INJECTIONS

KELOID—EAR LOBE

(Sources of photos: *Lichenification*—Hall JC. Sauer's Manual of Skin Diseases, 9th ed. Philadelphia, Lippincott Williams & Wilkins, 2006; *Ichthyosis, Dry Skin, Hypertrophic Scar, Keloids*—Goodheart HP. Goodheart's Photoguide of Common Skin Disorders: Diagnosis and Management, 2nd ed. Philadelphia, Lippincott Williams & Wilkins, 2003.)

TABLE
6-6

Secondary Skin Lesions—Depressed

Erosion—Nonscarring loss of the superficial epidermis; surface is moist but does not bleed

> *Example:* Aphthous stomatitis, moist area after the rupture of a vesicle, as in chickenpox

Excoriation—Linear or punctate erosions caused by scratching

> *Example:* Cat scratches

Fissure—A linear crack in the skin, often resulting from excessive dryness

> *Example:* Athlete's foot

Ulcer—A deeper loss of epidermis and dermis; may bleed and scar

> *Examples:* Stasis ulcer of venous insufficiency, syphilitic chancre

(Sources of photos: *Erosion, Excoriation, Fissure*—Goodheart HP. Goodheart's Photoguide of Common Skin Disorders: Diagnosis and Management, 2nd ed. Philadelphia, Lippincott Williams & Wilkins, 2003; *Ulcer*—Hall JC. Sauer's Manual of Skin Diseases, 8th ed. Philadelphia, Lippincott Williams & Wilkins, 2000)

TABLE
6-7

Acne Vulgaris—Primary and Secondary Lesions

Acne vulgaris is the most common cutaneous disorder in the United States, affecting more than 85% of adolescents.[18] Acne is a disorder of the pilosebaceous follicle that involves proliferation of the keratinocytes at the opening of the follicle; increased production of sebum, stimulated by androgens, which combines with keratinocytes to plug the follicular opening; growth of *Propionibacterium acnes*, an anaerobic diphtheroid normally found on the skin; and inflammation from bacterial activity and release of free fatty acids and enzymes from activated neutrophils.[18] Cosmetics, humidity, heavy sweating, and stress are contributing factors.

Lesions appear in areas with the greatest number of sebaceous glands, namely the face, neck, chest, upper back, and upper arms. They may be primary, secondary, or mixed.

Primary Lesions

Mild Acne

Open and closed comedones, occasional papules

Moderate Acne

Comedones, papules, pustules

Severe Cystic Acne

Secondary Lesions

Acne With Pitting and Scars

TABLE
6-8

Vascular and Purpuric Lesions of the Skin

Vascular Lesions

	Spider Angioma*	Spider Vein*	Cherry Angioma
			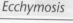
Color and Size	Fiery red. From very small to 2 cm	Bluish. Size variable, from very small to several inches	Bright or ruby red; may become brownish with age. 1–3 mm
Shape	Central body, sometimes raised, surrounded by erythema and radiating legs	Variable. May resemble a spider or be linear, irregular, cascading	Round, flat or sometimes raised, may be surrounded by a pale halo
Pulsatility and Effect of Pressure	Often seen in center of the spider, when pressure with a glass slide is applied. Pressure on the body causes blanching of the spider.	Absent. Pressure over the center does not cause blanching, but diffuse pressure blanches the veins.	Absent. May show partial blanching, especially if pressure applied with edge of a pinpoint
Distribution	Face, neck, arms, and upper trunk; almost never below the waist	Most often on the legs, near veins; also on the anterior chest	Trunk; also extremities
Significance	Liver disease, pregnancy, vitamin B deficiency; also occurs normally in some people	Often accompanies increased pressure in the superficial veins, as in varicose veins	None; increases in size and numbers with aging

Purpuric Lesions

	Petechia/Purpura	Ecchymosis
Color and Size	Deep red or reddish purple, fading away over time. Petechia, 1–3 mm; purpura, larger	Purple or purplish blue, fading to green, yellow, and brown with time. Variable size, larger than petechiae, >3 mm
Shape	Rounded, sometimes irregular; flat	Rounded, oval, or irregular; may have a central subcutaneous flat nodule (a hematoma)
Pulsatility and Effect of Pressure	Absent. No effect from pressure	Absent. No effect from pressure
Distribution	Variable	Variable
Significance	Blood outside the vessels; may suggest a bleeding disorder or, if petechiae, emboli to skin; palpable purpura in *vasculitis*	Blood outside the vessels; often secondary to bruising or trauma; also seen in bleeding disorders

*These are telangiectasias, or dilated small vessels that look red or bluish.

(Sources of photos: *Spider Angioma*—Marks R. Skin Disease in Old Age. Philadelphia, JB Lippincott, 1987; *Petechia/Purpura*—Kelley WN. Textbook of Internal Medicine. Philadelphia, JB Lippincott, 1989.)

TABLE
6-9

Skin Tumors

Actinic Keratosis

Superficial, flattened papules covered by a dry scale. Often multiple; can be round or irregular; pink, tan, or grayish. Appear on sun-exposed skin of older, fair-skinned people. Though benign, 1 of every 1000 per year develop into squamous cell carcinoma (suggested by rapid growth, induration, redness at the base, and ulceration). Keratoses on face and hand, typical locations, are shown.

Seborrheic Keratosis

Common, benign, yellowish to brown raised lesions that feel slightly greasy and velvety or warty and have a "stuck on" appearance. Typically multiple and symmetrically distributed on the trunk of older people, but may also appear on the face and elsewhere. In black people, often younger women, may appear as small, deeply pigmented papules on the cheeks and temples (dermatosis papulosa nigra).

Basal Cell Carcinoma

A basal cell carcinoma, though malignant, grows slowly and seldom metastasizes. It is most common in fair-skinned adults 40 years or older, and usually appears on the face. An initial translucent nodule spreads, leaving a depressed center and a firm, elevated border. Telangiectatic vessels are often visible.

Squamous Cell Carcinoma

Usually appears on sun-exposed skin of fair-skinned adults older than 60 years. May develop in an actinic keratosis. Usually grows more quickly than a basal cell carcinoma, is firmer, and looks redder. The face and the back of the hand are often affected, as shown here.

(Sources of photos: *Basal Cell Carcinoma*—Rapini R. *Squamous Cell Carcinoma, Actinic Keratosis, Seborrheic Keratosis*—Hall JC. Sauer's Manual of Skin Diseases, 9th ed. Philadelphia, Lippincott, Williams & Wilkins, 2006.)

TABLE
6-10

Benign and Malignant Nevi

Benign Nevus

The *benign nevus*, or common mole, usually appears in the first few decades. Several nevi may arise at the same time, but their appearance usually remains unchanged. Note the following typical features and contrast them with those of atypical nevi and melanoma:

- Round or oval shape   ← ABCDs
- Sharply defined borders
- Uniform color, especially tan or brown
- Diameter <6 mm
- Flat or raised surface

Changes in these features raise the the spectre of *atypical (dysplastic) nevi,* or melanoma. Atypical nevi are varied in color but often dark and larger than 6 mm, with irregular borders that fade into the surrounding skin. Look for atypical nevi primarily on the trunk. They may number more than 50 to 100.

A

Malignant Melanoma

Learn the **ABCDs** of melanoma from these reference standard photographs from the American Cancer Society:

- *Asymmetry* (Fig. A)
- Irregular *Borders*, especially notching (Fig. B)
- Variation in *Color*, especially mixtures of black, blue, and red (Figs. B, C)
- *Diameter* >6 mm (Fig. C)

Review *melanoma risk factors* such as intense year-round sun exposure, blistering sunburns in childhood, fair skin that freckles or burns easily (especially if blond or red hair), family history of melanoma, and nevi that are changing or atypical, especially if the patient is older than 50 years. Changing nevi may have new swelling or redness beyond the border, scaling, oozing, or bleeding, or sensations such as itching, burning, or pain.

On darker skin, look for melanomas under the nails, on the hands, or on the soles of the feet.

B

C

(Source: Courtesy of American Cancer Society; American Academy of Dermatology)

TABLE
6-11

Skin Lesions in Context

This table shows a variety of primary and secondary skin lesions. Try to identify them, including those indicated by letters, before reading the accompanying text.

Macules on the dorsum of the hand, wrist, and forearm (*actinic lentigines*)

Papules and pustules (in hot tub folliculitis from *Pseudomonas*)

Pustules on the palm (*pustular psoriasis*)

Vesicles (*chickenpox*)

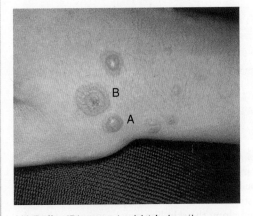

(A) Bulla, (B) target (or iris) lesion (in *erythema multiforme*)

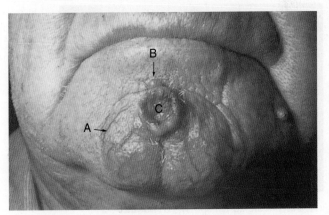

(A) Telangiectasia, (B) nodule, (C) ulcer (in *squamous cell carcinoma*)

(*table continues on page 188*)

TABLE 6-11

Skin Lesions in Context (continued)

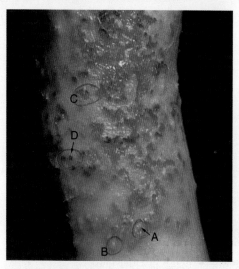

(A) Vesicle, (B) pustule, (C) erosions, (D) crust, on the back of a knee (in *infected atopic dermatitis*)

(A) Excoriation, (B) lichenification on the leg (in *atopic dermatitis*)

Wheals (*urticaria*) in a drug eruption in an infant

Plaques with scales on knee (*psoriasis*) and legs

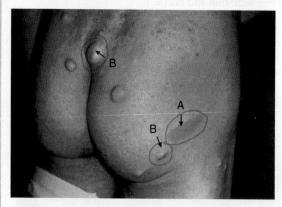

(A) Patch (café-au-lait spots), (B) nodules—a combination typical of neurofibromatosis.

Kaposi's sarcoma in AIDS: This malignant tumor may appear in many forms: macules, papules, plaques, or nodules almost anywhere on the body. Lesions are often multiple and may involve internal structures. On left: ovoid, pinkish red plaques that typically lengthen along the skin line may become pigmented. On right: a purplish red nodule on the foot.

(Sources of photos: Hall JC. Sauer's Manual of Skin Diseases, 9th ed. Philadelphia, Lippincott Williams & Wilkins, 2006; *Kaposi's Sarcoma in AIDS*—DeVita VT Jr, Hellman S, Rosenberg SA [eds]: AIDS: Etiology, Diagnosis, Treatment, and Prevention. Philadelphia, JB Lippincott, 1985; *Psoriasis, Papules, Vesicles [chickenpox]*—Goodheart HP. Goodheart's Photoguide of Common Skin Disorders: Diagnosis and Management, 2nd ed. Philadelphia, Lippincott Williams & Wilkins, 2003.)

TABLE
6-12

Diseases and Related Skin Conditions

Addison's disease	Hyperpigmentation of skin and mucous membranes
AIDS	*Hairy leukoplakia, Kaposi's sarcoma,* herpes simplex virus (HSV), human papillomavirus (HPV), cytomegalovirus (CMV), molluscum contagiosum, mycobacterial skin infections, candidiasis and other cutaneous fungal infections, oral and anal squamous cell carcinoma, acquired ichthyosis, bacterial abscesses, *psoriasis* (often severe), erythroderma, seborrheic dermatitis (often severe)
Chronic renal disease	Pallor, xerosis, pruritus, hyperpigmentation, uremic frost, metastatic calcification in the skin, calciphylaxis, "half and half" nails, hemodialysis-related skin disease
CREST syndrome	Calcinosis, Raynaud's phenomenon, sclerodactyly, *telangiectasias*
Crohn's disease	Erythema nodosum, pyoderma gangrenosum, enterocutaneous fistulas, aphthous ulcers
Cushing's disease	Striae, skin atrophy, purpura, ecchymoses, telangiectasias, acne, moon facies, buffalo hump, hypertrichosis
Dermatomyositis	Heliotrope rash, Gottron's papules, periungual telangiectasias, alopecia, poikiloderma in sun-exposed areas, Raynaud's phenomenon
Diabetes	Necrobiosis lipoidica diabeticorum, diabetic bullae, diabetic dermopathy, granuloma annulare, acanthosis nigricans, candidiasis, neuropathic ulcers, eruptive xanthomas, peripheral vascular disease
Disseminated intravascular coagulation	Skin necrosis, petechiae, ecchymoses, hemorrhagic bullae, purpura fulminans
Dyslipidemias	Xanthomas (tendon, eruptive, and tuberous), xanthelasma (may occur in healthy people)
Gonococcemia	Erythematous macules to hemorrhagic pustules; lesions in acral distribution that can involve palms and soles
Hemochromatosis	Skin bronzing and hyperpigmentation
Hypothyroidism	Dry, rough, and pale skin; coarse and brittle hair; myxedema; alopecia (lateral third of the eyebrows to diffuse); skin cool to touch; thin and brittle nails
Hyperthyroidism	Warm, moist, soft, and velvety skin; thin and fine hair; alopecia; vitiligo; pretibial myxedema (in Graves' disease); hyperpigmentation (local or generalized)
Infective endocarditis	Janeway lesions, Osler nodes, splinter hemorrhages, petechiae
Kawasaki disease	Mucosal erythema (lips, tongue, and pharynx), strawberry tongue, cherry red lips, polymorphous rash (primarily on trunk), erythema of palms and soles with later desquamation of fingertips
Liver disease	*Jaundice, spider angiomas* and other telangiectasias, palmar erythema, *Terry's nails,* pruritus, purpura, caput medusae
Leukemia/lymphoma	Pallor, exfoliative erythroderma, nodules, *petechiae,* ecchymoses, pruritus, vasculitis, pyoderma gangrenosum, bullous diseases
Meningococcemia	Pink macules and papules, *petechiae,* hemorrhagic petechiae, hemorrhagic bullae, purpura fulminans
Neurofibromatoses 1 (von Recklinghausen's syndrome)	*Neurofibromas,* café au lait, freckling in the axillary and inguinal areas, plexiform neurofibroma

(table continues on page 190)

Pancreatitis (hemorrhagic)	Grey Turner sign, Cullen's sign, panniculitis
Pancreatic carcinoma	Panniculitis, migratory thrombophlebitis
Peripheral vascular disease	Dry, scaly, shiny atrophic skin; dystrophic, brittle toenails; cool skin; hairless shins; ulcers; pallor; cyanosis; gangrene
Pregnancy (physiologic changes)	Melasma, increased pigmentation of areolae, linea nigra, palmar erythema, varicose veins, striae, *spider angiomas*, hirsutism, pyogenic granuloma
Reiter's syndrome	Psoriasis-like skin and mucous membrane lesions, keratoderma blennorrhagicum, balanitis circinata
Rheumatoid arthritis	Vasculitis, *Raynaud's phenomenon*, rheumatoid nodules, pyoderma gangrenosum, rheumatoid papules, erythematous to salmon-colored rashes
Rocky Mountain spotted fever	Erythematous rash that begins on wrists and ankles, then spreads to palms and soles; becomes more purpuric as it generalizes
Scleroderma	Thickened, taut, and shiny skin; ulcerations and pitted scars on fingertips; sclerodactyly; telangiectasias; Raynaud's phenomenon
Sickle cell	Jaundice, *leg ulcers* (malleolar regions), pallor
Syphilis	*1°: Chancre* (painless) (see p. 516) *2°:* Rash ("the great imitator")—ham- to bronze-colored, generalized, maculopapular rash that involves the palms and soles, pustules, condylomata lata, alopecia ("moth-eaten"), white plaques on oral and genital mucosa *3°:* Gummas, granulomas
Systemic lupus erythematosus	Photosensitivity, malar (butterfly) rash, discoid rash, alopecia, vasculitis, oral ulcers, Raynaud's phenomenon
Thrombocytopenic purpura	*Petechiae, ecchymoses*
Tuberous sclerosis	Adenoma sebaceum (angiofibromas), ash-leaf spots, shagreen patch, perungual fibromas
Ulcerative colitis	*Erythema nodosum*, pyoderma gangrenosum
Viral exanthems	
Coxsackie A (hand, foot, and mouth)	Oral ulcers; macules, papules, and vesicles on hands, feet, and buttocks
Erythema infectiosum (fifth disease)	Erythema of cheeks ("slapped cheeks") followed by erythematous, pruritic, reticulated (net-like) rash that starts on trunk and proximal extremities (rash worsens with sun, fever, and temperature changes)
Roseola infantum (HSV 6)	Erythematous, maculopapular, discrete rash (often fever present) that begins on head and spreads to involve trunk and extremities, petechiae on soft palate
Rubella (German measles)	Erythematous, maculopapular, discrete rash (often fever present) that begins on head and spreads to involve trunk and extremities, petechiae on soft palate
Rubeola (measles)	Erythematous, maculopapular rash that begins on head and spreads to involve trunk and extremities (lesions become confluent on face and trunk, but are discrete on extremities), Koplik spots on buccal mucosa
Varicella (chickenpox)	Generalized, pruritic, vesicular (vesicles on an erythematous base, "dewdrop on a rose petal") rash begins on trunk and spreads peripherally, lesions appear in crops and are in different stages of healing
Herpes zoster (shingles)	Pruritic, vesicular rash (vesicles on an erythematous base) in a dermatomal distribution

Pressure Ulcers

Pressure (*decubitus*) ulcers usually develop over bony prominences subject to unrelieved pressure, resulting in ischemic damage to underlying tissue. Prevention is important: inspect the skin thoroughly for *early warning signs of erythema that blanches with pressure*, especially in patients with risk factors.

(does not)

Pressure ulcers form most commonly over the sacrum, ischial tuberosities, greater trochanters, and heels. A commonly applied staging system, based on depth of destroyed tissue, is illustrated below. Note that necrosis or eschar must be débrided before ulcers can be staged. Ulcers may not progress sequentially through the four stages.

or "unstage-able"

Inspect ulcers for signs of infection (drainage, odor, cellulitis, or necrosis). Fever, chills, and pain suggest underlying **osteomyelitis**. Address the patient's overall health, including *comorbid conditions* such as vascular disease, diabetes, immune deficiencies, collagen vascular disease, malignancy, psychosis, or depression; nutritional status; pain and level of analgesia; risk for recurrence; psychosocial factors such as learning ability, social supports, and lifestyle; and evidence of polypharmacy, overmedication, or abuse of alcohol, tobacco, or illicit drugs.

Risk Factors for Pressure Ulcers

- Decreased mobility, especially if accompanied by increased pressure or movement causing friction or shear stress
- Decreased sensation, from brain or spinal cord lesions or peripheral nerve disease

- Decreased blood flow from hypotension or microvascular disease such as diabetes or atherosclerosis
- Fecal or urinary incontinence
- Presence of fracture
- Poor nutritional status or low albumin

Stage I

Pressure-related alteration of intact skin, with changes in temperature (warmth or coolness), consistency (firm or boggy), sensation (pain or itching), or color (red, blue, or purple on darker skin; red on lighter skin)

Stage II

Partial-thickness skin loss or ulceration involving the epidermis, dermis, or both

Stage III

Full-thickness skin loss, with damage to or necrosis of subcutaneous tissue that may extend to, but not through, underlying muscle

Stage IV

Full-thickness skin loss, with destruction, tissue necrosis, or damage to underlying muscle, bone, or supporting structures

(Source: National Pressure Ulcer Advisory Panel, Reston, VA)

TABLE	
6-14	**Hair Loss**

Alopecia Areata

Clearly demarcated round or oval patches of hair loss, usually affecting young adults and children. There is no visible scaling or inflammation.

Trichotillomania

Hair loss from pulling, plucking, or twisting hair. Hair shafts are broken and of varying lengths. More common in children, often in settings of family or psychosocial stress.

Tinea Capitis ("Ringworm")

Round scaling patches of alopecia. Hairs are broken off close to the surface of the scalp. Usually caused by fungal infection from *tinea tonsurans*. Mimics seborrheic dermatitis.

(Sources of photos: *Alopecia Areata [left], Trichotillomania [top]*—Hall JC. Sauer's Manual of Skin Diseases, 9th ed. Philadelphia, Lippincott Williams & Wilkins, 2006; *Alopecia Areata [bottom], Tinea Capitis*—Goodheart HP. Goodheart's Photoguide of Common Skin Disorders: Diagnosis and Management, 2nd ed. Philadelphia, Lippincott Williams & Wilkins, 2003; *Trichotillomania [bottom]*—Ostler HB, Mailbach HI, Hoke AW, Schwab IR. Diseases of the Eye and Skin: A Color Atlas. Philadelphia, Lippincott Williams & Wilkins, 2004.)

Findings in or Near the Nails

Paronychia

A superficial infection of the proximal and lateral nail folds adjacent to the nail plate. The nail folds are often red, swollen, and tender. Represents the most common infection of the hand, usually from *Staphylococcus aureus* or *Streptococcus* species, and may spread until it completely surrounds the nail plate. Creates a felon if it extends into the pulp space of the finger. Arises from local trauma due to nail biting, manicuring, or frequent hand immersion in water.

Clubbing of the Fingers

Clinically a bulbous swelling of the soft tissue at the nail base, with loss of the normal angle between the nail and the proximal nail fold. The angle increases to 180° or more, and the nail bed feels spongy or floating. The mechanism is still unknown but involves vasodilatation with increased blood flow to the distal portion of the digits and changes in connective tissue, possibly from hypoxia, changes in innervation, genetics, or a platelet-derived growth factor from fragments of platelet clumps. Seen in congenital heart disease, interstitial lung disease and lung cancer, inflammatory bowel diseases, and malignancies.[19]

Onycholysis

A painless separation of the whitened opaque nail plate from the pinker translucent nail bed. Starts distally and progresses proximally, enlarging the free edge of the nail. Local causes include trauma from excess manicuring, psoriasis, fungal infection, and allergic reactions to nail cosmetics. Systemic causes include diabetes, anemia, photosensitive drug reactions, hyperthyroidism, peripheral ischemia, bronchiectasis, and syphilis.

Terry's Nails

Nail plate turns white with a ground-glass appearance, a distal band of reddish brown, and obliteration of the lunula. Commonly affects all fingers, although may appear in only one finger. Seen in liver disease, usually cirrhosis, congestive heart failure, and diabetes. May arise from decreased vascularity and increased connective tissue in nail bed.

(table continues on page 194)

White Spots (Leukonychia)

Trauma to the nails is commonly followed by nonuniform white spots that grow slowly out with the nail. Spots in the pattern illustrated are typical of overly vigorous and repeated manicuring. The curves in this example resemble the curve of the cuticle and proximal nail fold.

Transverse White Bands (Mees' Lines)

Curving transverse white bands that cross the nail parallel to the lunula. Arising from the disrupted matrix of the proximal nail, they vary in width and move distally as the nail grows out. Seen in arsenic poisoning, heart failure, Hodgkin's disease, chemotherapy, carbon monoxide poisoning, and leprosy.[20]

Transverse Linear Depressions (Beau's Lines)

Transverse depressions of the nail plates, usually bilateral, resulting from temporary disruption of proximal nail growth from systemic illness. As with Mees' lines, timing of the illness may be estimated by measuring the distance from the line to the nail bed (nails grow approximately 1 mm every 6 to 10 days). Seen in severe illness, trauma, and cold exposure if Raynaud's disease is present.[20,21]

Pitting

Punctate depressions of the nail plate caused by defective layering of the superficial nail plate by the proximal nail matrix. Usually associated with psoriasis but also seen in Reiter's syndrome, sarcoidosis, alopecia areata, and localized atopic or chemical dermatitis.[20]

(Sources of photos: *Clubbing of the Fingers, Paronychia, Onycholysis, Terry's Nails*—Habif TP. Clinical Dermatology: A Color Guide to Diagnosis and Therapy, 2nd ed. St. Louis, CV Mosby, 1990; *White Spots, Transverse White Lines, Psoriasis, Beau's Lines*—Sams WM Jr, Lynch PJ. Principles and Practice of Dermatology. New York, Churchill Livingstone, 1990.)

The Head and Neck

GUIDE TO NEW ORGANIZATION OF THIS CHAPTER

Numerous critical structures like the cranial nerves, the major senses of vision, hearing, smell, and taste, and many common clinical conditions arise in the head and neck. In this edition, this chapter has been reorganized to strengthen the links between anatomy and physiology and related skills of physical examination as you learn to conduct this important regional assessment.

Because many head and neck symptoms and prevention strategies are interrelated, the Health History and the Health Promotion and Counseling sections remain unified as in prior editions. For these two sections, "HEENT" (Head, Eyes, Ears, Nose, and Throat) information is grouped together. To facilitate student learning, however, Anatomy and Physiology is now grouped with the relevant Techniques of Examination in separate sections for the Head, the Eyes, the Ears, the Nose, the Throat, and the Neck, as outlined below.

OVERVIEW: NEW FORMAT OF THIS CHAPTER

- Health History
- Health Promotion and Counseling
- Examination of the Head and Neck: Anatomy and Physiology and Techniques of Examination are now combined for:

  Head—pp. 204–205
  Eyes—pp. 205–222
  Ears—pp. 222–227
  Nose—pp. 228–231
  Throat—pp. 231–236
  Neck—pp. 236–243

THE HEALTH HISTORY

Common or Concerning Symptoms

- Headache
- Change in vision: hyperopia, presbyopia, myopia, scotomas
- Double vision, or diplopia
- Hearing loss, earache, tinnitus
- Vertigo
- Nosebleed, or epistaxis
- Sore throat, hoarseness
- Swollen glands
- Goiter

THE HEAD

Headache is one of the most common symptoms in clinical practice, with a lifetime prevalence of 30% in the general population.[1,2] Migraine headaches are by far the most frequent cause of headaches seen in office practice, approaching 80% with careful diagnosis. Nevertheless, every headache warrants careful evaluation for life-threatening causes such as meningitis, subdural or intracranial hemorrhage, or mass lesion. It is important to elicit a full description of the headache and all seven attributes of the patient's pain (see p. 65). Is the headache one-sided or bilateral? Severe with sudden onset? Steady or throbbing? Continuous or intermittent (comes and goes)?

Look for "red flags" that raise suspicion of worrisome secondary causes: recent onset (less than 6 months); onset after 50 years; acute onset like a "thunderclap," or "the worst headache of my life"; markedly elevated blood pressure; presence of rash or signs of infection; presence of cancer, HIV, or pregnancy; vomiting; recent head trauma; or persisting neurologic deficits.

The most important attributes of headache are its *severity* and *chronologic pattern.* Is the headache severe and of sudden onset? Does it intensify over several hours? Is it episodic? Chronic and recurring? Is there a recent change in pattern? Does the headache recur at the same time every day?

See Table 7-1, Primary Headaches, p. 249, and Table 7-2, Secondary Headaches; Cranial Neuralgias pp. 250–251.

Primary headaches have no identifiable underlying cause. *Secondary headaches* arise from other conditions—some of these may endanger the patient's life.[3]

If headache is severe and of sudden onset, consider *subarachnoid hemorrhage* or *meningitis.*

Migraine and *tension headaches* are episodic and tend to peak over several hours. New and persisting, progressively severe headaches raise concerns of *tumor, abscess,* or *mass lesion.*

After your usual open-ended assessment, it is helpful to ask the patient to *point to the area of pain or discomfort.*

Unilateral headache in *migraine and cluster headaches.*[1,3] Tension headaches often arise in the temporal areas; cluster headaches may be retro-orbital.

Ask about associated symptoms such as nausea and vomiting.

? Pregnancy?

Nausea and vomiting are common with *migraine* but also occur with *brain tumors* and *subarachnoid hemorrhage.*

Is there a prodrome of unusual feelings such as euphoria, craving for food, fatigue, or dizziness? Does the patient report an aura with neurologic symptoms, such as change in vision or numbness or weakness in an arm or leg?

Approximately 60% to 70% of patients with migraine have a prodrome prior to onset; 20% experience an aura, including photophobia, scintillating scotomata, or reversible visual and sensory symptoms.

Ask whether coughing, sneezing, or changing the position of the head has any effect (better, worse, or none) on the headache.

Such maneuvers may increase pain from brain tumor and acute sinusitis.

Is there a history of overuse of analgesics, ergotamine, or triptans?

Consider medication overuse in patients with chronic daily headache taking symptomatic medications more than 2 days a week.[1,4]

Ask about family history.

Family history may be positive in patients with migraine.

THE EYES

Start your inquiry about eye and vision problems with open-ended questions such as "How is your vision?" and "Have you had any trouble with your eyes?" If the patient reports a change in vision, pursue the related details.[5]

● Is the problem worse during close work or at distances?

Difficulty with close work suggests *hyperopia* (farsightedness) or *presbyopia* (aging vision); with distances, *myopia* (nearsightedness).

● Is there blurred vision? If yes, is the onset sudden or gradual? If sudden and unilateral, is the visual loss painless or painful?

If sudden *unilateral* visual loss is *painless,* consider vitreous hemorrhage from diabetes or trauma, *macular degeneration, retinal detachment, retinal vein occlusion,* or *central retinal artery occlusion.* If *painful,* causes are usually in the cornea and anterior chamber as in *corneal ulcer, uveitis, traumatic hyphema,* and *acute glaucoma. Optic neuritis* from multiple sclerosis may also be painful.[6] Immediate referral may be warranted.[7]

- Sudden bilateral visual loss is rare.

If *bilateral and painless,* medications that change refraction such as cholinergics, anticholinergics, and steroids may contribute. If bilateral and painful, consider chemical or radiation exposures.

- Is the onset of bilateral visual loss gradual?

This usually arises from *cataracts* or *macular degeneration.*

- Location of visual loss may also be helpful. Is there blurring of the entire field of vision or only parts of it?

- If the visual field defect is partial, is it central, peripheral, or on only one side?

Slow central loss in nuclear cataract (p. 258), *macular degeneration*[8] (p. 267); peripheral loss in advanced *open-angle glaucoma* (p. 257); one-sided loss in *hemianopsia* and *quadrantic defects* (p. 254)

- Are there specks in the vision or areas where the patient cannot see (*scotomas*)? If so, do they move around in the visual field with shifts in gaze or are they fixed?

Moving specks or strands suggest vitreous floaters; fixed defects (*scotomas*) suggest lesions in the retina or visual pathways.

- Has the patient seen lights flashing across the field of vision? Vitreous floaters may accompany this symptom.

Flashing lights or new vitreous floaters suggest detachment of vitreous from retina. Prompt eye consultation is indicated.

- Does the patient wear glasses?

Ask about *pain* in or around the eyes, *redness,* and *excessive tearing or watering* (see p. 257).

Check for *diplopia,* or double vision. If present, find out whether the images are side by side (horizontal diplopia) or on top of each other (vertical diplopia). Does diplopia persist with one eye closed? Which eye is affected?

One kind of horizontal diplopia is physiologic. Hold one finger upright approximately 6 inches in front of your face, a second at arm's length. When you focus on either finger, the image of the other is double. A patient who notices this phenomenon can be reassured.

Diplopia in adults may arise from a lesion in the brainstem or cerebellum, or from weakness or paralysis of one or more extraocular muscles, as in horizontal diplopia from palsy of CN III or VI, or vertical diplopia from palsy of CN III or IV. Diplopia in one eye, with the other closed, suggests a problem in the cornea or lens.

THE EARS

Opening questions are "How is your hearing?" and "Have you had any trouble with your ears?" If the patient has noticed a *hearing loss*, does it involve one or both ears? Did it start suddenly or gradually? What are the associated symptoms, if any? (See p. 65.)

Try to distinguish between two basic types of hearing impairment: *conductive loss*, which results from problems in the external or middle ear, and *sensorineural loss*, from problems in the inner ear, the cochlear nerve, or its central connections in the brain. Two questions may be helpful: Does the patient have special difficulty understanding people as they talk? What difference does a noisy environment make?

Symptoms associated with hearing loss, such as earache or vertigo, help you to assess likely causes. In addition, inquire specifically about medications that might affect hearing and ask about sustained exposure to loud noise.

Complaints of *earache*, or *pain in the ear*, are especially common. Ask about associated fever, sore throat, cough, and concurrent upper respiratory infection.

Ask about *discharge from the ear*, especially if associated with earache or trauma.

Tinnitus is a perceived sound that has no external stimulus—commonly a musical ringing or a rushing or roaring noise. It can involve one or both ears. Tinnitus may accompany hearing loss and often remains unexplained. Occasionally, popping sounds originate in the temporomandibular joint, or vascular noises from the neck may be audible.

Vertigo refers to the perception that the patient or the environment is rotating or spinning. These sensations point primarily to a problem in the labyrinths of the inner ear, peripheral lesions of CN VIII, or lesions in its central pathways or nuclei in the brain.

Hearing loss may also be congenital, from single gene mutations.[9]

People with sensorineural loss have particular trouble understanding speech, often complaining that others mumble; noisy environments make hearing worse. In conductive loss, noisy environments may help.

Medications that affect hearing include aminoglycosides, aspirin, NSAIDs, quinine, furosemide, and others.

Pain suggests a problem in the external ear, such as *otitis externa,* or, if associated with symptoms of respiratory infection, in the inner ear, as in *otitis media.*[10] It may also be referred from other structures in the mouth, throat, or neck.

Unusually soft wax, debris from inflammation or rash in the ear canal, or discharge through a perforated eardrum may be secondary to *acute* or *chronic otitis media.*

Tinnitus is a common symptom, increasing in frequency with age. When associated with hearing loss and vertigo, it suggests *Ménière's disease.*

See Table 7-3, Dizziness and Vertigo, p. 252.

Vertigo is a challenging symptom for you as a clinician, because patients differ widely in what they mean by the word "dizzy." "Are there times when you feel dizzy?" is an appropriate first question, but patients often find it difficult to be more specific. Ask "Do you feel unsteady, as if you are going to fall or black out? . . . Or do you feel the room is spinning (true vertigo)?" Get the story without biasing it. You may need to offer the patient several choices of wording. Ask if the patient feels pulled to the ground or off to one side, and if the dizziness is related to a change in body position. Pursue any associated feelings of clamminess or flushing, nausea, or vomiting. Check if any medications may be contributing.

Feeling unsteady, lightheaded, or "dizzy in the legs" sometimes suggests a cardiovascular etiology. A feeling of being pulled suggests true vertigo from an inner ear problem or a central or peripheral lesion of CN VIII.

THE NOSE AND SINUSES

Rhinorrhea refers to drainage from the nose and is often associated with *nasal congestion,* a sense of stuffiness or obstruction. These symptoms are frequently accompanied by sneezing, watery eyes, and throat discomfort, and also by itching in the eyes, nose, and throat.[11]

Causes include viral infections, *allergic rhinitis* ("hay fever"), and *vasomotor rhinitis.* Itching favors an allergic cause.

Assess the chronology of the illness. Does it last for a week or so, especially when common colds and related syndromes are prevalent, or does it occur seasonally when pollens are in the air? Is it associated with specific contacts or environments? What remedies has the patient used? For how long? And how well do they work?

Relation to seasons or environmental contacts suggests allergy.[11]

Excessive use of decongestants can worsen symptoms, causing *rhinitis medicamentosa.*

Did symptoms appear after a URI? Is there pain on bending forward or maxillary toothache? Fever or local headache? Tenderness over the sinuses?

Together these suggest *acute bacterial sinusitis.* Sensitivity and specificity are highest for symptoms appearing after a URI (~90% and ~80%).[12–14]

Inquire about drugs that might cause stuffiness.

Oral contraceptives, reserpine, guanethidine, and alcohol

Is the patient's nasal congestion limited to one side? If so, you may be dealing with a different problem that requires careful physical examination.

Consider a deviated nasal septum, foreign body, or tumor.

Epistaxis means bleeding from the nose. The blood usually originates from the nose itself, but may come from a paranasal sinus or the nasopharynx. The history is usually quite graphic! However, in patients who are lying down or have bleeding that originates in posterior structures, blood may pass into the throat instead of out the nostrils. You must identify the source of the bleeding carefully—is it from the nose, or has it been coughed up or vomited? Assess the site of bleeding, its severity, and associated symptoms. Carefully differentiate epistaxis from *hemoptysis* or *hematemesis,* because each has different causes. Is it a recurrent problem? Has there been easy bruising or bleeding elsewhere in the body?

Local causes of epistaxis include trauma (especially nose picking), inflammation, drying and crusting of the nasal mucosa, tumors, and foreign bodies.

Bleeding disorders may contribute to epistaxis.

THE MOUTH, THROAT, AND NECK

Sore throat is a frequent complaint, usually associated with acute upper respiratory symptoms.

Fever, pharyngeal exudates, and anterior lymphadenopathy, especially in the absence of cough, suggest *streptococcal pharyngitis,* or *strep throat* (p. 274).[15,16]

A *sore tongue* may result from local lesions as well as systemic illness.

Aphthous ulcers (p. 234); sore smooth tongue of nutritional deficiency (p. 279).

Bleeding from the gums is a common symptom, especially when brushing teeth. Ask about local lesions and any tendency to bleed or bruise elsewhere.

Bleeding gums are most often caused by *gingivitis* (p. 277).

Hoarseness refers to an altered quality of the voice, often described as husky, rough, or harsh. The pitch may be lower than before. Hoarseness usually arises from disease of the larynx but may also develop as extralaryngeal lesions press on the laryngeal nerves. Check for overuse of the voice, allergy, smoking or other inhaled irritants, and any associated symptoms. Is the problem acute or chronic? If hoarseness lasts more than 2 weeks, visual examination of the larynx by indirect or direct laryngoscopy is advisable.

Overuse of the voice (as in cheering) and acute infections are the most likely causes.

Causes of chronic hoarseness include smoking, allergy, voice abuse, *hypothyroidism,* chronic infections such as *tuberculosis,* and *tumors.*

Ask "Have you noticed any swollen glands or lumps in your neck?" because patients are more familiar with the lay terms than with "*lymph nodes.*"

Enlarged tender lymph nodes commonly accompany *pharyngitis.*

Assess thyroid function and ask about any evidence of an enlarged thyroid gland or *goiter*. To evaluate thyroid function, ask about *temperature intolerance* and *sweating*. Opening questions include "Do you prefer hot or cold weather?" "Do you dress more warmly or less warmly than other people?" "What about blankets . . . do you use more or fewer than others at home?" "Do you perspire more or less than others?" "Any new palpitations or change in weight?" Note that as people grow older, they sweat less, have less tolerance for cold, and tend to prefer warmer environments.

With *goiter,* thyroid function may be increased, decreased, or normal.

Intolerance to cold, preference for warm clothing and many blankets, and decreased sweating suggest *hypothyroidism;* the opposite symptoms, palpitations, and involuntary weight loss suggest *hyperthyroidism* (p. 281).

HEALTH PROMOTION AND COUNSELING

Important Topics for Health Promotion and Counseling

- Changes in vision: cataracts, macular degeneration, glaucoma
- Hearing loss
- Oral health

Vision and hearing, critical senses for experiencing the world around us, are two areas of special importance for health promotion and counseling. Oral health, often overlooked, also merits clinical attention.

Changes in Vision.   Disorders of vision shift with age. Healthy young adults generally have refractive errors. Up to 25% of adults older than 65 years have refractive errors; however, cataracts, macular degeneration, and glaucoma become more prevalent.[17] These disorders reduce awareness of the social and physical environment and contribute to falls and injuries. To improve detection of visual defects, test visual acuity with a Snellen chart or hand-held card (p. 211). Examine the lens and fundi for clouding of the lens (*cataracts*); mottling of the *macula;* variations in the retinal pigmentation; subretinal hemorrhage or exudate (*macular degeneration*); and change in size and color of the optic cup (*glaucoma*). After diagnosis, review effective treatments—corrective lenses, cataract surgery, photocoagulation for choroidal neovascularization in macular degeneration, and topical medications for glaucoma.

Risk factor surveillance for primary open-angle glaucoma (POAG) is especially important; however, in 2005 the U.S. Preventive Services Task Force found insufficient evidence for general screening because of the complexities of diagnosis and treatment.[18] Glaucoma is the leading cause of blindness in African Americans and the second leading cause of blindness overall. Approximately 2.5 million Americans are affected, and more than half are unaware of having the disease. In POAG there is gradual loss of vision as a result of the loss of retinal ganglion cell axons, initial loss of peripheral visual fields, and pallor and increasing size of the optic cup, which enlarges to more than half the diameter of the optic disc. Blindness occurs in 5% of those with the disease. Risk factors include age older than 65 years, family history, African-American descent, diabetes, myopia, and ocular hypertension (IOP ≥21 mm Hg). Not all people with POAG have elevated IOP, however, so tonometry is no longer recommended for screening. In addition, some with POAG have either minimal or no progression of visual field defects, and predicting which patients will progress is difficult. Diagnosis of optic disc enlargement is variable, even among experts, and the benefits of treatment, which may cause cataract formation, are unclear. Attention to risk factors and referral to eye specialists remain important tools for clinical care, but use of tonometry for screening is now of uncertain value.

Hearing Loss.   Hearing loss can also trouble the later years.[19,20] More than a third of adults older than 65 years have detectable hearing deficits, contributing to emotional isolation and social withdrawal. These losses may go undetected—unlike vision prerequisites for driving, there is no mandate for widespread testing of hearing, and many seniors avoid use of hearing aids. Questionnaires and hand-held audioscopes work well for periodic screening. Less sensitive are the clinical "whisper test," rubbing fingers, or use of the tuning fork. Groups at risk are those with a history of congenital or familial hearing loss, syphilis, rubella, meningitis, or exposure to hazardous noise levels at work or on the battlefield.

Oral Health. Clinicians should play an active role in promoting oral health: up to half of all children 5 to 17 years have from one to eight cavities, and the average U.S. adult has 10 to 17 teeth that are decayed, missing, or filled.[21] In adults, the prevalence of gingivitis and periodontal disease is 50% and 80%, respectively. In the United States, more than half of all adults older than 65 years have no teeth at all! Effective screening begins with careful examination of the mouth. Inspect the oral cavity for decayed or loose teeth, inflammation of the gingiva, and signs of periodontal disease (bleeding, pus, recession of the gums, and bad breath). Inspect the mucous membranes, the palate, the oral floor, and the surfaces of the tongue for ulcers and leukoplakia, warning signs for oral cancer and HIV disease.

To improve oral health, counsel patients to adopt daily hygiene measures. Use of fluoride-containing toothpastes reduces tooth decay, and brushing and flossing retard periodontal disease by removing bacterial plaques. Urge patients to seek dental care at least annually to receive the benefits of more specialized preventive care such as scaling, planing of roots, and topical fluorides.

Diet, tobacco and alcohol use, changes in salivary flow from medication, and proper use of dentures should also be addressed. As with children, adults should avoid excessive intake of foods high in refined sugars such as sucrose, which enhance attachment and colonization of cariogenic bacteria. Use of all tobacco products and excessive alcohol, the principal risk factors for oral cancers, should be avoided.

Saliva cleanses and lubricates the mouth. Many medications reduce salivary flow, increasing risk for tooth decay, mucositis, and gum disease from xerostomia, especially for the elderly. For those wearing dentures, be sure to counsel removal and cleaning each night to reduce bacterial plaque and risk of malodor. Regular massage of the gums relieves soreness and pressure from dentures on the underlying soft tissue.

ANATOMY AND PHYSIOLOGY AND TECHNIQUES OF EXAMINATION

THE HEAD

Anatomy and Physiology

Regions of the head take their names from the underlying bones of the skull, for example, the frontal area. Knowing this anatomy helps to locate and describe physical findings.

Two paired salivary glands lie near the mandible: the *parotid gland*, superficial to and behind the mandible (both visible and palpable when enlarged), and the *submandibular gland*, located deep to the mandible. Feel for the latter as you bow and press your tongue against your lower incisors. Its lobular surface can often be felt against the tightened muscle. The openings of the parotid and submandibular ducts are visible within the oral cavity (see p. 233).

The *superficial temporal artery* passes upward just in front of the ear, where it is readily palpable. In many normal people, especially thin and elderly ones, the tortuous course of one of its branches can be traced across the forehead.

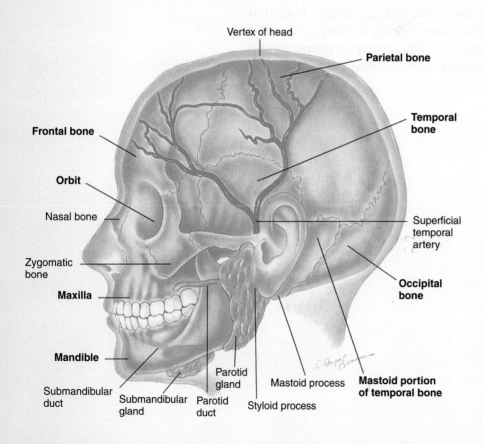

Vertex of head

Parietal bone

Temporal bone

Frontal bone

Orbit

Nasal bone

Superficial temporal artery

Zygomatic bone

Maxilla

Occipital bone

Mandible

Submandibular duct

Submandibular gland

Parotid duct

Parotid gland

Styloid process

Mastoid process

Mastoid portion of temporal bone

Techniques of Examination

Because abnormalities covered by the hair are easily missed, ask if the patient has noticed anything wrong with the scalp or hair. If you detect a hairpiece or wig, ask the patient to remove it.

Examine:

The Hair. Note its quantity, distribution, texture, and pattern of loss, if any. You may see loose flakes of dandruff.

Fine hair accompanies *hyperthyroidism;* coarse hair is found with *hypothyroidism.* Tiny white ovoid granules that adhere to hairs may be nits (eggs of lice).

The Scalp. Part the hair in several places and look for scaliness, lumps, nevi, or other lesions.

Redness and scaling may indicate *seborrheic dermatitis, psoriasis;* soft lumps of *pilar cysts* (wens); pigmented nevi.

The Skull. Observe the general size and contour of the skull. Note any deformities, depressions, lumps, or tenderness. Learn to recognize the irregularities in a normal skull, such as those near the suture lines between the parietal and occipital bones.

Enlarged skull may signify *hydrocephalus* or *Paget's disease* of bone. Tenderness or step-offs are common after trauma.

The Face. Note the patient's facial expression and contours. Observe for asymmetry, involuntary movements, edema, and masses.

See Table 7-4, Selected Facies (p. 253).

The Skin. Observe the skin, noting its color, pigmentation, texture, thickness, hair distribution, and any lesions.

Acne is found in many adolescents. *Hirsutism* (excessive facial hair) occurs in some women with *polycystic ovary syndrome.*

THE EYES

Anatomy and Physiology

Begin by identifying the structures illustrated on this page. Note that the upper eyelid covers a portion of the iris but does not normally overlay the pupil. The opening between the eyelids is called the *palpebral fissure.* The white sclera may look somewhat buff-colored at its periphery. Do not mistake this color for jaundice, which is a deeper yellow.

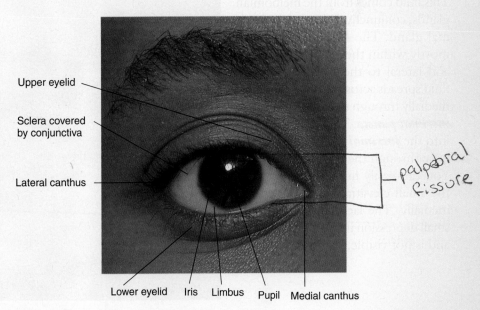

Upper eyelid

Sclera covered by conjunctiva

Lateral canthus

palpebral fissure

Lower eyelid   Iris   Limbus   Pupil   Medial canthus

The *conjunctiva* is a clear mucous membrane with two easily visible components. The *bulbar conjunctiva* covers most of the anterior eyeball, adhering loosely to the underlying tissue. It meets the cornea at the *limbus*. The *palpebral conjunctiva* lines the eyelids. The two parts of the conjunctiva merge in a folded recess that permits movement of the eyeball.

Within the eyelids lie firm strips of connective tissue called *tarsal plates*. Each plate contains a parallel row of *meibomian glands*, which open on the lid margin. The *levator palpebrae,* the muscle that raises the upper eyelid, is innervated by the oculomotor nerve, Cranial Nerve III. Smooth muscle, innervated by the sympathetic nervous system, also contributes to lid elevation.

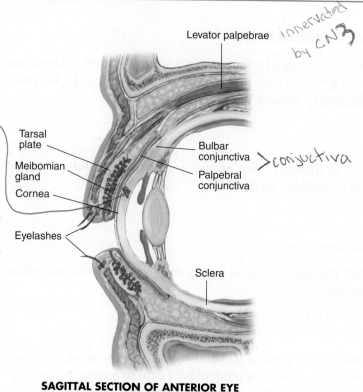

[handwritten: innervated by CN3]

Levator palpebrae

Tarsal plate

Meibomian gland

Cornea

Bulbar conjunctiva

Palpebral conjunctiva

[handwritten: conjunctiva]

Eyelashes

Sclera

SAGITTAL SECTION OF ANTERIOR EYE WITH LIDS CLOSED

A film of tear fluid protects the conjunctiva and cornea from drying, inhibits microbial growth, and gives a smooth optical surface to the cornea. This fluid comes from the meibomian glands, conjunctival glands, and lacrimal gland. The *lacrimal gland* lies mostly within the bony orbit, above and lateral to the eyeball. The tear fluid spreads across the eye and drains medially through two tiny holes called *lacrimal puncta*. The tears then pass into the *lacrimal sac* and on into the nose through the *nasolacrimal duct*. You can easily find a *punctum* atop the small elevation of the lower lid medially. The lacrimal sac rests in a small depression inside the bony orbit and is not visible.

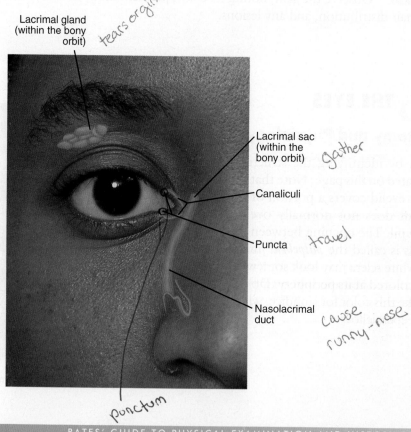

Lacrimal gland (within the bony orbit)

[handwritten: tears originate]

Lacrimal sac (within the bony orbit)

[handwritten: gather]

Canaliculi

Puncta

[handwritten: travel]

Nasolacrimal duct

[handwritten: cause runny-nose]

[handwritten: punctum]

The eyeball is a spherical structure that focuses light on the neurosensory elements within the retina. The muscles of the iris control pupillary size. Muscles of the *ciliary body* control the thickness of the lens, allowing the eye to focus on near or distant objects.

A clear liquid called *aqueous humor* fills the anterior and posterior chambers of the eye. Aqueous humor is produced by the *ciliary body*, circulates from the posterior chamber through the pupil into the anterior chamber, and drains out through the *canal of Schlemm*. This circulatory system helps to control the pressure inside the eye.

[handwritten annotations: eye pressure; makes clear liquid...aqueous humor; = control; exit aqueous humor; see far/near; down here enters eye.; drains]

Anterior chamber
Cornea
Anterior chamber
Canal of Schlemm
Ciliary body
Lens
Posterior chamber

CIRCULATION OF AQUEOUS HUMOR

[handwritten: Fundus]

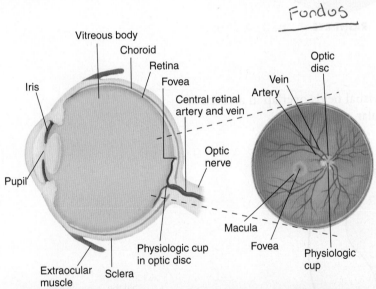

Vitreous body
Choroid
Retina
Fovea
Central retinal artery and vein
Iris
Optic nerve
Pupil
Extraocular muscle
Sclera
Physiologic cup in optic disc

Optic disc
Vein
Artery
Macula
Fovea
Physiologic cup

CROSS SECTION OF THE RIGHT EYE SHOWING A PORTION OF THE FUNDUS COMMONLY SEEN WITH THE OPHTHALMOSCOPE

The posterior part of the eye that is seen through an ophthalmoscope is often called the *fundus* of the eye. Structures here include the retina, choroid, fovea, macula, optic disc, and retinal vessels. The optic nerve with its retinal vessels enters the eyeball posteriorly. You can find it with an ophthalmoscope at the *optic disc*. Lateral and slightly inferior to the disc, there is a small depression in the retinal surface that marks the point of central vision. Around it is a darkened circular area called the *fovea*. The roughly circular *macula* (named for a microscopic yellow spot) surrounds the fovea but has no discernible margins. You do not usually see the normal *vitreous body*, a transparent mass of gelatinous material that fills the eyeball behind the lens. It helps to maintain the shape of the eye.

Visual Fields.   A *visual field* is the entire area seen by an eye when it looks at a central point. Fields are conventionally diagrammed on circles from the patient's point of view. The center of the circle represents the focus of gaze. The circumference is 90° from the line of gaze. Each visual field, shown by the white areas below, is divided into quadrants. Note that the fields extend farthest on the temporal sides. Visual fields are normally limited by the brows above, the cheeks below, and the nose medially. A lack of retinal receptors at the optic disc produces an oval blind spot in the normal field of each eye, 15° temporal to the line of gaze.

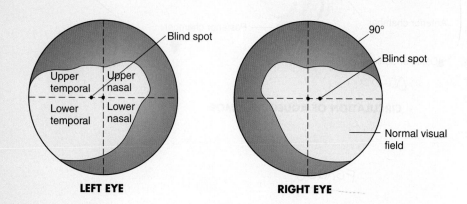

When a person is using both eyes, the two visual fields overlap in an area of binocular vision. Laterally, vision is monocular.

Visual Pathways.   To see an image, light reflected from the image must pass through the pupil and be focused on sensory neurons in the retina. The image projected there is upside down and reversed right to left. An image from the upper nasal visual field thus strikes the lower temporal quadrant of the retina.

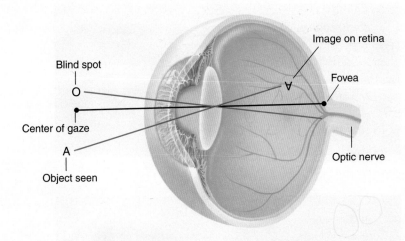

Nerve impulses, stimulated by light, are conducted through the retina, optic nerve, and optic tract on each side, then on through a curving tract called the *optic radiation*. This ends in the visual cortex, a part of the occipital lobe.

Pupillary Reactions. Pupillary size changes in response to light and to the effort of focusing on a near object.

The Light Reaction. A light beam shining onto one retina causes pupillary constriction in both that eye, termed the *direct reaction* to light, and in the opposite eye, the *consensual reaction*. The initial sensory pathways are similar to those described for vision: retina, optic nerve, and optic tract. The pathways diverge in the midbrain, however, and impulses are transmitted through the oculomotor nerve, CN III, to the constrictor muscles of the iris of each eye.

PATHWAYS OF THE LIGHT REACTION

The Near Reaction. When a person shifts gaze from a far object to a near one, the pupils constrict. This response, like the light reaction, is mediated by the oculomotor nerve (CN III). Coincident with this *pupillary constriction*, but not part of it, are (1) *convergence* of the eyes, an extraocular movement; and (2) *accommodation*, an increased convexity of the lenses caused by contraction of the ciliary muscles. This change in shape of the lenses brings near objects into focus but is not visible to the examiner.

Autonomic Nerve Supply to the Eyes. Fibers travelling in the oculomotor nerve (CN III) and producing pupillary constriction are part of the parasympathetic nervous system. The iris is also supplied by sympathetic fibers. When these are stimulated, the pupil dilates, and the upper eyelid rises a little, as if from fear. The sympathetic pathway starts in the hypothalamus and passes down through the brainstem and cervical cord into the neck. From there, it follows the carotid artery or its branches into the orbit. A lesion anywhere along this pathway may impair sympathetic effects that dilate the pupil.

VISUAL PATHWAYS FROM THE RETINA TO THE VISUAL CORTEX

Extraocular Movements. The coordinated action of six muscles, the four rectus and two oblique, control the eye. You can test the function of each muscle and the nerve that supplies it by asking the patient to move the eye in the direction controlled by that muscle. There are six such *cardinal directions,* indicated by the lines on the figure below. When a person looks down and to the right, for example, the right inferior rectus (CN III) is principally responsible for moving the right eye, whereas the left superior oblique (CN IV) is principally responsible for moving the left. If one of these muscles is paralyzed, the eye will deviate from its normal position in that direction of gaze and the eyes will no longer appear conjugate, or parallel.

CARDINAL DIRECTIONS OF GAZE

Techniques of Examination

Important Areas of Examination

- Visual acuity
- Visual fields
- Conjunctiva and sclera
- Cornea, lens, and pupils
- Extraocular movements

- Fundi, including:
  Optic disc and cup
  Retina
  Retinal vessels

Visual Acuity. To test the acuity of central vision, use a Snellen eye chart, if possible, and light it well. Position the patient 20 feet from the chart. Patients who use glasses other than for reading should put them on. Ask the patient to cover one eye with a card (to prevent peeking through the fingers) and to read the smallest line of print possible. Coaxing to attempt the next line may improve performance. A patient who cannot read the largest letter should be positioned closer to the chart; note the intervening distance. Determine the smallest line of print from which the patient can identify more than half the letters. Record the visual acuity designated at the side of this line, along with use of glasses, if any. Visual acuity is expressed as two numbers (e.g., 20/30): the first indicates the distance of the patient from the chart, and the second, the distance at which a normal eye can read the line of letters.

Testing near vision with a special hand-held card helps identify the need for reading glasses or bifocals in patients older than 45 years. You can also use this

Vision of 20/200 means that at 20 feet the patient can read print that a person with normal vision could read at 200 feet. The larger the second number, the worse the vision. "20/40 corrected" means the patient could read the 40 line with glasses (a correction).

Myopia is impaired far vision.

Presbyopia is the impaired near vision, found in middle-aged and card to test visual acuity at the bedside. Held 14 inches from the patient's eyes, the card simulates a Snellen chart. You may, however, let patients choose their own distance.

If you have no charts, screen visual acuity with any available print. If patients cannot read even the largest letters, test their ability to count your upraised fingers and distinguish light (such as your flashlight) from dark.

older people. A presbyopic person often sees better when the card is farther away.

In the United States, a person is usually considered legally blind when vision in the better eye, corrected by glasses, is 20/200 or less. Legal blindness also results from a constricted field of vision: 20° or less in the better eye.

Visual Fields by Confrontation

Screening.   Screening starts in the temporal fields because most defects involve these areas. Imagine the patient's visual fields projected onto a glass bowl that encircles the front of the patient's head. Ask the patient to look

Field defects that are all or partly temporal include:

Homonymous hemianopsia

Bitemporal hemianopsia

Quadrantic defects

Review these patterns in Table 7-5, Visual Field Defects, p. 254.

with both eyes into your eyes. While you return the patient's gaze, place your hands about 2 feet apart, lateral to the patient's ears. Instruct the patient to point to your fingers as soon as they are seen. Then slowly move the wiggling fingers of both your hands along the imaginary bowl and toward the line of gaze until the patient identifies them. Repeat this pattern in the upper and lower temporal quadrants. Usually a person sees both sets of fingers at the same time. If so, fields are usually normal.

Further Testing.   If you find a defect, try to establish its boundaries. Test one eye at a time. If you suspect a temporal defect in the left visual field, for example, ask the patient to cover the right eye and, with the left one,

When the patient's left eye repeatedly does not see your fingers until they have crossed the line of to look into your eye directly opposite. Then slowly move your wiggling fingers from the defective area toward the better vision, noting where the patient first responds. Repeat this at several levels to define the border.

A temporal defect in the visual field of one eye suggests a nasal defect in the other eye. To test this hypothesis, examine the other eye in a similar way, again moving from the anticipated defect toward the better vision.

Small visual field defects and enlarged blind spots require a finer stimulus. Using a small red object such as a red-headed matchstick or the red eraser on a pencil, test one eye at a time. As the patient looks into your eye directly opposite, move the object about in the visual field. The normal blind spot can be found 15° temporal to the line of gaze—the small red object disappears. (Find your own blind spots for practice.)

Position and Alignment of the Eyes. Stand in front of the patient and survey the eyes for position and alignment. If one or both eyes seem to protrude, assess them from above (see p. 243).

Eyebrows. Inspect the eyebrows, noting their quantity and distribution and any scaliness of the underlying skin.

Eyelids. Note the position of the lids in relation to the eyeballs. Inspect for the following:

● Width of the palpebral fissures

● Edema of the lids

● Color of the lids

gaze, a left *temporal hemianopsia* is present. It is diagrammed from the patient's viewpoint.

A left *homonymous hemianopsia* may thus be established.

An enlarged blind spot occurs in conditions affecting the optic nerve such as *glaucoma, optic neuritis,* and *papilledema.*[7]

Inward or outward deviation of the eyes; abnormal protrusion in *Graves' disease* or ocular tumors

Scaliness in *seborrheic dermatitis;* lateral sparseness in *hypothyroidism*

See Table 7-6, Variations and Abnormalities of the Eyelids (p. 255).

Upstarting palpebral fissures in *Down syndrome*

Red inflamed lid margins in *blepharitis,* often with crusting

- Lesions

- Condition and direction of the eyelashes

- Adequacy with which the eyelids close. Look for this especially when the eyes are unusually prominent, when there is facial paralysis, or when the patient is unconscious.

Failure of the eyelids to close exposes the corneas to serious damage.

Lacrimal Apparatus. Briefly inspect the regions of the lacrimal gland and lacrimal sac for swelling.

Look for excessive tearing or dryness of the eyes. Assessment of dryness may require special testing by an ophthalmologist. To test for nasolacrimal duct obstruction, see p. 243.

See Table 7-7, Lumps and Swellings in and Around the Eyes (p. 256).

Excessive tearing may be from increased production or impaired drainage of tears. In the first group, causes include *conjunctival inflammation* and *corneal irritation*; in the second, *ectropion* (p. 255) and *nasolacrimal duct obstruction*.

Conjunctiva and Sclera. Ask the patient to look up as you depress both lower lids with your thumbs, exposing the sclera and conjunctiva. Inspect the sclera and palpebral conjunctiva for color, and note the vascular pattern against the white scleral background. Look for any nodules or swelling.

A yellow sclera indicates jaundice.

If you need a fuller view of the eye, rest your thumb and finger on the bones of the cheek and brow, respectively, and spread the lids.

Ask the patient to look to each side and down. This technique gives you a good view of the sclera and bulbar conjunctiva, but not of the palpebral conjunctiva of the upper lid. For this purpose, you need to evert the lid (see pp. 243–244).

The local redness below is from *nodular episcleritis,* often self-limiting in younger adults; also seen in *rheumatoid arthritis* and *SLE.*

For comparisons, see Table 7-8, Red Eyes (p. 257).

Cornea and Lens. With oblique lighting, inspect the cornea of each eye for opacities and note any opacities in the lens that may be visible through the pupil.

See Table 7-9, Opacities of the Cornea and Lens (p. 258).

Iris. At the same time, inspect each iris. The markings should be clearly defined. With your light shining directly from the temporal side, look for a crescentic shadow on the medial side of the iris. Because the iris is normally fairly flat and forms a relatively open angle with the cornea, this lighting casts no shadow.

Occasionally the iris bows abnormally far forward, forming a very narrow angle with the cornea. The light then casts a crescentic shadow.

This narrow angle increases the risk for acute *narrow-angle glaucoma*—a sudden increase in intraocular pressure when drainage of the aqueous humor is blocked.

In *open-angle glaucoma*—the common form of glaucoma—the normal spatial relation between iris and cornea is preserved and the iris is fully lit.

Pupils. Inspect the *size*, *shape*, and *symmetry* of the pupils. If the pupils are large (>5 mm), small (<3 mm), or unequal, measure them. A card with black circles of varying sizes facilitates measurement.

Miosis refers to constriction of the pupils, *mydriasis* to dilation.

1   2   3   4   5   6   7 mm

Pupillary inequality of less than 0.5 mm (*anisocoria*) is visible in approximately 20% of normal people. If pupillary reactions are normal, anisocoria is considered benign.

Compare benign anisocoria with *Horner's syndrome, oculomotor nerve paralysis,* and *tonic pupil.* See Table 7-10, Pupillary Abnormalities (p. 259).

Test the *pupillary reaction to light.* Ask the patient to look into the distance, and shine a bright light obliquely into each pupil in turn. (Both the distant gaze and the oblique lighting help to prevent a near reaction.) Look for:

● The *direct reaction* (pupillary constriction in the same eye)

● The *consensual reaction* (pupillary constriction in the opposite eye)

Always darken the room and use a bright light before deciding that a light reaction is absent.

If the reaction to light is impaired or questionable, test the *near reaction* in normal room light. Testing one eye at a time makes it easier to concentrate on pupillary responses, without the distraction of extraocular movement. Hold your finger or pencil about 10 cm from the patient's eye. Ask the patient to look alternately at it and into the distance directly behind it. Watch for pupillary constriction with near effort.

Testing the near reaction is helpful in diagnosing *Argyll Robertson* and *tonic (Adie's) pupils* (see p. 259).

Extraocular Muscles.   From about 2 feet directly in front of the patient, shine a light onto the patient's eyes and ask the patient to look at it. *Inspect the reflections in the corneas.* They should be visible slightly nasal to the center of the pupils.

Asymmetry of the corneal reflections indicates a deviation from normal ocular alignment. A temporal light reflection on one cornea, for example, indicates a nasal deviation of that eye. See Table 7-11, Dysconjugate Gaze (p. 260).

A *cover–uncover test* may reveal a slight or latent muscle imbalance not otherwise seen (see p. 260).

Now *assess the extraocular movements,* looking for:

- The normal *conjugate movements* of the eyes in each direction, or any *deviation* from normal

See Table 7-11, Dysconjugate Gaze (p. 260).

- *Nystagmus,* a fine rhythmic oscillation of the eyes. A few beats of nystagmus on extreme lateral gaze are normal. If you see it, bring your finger in to within the field of binocular vision and look again.

Sustained nystagmus within the binocular field of gaze is seen with various neurologic conditions. See Table 17-6, Nystagmus (pp. 723–724).

- *Lid lag* as the eyes move from up to down.

In lid lag of *hyperthyroidism,* a rim of sclera is visible above the iris with downward gaze

To test the six extra-ocular movements (EOMs), ask the patient to follow your finger or pencil as you sweep through the six cardinal directions of gaze. Making a wide H in the air, lead the patient's gaze (1) to the patient's extreme right, (2) to the right and upward, and (3) down on the right; then (4) without pausing in the middle, to the extreme left, (5) to the left and upward, and (6) down on the left. Pause during upward and lateral gaze to detect nystagmus. Move your finger or pencil at a comfortable distance from the patient. Because middle-aged or older people may have difficulty focusing on near objects, make this distance greater for them than for young people. Some patients move their heads to follow your finger. If necessary, hold the head in the proper midline position.

In paralysis of the CN VI, illustrated below, the eyes are conjugate in right lateral gaze but not in left lateral gaze.

LOOKING RIGHT

LOOKING LEFT

If you suspect lid lag or hyperthyroidism, ask the patient to follow your finger again as you move it slowly from up to down in the midline. The lid should overlap the iris slightly throughout this movement.

Note the rim of sclera from *proptosis*, an abnormal protrusion of the eyeball in *hyperthyroidism*, leading to a characteristic "stare" on frontal gaze.

Finally, test for *convergence*. Ask the patient to follow your finger or pencil as you move it in toward the bridge of the nose. The converging eyes normally follow the object to within 5 cm to 8 cm of the nose.

CONVERGENCE

Ophthalmoscopic Examination. In general health care, you should usually examine your patients' eyes *without dilating their pupils*. Your view is therefore limited to the posterior structures of the retina. To see more peripheral structures, to evaluate the macula well, or to investigate unexplained visual loss, ophthalmologists dilate the pupils with mydriatic drops unless this is contraindicated.

At first, using the ophthalmoscope may seem awkward, and it may be difficult to visualize the fundus. With patience and practice of proper technique, the fundus will come into view, and you will be able to assess important structures such as the optic disc and the retinal vessels. Remove your glasses unless you have marked nearsightedness or severe astigmatism. (If the patient's refractive errors make it difficult to focus on the fundi, however, it may be easier to keep your glasses on.)

Aperture

Indicator of diopters

Lens disc

Contraindications for mydriatic drops include (1) head injury and coma, in which continuing observations of pupillary reactions are essential, and (2) any suspicion of narrow-angle glaucoma.

Review the components of the ophthalmoscope pictured above. Then follow the steps for using the ophthalmoscope, and your examination skills will improve over time.

EXAMINER AT 15° ANGLE FROM PATIENT'S LINE OF VISION, ELICITING RED REFLEX

STEPS FOR USING THE OPHTHALMOSCOPE

- Darken the room. Switch on the ophthalmoscope light and turn the lens disc until you see the large round beam of white light.* Shine the light on the back of your hand to check the type of light, its desired brightness, and the electrical charge of the ophthalmoscope.

- Turn the lens disc to the 0 diopter (a diopter is a unit that measures the power of a lens to converge or diverge light). At this diopter, the lens neither converges nor diverges light. Keep your finger on the edge of the lens disc so you can turn the disc to focus the lens when you examine the fundus.

- Remember, hold the ophthalmoscope *in your right hand* to examine *the patient's right eye;* hold it *in your left hand* to examine *the patient's left eye*. This keeps you from bumping the patient's nose and gives you more mobility and closer range for visualizing the fundus. At first, you may have difficulty using the nondominant eye, but this will abate with practice.

- Hold the ophthalmoscope firmly braced against the medial aspect of your bony orbit, with the handle tilted laterally at about a 20° slant from the vertical. Check to make sure you can see clearly through the aperture. Instruct the patient to look slightly up and over your shoulder at a point directly ahead on the wall.

- Place yourself about 15 inches away from the patient and at an angle *15° lateral to the patient's line of vision*. Shine the light beam on the pupil and look for the orange glow in the pupil—the *red reflex*. Note any opacities interrupting the red reflex.

- Now, place the thumb of your other hand across the patient's eyebrow (this technique helps keep you steady but is not essential). Keeping the light beam focused on the red reflex, move in with the ophthalmoscope on the 15° angle toward the pupil until you are very close to it, almost touching the patient's eyelashes.

    Try to keep both eyes open and relaxed, as if gazing into the distance, to help minimize any fluctuating blurriness as your eyes attempt to accommodate.

    You may need to lower the brightness of the light beam to make the examination more comfortable for the patient, avoid *hippus* (spasm of the pupil), and improve your observations.

*Some clinicians like to use the large round beam for large pupils, the small round beam for small pupils. The other beams are rarely helpful. The slitlike beam is sometimes used to assess elevations or concavities in the retina, the green (or red-free) beam to detect small red lesions, and the grid to make measurements. Ignore the last three lights and practice with the large or small round white beam.

Absence of a *red reflex* suggests an opacity of the lens (cataract) or possibly of the vitreous. Less commonly, a *detached retina* or, in children, a *retinoblastoma* may obscure this reflex. Do not be fooled by an artificial eye, which has no red reflex.

Now you are ready to inspect the *optic disc* and the *retina*. You should be seeing the optic disc—a yellowish orange to creamy pink oval or round structure that may fill your field of gaze or even exceed it. Of interest, the ophthalmoscope magnifies the normal retina about 15 times and the normal iris about 4 times. The optic disc actually measures about 1.5 mm. Follow the next steps for this important segment of the physical examination.

When the lens has been removed surgically, its magnifying effect is lost. Retinal structures then look much smaller than usual, and you can see a much larger expanse of the fundus.

STEPS FOR EXAMINING THE OPTIC DISC AND THE RETINA

The Optic Disc

- First, *locate the optic disc.* Look for the round yellowish-orange structure described on the previous page. If you do not see it at first, follow a blood vessel centrally until you do. You can tell which direction is central by noting the angles at which vessels branch—the vessel size becomes progressively larger at each junction as you approach the disc.

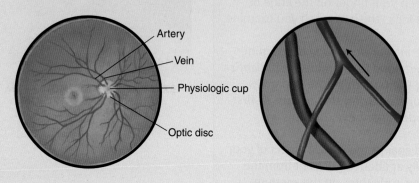

Artery

Vein

Physiologic cup

Optic disc

- Now, *bring the optic disc into sharp focus* by adjusting the lens of your ophthalmoscope. If both you and the patient have no refractive errors, the retina should be in focus at 0 diopters. If structures are blurred, rotate the lens disc until you find the sharpest focus.

  For example, if the patient is myopic (nearsighted), rotate the lens disc counterclockwise to the minus diopters; in a hyperopic (farsighted) patient, move the disc clockwise to the plus diopters. You can correct your own refractive error in the same way.

- *Inspect the optic disc.* Note the following features:
  - *The sharpness or clarity of the disc outline.* The nasal portion of the disc margin may be somewhat blurred, a normal finding.
  - *The color of the disc,* normally yellowish orange to creamy pink. White or pigmented crescents may ring the disc, a normal finding.
  - *The size of the central physiologic cup,* if present. It is usually yellowish white. The horizontal diameter is usually less than half the horizontal diameter of the disc.
  - *The comparative symmetry* of the eyes and findings in the fundi.

Detecting Papilledema. *Papilledema* describes swelling of the optic disc and anterior bulging of the physiologic cup. Increased intracranial pressure is transmitted to the optic nerve, causing stasis of axoplasmic flow, intra-axonal edema, and swelling of the optic nerve head. Papilledema often signals serious disorders of the brain, such as meningitis, subarachnoid hemorrhage, trauma, and mass lesions, so searching for this important disorder is a priority during all your fundoscopic examinations.

In a *refractive error,* light rays from a distance do not focus on the retina. In *myopia,* they focus anterior to it; in *hyperopia,* posterior to it. Retinal structures in a myopic eye look larger than normal.

See Table 7-12, Normal Variations of the Optic Disc (p. 261), and Table 7-13, Abnormalities of the Optic Disc (p. 262).

An enlarged cup suggests *chronic open-angle glaucoma.*

PAPILLEDEMA

(continued)

STEPS FOR EXAMINING THE OPTIC DISC AND THE RETINA (CONTINUED)

The presence or absence of spontaneous venous pulsations (SVP) can be used when trying to determine if a patient has papilledema. SVP are a common occurrence in normal eyes (seen in up to 75% or more of patients) and indicate that the intracranial pressure is probably normal. However, SVP is absent in a minority of normal patients.

Loss of venous pulsations in pathologic conditions like head trauma, *meningitis,* or mass lesions may be an early sign of elevated intracranial pressure.

The Retina—Arteries, Veins, Fovea, and Macula

- *Inspect the retina,* including arteries and veins as they extend to the periphery, arteriovenous crossings, the fovea, and the macula. Distinguish arteries from veins based on the features listed below.

	Arteries	Veins
Color	Light red	Dark red
Size	Smaller (²⁄₃ to ⁴⁄₅ the diameter of veins)	Larger
Light Reflex (*reflection*)	Bright	Inconspicuous or absent

- *Follow the vessels peripherally in each of four directions,* noting their relative sizes and the character of the arteriovenous crossings.

  Identify any lesions of the surrounding *retina* and note their size, shape, color, and distribution. As you search the retina, *move your head and instrument as a unit,* using the patient's pupil as an imaginary fulcrum. At first, you may repeatedly lose your view of the retina because your light falls out of the pupil. You will improve with practice.

  Lesions of the retina can be measured in terms of "disc diameters" from the optic disc.

Sequence of inspection from disc to macula
LEFT EYE

See Table 7-14, Retinal Arteries and Arteriovenous Crossings: Normal and Hypertensive (p. 263); Table 7-15, Red Spots and Streaks in the Fundi (p. 264); Table 7-16, Ocular Fundi: Normal and Hypertensive Retinopathy; Table 7-17, Ocular Fundi: Diabetic Retinopathy (p. 266); Table 7-18, Light-Colored Spots in the Fundi (p. 267).

COTTON-WOOL PATCHES

Note the irregular patches between 11 and 12 o'clock, 1 to 2 disc diameters from the disc. Each measures about one-half by one-half disc diameters.

(continued)

STEPS FOR EXAMINING THE OPTIC DISC AND THE RETINA (CONTINUED)

- Inspect the *fovea* and surrounding *macula*. Direct your light beam laterally or by asking the patient to look directly into the light. Except in older people, the tiny bright reflection at the center of the fovea helps to orient you. Shimmering light reflections in the macular area are common in young people.

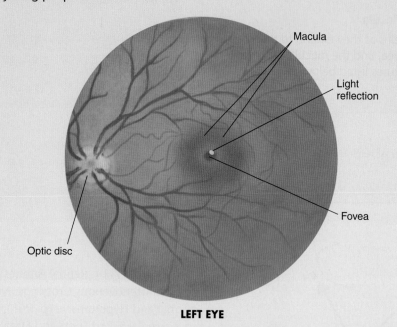

LEFT EYE

- *Inspect the anterior structures.* Look for opacities in the *vitreous* or *lens* by rotating the lens disc progressively to diopters of around +10 or +12. This technique allows you to focus on the more anterior structures in the eye.

Macular degeneration is an important cause of poor central vision in the elderly. Types include *dry atrophic* (more common but less severe) and *wet exudative,* or neovascular. Undigested cellular debris, called *drusen,* may be hard and sharply defined, as seen below, or soft and confluent with altered pigmentation (see p. 267).

Photo from Tasman W, Jaeger E (eds). The Wills Eye Hospital Atlas of Clinical Ophthalmology, 2nd ed. Philadelphia, Lippincott Williams & Wilkins, 2001.

Vitreous floaters may be seen as dark specks or strands between the fundus and the lens. Cataracts are densities in the lens (see p. 258).

THE EAR

Anatomy and Physiology

The ear has three compartments: the external ear, the middle ear, and the inner ear.

The *external ear* comprises the auricle and ear canal. The *auricle* consists chiefly of cartilage covered by skin and has a firm elastic consistency. Its prominent curved outer ridge is the *helix*. Parallel and anterior to the helix is another curved prominence, the *antihelix*. Inferiorly lies the fleshy projection of the earlobe, or *lobule*. The ear canal opens behind the *tragus,* a nodular eminence that points backward over the entrance to the canal.

The *ear canal* curves inward and is approximately 24 mm long. Cartilage surrounds its outer portion. The skin in this portion is hairy and contains glands that produce cerumen (wax). The inner portion of the canal is surrounded by bone and lined by thin, hairless skin. Pressure on this latter area causes pain—a point to remember when you examine the ear.

Behind and below the ear canal is the mastoid part of the temporal bone. The lowest portion of this bone, the *mastoid process,* is palpable behind the lobule.

At the end of the ear canal lies the *tympanic membrane,* or eardrum, marking the lateral limits of the middle ear. The *middle ear* is an air-filled cavity that transmits sound by way of three tiny bones, the *ossicles.* It is connected by the *eustachian tube* to the nasopharynx.

The eardrum is an oblique membrane held inward at its center by the *malleus,* one of its three ossicles. Find the *handle* and the *short process* of the malleus—the two chief landmarks. From the *umbo,* where the eardrum meets the tip of the malleus, a light reflection called the *cone of light* fans downward and anteriorly. Above the short process lies a small portion of the eardrum called the *pars flaccida.* The remainder of the drum is the *pars tensa.* Anterior and posterior malleolar folds, which extend obliquely upward from the short process, separate the pars flaccida from the pars tensa but are usually invisible unless the eardrum is retracted. A second ossicle, the *incus,* can sometimes be seen through the drum.

Pars flaccida

Short process of malleus

Incus

Handle of malleus

Pars tensa

Umbo

Cone of light

RIGHT EARDRUM

Much of the middle ear and all of the inner ear are inaccessible to direct examination. Some inferences concerning their condition can be made, however, by testing auditory function.

Pathways of Hearing. Vibrations of sound pass through the air of the external ear and are transmitted through the eardrum and ossicles of the middle ear to the *cochlea,* a part of the inner ear. The cochlea senses and codes the vibrations, and nerve impulses are sent to the brain through the cochlear nerve. The first part of this pathway—from the external ear through the middle ear—is known as the *conductive* phase, and a disorder here causes *conductive hearing loss.* The second part of the pathway, involving the cochlea and the cochlear nerve, is called the *sensorineural* phase; a disorder here causes *sensorineural hearing loss.*

Sensorineural

Air conduction

Bone conduction

Air conduction describes the normal first phase in the hearing pathway. An alternate pathway, known as *bone conduction,* bypasses the external and middle ear and is used for testing purposes. A vibrating tuning fork, placed on the head, sets the bone of the skull into vibration and stimulates the cochlea directly. In a normal person, air conduction is more sensitive than bone conduction.

Equilibrium. The labyrinth within the inner ear senses the position and movements of the head and helps to maintain balance.

Techniques of Examination

The Auricle.   Inspect the auricle and surrounding tissue for deformities, lumps, or skin lesions.

If ear pain, discharge, or inflammation is present, move the auricle up and down, press the tragus, and press firmly just behind the ear.

Ear Canal and Drum.   To see the ear canal and drum, use an otoscope with the largest ear speculum that the canal will accommodate. Position the patient's head so that you can see comfortably through the instrument. To straighten the ear canal, grasp the auricle firmly but gently and pull it upward, backward, and slightly away from the head.

Holding the otoscope handle between your thumb and fingers, brace your hand against the patient's face. Your hand and instrument thus follow unexpected movements by the patient. (If you are uncomfortable switching hands for the left ear, as shown below, you may reach over that ear to pull it up and back with your left hand and rest your otoscope-holding right hand on the head behind the ear.)

Insert the speculum gently into the ear canal, directing it somewhat down and forward and through the hairs, if any.

See Table 7-19, Lumps on or Near the Ear (p. 268).

Movement of the auricle and tragus (the "tug test") is painful in acute *otitis externa* (inflammation of the ear canal), but not in *otitis media* (inflammation of the middle ear). Tenderness behind the ear may be present in *otitis media.*

Nontender nodular swellings covered by normal skin deep in the ear canals suggest *exostoses.* These are nonmalignant overgrowths, which may obscure the drum.

Inspect the ear canal, noting any discharge, foreign bodies, redness of the skin, or swelling. Cerumen, which varies in color and consistency from yellow and flaky to brown and sticky or even to dark and hard, may wholly or partly obscure your view.

RIGHT EARDRUM

(labels: Pars flaccida, Incus, Pars tensa, Short process of malleus, Handle of malleus, Umbo, Cone of light)

In acute *otitis externa,* shown below, the canal is often swollen, narrowed, moist, pale, and tender. It may be reddened.

Inspect the eardrum, noting its color and contour. The cone of light—usually easy to see—helps to orient you.

In *chronic otitis externa,* the skin of the canal is often thickened, red, and itchy.

Red bulging drum of acute purulent *otitis media*[10]; amber drum of a serous effusion. See Table 7-20, Abnormalities of the Eardrum (pp. 269–270).

Identify the *handle of the malleus,* noting its position, and inspect the *short process of the malleus.*

An unusually prominent short process and a prominent handle that looks more horizontal suggest a retracted drum.

Gently move the speculum so that you can see as much of the drum as possible, including the *pars flaccida* superiorly and the margins of the *pars tensa.* Look for any perforations. The anterior and inferior margins of the drum may be obscured by the curving wall of the ear canal.

Mobility of the eardrum can be evaluated with a pneumatic otoscope.

A serous effusion, a thickened drum, or purulent *otitis media* may decrease mobility.

why?

Auditory Acuity. To estimate hearing, test one ear at a time. Ask the patient to occlude one ear with a finger, or better still, occlude it yourself. When auditory acuity on the two sides is different, move your finger rapidly, but gently, in the occluded canal. This noise helps prevent the occluded ear from doing the work of the ear you wish to test. Then, standing 1 or 2 feet away, exhale fully (so as to minimize the intensity of your voice) and whisper softly toward the unoccluded ear. Choose numbers or other words with two equally accented syllables, such as "nine-four," or "baseball." If necessary, increase the intensity of your voice to a medium whisper, a loud whisper, and then a soft, medium, and loud voice. To make sure the patient does not read your lips, cover your mouth or obstruct the patient's vision.

Air and Bone Conduction. If hearing is diminished, *try to distinguish conductive from sensorineural hearing loss.* You need a quiet room and a tuning fork, preferably of 512 Hz or possibly 1024 Hz. These frequencies fall within the range of human speech (300 Hz to 3000 Hz)—functionally the most important range. Forks with lower pitches may lead to overestimating bone conduction and can also be felt as vibration.

Set the fork into light vibration by briskly stroking it between the thumb and index finger (——⊃) or by tapping it on your knuckles.

● *Test for lateralization* (Weber test). Place the base of the lightly vibrating tuning fork firmly on top of the patient's head or on the midforehead.

In unilateral *conductive hearing loss,* sound is heard in (lateralized to) the impaired ear. Visible explanations include *acute otitis media,* perforation of the eardrum, and obstruction of the ear canal, as by cerumen. See Table 7-21, Patterns of Hearing Loss (p. 271).

Ask where the patient hears it: on one or both sides? Normally the sound is heard in the midline or equally in both ears. If nothing is heard, try again, pressing the fork more firmly on the head. Because patients with normal hearing may lateralize, this test should be restricted to those with hearing loss.

In unilateral *sensorineural hearing loss,* sound is heard in the good ear.

● *Compare air conduction (AC) and bone conduction (BC)* (Rinne test). Place the base of a lightly vibrating tuning fork on the mastoid bone, behind the ear and level with the canal. When the patient can no longer hear the sound, quickly place the fork close to the ear canal and ascertain whether the sound can be heard again. Here the "U" of the fork should face forward, thus maximizing its sound for the patient. Normally the sound is heard longer through air than through bone (AC > BC).

In *conductive hearing loss,* sound is heard through bone as long as or longer than it is through air (BC = AC or BC > AC). In *sensorineural hearing loss,* sound is heard longer through air (AC > BC).

THE NOSE AND PARANASAL SINUSES

Anatomy and Physiology

Review the terms used to describe the external anatomy of the nose.

Approximately the upper third of the nose is supported by bone, the lower two thirds by cartilage. Air enters the nasal cavity by way of the *anterior naris* on either side, then passes into a widened area known as the *vestibule* and on through the narrow nasal passage to the nasopharynx.

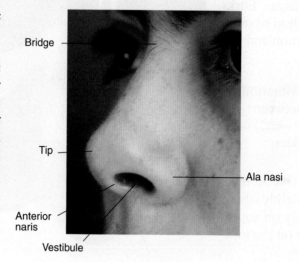

Bridge
Tip
Ala nasi
Anterior naris
Vestibule

The medial wall of each nasal cavity is formed by the *nasal septum*, which, like the external nose, is supported by both bone and cartilage. It is covered by a mucous membrane well supplied with blood. The vestibule, unlike the rest of the nasal cavity, is lined with hair-bearing skin, not mucosa.

Laterally, the anatomy is more complex. Curving bony structures, the *turbinates,* covered by a highly vascular mucous membrane, protrude into the nasal cavity. Below each turbinate is a groove, or meatus, each named according to the turbinate above it. The nasolacrimal duct drains into the inferior meatus; into the middle meatus drain most of the paranasal sinuses. Their openings are not usually visible.

The additional surface area provided by the turbinates and the mucosa covering them aids the nasal cavities in their principal functions: cleansing, humidification, and temperature control of inspired air.

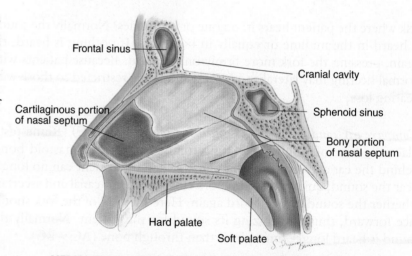

Frontal sinus
Cranial cavity
Cartilaginous portion of nasal septum
Sphenoid sinus
Bony portion of nasal septum
Hard palate
Soft palate

MEDIAL WALL—LEFT NASAL CAVITY (MUCOSA REMOVED)

Frontal sinus
Cranial cavity
Superior turbinate
sphenoid sinus
Middle turbinate
Inferior turbinate
Vestibule
Nasopharynx
Opening to eustachian tube
Hard palate
Soft palate

LATERAL WALL—NASAL CAVITY

The *paranasal sinuses* are air-filled cavities within the bones of the skull. Like the nasal cavities into which they drain, they are lined with mucous membrane. Their locations are diagrammed below. Only the frontal and maxillary sinuses are readily accessible to clinical examination.

infection c̄ mucosal membrane cause sinititis!

Frontal sinus

Orbit

Ethmoid sinus

Middle meatus

Inferior meatus

Middle turbinate

Maxillary sinus

Inferior turbinate

CROSS SECTION OF NASAL CAVITY—ANTERIOR VIEW

Frontal sinus

Maxillary sinus

Techniques of Examination

Inspect the anterior and inferior surfaces of the nose. Gentle pressure on the tip of the nose with your thumb usually widens the nostrils and, with the aid of a penlight or otoscope light, you can get a partial view of each nasal *vestibule.* If the tip is tender, be particularly gentle and manipulate the nose as little as possible.

Note any asymmetry or deformity of the nose.

Test for nasal obstruction, if indicated, by pressing on each ala nasi in turn and asking the patient to breathe in.

Tenderness of the nasal tip or alae suggests local infection such as a furuncle.

Vestibule

Inspect the inside of the nose with an otoscope and the largest ear speculum available.‡ Tilt the patient's head back a bit and insert the speculum gently into the vestibule of each nostril, avoiding contact with the sensitive nasal septum. Hold the otoscope handle to one side to avoid the patient's chin and improve your mobility. By directing the speculum posteriorly, then upward in small steps, try to see the inferior and middle turbinates, the nasal septum, and the narrow nasal passage between them. Some asymmetry of the two sides is normal.

Deviation of the lower septum is common and may be easily visible, as illustrated in previous photo. Deviation seldom obstructs air flow.

Middle turbinate

Nasal passage

Septum

Inferior turbinate

Observe the nasal mucosa, the nasal septum, and any abnormalities.

● The *nasal mucosa* that covers the septum and turbinates. Note its color and any swelling, bleeding, or exudate. If exudate is present, note its character: clear, mucopurulent, or purulent. The nasal mucosa is normally somewhat redder than the oral mucosa.

In *viral rhinitis* the mucosa is reddened and swollen; in *allergic rhinitis* it may be pale, bluish, or red.

● The *nasal septum*. Note any deviation, inflammation, or perforation of the septum. The lower anterior portion of the septum (where the patient's finger can reach) is a common source of *epistaxis* (nosebleed).

Fresh blood or crusting may be seen. Causes of septal perforation include trauma, surgery, and the intranasal use of cocaine or amphetamines.

● Any *abnormalities* such as ulcers or polyps.

Polyps are pale, semitranslucent masses that usually come from the middle meatus. Ulcers may result from nasal use of cocaine.

Inspection of the nasal cavity through the anterior naris is usually limited to the vestibule, the anterior portion of the septum, and the lower and middle turbinates. Examination with a nasopharyngeal mirror is required for detection of posterior abnormalities. This technique is beyond the scope of this book.

---

‡A nasal illuminator, equipped with a short wide nasal speculum but lacking an otoscope's magnification, may also be used, but structures look much smaller. Otolaryngologists use special equipment not widely available to others.

Make it a habit to place all nasal and ear specula outside your instrument case after use. Then discard them or clean and disinfect them appropriately. (Check the policies of your institution.)

Palpate for sinus tenderness. Press up on the *frontal sinuses* from under the bony brows, avoiding pressure on the eyes. Then press up on the *maxillary sinuses.*

Local tenderness, together with symptoms such as pain, fever, and nasal discharge, suggest *acute sinusitis* involving the frontal or maxillary sinuses.[12–14] Transillumination may be diagnostically useful. For this technique, see pp. 244–245.

MOUTH AND PHARYNX

Anatomy and Physiology

The *lips* are muscular folds that surround the entrance to the mouth. When opened, the gums (gingiva) and teeth are visible. Note the scalloped shape of the *gingival margins* and the pointed *interdental papillae.*

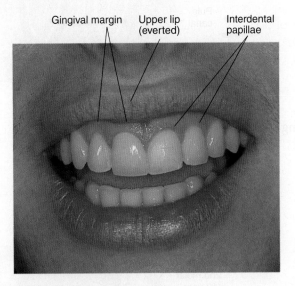

Gingival margin   Upper lip (everted)   Interdental papillae

The *gingiva* is firmly attached to the teeth and to the maxilla or mandible in which they are seated. In lighter-skinned people, the gingiva is pale or coral pink and lightly stippled. In darker-skinned people, it may be diffusely or partly brown, as shown on the following page. A midline mucosal fold, called a *labial frenulum,* connects each lip with the gingiva. A shallow *gingival sulcus* between the gum's thin margin and each tooth is not readily visible (but is probed and measured by dentists). Adjacent to the gingiva is the *alveolar mucosa,* which merges with the *labial mucosa* of the lip.

Gingiva

Alveolar mucosa

Labial frenulum

Labial mucosa

Each tooth, composed chiefly of dentin, lies rooted in a bony socket with only its enamel-covered crown exposed. Small blood vessels and nerves enter the tooth through its apex and pass into the pulp canal and pulp chamber.

Crown

Gingival margin

Gingiva

Pulp chamber

Bone

Root

Pulp canal

Apex

Enamel

Gingival sulcus

Dentin

Note the terms designating the 32 adult teeth, 16 in each jaw.

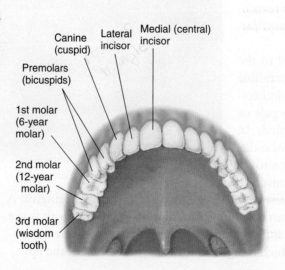

Canine (cuspid)

Lateral incisor

Medial (central) incisor

Premolars (bicuspids)

1st molar (6-year molar)

2nd molar (12-year molar)

3rd molar (wisdom tooth)

The dorsum of the *tongue* is covered with papillae, giving it a rough surface. Some of these papillae look like red dots, which contrast with the thin white coat that often covers the tongue. The undersurface of the tongue has no papillae. Note the midline *lingual frenulum* that connects the tongue to the floor of the mouth. At the base of the tongue the *ducts of the submandibular gland* (Wharton's ducts) pass forward and medially. They open on papillae that lie on each side of the lingual frenulum.

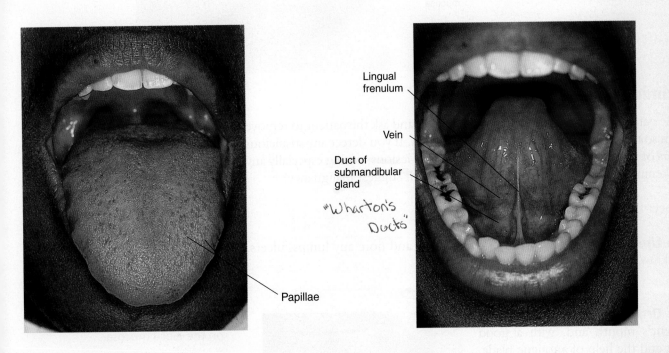

Lingual frenulum

Vein

Duct of submandibular gland

"Wharton's Ducts"

Papillae

Above and behind the tongue rises an arch formed by the *anterior* and *posterior pillars,* the *soft palate,* and the *uvula.* A meshwork of small blood vessels may web the soft palate. The *pharynx* is visible in the recess behind the soft palate and tongue.

In the adjacent photograph, note the right tonsil protruding from the hollowed *tonsillar fossa,* or cavity, between the anterior and posterior pillars. In adults, tonsils are often small or absent, as in the empty left tonsillar fossa here.

Posterior pillar

Anterior pillar

Right tonsil

Hard palate

Soft palate

Uvula

Pharynx

Tongue

The *buccal mucosa* lines the cheeks. Each *parotid duct,* sometimes termed *Stenson's duct,* opens onto the buccal mucosa near the upper second molar. Its location is frequently marked by its own small papilla.

"Stenson's Duct"

Opening of the parotid duct

Papilla

Upper lip (retracted)

Buccal mucosa

Techniques of Examination

If the patient wears dentures, offer a paper towel and ask the patient to remove them so that you can see the mucosa underneath. If you detect any suspicious ulcers or nodules, put on a glove and palpate any lesions, noting especially any thickening or infiltration of the tissues that might suggest malignancy.

Bright red edematous mucosa underneath a denture suggests denture sore mouth. There may be ulcers or papillary granulation tissue.

Inspect the following:

The Lips.   Observe their color and moisture, and note any lumps, ulcers, cracking, or scaliness.

Cyanosis, pallor. See Table 7-22, Abnormalities of the Lips (pp. 272–273).

The Oral Mucosa.   Look into the patient's mouth and, with a good light and the help of a tongue blade, inspect the oral mucosa for color, ulcers, white patches, and nodules. The wavy white line on this buccal mucosa developed where the upper and lower teeth meet. Irritation from sucking or chewing may cause or intensify it.

This patient has an *aphthous ulcer* on the labial mucosa.

See Table 7-23, Findings in the Pharynx, Palate, and Oral Mucosa (pp. 274–276).

The Gums and Teeth.   Note the color of the gums, normally pink. Patchy brownness may be present, especially but not exclusively in black people.

Inspect the gum margins and the interdental papillae for swelling or ulceration.

Redness of *gingivitis,* black line of *lead poisoning*

Swollen interdental papillae in *gingivitis.* See Table 7-24, Findings in the Gums and Teeth (pp. 277–278).

Inspect the teeth. Are any of them missing, discolored, misshapen, or abnormally positioned? You can check for looseness with your gloved thumb and index finger.

The Roof of the Mouth. Inspect the color and architecture of the hard palate.

Torus palatinus, a benign midline lump (see p. 275)

The Tongue and the Floor of the Mouth. Ask the patient to put out his or her tongue. Inspect it for symmetry—a test of the hypoglossal nerve (Cranial Nerve XII).

Asymmetric protrusion suggests a lesion of CN XII, as shown below.

Note the color and texture of the dorsum of the tongue.

Inspect the sides and undersurface of the tongue and the floor of the mouth. These are the areas where cancer most often develops. Note any white or reddened areas, nodules, or ulcerations. Because cancer of the tongue is more common in men older than 50 years, especially in smokers and drinkers of alcohol, palpation is indicated.[22] Explain what you plan to do and put on gloves. Ask the patient to protrude his tongue. With your right hand, grasp the tip of the tongue with a square of gauze and gently pull it to the patient's left. Inspect the side of the tongue, and then palpate it with your gloved left hand, feeling for any induration (hardness).[22] Reverse the procedure for the other side.

Cancer of the tongue is the second most common cancer of the mouth, second only to cancer of the lip. Any persistent nodule or ulcer, red or white, must be suspect. Induration of the lesion further increases the possibility of malignancy. Cancer occurs most often on the side of the tongue, next most often at its base.

A carcinoma on the left side of a tongue:

(Photo reprinted by permission of the New England Journal of Medicine, 328: 186, 1993—arrows added)

See Table 7-25, Findings in or Under the Tongue (pp. 279–280).

The Pharynx.   Now, with the patient's mouth open but the tongue not protruded, ask the patient to say "ah" or yawn. This action may let you see the pharynx well. If not, press a tongue blade firmly down upon the midpoint of the arched tongue—far enough back to get good visualization of the pharynx but not so far that you cause gagging. Simultaneously, ask for an "ah" or a yawn. Note the rise of the soft palate—a test of Cranial Nerve X (the vagal nerve).

In CN X paralysis, the soft palate fails to rise and the uvula deviates to the opposite side.

Failure to rise

Deviated to left

Inspect the soft palate, anterior and posterior pillars, uvula, tonsils, and pharynx. Note their color and symmetry and look for exudate, swelling, ulceration, or tonsillar enlargement. If possible, palpate any suspicious area for induration or tenderness. Tonsils have crypts, or deep infoldings of squamous epithelium. Whitish spots of normal exfoliating epithelium may sometimes be seen in these crypts.

Discard your tongue blade after use.

See Table 7-23, Findings in the Pharynx, Palate, and Oral Mucosa (pp. 274–276).

THE NECK

Anatomy and Physiology

For descriptive purposes, divide each side of the neck into two triangles bounded by the sternomastoid muscle. Visualize the borders of the two triangles as follows:

- For the *anterior triangle:* the mandible above, the sternomastoid laterally, and the midline of the neck medially

- For the *posterior triangle:* the sternomastoid muscle, the trapezius, and the clavicle. Note that a portion of the omohyoid muscle crosses the lower portion of this triangle and can be mistaken for a lymph node or mass.

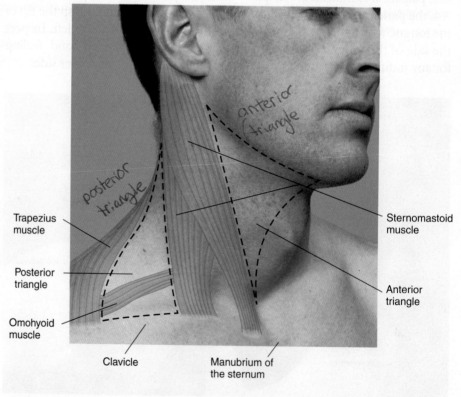

posterior triangle

anterior triangle

Trapezius muscle

Posterior triangle

Omohyoid muscle

Clavicle

Manubrium of the sternum

Sternomastoid muscle

Anterior triangle

Great Vessels. Deep to the sternomastoids run the great vessels of the neck: the *carotid artery* and the *internal jugular vein*. The *external jugular vein* passes diagonally over the surface of the sternomastoid and may be helpful when trying to identify the jugular venous pressure (see pp. 349–351).

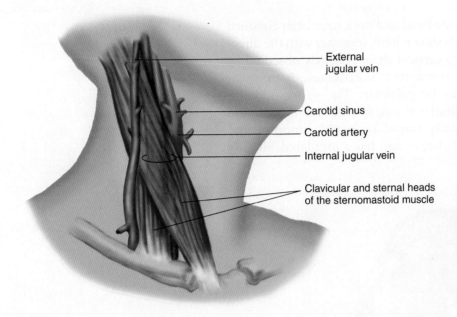

- External jugular vein
- Carotid sinus
- Carotid artery
- Internal jugular vein
- Clavicular and sternal heads of the sternomastoid muscle

Midline Structures and Thyroid Gland. Now identify the following midline structures: (1) the mobile *hyoid bone* just below the mandible, (2) the *thyroid cartilage*, readily identified by the notch on its superior edge, (3) the *cricoid cartilage*, (4) the *tracheal rings*, and (5) the *thyroid gland*.

- Thyroid cartilage
- **Cricoid cartilage**
- Thyroid lobe
- Thyroid isthmus
- Sternal notch
- Manubrium of sternum
- Hyoid bone
- Sternomastoid muscle
- Trachea
- Clavicle

The isthmus of the thyroid gland lies across the trachea below the cricoid. The lateral lobes of this gland curve posteriorly around the sides of the trachea and the esophagus. Except in the midline, the thyroid gland is covered by thin straplike muscles. Of these, only the sternomastoids are visible. Women have larger and more easily palpable glands than men.

Lymph Nodes. The *lymph nodes* of the head and neck have been classified in a variety of ways. One classification is shown here, together with the directions of lymphatic drainage. The deep cervical chain is largely obscured by the overlying sternomastoid muscle, but at its two extremes, the tonsillar node and supraclavicular nodes may be palpable. The submandibular nodes lie superficial to the submandibular gland, from which they should be differentiated. Nodes are normally round or ovoid, smooth, and smaller than this gland. The gland is larger and has a lobulated, slightly irregular surface (see p. 233).

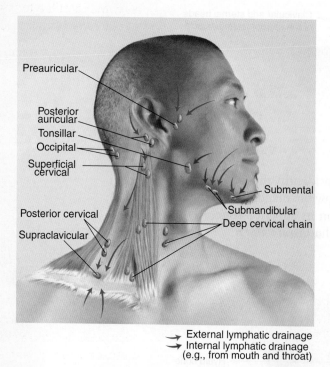

→ External lymphatic drainage
→ Internal lymphatic drainage
(e.g., from mouth and throat)

Note that the tonsillar, submandibular, and submental nodes drain portions of the mouth and throat as well as the face.

Knowledge of the lymphatic system is important to a sound clinical habit: whenever a malignant or inflammatory lesion is observed, look for involvement of the regional lymph nodes that drain it; whenever a node is enlarged or tender, look for a source such as infection in the area that it drains.

Techniques of Examination

Inspect the neck, noting its symmetry and any masses or scars. Look for enlargement of the parotid or submandibular glands, and note any visible lymph nodes.

A scar of past thyroid surgery is often a clue to unsuspected thyroid disease.

The Lymph Nodes. *Palpate the lymph nodes.* Using the pads of your index and middle fingers, move the skin over the underlying tissues in each area. The patient should be relaxed, with neck flexed slightly forward and, if needed, slightly toward the side being examined. You can usually examine both sides at once. For the submental node, however, it is helpful to feel with one hand while bracing the top of the head with the other.

Feel in sequence for the following nodes:

1. *Preauricular*—in front of the ear

2. *Posterior auricular*—superficial to the mastoid process

3. *Occipital*—at the base of the skull posteriorly

4. *Tonsillar*—at the angle of the mandible

5. *Submandibular*—midway between the angle and the tip of the mandible. These nodes are usually smaller and smoother than the lobulated submandibular gland against which they lie.

6. *Submental*—in the midline a few centimeters behind the tip of the mandible

7. *Superficial cervical*—superficial to the sternomastoid

8. *Posterior cervical*—along the anterior edge of the trapezius

9. *Deep cervical chain*—deep to the sternomastoid and often inaccessible to examination. Hook your thumb and fingers around either side of the sternomastoid muscle to find them.

10. *Supraclavicular*—deep in the angle formed by the clavicle and the sternomastoid

A "tonsillar node" that pulsates is really the carotid artery. A small, hard, tender "tonsillar node" high and deep between the mandible and the sternomastoid is probably a styloid process.

→ External lymphatic drainage
→ Internal lymphatic drainage
(e.g., from mouth and throat)

Enlargement of a supraclavicular node, especially on the left, suggests possible metastasis from a thoracic or an abdominal malignancy.

Note their size, shape, delimitation (discrete or matted together), mobility, consistency, and any tenderness. Small, mobile, discrete, nontender nodes, sometimes termed "shotty," are frequently found in normal people.

● Using the pads of the 2nd and 3rd fingers, palpate the *preauricular nodes* with a gentle rotary motion. Then examine the posterior auricular and occipital lymph nodes.

Tender nodes suggest inflammation; hard or fixed nodes suggest malignancy.

- Palpate the *anterior superficial and deep cervical chains,* located anterior and superficial to the sternomastoid. Then palpate the *posterior cervical chain* along the trapezius (anterior edge) and along the sternomastoid (posterior edge). Flex the patient's neck slightly forward toward the side being examined. Examine the supraclavicular nodes in the angle between the clavicle and the sternomastoid.

Enlarged or tender nodes, if unexplained, call for (1) reexamination of the regions they drain and (2) careful assessment of lymph nodes elsewhere so that you can distinguish between regional and generalized lymphadenopathy.

Diffuse lymphadenopathy raises the suspicion of HIV or AIDS.

Occasionally you may mistake a band of muscle or an artery for a lymph node. You should be able to roll a node in two directions: up and down, and side to side. Neither a muscle nor an artery will pass this test.

The Trachea and the Thyroid Gland. To orient yourself to the neck, identify the thyroid and cricoid cartilages and the trachea below them.

- *Inspect the trachea* for any deviation from its usual midline position. Then *feel for any deviation.* Place your finger along one side of the trachea and note the space between it and the sternomastoid. Compare it with the other side. The spaces should be symmetric.

Masses in the neck may push the trachea to one side. Tracheal deviation may also signify important problems in the thorax, such as a mediastinal mass, atelectasis, or a large pneumothorax (see pp. 320–321).

● *Inspect the neck for the thyroid gland.* Tip the patient's head back a bit. Using tangential lighting directed downward from the tip of the patient's chin, *inspect the region below the cricoid cartilage* for the gland. The lower shadowed border of each thyroid gland shown here is outlined by arrows.

The lower border of this large thyroid gland is outlined by tangential lighting. *Goiter* is a general term for an enlarged thyroid gland.[23,24]

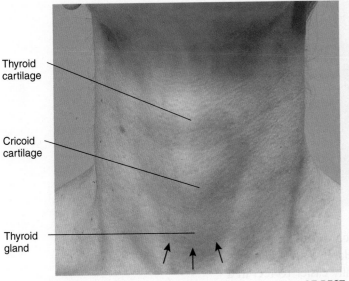

Thyroid cartilage

Cricoid cartilage

Thyroid gland

AT REST

Ask the patient to sip some water and to extend the neck again and swallow. Watch for upward movement of the thyroid gland, noting its contour and symmetry. The thyroid cartilage, the cricoid cartilage, and the thyroid gland all rise with swallowing and then fall to their resting positions.

With swallowing, the lower border of this large gland rises and looks less symmetric.

SWALLOWING

Until you become familiar with this examination, check your visual observations with your fingers from in front of the patient. This will orient you to the next step.

You are now ready to *palpate the thyroid gland*. This may seem difficult at first. Use the cues from visual inspection. Find your landmarks—the notched thyroid cartilage and the cricoid cartilage below it. Locate the *thyroid isthmus*, usually overlying the second, third, and fourth tracheal rings.

Cricoid cartilage

Adopt good technique, and follow the steps below, which outline the posterior approach (technique for the anterior approach is similar). With experience you will become more adept. The thyroid gland is usually easier to feel in a long slender neck than in a short stocky one. In shorter necks, added extension of the neck may help. In some people, however, the thyroid gland is partially or wholly substernal and not amenable to physical examination.

STEPS FOR PALPATING THE THYROID GLAND (POSTERIOR APPROACH)

- Ask the patient to flex the neck slightly forward to relax the sternomastoid muscles.
- Place the fingers of both hands on the patient's neck so that your index fingers are just below the cricoid cartilage.
- Ask the patient to sip and swallow water as before. Feel for the thyroid isthmus rising up under your finger pads. It is often but not always palpable.
- Displace the trachea to the right with the fingers of the left hand; with the right-hand fingers, palpate laterally for the right lobe of the thyroid in the space between the displaced trachea and the relaxed sternomastoid. Find the lateral margin. In similar fashion, examine the left lobe.

  The lobes are somewhat harder to feel than the isthmus, so practice is needed. The anterior surface of a lateral lobe is approximately the size of the distal phalanx of the thumb and feels somewhat rubbery.

- Note the *size, shape,* and *consistency* of the gland and identify any *nodules* or *tenderness*.

  If the thyroid gland is enlarged, listen over the lateral lobes with a stethoscope to detect a *bruit,* a sound similar to a cardiac murmur but of noncardiac origin.

Although physical characteristics of the thyroid gland, such as size, shape, and consistency, are diagnostically important, assessment of thyroid function depends upon symptoms, signs elsewhere in the body, and laboratory tests.[25] See Table 7-26, Thyroid Enlargement and Function (p. 281).

Soft in *Graves' disease;* firm in *Hashimoto's thyroiditis,* malignancy. Benign and malignant nodules,[26,27] tenderness in thyroiditis

A localized systolic or continuous bruit may be heard in *hyperthyroidism.*

The Carotid Arteries and Jugular Veins.   Defer a detailed examination of these vessels until the patient lies down for the cardiovascular examination. Jugular venous distention, however, may be visible in the sitting position and should not be overlooked. You should also be alert to unusually prominent arterial pulsations. See Chapter 9 for further discussion.

Note: Many clinicians would complete examination of the cranial nerves (see pp. 672–678) at this point.

SPECIAL TECHNIQUES

For Assessing Protruding Eyes (Proptosis or Exophthalmos).   For eyes that seem unusually prominent, stand behind the seated patient and inspect from above. Draw the upper lids gently upward, then compare the protrusion of the eyes and the relationship of the corneas to the lower lids. For objective measurement, use an exophthalmometer. This instrument measures the distance between the lateral angle of the orbit and an imaginary line across the most anterior point of the cornea. The upper limits of normal are 20 mm in whites and 22 mm in blacks.[28,29]

Exophthalmos is an abnormal protrusion of the eye.

When protrusion exceeds normal, further evaluation by ultrasound or computerized tomography scan often follows.[30]

For Nasolacrimal Duct Obstruction.   This test helps identify the cause of excessive tearing. Ask the patient to look up. Press on the lower lid close to the medial canthus, just inside the rim of the bony orbit—this compresses the lacrimal sac. Look for fluid regurgitated out of the puncta into the eye. Avoid this test if the area is inflamed and tender.

Discharge of mucopurulent fluid from the puncta suggests an obstructed nasolacrimal duct.

For Inspection of the Upper Palpebral Conjunctiva.   Adequate examination of the eye in search of a foreign body requires eversion of the upper eyelid. Follow these steps:

● Instruct the patient to look down. Get the patient to relax the eyes—by reassurance and by gentle, assured, and deliberate movements. Raise the upper eyelid slightly so that the eyelashes protrude, and then grasp the upper eyelashes and pull them gently down and forward.

● Place a small stick such as an applicator or a tongue blade at least 1 cm above the lid margin (and therefore at the upper border of the tarsal plate). Push down on the stick as you raise the edge of the lid, thus everting the eyelid or turning it "inside out." Do not press on the eyeball itself.

● Secure the upper lashes against the eyebrow with your thumb and inspect the palpebral conjunctiva. After your inspection, grasp the upper eyelashes and pull them gently forward. Ask the patient to look up. The eyelid will return to its normal position.

This view allows you to see the upper palpebral conjunctiva and look for a foreign body that might be lodged there.

Swinging Flashlight Test. The swinging flashlight test is a clinical test for functional impairment in the optic nerves. In dim light, note the size of the pupils. After asking the patient to gaze into the distance, swing the beam of a penlight first into one pupil, then into the other. Normally, each illuminated eye promptly becomes constricted. The opposite eye also constricts consensually.

Direct | Consensual | Consensual | "Dilation"
RIGHT | LEFT | RIGHT | LEFT
(optic nerve damage)

If left-sided optic nerve damage is present, the pupils will usually behave as follows: When the light is shown into the normal right eye, there is brisk pupillary constriction of both pupils (direct response on the right and a consensual response on the left). When the light is then swung over to the abnormal left eye, partial dilation of both pupils will occur. The afferent stimulus on the left is reduced; thus, the efferent signals to both pupils will also be reduced and a net dilation will occur. This demonstrates what is known as an afferent pupillary defect, sometimes also known as a *Marcus Gunn pupil*.

Transillumination of the Sinuses. When sinus tenderness or other symptoms suggest sinusitis, this test may be helpful but is not highly sensitive or specific for diagnosis. The room should be dark. Using a strong, narrow light source, place the light snugly deep under each brow, close to the nose. Shield the light with your hand. Look for a dim red glow as light is transmitted through the air-filled frontal sinus to the forehead.

Absence of glow on one or both sides suggests a thickened mucosa or secretions in the frontal sinus, but it may also result from developmental absence of one or both sinuses.

Ask the patient to tilt his or her head back with mouth opened wide. (An upper denture should first be removed.) Shine the light downward from just below the inner aspect of each eye. Look through the open mouth at the hard palate. A reddish glow indicates a normal air-filled maxillary sinus.

Absence of glow suggests thickened mucosa or secretions in the maxillary sinus. See p. 230 for an alternative method of transilluminating the maxillary sinuses.

RECORDING YOUR FINDINGS

Note that initially you may use sentences to describe your findings; later you will use phrases. The style below contains phrases appropriate for most write-ups.

Recording the Physical Examination—
The Head, Eyes, Ears, Nose, and Throat (HEENT)

HEENT: Head—The skull is normocephalic/atraumatic (NC/AT). Hair with average texture. *Eyes*—Visual acuity 20/20 bilaterally. Sclera white, conjunctiva pink. Pupils are 4 mm constricting to 2 mm, equally round and reactive to light and accommodations. Disc margins sharp; no hemorrhages or exudates, no arteriolar narrowing. *Ears*—Acuity good to whispered voice. Tympanic membranes (TMs) with good cone of light. Weber midline. AC > BC. *Nose*—Nasal mucosa pink, septum midline; no sinus tenderness. *Throat (or Mouth)*—Oral mucosa pink, dentition good, pharynx without exudates.

Neck—Trachea midline. Neck supple; thyroid isthmus palpable, lobes not felt.

Lymph Nodes—No cervical, axillary, epitrochlear, inguinal adenopathy.

OR

Head—The skull is normocephalic/atraumatic. Frontal balding. *Eyes*—Visual acuity 20/100 bilaterally. Sclera white; conjunctiva injected. Pupils constrict 3 mm to 2 mm, equally round and reactive to light and accommodation. Disc margins sharp; no hemorrhages or exudates. Arteriolar-to-venous ratio (AV ratio) 2:4; no A-V nicking. *Ears*—Acuity diminished to whispered voice; intact to spoken voice. TMs clear. *Nose*—Mucosa swollen with erythema and clear drainage. Septum midline. Tender over maxillary sinuses. *Throat*—Oral mucosa pink, dental caries in lower molars, pharynx erythematous, no exudates.

Neck—Trachea midline. Neck supple; thyroid isthmus midline, lobes palpable but not enlarged.

Lymph Nodes—Submandibular and anterior cervical lymph nodes tender, 1 × 1 cm, rubbery and mobile; no posterior cervical, epitrochlear, axillary, or inguinal lymphadenopathy.

Suggests myopia and mild arteriolar narrowing. Also upper respiratory infection.

BIBLIOGRAPHY

CITATIONS

1. Taylor FR. Diagnosis and classification of headache. Primary Care: Clinics in Office Practice 31(2):243–259, 2004.

2. Lipton RB, Stewart WF, Seymour D, et al. Prevalence and burden of migraine in the United States: data from the American Migraine Study II. Headache 41(7):646–657, 2001.

3. Lipton RB, Bigal ME, Steiner TJ, et al. Classification of primary headaches. Neurology 63(3):427–435, 2004.

4. Zwart JA, Dyb G, Hagen K, et al. Analgesic use: a predictor of chronic pain and medication overuse: the Head-HUNT Study. Neurology 61:160–164, 2003.

5. Shingleton BJ, O'Donoghue MW. Blurred vision. N Engl J Med 343(8):556–562, 2000.

6. Coleman AC. Glaucoma. Lancet 20:1803–1810, 1999.

7. Balcer LJ. Optic neuritis. N Engl J Med 354(12):1273–1280, 2006.

8. deJong PTVM. Age-related macular degeneration. N Engl J Med 355(14):1474–1485, 2006.

9. Willems PJ. Genetic causes of hearing loss. N Engl J Med 342(15):1101–1109, 2000.

10. Hendley JO. Otitis media. N Engl J Med 347(15):1169–1174, 2002.

11. Plaut M, Valentine MD. Allergic rhinitis. N Engl J Med 353(18):1934–1944, 2005.

12. Piccirillo JF. Acute bacterial sinusitis. N Engl J Med 351(9):902–910, 2004.

13. Spector SL, Bernstein IL, Li JT, et al. Parameters for the diagnosis and management of sinusitis. J Allergy Clin Immunol 102(6, Part 2):S107–S144, 1998.

14. Williams JW, Simel DL, Roberts L, et al. Clinical evaluation for sinusitis: making the diagnosis by history and physical examination. Ann Intern Med 117(9):705–710, 1992.

15. Cooper RJ, Hoffman JR, Bartlett JG, et al. Principles of appropriate antibiotic use for acute pharyngitis in adults: background. Ann Intern Med 134(6):509–517, 2001.

16. McGinn TG, Deluca J, Ahlawat SK, et al. Validation and modification of streptococcal pharyngitis clinical prediction rules. Mayo Clin Proc 78(3):289–293, 2003.

17. U.S. Preventive Services Task Force. Screening for visual impairment. In Guide to Clinical Preventive Services, 2nd ed. Baltimore: Williams & Wilkins, 1996:373–382.

18. U.S. Preventive Services Task Force. Screening for glaucoma: recommendation statement. AHRQ Publication No. 04-0548-A, March 2005. Rockville, MD, Agency for Healthcare Research and Quality, http://www.ahrq.gov/clinic/uspstf05/glaucoma/glaucrs.htm.

19. Jackler JK. A 73-year-old man with hearing loss. JAMA 289(12):1557–1565, 2003. Accessed August 28, 2007.

20. U.S. Preventive Services Task Force. Screening for hearing impairment. In Guide to Clinical Preventive Services, 2nd ed. Baltimore: Williams & Wilkins, 1996:393–405.

21. U.S. Preventive Services Task Force. Counseling to prevent dental and periodontal disease. In Guide to Clinical Preventive Services, 2nd ed. Baltimore: Williams & Wilkins, 1996:711–721.

22. Gupta R, Pery M. Digital examination for oral cancer. BMJ 319:1113–1114, 1999.

23. McGuirt WF. The neck mass. Med Clin N Am 83:219–234, 1989.

24. Siminoski K. Does this patient have a goiter? JAMA 273(10):813–817, 1995.

25. Surks MI, Ortiz E, Daniels GH, et al. Subclinical thyroid disease: scientific review and guidelines for diagnosis and management. JAMA 291(2):228–238, 2004.

26. Hegedus L. The thyroid nodule. N Engl J Med 351(17):1764–1771, 2004.

27. Castro MR, Gharib H. Controversies in the management of thyroid nodules. Ann Intern Med 142(11):926–931, 2005.

28. Gladstone GJ. Ophthalmologic aspects of thyroid-related orbitopathy. Endocrinol Metab Clin North Am 27:91–100, 1998.

29. Bartley GB, et al. Clinical features of Graves' ophthalmopathy in an incidence cohort. Am J Ophthalmol 121:284–290, 1996.

30. Hallin ES, Feldon SE. Graves' ophthalmopathy. II. Correlation of clinical signs with measures derived from computed tomography. Br J Ophthalmol 72:678–682, 1988.

31. Goadsby PJ, Lipton RB, Ferrari MD. Migraine: current understanding and treatment. N Engl J Med 346(4):257–270, 2002.

32. Smetana GW, Shmerling RH. Does this patient have temporal arteritis? JAMA 287(1):92–101, 2002.

33. Kroenke K, Lucas CA, Rosengerg ML, et al. Causes of persistent dizziness: a prospective study of 100 patients in ambulatory care. Ann Intern Med 117(11):898–904, 1992.

34. Kroenke K, Hoffman RM, Einstadter D. How common are various causes of dizziness? A critical review. South Med J 93(2):160–167, 2000.

35. Tusa RJ. Vertigo. Neurol Clin 19(1):23–55, 2001.

36. Branch W. Approach to the patient with dizziness. Available at: www.utdol.com. Accessed February 26, 2005.

37. Lockwood AH, Salvi RJ, Burkard RF. Tinnitus. N Engl J Med 347(12):904–910, 2002.

38. Matthies C, Samii M. Management of 1000 vestibular schwannomas (acoustic neuromas): clinical presentation. Neurosurgery 1:1–10, 1997.

39. Leibowitz HM. The red eye. N Engl J Med 342(5):345–351, 2000.

40. Wong TY, Mitchell P. Hypertensive retinopathy. N Engl J Med 351(22):2310–2317, 2004.

41. Frank RB. Diabetic retinopathy. N Engl J Med 350(1):48–58, 2004.

BIBLIOGRAPHY

ADDITIONAL REFERENCES

The Head

Bahra A, May A. Cluster headache: a prospective clinical study with diagnostic implications. Neurology 58(3):354–361, 2002.

Cady RK, Dodick DW, Levine HL, et al. Sinus headache: a neurology, otolaryngology, allergy, and primary care consensus on diagnosis and treatment. Mayo Clin Proc 80(7):908–916, 2005.

Evans RW. Headache case studies for the primary care physician. Med Clin North Am 87(3):589–607, 2003.

Franges EZ. When a headache is really a brain tumor. Nurse Pract 31(4):47–51, 2006.

Lipton RB, Bigal ME, Steiner TJ, et al. Classification of primary headaches. Neurology 63(3):427–435, 2004.

Paemeleire K, Bahra A, Evers S, et al. Medication-overuse headache in patients with cluster headache. Neurology 67(1):109–113, 2006.

Straus SE, Thorpe KE, Holroyd-Leduc J. How do I perform a lumbar puncture and analyze the results to diagnose bacterial meningitis? JAMA 296(16):2012–2022, 2006.

Van Gijn J, Kerr RS, Rinkel GJ. Subarachnoid haemorrhage. Lancet 369(9558):306–318, 2007.

Wong TY, Klein R, Sharrett AR, et al. Retinal arteriolar diameter and risk for hypertension. Ann Intern Med 140(4):248–255, 2004.

The Eye

Albert DM, Miller JW, Azar DT. Albert & Jakobiec's Principles and Practice of Ophthalmology, 3rd ed. Philadelphia: Saunders–Elsevier, 2008.

Congdon N, O'Colmain, Klaver CC, et al. Causes and prevalence of visual impairment among adults in the United States. Arch Ophthalmol 122(4):477–485, 2004.

Ehlers JP, Shah CP, Chirag P, et al., eds. The Wills Eye Manual: Office and Emergency Room Diagnosis and Treatment of Eye Disease. Philadelphia: Lippincott Williams & Wilkins, 2008.

Fong DS, Aiello LP, Ferris FL, et al. Diabetic retinopathy. Diabetes Care 27(10):2540–2553, 2004.

Gold DH, Weingeist TA. Color Atlas of the Eye in Systemic Disease. Philadelphia: Lippincott Williams & Wilkins, 2001.

McCluskey PJ, Towler HM, Lightman S. Management of chronic uveitis. BMJ 320(7234):555–558, 2000.

Mohamed Q, Gillies MC, Wong TY. Management of diabetic retinopathy. JAMA 298(8):902–916, 2007.

Ostler HB, Maibach HI, Hoke AW, et al. Diseases of the Eye and Skin: A Color Atlas. Philadelphia: Lippincott Williams & Wilkins, 2004.

Spoor TC, ed. Atlas of Neuro-ophthalmology. New York: Taylor & Francis, 2004.

Tasman W, Jaeger EA. The Wills Eye Hospital Atlas of Clinical Ophthalmology, 2nd ed. Philadelphia: Lippincott Williams & Wilkins, 2001.

Yanoff M, Duker JS. Ophthalmology, 2nd ed. St. Louis: Mosby, 2004.

The Ears, Nose, and Throat

Bagai A, Thavendiranathan P, Detsky AS. Does this patient have hearing impairment? JAMA 295(4):416–428, 2006.

Bevan Y, Shapiro N, MacLean CH, et al. Screening and management of adult hearing loss in primary care: scientific review. JAMA 289(15):1976–1985, 2003.

Bull TR. Color Atlas of ENT Diagnosis, 4th ed. New York: Thieme, 2003.

Cady RK, Dodick DW, Levine HL, et al. Sinus headache: a neurology, otolaryngology, allergy, and primary care consensus on diagnosis and treatment. Mayo Clin Proc 80(7):908–916, 2005.

Ebell MH, Smith MA, Barry HC, et al. Does this patient have strep throat? JAMA 284(22):2912–2918, 2000.

Hendley JO. Otitis media. N Engl J Med 347(15):1169–1174, 2002.

Kennedy DW. A 48-year-old man with recurrent sinusitis. JAMA 283(16):2143–2150, 2000.

O'Donoghue GM, Narula AA, Bates GJ. Clinical ENT: An Illustrated Textbook, 2nd ed. San Diego: Singular Publishing Group, 2000.

Patil SP, Schneider H, Schwartz AR, et al. Adult obstructive sleep apnea: pathophysiology and diagnosis. Chest 132(1):325–337, 2007.

Young T, Skatrud J, Peppard PE. Risk factors for obstructive sleep apnea in adults. JAMA 291(16):2013–2016, 2004.

The Mouth

Field EA, Longman L, Tyldesley WR, et al. Tyldesley's Oral Medicine, 5th ed. New York: Oxford University Press, 2003.

Langlais RP, Miller CS. Color Atlas of Common Oral Diseases, 3rd ed. Philadelphia: Lippincott Williams & Wilkins, 2003.

Newman MF, Carranza FA, Takei H, et al. Carranza's Clinical Periodontology, 10th ed. Philadelphia: Saunders–Elsevier, 2006.

Regezi JA, Sciubba JJ, Jordan RCK. Oral Pathology: Clinical Pathologic Correlations, 5th ed. St. Louis: Saunders–Elsevier, 2008.

The Neck

Bliss SJ, Flanders SA, Saint S. A pain in the neck. N Engl J Med 350(10):1037–1042, 2004.

Dorshimer GW, Kelly M. Cervical pain in the athlete: common conditions and treatment. Prim Care 32(1):231–243, 2005.

Henry PH, Long DL. Enlargement of the lymph nodes and spleen. In: Kasper DL, Fauci AS, Longo DL, et al., eds. Harrison's Principles of Internal Medicine, 16th ed. New York: McGraw-Hill, 2005:343–348.

Prisco MK. Evaluating neck masses. Nurse Pract 25(4):30–32, 35–36, 38, 2000.

Schwetschenau E, Kelley DJ. The adult neck mass. Am Fam Phys 67(6):1190, 1192, 1195, 2003.

The Bates' suite offers these additional resources to enhance learning and facilitate understanding of this chapter:

- *Bates' Pocket Guide to Physical Examination and History Taking,* 6th edition
- *Bates' Nursing Online*
- *Bates' Visual Guide to Physical Examination,* 4th edition
- thePoint online resources, http://thepoint.lww.com
- Student CD-ROM included with the book

TABLE
7-1

Primary Headaches[1, 3, 31]

	Migraines	Tension	Cluster
	• With aura • Without aura • Variants		
Process	Primary neuronal dysfunction, possibly of brainstem origin, causing imbalance of excitatory and inhibitory neurotransmitters and affecting craniovascular modulation	Unclear—muscle contraction or vasoconstriction unlikely	Unclear—possibly extracranial vasodilation from neural dysfunction with trigeminovascular pain
Location	Unilateral in ~70%; bifrontal or global in ~30%	Usually bilateral; may be generalized or localized to the back of the head and upper neck or to the frontotemporal area	Unilateral, usually behind or around the eye
Quality and Severity	Throbbing or aching, variable in severity.	Pressing or tightening pain; mild to moderate intensity	Deep, continuous, severe
Timing			
Onset	Fairly rapid, reaching a peak in 1–2 hours	Gradual	Abrupt; peaks within minutes
Duration	4–72 hours	Minutes to days	Up to 3 hours
Course	Peak incidence early to mid-adolescence; prevalence is ~6% in men and ~15% in women. Recurrent—usually monthly, but weekly in ~10%	Often recurrent of persistent over long periods; annual prevalence ~40%	Episodic, clustered in time, with several each day for 4–8 weeks and then relief for 6–12 months; prevalence <1%, more common in men.
Associated Factors	Nausea, vomiting, photophobia, phonophobia, visual auras flickering, zigzagging lines), motor auras affecting hand or arm, sensory auras (numbness, tingling usually precede attack)	Sometimes photophobia, phonophobia; nausea absent	Lacrimation, rhinorrhea, mioisis, ptosis, eyelid edema, conjunctival infection
Factors That Aggravate or Provoke	Alcohol, certain foods, or tension may provoke; more common premenstrually; aggravated by noise and bright light	Sustained muscle tension, as in driving or typing	During attack, sensitivity to alcohol may increase
Factors That Relieve	Quiet, dark room; sleep; sometimes transient relief from pressure on the involved artery, if early in the course	Possibly massage, relaxation	

Secondary Headaches[3]; Cranial Neuralgias

Type	Process	Location	Quality and Severity
Secondary Headaches			
Analgesic Rebound	Withdrawal of medication	Previous headache pattern	Variable
Headaches From Eye Disorders			
Errors of Refraction (farsightedness and astigmatism, but not nearsightedness)	Probably the sustained contraction of the extraocular muscles, and possibly of the frontal, temporal, and occipital muscles	Around and over the eyes; may radiate to the occipital area	Steady, aching, dull
Acute Glaucoma	Sudden increase in intraocular pressure (see p. 257)	In and around one eye	Steady, aching, often severe
Headache From Sinusitis	Mucosal inflammation of the paranasal sinuses	Usually above the eye (frontal sinus) or over the maxillary sinus	Aching or throbbing, variable in severity; consider possible migraine
Meningitis	Infection of the meninges surrounding the brain	Generalized	Steady or throbbing, very severe
Subarachnoid Hemorrhage	Bleeding, most often from a ruptured intracranial aneurysm	Generalized	Very severe, "the worst of my life"
Brain Tumor	Displacement of or traction on pain-sensitive arteries and veins or pressure on nerves	Varies with the location of the tumor	Aching, steady, variable in intensity
Giant Cell (Temporal) Arteritis[32]	Vasculitis from cell-mediated immune response to elastic lamina of artery	Localized near the involved artery, most often the temporal, but also the occipital; age related	Throbbing, generalized, persistent; often severe
Posttraumatic Headache	Mechanism unclear; episodes similar to tension-type and migraine without aura headaches[24]	May be localized to the injured area, but not necessarily	Generalized, dull, aching, constant
Cranial Neuralgias			
Trigeminal Neuralgia (CNV)	Compression of CN V, often by aberrant loop or artery of vein	Cheek, jaws, lips, or gums; trigeminal nerve divisions 2 and 3 > 1	Shocklike, stabbing, burning; severe

Note: Blanks appear in this table when the categories are not applicable or not usually helpful in assessing the problem.

Timing			Associated Factors	Factors That Aggravate or Provoke	Factors That Relieve
Onset	Duration	Course			
Variable	Depends on prior headache pattern	Depends on frequency of "mini-withdrawals"	Depends on prior headache pattern	Fever, carbon monoxide, hypoxia, withdrawal of caffeine, other headache triggers	Depends on cause
Gradual	Variable	Variable	Eye fatigue, "sandy" sensations in the eyes, redness of the conjunctiva	Prolonged use of the eyes, particularly for close work	Rest of the eyes
Often rapid	Variable, may depend on treatment	Variable, may depend on treatment	Diminished vision, sometimes nausea and vomiting	Sometimes provoked by drops that dilate the pupils	
Variable	Often several hours at a time, recurring over days or longer	Often recurrent in a repetitive daily pattern	Local tenderness, nasal congestion, discharge, and fever	May be aggravated by coughing, sneezing, or jarring the head	Nasal decongestants, antibiotics
Fairly rapid	Variable, usually days	A persistent headache in an acute illness	Fever, stiff neck		
Usually abrupt, severe; prodromal symptoms may occur	Variable, usually days	A persistent headache in an acute illness	Nausea, vomiting, possibly loss of consciousness, neck pain		
Variable	Often brief	Often intermittent but progressive	May be aggravated by coughing, sneezing, or sudden movements of the head		
Gradual or rapid	Variable	Recurrent or persistent over weeks to months	Tenderness of the adjacent scalp; fever (in ~50%), fatigue, weight loss; new headache (~60%), jaw claudication (~50%), visual loss or blindness (~15%–20%), polymyalgia rheumatica (~50%)	Movement of neck and shoulders	
Within hours to 1–2 days of the injury	Weeks, months, or even years	Tends to diminish over time	Poor concentration, problems with memory, vertigo, irritability, restlessness, fatigue	Mental and physical exertion, straining, stooping, emotional excitement, alcohol	Rest
Abrupt, paroxysmal	Each jab lasts seconds but recurs at intervals of seconds or minutes	May last for months, then disappear for months, but often recurs. It is uncommon at night.	Exhaustion from recurrent pain	Touching certain areas of the lower face or mouth; chewing, talking, brushing teeth	

TABLE
7-3

Dizziness and Vertigo[33-38]

"Dizziness" is a nonspecific term used by patients encompassing several disorders that clinicians must carefully sort out. A detailed history usually identifies the primary etiology. It is important to learn the specific meanings of the following terms or conditions:

- *Vertigo*—a spinning sensation accompanied by nystagmus and ataxia; usually from *peripheral vestibular dysfunction* (~40% of "dizzy" patients) but may be from a *central brainstem lesion* (~10%; causes include atherosclerosis, multiple sclerosis, vertebrobasilar migraine, or TIA)
- *Presyncope*—a near faint from "feeling faint or lightheaded"; causes include orthostatic hypotension, especially from medication, arrhythmias, and vasovagal attacks (~5%)
- *Dysequilibrium*—unsteadiness or imbalance when walking, especially in older patients (see p. 901); causes include fear of walking, visual loss, weakness from musculoskeletal problems, and peripheral neuropathy (up to 15%)
- *Psychiatric*—causes include anxiety, panic disorder, hyperventilation, depression, somatization disorder, alcohol, and substance abuse (~10%)
- *Multifactorial or unknown*—(up to 20%)

Peripheral and Central Vertigo

	Onset	Duration and Course	Hearing	Tinnitus	Additional Features
Peripheral Vertigo					
■ *Benign Positional Vertigo*	Sudden, on rolling onto affected side or tilting head up	Onset a few seconds to <1 minute. Lasts a few weeks, may recur	Not affected	Absent	Sometimes nausea, vomiting Nystagmus
■ *Vestibular Neuronitis (acute labyrinthitis)*	Sudden	Onset hours to up to 2 weeks. May recur over 12–18 months	Not affected	Absent	Nausea, vomiting, nystagmus
■ *Ménière's Disease*	Sudden	Onset several hours to ≥1 day. Recurrent	Sensorineural hearing loss—recurs, eventually progresses	Present, fluctuating	Pressure or fullness in affected ear; nausea, vomiting, nystagmus
■ *Drug Toxicity*	Insidious or acute—linked to loop diuretics, aminoglycosides, salicylates, alcohol	May or may not be reversible. Partial adaptation occurs	May be impaired	May be present	Nausea, vomiting
■ *Acoustic Neuroma*	Insidious from CN VIII compression, vestibular branch	Variable	Impaired, one side	Present	May involve CN V and VII
Central Vertigo	Often sudden (see causes above)	Variable but rarely continuous	Not affected	Absent	Usually with other brainstem deficits—dysarthria, ataxia, crossed motor and sensory deficits

Selected Facies

Facial Swelling

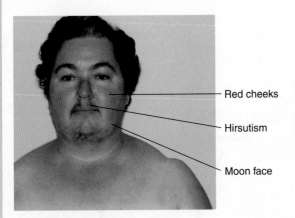

Red cheeks

Hirsutism

Moon face

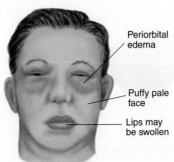

Periorbital edema

Puffy pale face

Lips may be swollen

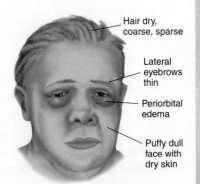

Hair dry, coarse, sparse

Lateral eyebrows thin

Periorbital edema

Puffy dull face with dry skin

Cushing's Syndrome
The increased adrenal cortisol production of Cushing's syndrome produces a round or "moon" face with red cheeks. Excessive hair growth may be present in the mustache and sideburn areas and on the chin.

Nephrotic Syndrome
The face is edematous and often pale. Swelling usually appears first around the eyes and in the morning. The eyes may become slitlike when edema is severe.

Myxedema
The patient with severe hypothyroidism (*myxedema*) has a dull, puffy facies. The edema, often pronounced around the eyes, does not pit with pressure. The hair and eyebrows are dry, coarse, and thinned. The skin is dry.

Other Facies

Swelling

Prominent brow

Enlarged soft tissues

Prominent jaw

Stare

Decreasd mobility

Parotid Gland Enlargement
Chronic bilateral asymptomatic parotid gland enlargement may be associated with obesity, diabetes, cirrhosis, and other conditions. Note the swellings anterior to the ear lobes and above the angles of the jaw. Gradual unilateral enlargement suggests neoplasm. Acute enlargement is seen in mumps.

Acromegaly
The increased growth hormone of acromegaly produces enlargement of both bone and soft tissues. The head is elongated, with bony prominence of the forehead, nose, and lower jaw. Soft tissues of the nose, lips, and ears also enlarge. The facial features appear generally coarsened.

Parkinson's Disease
Decreased facial mobility blunts expression. A masklike face may result, with decreased blinking and a characteristic stare. Since the neck and upper trunk tend to flex forward, the patient seems to peer upward toward the observer. Facial skin becomes oily, and drooling may occur.

TABLE
7-5
Visual Field Defects

Visual Field Defects

1 Horizontal Defect Occlusion of a branch of the central retinal artery may cause a horizontal (altitudinal) defect. Ischemia of the optic nerve also can produce a similar defect.

2 Blind Right Eye (right optic nerve) A lesion of the optic nerve, and of course of the eye itself, produces unilateral blindness.

3 Bitemporal Hemianopsia (optic chiasm) A lesion at the optic chiasm may involve only fibers crossing over to the opposite side. Since these fibers originate in the nasal half of each retina, visual loss involves the temporal half of each field.

4 Left Homonymous Hemianopsia (right optic tract) A lesion of the optic tract interrupts fibers originating on the same side of both eyes. Visual loss in the eyes is therefore similar (homonymous) and involves half of each field (hemianopsia).

5 Homonymous Left Superior Quadrantic Defect (right optic radiation, partial) A partial lesion of the optic radiation in the temporal lobe may involve only a portion of the nerve fibers, producing, for example, a homonymous quadrantic defect.

6 Left Homonymous Hemianopsia (right optic radiation) A complete interruption of fibers in the optic radiation produces a visual defect similar to that produced by a lesion of the optic tract.

TABLE
7-6

Variations and Abnormalities of the Eyelids

Ptosis

Ptosis is a drooping of the upper lid. Causes include myasthenia gravis, damage to the oculomotor nerve, and damage to the sympathetic nerve supply (*Horner's syndrome*). A weakened muscle, relaxed tissues, and the weight of herniated fat may cause senile ptosis. Ptosis may also be congenital.

Entropion

Entropion, more common in the elderly, is an inward turning of the lid margin. The lower lashes, which are often invisible when turned inward, irritate the conjunctiva and lower cornea. Asking the patient to squeeze the lids together and then open them may reveal an entropion that is not obvious.

Ectropion

In ectropion the margin of the lower lid is turned outward, exposing the palpebral conjunctiva. When the punctum of the lower lid turns outward, the eye no longer drains satisfactorily, and tearing occurs. Ectropion is more common in the elderly.

Lid Retraction and Exophthalmos

A wide-eyed stare suggests retracted eyelids. Note the rim of sclera between the upper lid and the iris. Retracted lids and a lid lag (p. 217) are often due to hyperthyroidism.

In exophthalmos the eyeball protrudes forward. When bilateral, it suggests the infiltrative ophthalmopathy of Graves' hyperthyroidism. Edema of the eyelids and conjunctival injection may be associated. Unilateral exophthalmos is seen in Graves' disease or a tumor or inflammation in the orbit.

(Source of photos: *Ptosis, Ectropion, Entropion*—Tasman W, Jaeger E, eds. The Wills Eye Hospital Atlas of Clinical Ophthalmology, 2nd ed. Philadelphia, Lippincott Williams & Wilkins, 2001.)

Lumps and Swellings in and Around the Eyes

Pinguecula

A harmless yellowish triangular nodule in the bulbar conjunctiva on either side of the iris. Appears frequently with aging, first on the nasal and then on the temporal side.

Episcleritis

A localized ocular redness from inflammation of the episcleral vessels. Vessels appear pink and are movable over the scleral surface. May be nodular, as shown, or may show only redness and dilated vessels.

Sty

A painful, tender red infection in a gland at the margin of the eyelid.

Chalazion

A subacute nontender and usually painless nodule involving a meibomian gland. May become acutely inflamed but, unlike a sty, usually points inside the lid rather than on the lid margin.

Xanthelasma

Slightly raised, yellowish, well-circumscribed plaques that appear along the nasal portions of one or both eyelids. May accompany lipid disorders.

Inflammation of the Lacrimal Sac (Dacryocystitis)

A swelling between the lower eyelid and nose. An *acute* inflammation (illustrated) is painful, red, and tender. *Chronic* inflammation is associated with obstruction of the nasolacrimal duct. Tearing is prominent, and pressure on the sac produces regurgitation of material through the puncta of the eyelids.

(Source of photos: Tasman W, Jaeger E, eds. The Wills Eye Hospital Atlas of Clinical Ophthalmology, 2nd ed. Philadelphia, Lippincott Williams & Wilkins, 2001.)

TABLE 7-8

Red Eyes[39]

Conjunctivitis

Subconjunctival Hemorrhage

	Conjunctivitis	Subconjunctival Hemorrhage
Pattern of Redness	Conjunctival injection: diffuse dilatation of conjunctival vessels with redness that tends to be maximal peripherally	Leakage of blood outside of the vessels, producing a homogeneous, sharply demarcated, red area that fades over days to yellow and then disappears
Pain	Mild discomfort rather than pain	Absent
Vision	Not affected except for temporary mild blurring due to discharge	Not affected
Ocular Discharge	Watery, mucoid, or mucopurulent	Absent
Pupil	Not affected	Not affected
Cornea	Clear	Clear
Significance	Bacterial, viral, and other infections; allergy; irritation	Often none. May result from trauma, bleeding disorders, or a sudden increase in venous pressure, as from cough

Corneal Injury or Infection

Acute Iritis

Glaucoma

	Corneal Injury or Infection	Acute Iritis	Glaucoma
Pattern of Redness	Ciliary injection: dilation of deeper vessels that are visible as radiating vessels or a reddish violet flush around the limbus. Ciliary injection is an important sign of these three conditions but may not be apparent. The eye may be diffusely red instead. Other clues of these more serious disorders are pain, decreased vision, unequal pupils, and a less than perfectly clear cornea.		
Pain	Moderate to severe, superficial	Moderate, aching, deep	Severe, aching, deep
Vision	Usually decreased	Decreased	Decreased
Ocular Discharge	Watery or purulent	Absent	Absent
Pupil	Not affected unless iritis develops	May be small and, with time, irregular	Dilated, fixed
Cornea	Changes depending on cause	Clear or slightly clouded	Steamy, cloudy
Significance	Abrasions, and other injuries; viral and bacterial infections	Associated with many ocular and systemic disorders	Acute increase in intraocular pressure—an emergency

TABLE
7-9

Opacities of the Cornea and Lens

Corneal Arcus. A thin grayish white arc or circle not quite at the edge of the cornea. Accompanies normal aging but also seen in younger people, especially African-Americans. In young people, suggests possible hyperlipoproteinemia. Usually benign.

Corneal Scar. A superficial grayish white opacity in the cornea, secondary to an old injury or to inflammation. Size and shape are variable. Do not confuse with the opaque lens of a cataract, visible on a deeper plane and only through the pupil.

Pterygium. A triangular thickening of the bulbar conjunctiva that grows slowly across the outer surface of the cornea, usually from the nasal side. Reddening may occur. May interfere with vision as it encroaches on the pupil.

Cataracts. Opacities of the lenses visible through the pupil; most common in old age.

Nuclear cataract. A nuclear cataract looks gray when seen by a flashlight. If the pupil is widely dilated, the gray opacity is surrounded by a black rim.

Peripheral cataract. Produces spokelike shadows that point inward—gray against black, as seen with a flashlight, or black against red with an ophthalmoscope. A dilated pupil, as shown here, facilitates this observation.

Pupillary Abnormalities

Unequal Pupils *(Anisocoria)*—When anisocoria is greater in bright light than in dim light, the larger pupil cannot constrict properly. Causes include blunt trauma to the eye, open-angle glaucoma (p. 257), and impaired parasympathetic nerve supply to the iris, as in tonic pupil and oculomotor nerve paralysis. When anisocoria is greater in dim light, the smaller pupil cannot dilate properly, as in Horner's syndrome, caused by an interruption of the sympathetic nerve supply. See also Table 17-12, Pupils in Comatose Patients, p. 732.

Tonic Pupil *(Adie's Pupil).* Pupil is large, regular, and usually unilateral. Reaction to light is severely reduced and slowed, or even absent. Near reaction, although very slow, is present. Slow accommodation causes blurred vision. Deep tendon reflexes are often decreased.

Oculomotor Nerve (CN III) Paralysis. The dilated pupil is fixed to light and near effort. Ptosis of the upper eyelid and lateral deviation of the eye are almost always present.

Horner's Syndrome. The affected pupil, though small, reacts briskly to light and near effort. Ptosis of the eyelid is present, perhaps with loss of sweating on the forehead. In congenital Horner's syndrome, the involved iris is lighter in color than its fellow (*heterochromia*).

Small, Irregular Pupils. Small, irregular pupils that accommodate but do not react to light indicate *Argyll Robertson pupils*. Seen in central nervous system syphilis.

Equal Pupils and One Blind Eye. Unilateral blindness does not cause anisocoria as long as the sympathetic and parasympathetic innervation to both irises is normal. A light directed into the seeing eye produces a direct reaction in that eye and a consensual reaction in the blind eye. A light directed into the blind eye, however, causes no response in either eye.

Blind eye

Light

Blind eye

Light

TABLE 7-11

Dysconjugate Gaze

There are a variety of gaze abnormality patterns that give clinicians clues about developmental disorders and cranial nerve abnormalities.

Developmental Disorders

Developmental dysconjugate gaze is caused by an imbalance in ocular muscle tone. This imbalance has many causes, may be hereditary, and usually appears in early childhood. These gaze deviations are classified according to direction:

Esotropia *Exotropia*

Cover–Uncover Test

A cover–uncover test may be helpful. Here is what you would see in the right monocular esotropia illustrated above.

Corneal reflections are asymmetric.

COVER

The right eye moves outward to fix on the light. (The left eye is not seen but moves inward to the same degree.)

UNCOVER

The left eye moves outward to fix on the light. The right eye deviates inward again.

Disorders of Cranial Nerves

New onset of dysconjugate gaze in adult life is usually the result of cranial nerve injuries, lesions, or abnormalities from such causes as trauma, multiple sclerosis, syphilis, and others.

A Left Cranial Nerve VI Paralysis

LOOKING TO THE RIGHT

Eyes are conjugate.

LOOKING STRAIGHT AHEAD

Esotropia appears.

LOOKING TO THE LEFT

Esotropia is maximum.

A Left Cranial Nerve IV Paralysis

LOOKING DOWN AND TO THE RIGHT

The left eye cannot look down when turned inward. Deviation is maximum in this direction.

A Left Cranial Nerve III Paralysis

LOOKING STRAIGHT AHEAD

The eye is pulled outward by action of the 6th nerve. Upward, downward, and inward movements are impaired or lost. Ptosis and pupillary dilation may be associated.

TABLE
7-12

Normal Variations of the Optic Disc

Physiologic Cupping

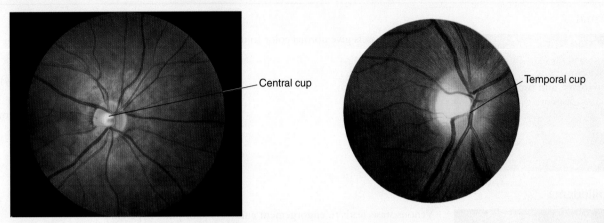

The physiologic cup is a small whitish depression in the optic disc, from which the retinal vessels appear to emerge. Although sometimes absent, the cup is usually visible either centrally or toward the temporal side of the disc. Grayish spots are often seen at its base.

Rings and Crescents

Rings and crescents are often seen around the optic disc. These are developmental variations in which you can glimpse either white sclera, black retinal pigment, or both, especially along the temporal border of the disc. Rings and crescents are not part of the disc itself and should not be included in your estimates of disc diameters.

Medullated Nerve Fibers

Medullated nerve fibers are a much less common but dramatic finding. Appearing as irregular white patches with feathered margins, they obscure the disc edge and retinal vessels. They have no pathologic significance.

TABLE
7-13

Abnormalities of the Optic Disc

	Process	Appearance

Normal

Tiny disc vessels give normal color to the disc.

Color yellowish orange to creamy pink

Disc vessels tiny

Disc margins sharp (except perhaps nasally)

The physiologic cup is located centrally or somewhat temporally. It may be conspicuous or absent. Its diameter from side to side is usually less than half that of the disc.

Papilledema

Venous stasis leads to engorgement and swelling.

Color pink, hyperemic

Often with loss of venous pulsations

Disc vessels more visible, more numerous, curve over the borders of the disc

Disc swollen with margins blurred

The physiologic cup is not visible.

Glaucomatous Cupping

Increased pressure within the eye leads to increased cupping (backward depression of the disc) and atrophy.

The base of the enlarged cup is pale.

The physiologic cup is enlarged, occupying more than half of the disc's diameter, at times extending to the edge of the disc. Retinal vessels sink in and under it, and may be displaced nasally.

Optic Atrophy

Death of optic nerve fibers leads to loss of the tiny disc vessels.

Color white

Tiny disc vessels absent

(Sources of photos for *Normal*—Tasman W, Jaeger E, eds. The Wills Eye Hospital Atlas of Clinical Ophthalmology, 2nd ed. Philadelphia, Lippincott Williams & Wilkins, 2001; *Papilledema, Glaucomatous Cupping, Optic Atrophy*—Courtesy of Ken Freedman, MD.)

TABLE
7-14

Retinal Arteries and Arteriovenous Crossings: Normal and Hypertensive

Normal Retinal Artery and Arteriovenous (A-V) Crossing

- Arterial wall (invisible)
- Column of blood
- Light reflex

The normal arterial wall is transparent. Only the column of blood within it can usually be seen. The normal light reflex is *narrow—about one fourth the diameter of the blood column.* Because the arterial wall is transparent, a vein crossing beneath the artery can be seen right up to the column of blood on either side.

- Vein
- Arterial wall
- Artery

Retinal Arteries in Hypertension

- Focal narrowing
- Narrowed column of blood
- Narrowed light reflex

In hypertension, the arteries may show areas of focal or generalized narrowing. The light reflex is also narrowed. The arterial wall thickens and becomes less transparent.

Copper Wiring

Sometimes the arteries, especially those close to the disc, become full and somewhat tortuous and develop an increased light reflex with a bright coppery luster.

Silver Wiring

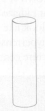

Occasionally a portion of a narrowed artery develops such an opaque wall that no blood is visible within it. It is then called a silver wire artery.

Arteriovenous Crossing

When the arterial walls lose their transparency, changes appear in the arteriovenous crossings. Decreased transparency of the retina probably also contributes to the first two changes shown below.

CONCEALMENT OR A-V NICKING

The vein appears to stop abruptly on either side of the artery.

TAPERING AND BANKING

Tapering. The vein appears to taper down on either side of the artery.

BANKING

Banking. The vein is twisted on the distal side of the artery and forms a dark, wide knuckle.

TABLE 7-15

Red Spots and Streaks in the Fundi

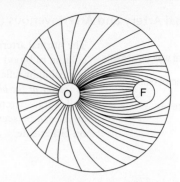

Superficial Retinal Hemorrhages—Small, linear, flame-shaped, red streaks in the fundi, shaped by the superficial bundles of nerve fibers that radiate from the optic disc in the pattern illustrated (O = optic disc; F = fovea). Sometimes the hemorrhages occur in clusters and look like a larger hemorrhage, but can be identified by the linear streaking at the edges. Superficial hemorrhages are seen in severe hypertension, papilledema, and occlusion of the retinal vein, among other conditions. An occasional superficial hemorrhage has a white center consisting of fibrin. White-centered retinal hemorrhages have many causes.

Preretinal Hemorrhage—Develops when blood escapes into the potential space between the retina and vitreous. This hemorrhage is typically larger than retinal hemorrhages. Because it is anterior to the retina, it obscures any underlying retinal vessels. In an erect patient, red cells settle, creating a horizontal line of demarcation between plasma above and cells below. Causes include a sudden increase in intracranial pressure.

Deep Retinal Hemorrhages—Small, rounded, slightly irregular red spots that are sometimes called dot or blot hemorrhages. They occur in a deeper layer of the retina than flame-shaped hemorrhages. Diabetes is a common cause.

Neovascularization—Refers to the formation of new blood vessels. They are more numerous, more tortuous, and narrower than other blood vessels in the area and form disorderly looking red arcades. A common cause is the late, proliferative stage of diabetic retinopathy. The vessels may grow into the vitreous, where retinal detachment or hemorrhage may cause loss of vision.

Microaneurysms—Tiny, round, red spots seen commonly but not exclusively in and around the macular area. They are minute dilatations of very small retinal vessels, but the vascular connections are too small to be seen ophthalmoscopically. They arise from diabetic retinopathy but have other causes.

(Source of photos: Tasman W, Jaeger E, eds. The Wills Eye Hospital Atlas of Clinical Ophthalmology, 2nd ed. Philadelphia, Lippincott Williams & Wilkins, 2001.)

TABLE
7-16

Ocular Fundi: Normal and Hypertensive Retinopathy[40]

Normal Fundus of a Fair-Skinned Person

Inspect the optic disc. Follow the major vessels in four directions, noting their relative sizes and any arteriovenous crossings—both normal here. Inspect the macular area. The slightly darker fovea is just discernible; no light reflex is visible in this subject. Look for any lesions in the retina. Note the striped, or tessellated, character of the fundus, especially in the lower field, that comes from normal underlying choroidal vessels.

Normal Fundus of a Dark-Skinned Person

Again, inspect the disc, vessels, macula, and retina. The ring around the fovea is a normal light reflection. The color of the fundus has a grayish brown, almost purplish cast, which comes from pigment in the retina and the choroid that characteristically obscures the choroidal vessels no; tessellation is visible. The fundus of a light-skinned person with brunette coloring is redder.

Hypertensive Retinopathy[40]

Marked arteriolar-venous crossing changes are seen, especially along the inferior vessels. Copper wiring of the arterioles is present. A cotton-wool spot is seen just superior to the disc. Incidental disc drusen are also present but are unrelated to hypertension.

Hypertensive Retinopathy With Macular Star

Punctate exudates are readily visible: some are scattered; others radiate from the fovea to form a macular star. Note the two small, soft exudates about 1 disc diameter from the disc. Find the flame-shaped hemorrhages sweeping toward 7 o'clock and 8 o'clock; a few more may be seen toward 10 o'clock. These fundi show changes typical of accelerated (malignant) hypertension and are often accompanied by a papilledema (p. 220).

(Source of photos: *Hypertensive Retinopathy, Hypertensive Retinopathy With Macular Star*—Tasman W, Jaeger E, eds. The Wills Eye Hospital Atlas of Clinical Ophthalmology, 2nd ed. Philadelphia, Lippincott Williams & Wilkins, 2001.)

TABLE
7-17

Ocular Fundi: Diabetic Retinopathy[41]

Diabetic Retinopathy

Study carefully the fundi in the series of photographs below. They represent a national standard used by ophthalmologists to assess diabetic retinopathy.

Nonproliferative Retinopathy, Moderately Severe

Note tiny red dots or microaneurysms. Note also the ring of hard exudates (white spots) located superotemporally. Retinal thickening or edema in the area of the hard exudates can impair visual acuity if it extends into the center of the macula (detection requires specialized stereoscopic examination).

Nonproliferative Retinopathy, Severe

In the superior temporal quadrant, note the large retinal hemorrhage between two cotton-wool patches, beading of the retinal vein just above them, and tiny tortuous retinal vessels above the superior temporal artery.

Proliferative Retinopathy, With Neovascularization

Note new preretinal vessels arising on the disc and extending across the disc margins. Visual acuity is still normal, but the risk for visual loss is high (photocoagulation reduces this risk by >50%).

Proliferative Retinopathy, Advanced

This is the same eye, but 2 years later and without treatment. Neovascularization has increased, now with fibrous proliferations, distortion of the macula, and reduced visual acuity.

(Source of photos: *Nonproliferative Retinopathy, Moderately Severe; Proliferative Retinopathy, With Neovascularization; Nonproliferative Retinopathy, Severe; Proliferative Retinopathy, Advanced*—Early Treatment Diabetic Retinopathy Study Research Group. Courtesy of MF Davis, MD, University of Wisconsin, Madison.)

TABLE
7-18

Light-Colored Spots in the Fundi

Soft Exudates: Cotton-Wool Patches

Cotton-wool patches are white or grayish, ovoid lesions with irregular "soft" borders. They are moderate in size but usually smaller than the disc. They result from infarcted nerve fibers and are seen in hypertension and many other conditions.

Hard Exudates

Hard exudates are creamy or yellowish, often bright lesions with well-defined "hard" borders. They are small and round but may coalesce into larger irregular spots. They often occur in clusters or in circular, linear, or star-shaped patterns. Causes include diabetes and hypertension.

Drusen

Drusen are yellowish round spots that vary from tiny to small. The edges may be soft, as here, or hard (p. 222). They are haphazardly distributed but may concentrate at the posterior pole. Drusen appear with normal aging but may also accompany various conditions, including age-related macular degeneration.

Healed Chorioretinitis

Here inflammation has destroyed the superficial tissues to reveal a well-defined, irregular patch of white sclera marked with dark pigment. Size varies from small to very large. *Toxoplasmosis* is illustrated. Multiple, small, somewhat similar-looking areas may be due to laser treatments. Here there is also a temporal scar near the macula.

(Source of photos: *Cotton-Wool Patches, Drusen, Healed Chorioretinitis*—Tasman W, Jaeger E, eds. The Wills Eye Hospital Atlas of Clinical Ophthalmology, 2nd ed. Philadelphia, Lippincott Williams & Wilkins, 2001; *Hard Exudates*—Courtesy of Ken Freedman, MD.)

TABLE
7-19

Lumps on or Near the Ear

Keloid. A firm, nodular, hypertrophic mass of scar tissue extending beyond the area of injury. It may develop in any scarred area but is most common on the shoulders and upper chest. A keloid on a pierced earlobe may have troublesome cosmetic effects. Keloids are more common in darker-skinned people. Recurrence may follow treatment.

Chondrodermatitis Helicis. This chronic inflammatory lesion starts as a painful, tender papule on the helix or antihelix. Here the upper lesion is at a later stage of ulceration and crusting. Reddening may occur. Biopsy is needed to rule out carcinoma.

Tophi. A deposit of uric acid crystals characteristic of chronic tophaceous gout. It appears as hard nodules in the helix or antihelix and may discharge chalky white crystals through the skin. It also may appear near the joints, hands (p. 649), feet, and other areas. It usually develops after chronic sustained high blood levels of uric acid.

Basal Cell Carcinoma. This raised nodule shows the lustrous surface and telangiectatic vessels of basal cell carcinoma, a common slow-growing malignancy that rarely metastasizes. Growth and ulceration may occur. These are more frequent in fair-skinned people overexposed to sunlight.

Cutaneous Cyst. Formerly called a *sebaceous cyst,* a dome-shaped lump in the dermis forms a benign closed firm sac attached to the epidermis. A dark dot (blackhead) may be visible on its surface. Histologically, it is usually either (1) an *epidermoid* cyst, common on the face and neck, or (2) a *pilar (trichilemmal)* cyst, common in the scalp. Both may become inflamed.

Rheumatoid Nodules. In chronic rheumatoid arthritis, look for small lumps on the helix or antihelix and additional nodules elsewhere on the hands, along the surface of the ulna distal to the elbow (p. 648), and on the knees and heels. Ulceration may result from repeated injuries. Such nodules may antedate the arthritis.

(Sources of photos: *Keloid*—Sams WM Jr, Lynch PJ, eds. Principles and Practice of Dermatology. Edinburgh, Churchill Livingstone, 1990; *Tophi*—du Vivier A. Atlas of Clinical Dermatology, 2nd ed. London, UK: Gower Medical Publishing, 1993; *Cutaneous Cyst, Chondrodermatitis Helicis*—Young EM, Newcomer VD, Kligman AM. Geriatric Dermatology: Color Atlas and Practitioner's Guide. Philadelphia, Lea & Febiger, 1993; *Basal Cell Carcinoma*—N Engl J Med, 326:169–170, 1992; *Rheumatoid Nodules*—Champion RH, Burton JL, Ebling FJG, eds. Rook/Wilkinson/Ebling Textbook of Dermatology, 5th ed. Oxford, UK: Blackwell Scientific, 1992.)

TABLE
7-20

Abnormalities of the Eardrum

Normal Eardrum (Right)

This normal right eardrum (tympanic membrane) is pinkish gray. Note the malleus lying behind the upper part of the drum. Above the short process lies the *pars flaccida*. The remainder of the drum is the *pars tensa*. From the umbo, the bright cone of light fans anteriorly and downward. Posterior to the malleus, part of the incus is visible behind the drum. The small blood vessels along the handle of the malleus are normal.

Perforation of the Drum

Perforations are holes in the eardrum that usually result from purulent infections of the middle ear. They are classified as *central* perforations, which do not extend to the margin of the drum, and *marginal* perforations, which do involve the margin.

The more common central perforation is illustrated here. A reddened ring of granulation tissue surrounds the perforation, indicating chronic infection. The eardrum itself is scarred, and no landmarks are visible. Discharge from the infected middle ear may drain out through such a perforation. A perforation often closes in the healing process, as in the next photo. The membrane covering the hole may be exceedingly thin and transparent.

Tympanosclerosis

In the inferior portion of this left eardrum, there is a large, chalky white patch with irregular margins. It is typical of tympanosclerosis: a deposition of hyaline material within the layers of the tympanic membrane that sometimes follows a severe episode of otitis media. It does not usually impair hearing and is seldom clinically significant.

Other abnormalities in this eardrum include a *healed perforation* (the large oval area in the upper posterior drum) and signs of a *retracted drum*. A retracted drum is pulled medially, away from the examiner's eye, and the malleolar folds are tightened into sharp outlines. The short process often protrudes sharply, and the handle of the malleus, pulled inward at the umbo, looks foreshortened and more horizontal.

(Sources of photos: *Normal Eardrum*—Hawke M, Keene M, Alberti PW. Clinical Otoscopy: A Text and Colour Atlas. Edinburgh, Churchill Livingstone, 1984; *Perforation of the Drum, Tympanosclerosis*—Courtesy of Michael Hawke, MD, Toronto, Canada.)

(table continues on page 270)

TABLE
7-20

Abnormalities of the Eardrum (continued)

Serous Effusion

Serous effusions are usually caused by viral upper respiratory infections (*otitis media with serous effusion*) or by sudden changes in atmospheric pressure as from flying or diving (*otitic barotrauma*). The eustachian tube cannot equalize the air pressure in the middle ear with that of the outside air. Air is partly or completely absorbed from the middle ear into the bloodstream, and serous fluid accumulates there instead. Symptoms include fullness and popping sensations in the ear, mild conduction hearing loss, and perhaps some pain.

Amber fluid behind the eardrum is characteristic, as in this patient with otitic barotrauma. A fluid level, a line between air above and amber fluid below, can be seen on either side of the short process. Air bubbles (not always present) can be seen here within the amber fluid.

Acute Otitis Media With Purulent Effusion

Acute otitis media with purulent effusion is caused by bacterial infection. Symptoms include earache, fever, and hearing loss. The eardrum reddens, loses its landmarks, and bulges laterally, toward the examiner's eye.

Here the eardrum is bulging, and most landmarks are obscured. Redness is most obvious near the umbo, but dilated vessels can be seen in all segments of the drum. A diffuse redness of the entire drum often develops. Spontaneous rupture (perforation) of the drum may follow, with discharge of purulent material into the ear canal.

Hearing loss is of the conductive type. Acute purulent otitis media is much more common in children than in adults.

Bullous Myringitis

Bullous myringitis is a viral infection characterized by painful hemorrhagic vesicles that appear on the tympanic membrane, the ear canal, or both. Symptoms include earache, blood-tinged discharge from the ear, and hearing loss of the conductive type.

In this right ear, at least two large vesicles (bullae) are discernible on the drum. The drum is reddened, and its landmarks are obscured.

Several different viruses may cause this condition, including mycoplasma.

(Sources of photos: *Serous Effusion*—Hawke M, Keene M, Alberti PW. Clinical Otoscopy: A Text and Colour Atlas. Edinburgh, Churchill Livingstone, 1984; *Acute Otitis Media, Bullous Myringitis*—The Wellcome Trust, National Medical Slide Bank, London, UK.)

Patterns of Hearing Loss

	Conductive Loss	Sensorineural Loss
Pathophysiology	External or middle ear disorder impairs sound conduction to inner ear. Causes include foreign body, *otitis media,* perforated eardrum, and otosclerosis of ossicles.	Inner ear disorder involves cochlear nerve and neuronal impulse transmission to the brain. Causes include loud noise exposure, inner ear infections, trauma, tremors, congenital and familial disorders, and aging.
Usual Age of Onset	Childhood and young adulthood, up to age 40	Middle or later years
Ear Canal and Drum	Abnormality usually visible, except in otosclerosis	Problem not visible
Effects	• Little effect on sound • Hearing seems to improve in noisy environment • Voice becomes soft because inner ear and cochlear nerve are intact	• Higher registers are lost, so sound may be distorted. • Hearing worsens in noisy environment • Voice may be loud because hearing is difficult.
Weber Test (*in unilateral hearing loss*)	• Tuning fork at vertex • Sound lateralizes to *impaired ear*—room noise not well heard, so detection of vibrations *improves.*	• Tuning fork at vertex • Sound lateralizes to *good ear*—inner ear or cochlear nerve damage impairs transmission to affected ear.
Rinne Test	• Tuning fork at external auditory meatus then on mastoid bone • Bone conduction longer than or equal to air conduction (BC ≥ AC). While air conduction through the external or middle ear is impaired, vibrations through bone bypass the problem to reach the cochlea.	• Tuning fork at external auditory meatus then on mastoid bone • Air conduction longer than bone conduction (AC > BC). The inner ear or cochlear nerve is less able to transmit impulses regardless of how the vibrations reach the cochlea. The normal pattern prevails.

TABLE
7-22

Abnormalities of the Lips

Angular Cheilitis

Angular cheilitis starts with softening of the skin at the angles of the mouth, followed by fissuring. It may be due to nutritional deficiency or, more commonly, to overclosure of the mouth, as in people with no teeth or with ill-fitting dentures. Saliva wets and macerates the infolded skin, often leading to secondary infection with *Candida,* as seen here.

Actinic Cheilitis

Actinic cheilitis results from excessive exposure to sunlight and affects primarily the lower lip. Fair-skinned men who work outdoors are most often affected. The lip loses its normal redness and may become scaly, somewhat thickened, and slightly everted. Because solar damage also predisposes to carcinoma of the lip, be alert to this possibility.

Herpes Simplex *(Cold Sore, Fever Blister)*

The herpes simplex virus (HSV) produces recurrent and painful vesicular eruptions of the lips and surrounding skin. A small cluster of vesicles first develops. As these break, yellow-brown crusts form, and healing ensues within 10 to 14 days. Both of these stages are visible here.

Angioedema

Angioedema is a diffuse, nonpitting, tense swelling of the dermis and subcutaneous tissue. It develops rapidly, and typically disappears over subsequent hours or days. Although usually allergic in nature and sometimes associated with hives, angioedema does not itch.

(Sources of photos: *Angular Cheilitis, Herpes Simplex, Angioedema*—Neville B, et al. Color Atlas of Clinical Oral Pathology. Philadelphia, Lea & Febiger, 1991; Used with permission; *Actinic Cheilitis*—Langlais RP, Miller CS. Color Atlas of Common Oral Diseases. Philadelphia, Lea & Febiger, 1992. Used with permission.)

(table continues on page 273)

Hereditary Hemorrhagic Telangiectasia

Multiple small red spots on the lips strongly suggest hereditary hemorrhagic telangiectasia. Spots may also be visible on the face and hands and in the mouth. The spots are dilated capillaries and may bleed when traumatized. Affected people often have nosebleeds and gastrointestinal bleeding.

Peutz-Jeghers Syndrome

When pigmented spots on the lips are more prominent than freckling of the surrounding skin, suspect this syndrome. Pigment in the buccal mucosa helps to confirm the diagnosis. Pigmented spots may also be found on the face and hands. Multiple intestinal polyps are often associated.

Chancre of Syphilis

This lesion of primary syphilis may appear on the lip rather than on the genitalia. It is a firm, buttonlike lesion that ulcerates and may become crusted. A chancre may resemble a carcinoma or a crusted cold sore. Because it is infectious, use gloves to feel any suspicious lesion.

Carcinoma of the Lip

Like actinic cheilitis, carcinoma usually affects the lower lip. It may appear as a scaly plaque, as an ulcer with or without a crust, or as a nodular lesion, illustrated here. Fair skin and prolonged exposure to the sun are common risk factors.

(Sources of photos: *Hereditary Hemorrhagic Telangiectasia*—Langlais RP, Miller CS. Color Atlas of Common Oral Diseases. Philadelphia, Lea & Febiger, 1992; Used with permission; *Peutz-Jeghers Syndrome*—Robinson HBG, Miller AS. Colby, Kerr, and Robinson's Color Atlas of Oral Pathology. Philadelphia, JB Lippincott, 1990; *Chancre of Syphilis*—Wisdom A. A Colour Atlas of Sexually Transmitted Diseases, 2nd ed. London, Wolfe Medical Publications, 1989; *Carcinoma of the Lip*—Tyldesley WR. A Colour Atlas of Orofacial Diseases, 2nd ed. London, Wolfe Medical Publications, 1991.)

TABLE
7-23

Findings in the Pharynx, Palate, and Oral Mucosa

Large Normal Tonsils

Normal tonsils may be large without being infected, especially in children. They may protrude medially beyond the pillars and even to the midline. Here they touch the sides of the uvula and obscure the pharynx. Their color is pink. The white marks are light reflections, not exudate.

Exudative Tonsillitis

This red throat has a white exudate on the tonsils. This, together with fever and enlarged cervical nodes, increases the probability of *group A streptococcal infection* or *infectious mononucleosis*. Anterior cervical lymph nodes are usually enlarged in the former, posterior nodes in the latter.

Pharyngitis

These two photos show reddened throats without exudate.

In **A**, redness and vascularity of the pillars and uvula are mild to moderate.

A

In **B**, redness is diffuse and intense. Each patient would probably complain of a sore throat, or at least a scratchy one. Possible causes include several kinds of viruses and bacteria. If the patient has no fever, exudate, or enlargement of cervical lymph nodes, the chances of infection by either of two common causes—*group A streptococci* and *Epstein-Barr virus* (infectious mononucleosis)—are very small.

B

(Sources of photos: *Large Normal Tonsils, Exudative Tonsillitis, Pharyngitis [A and B]*—The Wellcome Trust, National Medical Slide Bank, London, UK.)

(table continues on page 275)

Diphtheria

Diphtheria (an acute infection caused by *Corynebacterium diphtheriae*) is now rare but still important. Prompt diagnosis may lead to life-saving treatment. The throat is dull red, and a gray exudate (pseudomembrane) is present on the uvula, pharynx, and tongue. The airway may become obstructed.

Thrush on the Palate (Candidiasis)

Thrush is a yeast infection due to *Candida*. Shown here on the palate, it may appear elsewhere in the mouth (see p. 279). Thick, white plaques are somewhat adherent to the underlying mucosa. Predisposing factors include (1) prolonged treatment with antibiotics or corticosteroids and (2) AIDS.

Kaposi's Sarcoma in AIDS

The deep purple color of these lesions, although not necessarily present, strongly suggests Kaposi's sarcoma. The lesions may be raised or flat. Among people with AIDS, the palate, as illustrated here, is a common site for this tumor.

Torus Palatinus

A torus palatinus is a midline bony growth in the hard palate that is fairly common in adults. Its size and lobulation vary. Although alarming at first glance, it is harmless. In this example, an upper denture has been fitted around the torus.

(Sources of photos: *Diphtheria*—Harnisch JP, et al. Diphtheria among alcoholic urban adults. Ann Intern Med 1989;111:77; *Thrush on the Palate*—The Wellcome Trust, National Medical Slide Bank, London, UK; *Kaposi's Sarcoma in AIDS*—Ioachim HL. Textbook and Atlas of Disease Associated With Acquired Immune Deficiency Syndrome. London, UK, Gower Medical Publishing, 1989.)

(table continues on page 276)

Fordyce Spots *(Fordyce Granules)*

Fordyce spots are normal sebaceous glands that appear as small yellowish spots in the buccal mucosa or on the lips. A worried person who has suddenly noticed them may be reassured. Here they are seen best anterior to the tongue and lower jaw. These spots are usually not so numerous.

Koplik's Spots

Koplik's spots are an early sign of measles (rubeola). Search for small white specks that resemble grains of salt on a red background. They usually appear on the buccal mucosa near the first and second molars. In this photo, look also in the upper third of the mucosa. The rash of measles appears within a day.

Petechiae

Petechiae are small red spots that result when blood escapes from capillaries into the tissues. Petechiae in the buccal mucosa, as shown, are often caused by accidentally biting the cheek. Oral petechiae may be due to infection or decreased platelets, as well as to trauma.

Leukoplakia

A thickened white patch (*leukoplakia*) may occur anywhere in the oral mucosa. The extensive example shown on this buccal mucosa resulted from frequent chewing of tobacco, a local irritant. This kind of irritation may lead to cancer.

(Sources of photos: *Fordyce Spots*—Neville B, et al. Color Atlas of Clinical Oral Pathology. Philadelphia, Lea & Febiger, 1991; Used with permission; *Koplik's Spots, Petechiae*—The Wellcome Trust, National Medical Slide Bank, London, UK; *Leukoplakia*—Robinson HBG, Miller AS. Colby, Kerr, and Robinson's Color Atlas of Oral Pathology. Philadelphia, JB Lippincott, 1990.)

TABLE
7-24

Findings in the Gums and Teeth

Marginal Gingivitis

Marginal gingivitis is common among teenagers and young adults. The gingival margins are reddened and swollen, and the interdental papillae are blunted, swollen, and red. Brushing the teeth often makes the gums bleed. *Plaque*—the soft white film of salivary salts, protein, and bacteria that covers the teeth and leads to gingivitis—is not readily visible.

Acute Necrotizing Ulcerative Gingivitis

This uncommon form of gingivitis occurs suddenly in adolescents and young adults and is accompanied by fever, malaise, and enlarged lymph nodes. Ulcers develop in the interdental papillae. Then the destructive (necrotizing) process spreads along the gum margins, where a grayish pseudomembrane develops. The red, painful gums bleed easily; the breath is foul.

Gingival Hyperplasia

Gums enlarged by hyperplasia are swollen into heaped-up masses that may even cover the teeth. The redness of inflammation may coexist, as in this example. Causes include dilantin therapy (as in this case), puberty, pregnancy, and leukemia.

Pregnancy Tumor (Epulis, Pyogenic Granuloma)

Gingival enlargement may be localized, forming a tumorlike mass that usually originates in an interdental papilla. It is red and soft and usually bleeds easily. The estimated incidence of this lesion in pregnancy is about 1%. Note the accompanying gingivitis in this example.

(Sources of photos: *Marginal Gingivitis, Acute Necrotizing Ulcerative Gingivitis*—Tyldesley WR. A Colour Atlas of Orofacial Diseases, 2nd ed. London, Wolfe Medical Publications, 1991; *Gingival Hyperplasia*—Courtesy of Dr. James Cottone; *Pregnancy Tumor*—Langlais RP, Miller CS. Color Atlas of Common Oral Diseases. Philadelphia, Lea & Febiger, 1992. Used with permission.)

(table continues on page 278)

TABLE 7-24

Findings in the Gums and Teeth (continued)

Attrition of Teeth; Recession of Gums

In many elderly people, the chewing surfaces of the teeth have been worn down by repetitive use so that the yellow-brown dentin becomes exposed—a process called *attrition*. Note also the *recession of the gums*, which has exposed the roots of the teeth, giving a "long in the tooth" appearance.

Erosion of Teeth

Teeth may be eroded by chemical action. Note here the erosion of the enamel from the lingual surfaces of the upper incisors, exposing the yellow-brown dentin. This results from recurrent regurgitation of stomach contents, as in bulimia.

Abrasion of Teeth With Notching

The biting surface of the teeth may become abraded or notched by recurrent trauma, such as holding nails or opening bobby pins between the teeth. Unlike Hutchinson's teeth, the sides of these teeth show normal contours; size and spacing of the teeth are unaffected.

Hutchinson's Teeth

Hutchinson's teeth are smaller and more widely spaced than normal and are notched on their biting surfaces. The sides of the teeth taper toward the biting edges. The upper central incisors of the permanent (not the deciduous) teeth are most often affected. These teeth are a sign of congenital syphilis.

(Sources of photos: *Attrition of Teeth, Erosion of Teeth*—Langlais RP, Miller CS. Color Atlas of Common Oral Diseases. Philadelphia, Lea & Febiger, 1992. Used with permission; *Abrasion of Teeth*, *Hutchinson's Teeth*—Robinson HBG, Miller AS. Colby, Kerr, and Robinson's Color Atlas of Oral Pathology. Philadelphia, JB Lippincott, 1990.)

Geographic Tongue. In this benign condition, the dorsum shows scattered smooth red areas denuded of papillae. Together with the normal rough and coated areas, they give a maplike pattern that changes over time.

Hairy Tongue. Note the "hairy" yellowish to brown or black elongated papillae on the tongue's dorsum. This benign condition may follow antibiotic therapy; it also may occur spontaneously.

Fissured Tongue. Fissures appear with increasing age, sometimes termed *scrotal tongue*. Food debris may accumulate in the crevices and become irritating, but a fissured tongue is benign.

Smooth Tongue (Atrophic Glossitis). A smooth and often sore tongue that has lost its papillae suggests a deficiency in riboflavin, niacin, folic acid, vitamin B_{12}, pyridoxine, or iron, or treatment with chemotherapy.

Candidiasis. Note the thick white coating from *Candida* infection. The raw red surface is where the coat was scraped off. Infection may also occur without the white coating. It is seen in immunosuppressed conditions.

Hairy Leukoplakia. These whitish raised areas with a feathery or corrugated pattern most often affect the sides of the tongue. Unlike candidiasis, these areas cannot be scraped off. They are seen with HIV and AIDS.

(table continues on page 280)

TABLE
7-25

Findings in or Under the Tongue (continued)

Varicose Veins. Small purplish or blue-black round swellings appear under the tongue with age. These dilatations of the lingual veins have no clinical significance.

Aphthous Ulcer (Canker Sore). A painful, round or oval ulcer that is white or yellowish gray and surrounded by a halo of reddened mucosa. It may be single or multiple. It heals in 7–10 days, but may recur.

Mucous Patch of Syphilis. This painless lesion in the secondary stage of syphilis is highly infectious. It is slightly raised, oval, and covered by a grayish membrane. It may be multiple and occur elsewhere in the mouth.

Leukoplakia. With this persisting painless white patch in the oral mucosa, the undersurface of the tongue appears painted white. Patches of any size raise the possibility of malignancy and require a biopsy.

Tori Mandibulares. Rounded bony growths on the inner surfaces of the mandible are typically bilateral, asymptomatic, and harmless.

Carcinoma, Floor of the Mouth. This ulcerated lesion is in a common location for carcinoma. Medially, note the reddened area of mucosa, called *erythroplakia*, suggesting possible malignancy.

Thyroid Enlargement and Function

Diffuse Enlargement. Includes the isthmus and lateral lobes; there are no discretely palpable nodules. Causes include Graves' disease, Hashimoto's thyroiditis, and endemic goiter.

Single Nodule. May be a cyst, a benign tumor, or one nodule within a multinodular gland. It raises the question of malignancy. Risk factors are prior irradiation, hardness, rapid growth, fixation to surrounding tissues, enlarged cervical nodes, and occurrence in males.[2c6]

Multinodular Goiter. An enlarged thyroid gland with two or more nodules suggests a metabolic rather than a neoplastic process. Positive family history and continuing nodular enlargement are additional risk factors for malignancy.

Symptoms and Signs of Thyroid Dysfunction[25,28–30]

	Hyperthyroidism	Hypothyroidism
Symptoms	Nervousness Weight loss despite increased appetite Excessive sweating and heat intolerance Palpitations Frequent bowel movements Muscular weakness of the proximal type and tremor	Fatigue, lethargy Modest weight gain with anorexia Dry, coarse skin and cold intolerance Swelling of face, hands, and legs Constipation Weakness, muscle cramps, arthralgias, paresthesias, impaired memory and hearing
Signs	Warm, smooth, moist skin With Graves' disease, eye signs such as stare, lid lag, and exophthalmos Increased systolic and decreased diastolic blood pressures Tachycardia or atrial fibrillation Hyperdynamic cardiac pulsations with an accentuated S_1 Tremor and proximal muscle weakness	Dry, coarse, cool skin, sometimes yellowish from carotene, with nonpitting edema and loss of hair Periorbital puffiness Decreased systolic and increased diastolic blood pressures Bradycardia and, in late stages, hypothermia Intensity of heart sounds sometimes decreased Impaired memory, mixed hearing loss, somnolence, peripheral neuropathy, carpal tunnel syndrome

The Thorax and Lungs

ANATOMY AND PHYSIOLOGY

Study the *anatomy of the chest wall,* identifying the structures illustrated.
Note that an interspace between two ribs is numbered by the rib above it.

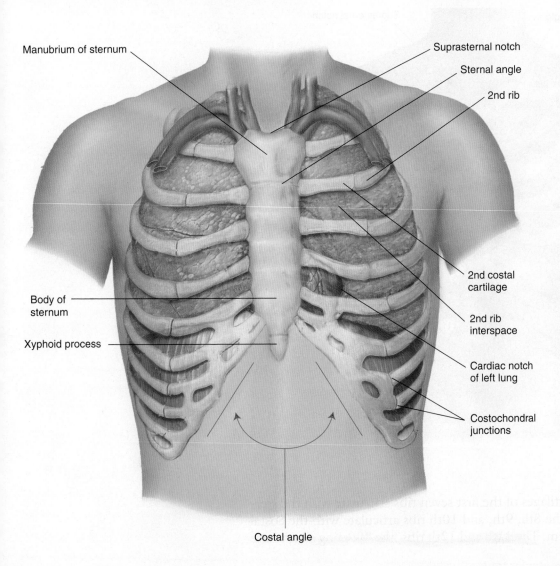

Manubrium of sternum

Suprasternal notch

Sternal angle

2nd rib

Body of
sternum

Xyphoid process

2nd costal
cartilage

2nd rib
interspace

Cardiac notch
of left lung

Costochondral
junctions

Costal angle

Locating Findings on the Chest.   Describe abnormalities of the chest in two dimensions: *along the vertical axis* and *around the circumference of the chest*.

To make *vertical* locations, you must be able to count the ribs and interspaces. The *sternal angle,* also termed the angle of Louis, is the best guide: place your finger in the hollow curve of the suprasternal notch, then move your finger down approximately 5 cm to the horizontal bony ridge joining the manubrium to the body of the sternum. Then move your finger laterally and find the adjacent 2nd rib and costal cartilage. From here, using two fingers, "walk down" the interspaces, one space at a time, on an oblique line, illustrated by the red numbers below. Do not try to count interspaces along the lower edge of the sternum; the ribs there are too close together. In a woman, to find the interspaces, either displace the breast laterally or palpate a little more medially than illustrated. Avoid pressing too hard on tender breast tissue.

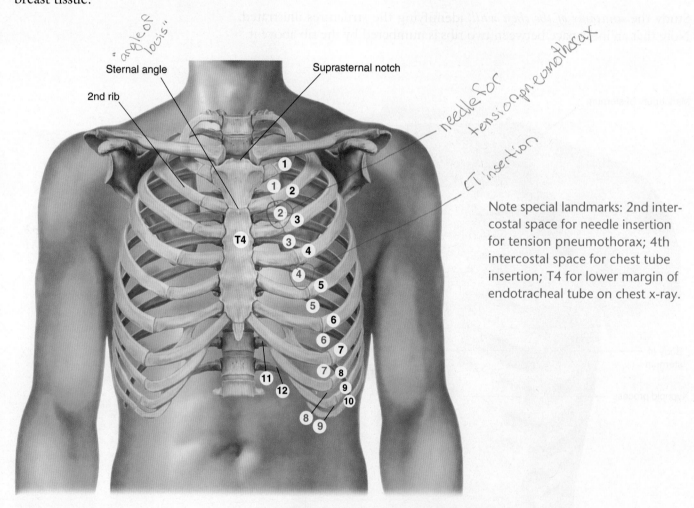

Note special landmarks: 2nd intercostal space for needle insertion for tension pneumothorax; 4th intercostal space for chest tube insertion; T4 for lower margin of endotracheal tube on chest x-ray.

Note that the costal cartilages of the first seven ribs articulate with the sternum; the cartilages of the 8th, 9th, and 10th ribs articulate with the costal cartilages just above them. The 11th and 12th ribs, the "floating ribs," have no anterior attachments. The cartilaginous tip of the 11th rib usually can be felt laterally, and the 12th rib may be felt posteriorly. On palpation, costal cartilages and ribs feel identical.

Posteriorly, the 12th rib is another possible starting point for counting ribs and interspaces: it helps locate findings on the lower posterior chest and provides an option when the anterior approach is unsatisfactory. With the fingers of one hand, press in and up against the lower border of the 12th rib, then "walk up" the interspaces numbered in red below, or follow a more oblique line up and around to the front of the chest.

The inferior tip of the scapula is another useful bony landmark—it usually lies at the level of the 7th rib or interspace.

Spinous process of C7

Spinous process of T1

7th rib

Note T7–8 interspace as landmark for thoracentesis.

Inferior angle of scapula

The spinous processes of the vertebrae are also useful anatomical landmarks. When the neck is flexed forward, the most protruding process is usually the vertebra of C7. If two processes are equally prominent, they are C7 and T1. You can often palpate and count the processes below them, especially when the spine is flexed.

To locate findings around the *circumference of the chest*, use a series of vertical lines, shown in the adjacent illustrations. The *midsternal* and *vertebral lines* are precise; the others are estimated. The *midclavicular line* drops vertically from the midpoint of the clavicle. To find it, you must identify both ends of the clavicle accurately (see p. 588).

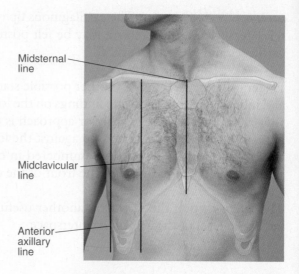

Midsternal line

Midclavicular line

Anterior axillary line

The *anterior* and *posterior axillary lines* drop vertically from the anterior and posterior axillary folds, the muscle masses that border the axilla. The *midaxillary line* drops from the apex of the axilla.

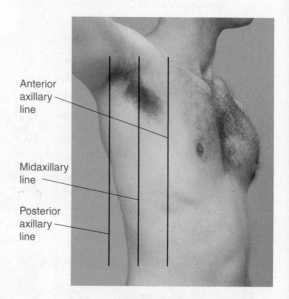

Anterior axillary line

Midaxillary line

Posterior axillary line

Posteriorly, the *vertebral line* overlies the spinous processes of the vertebrae. The scapular line drops from the inferior angle of the scapula.

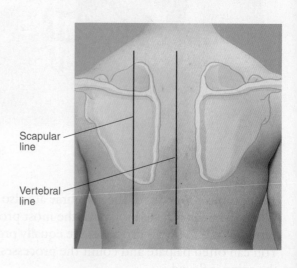

Scapular line

Vertebral line

Lungs, Fissures, and Lobes.   Picture the lungs and their fissures and lobes on the chest wall. Anteriorly, the apex of each lung rises approximately 2 cm to 4 cm above the inner third of the clavicle. The lower border of the lung crosses the 6th rib at the midclavicular line and the 8th rib at the midaxillary line. Posteriorly, the lower border of the lung lies at about the level of the T10 spinous process. On inspiration, it descends farther.

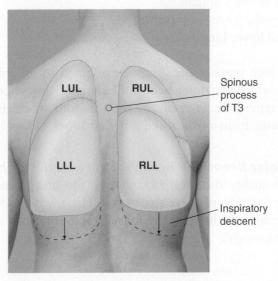

Each lung is divided roughly in half by an *oblique (major) fissure*. This fissure may be approximated by a string that runs from the T3 spinous process obliquely down and around the chest to the 6th rib at the midclavicular line. The right lung is further divided by the *horizontal (minor) fissure*. Anteriorly, this fissure runs close to the 4th rib and meets the oblique fissure in the midaxillary line near the 5th rib. The *right lung* is thus divided into *upper, middle,* and *lower lobes*. The *left lung* has only *two lobes*, upper and lower.

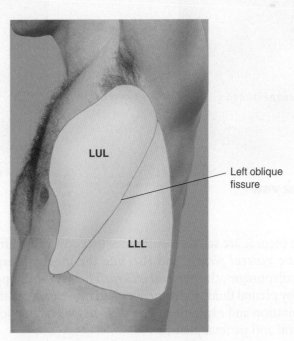

Locations on the Chest. Learn the general anatomical terms used to locate chest findings, such as:

Supraclavicular—above the clavicles
Infraclavicular—below the clavicles
Interscapular—between the scapulae
Infrascapular—below the scapulae
Bases of the lungs—the lowermost portions
Upper, middle, and lower lung fields

You may then infer which parts of the lungs are affected by an abnormal process. Signs in the right upper lung field, for example, almost certainly originate in the right upper lobe. Signs in the right middle lung field laterally, however, could come from any of three different lobes.

The Trachea and Major Bronchi. Breath sounds over the trachea and bronchi have a different quality than breath sounds over the lung parenchyma. Be sure you know the location of these structures. The trachea bifurcates into its mainstem bronchi at the levels of the sternal angle anteriorly and the T4 spinous process posteriorly.

ANTERIOR VIEW

POSTERIOR VIEW

The Pleurae. The pleurae are serous membranes that cover the outer surface of each lung, the *visceral pleura,* and also line the inner rib cage and upper surface of the diaphragm, the *parietal pleura.* Their smooth opposing surfaces, lubricated by pleural fluid, allow the lungs to move easily within the rib cage during inspiration and expiration. The *pleural space* is the potential space between visceral and parietal pleurae.

Breathing.   Breathing is largely an automatic act, controlled in the brainstem and mediated by the muscles of respiration. The dome-shaped *diaphragm* is the primary muscle of inspiration. When it contracts, it descends in the chest and enlarges the thoracic cavity. At the same time, it compresses the abdominal contents, pushing the abdominal wall outward. Muscles in the rib cage and neck expand the thorax during inspiration, especially the *parasternals,* which run obliquely from sternum to ribs, and the *scalenes,* which run from the cervical vertebrae to the first two ribs.

During inspiration, as these muscles contract, the thorax expands. Intrathoracic pressure decreases, drawing air through the tracheobronchial tree into the *alveoli,* or distal air sacs, and expanding the lungs. Oxygen diffuses into the blood of adjacent pulmonary capillaries, and carbon dioxide diffuses from the blood into the alveoli.

After inspiratory effort stops, the expiratory phase begins. The chest wall and lungs recoil, the diaphragm relaxes and rises passively, air flows outward, and the chest and abdomen return to their resting positions.

Normal breathing is quiet and easy—barely audible near the open mouth as a faint whish. When a healthy person lies supine, the breathing movements of the thorax are relatively slight. In contrast, the abdominal movements are usually easy to see. In the sitting position, movements of the thorax become more prominent.

During exercise and in certain diseases, extra work is required to breathe, and accessory muscles join the inspiratory effort. The sternomastoids are the most important of these, and the scalenes may become visible. Abdominal muscles assist in expiration.

Sternal head ⎫
                ⎬ of the sternomastoid muscle
Clavicular head ⎭

THE HEALTH HISTORY

Common or Concerning Symptoms

- Chest pain
- Shortness of breath (dyspnea)
- Wheezing
- Cough
- Blood-streaked sputum (hemoptysis)

Chest Pain. Complaints of *chest pain* or *chest discomfort* raise concern about heart disease but often arise from structures in the thorax and lung as well. To assess this symptom, you must pursue a dual investigation of both thoracic and cardiac causes. Sources of chest pain are listed below. For this important symptom, you must keep all of these in mind:

- The myocardium

  Angina pectoris, myocardial infarction

- The pericardium

  Pericarditis

- The aorta

  Dissecting aortic aneurysm

- The trachea and large bronchi

  Bronchitis

- The parietal pleura

  Pericarditis, pneumonia

- The chest wall, including the musculoskeletal system and skin

  Costochondritis, herpes zoster

- The esophagus

  Reflux esophagitis, esophageal spasm

- Extrathoracic structures such as the neck, gallbladder, and stomach.

  Cervical arthritis, biliary colic, gastritis

This section focuses on *pulmonary complaints*, including general questions about chest symptoms, dyspnea, wheezing, cough, and hemoptysis. For health history questions about exertional chest pain, palpitations, orthopnea, paroxysmal nocturnal dyspnea, and edema, see Chapter 9, The Cardiovascular System.

Your initial questions should be as broad as possible. "Do you have any discomfort or unpleasant feelings in your chest?" As you proceed to the full history, ask the patient to point to where the pain is in the chest. Watch for any

See Table 8-1. Chest Pain, pp. 312–313.

A clenched fist over the sternum suggests *angina pectoris;* a finger pointing to a tender area on the gestures as the patient describes the pain. You should elicit all seven attributes of this symptom (see p. 65) to distinguish among the various causes of chest pain.

chest wall suggests *musculo-skeletal pain*; a hand moving from neck to epigastrum suggests *heartburn.*

Lung tissue itself has no pain fibers. Pain in lung conditions such as pneumonia or pulmonary infarction usually arises from inflammation of the adjacent parietal pleura. Muscle strain from prolonged recurrent coughing may also be responsible. The pericardium also has few pain fibers—the pain of pericarditis stems from inflammation of the adjacent parietal pleura. (Chest pain is commonly associated with anxiety, too, but the mechanism remains obscure.)

Anxiety is the most frequent cause of chest pain in children; *costochondritis* is also common.

Shortness of Breath (Dyspnea) and Wheezing. *Dyspnea* is a nonpainful but uncomfortable awareness of breathing that is inappropriate to the level of exertion, commonly termed *shortness of breath.*[1] This serious symptom warrants a full explanation and assessment because dyspnea commonly results from cardiac or pulmonary disease.

See Table 8-2, Dyspnea, pp. 314–315.

Ask "Have you had any difficulty breathing?" Find out when the symptom occurs, at rest or with exercise, and how much effort produces onset. Because of variations in age, body weight, and physical fitness, there is no absolute scale for quantifying dyspnea. Instead, make every effort *to determine its severity based on the patient's daily activities.* How many steps or flights of stairs can the patient climb before pausing for breath? What about work such as carrying bags of groceries, mopping the floor, or making the bed? Has dyspnea altered the patient's lifestyle and daily activities? How? Carefully elicit the timing and setting of dyspnea, any associated symptoms, and relieving or aggravating factors.

Most patients with dyspnea relate shortness of breath to their level of activity. Anxious patients present a different picture. They may describe difficulty taking a deep enough breath, or a smothering sensation with inability to get enough air, along with *paresthesias,* or sensations of tingling or "pins and needles" around the lips or in the extremities.

Anxious patients may have episodic dyspnea during both rest and exercise, and *hyperventilation,* or rapid, shallow breathing. At other times, they may sigh frequently.

Wheezes are musical respiratory sounds that may be audible to the patient and to others.

Wheezing suggests partial airway obstruction from secretions, tissue inflammation, or a foreign body.

Cough. *Cough* is a common symptom that ranges in significance from trivial to ominous. Typically, cough is a reflex response to stimuli that irritate receptors in the larynx, trachea, or large bronchi. These stimuli include mucus, pus, and blood, as well as external agents such as dust, foreign bodies, or even extremely hot or cold air. Other causes include inflammation of the respiratory mucosa and pressure or tension in the air passages from a tumor or enlarged peribronchial lymph nodes. Although cough typically signals a problem in the respiratory tract, it may also be cardiovascular in origin.

See Table 8-3, Cough and Hemoptysis, p. 316.

Cough can be a symptom of *left-sided heart failure.*

For complaints of cough, a thorough assessment is in order. Duration of the cough is important: is the cough *acute*, or lasting less than 3 weeks; *subacute*, or 3 to 8 weeks; or *chronic*, more than 8 weeks?[2]

Viral upper respiratory infections are the most common cause of *acute cough;* also consider acute bronchitis, pneumonia, left ventricular heart failure, asthma, foreign body. Postinfectious cough, bacterial sinusitis, asthma in *subacute cough;* postnasal drip, asthma, gastroesophageal reflux, chronic bronchitis, bronchiectasis in *chronic cough.*[2-4]

Ask whether the cough is dry or produces sputum, or phlegm.

Mucoid sputum is translucent, white, or gray; *purulent* sputum is yellowish or greenish.

Ask the patient to describe the volume of any sputum and its color, odor, and consistency.

Foul-smelling sputum in anaerobic *lung abscess;* tenacious sputum in cystic fibrosis

To help patients quantify volume, a multiple-choice question may be helpful. "How much do you think you cough up in 24 hours: a teaspoon, tablespoon, quarter cup, half cup, cupful?" If possible, ask the patient to cough into a tissue; inspect the phlegm and note its characteristics. The symptoms associated with a cough often lead you to its cause.

Large volumes of purulent sputum in *bronchiectasis* or *lung abscess*

Diagnostically helpful symptoms include fever, chest pain, dyspnea, orthopnea, and wheezing.

Hemoptysis. *Hemoptysis* is the coughing up of blood from the lungs; it may vary from blood-streaked phlegm to frank blood. For patients reporting hemoptysis, assess the volume of blood produced as well as the other sputum attributes; ask about the related setting and activity and any associated symptoms.

See Table 8-3, Cough and Hemoptysis, p. 316. Hemoptysis is rare in infants, children, and adolescents; it is seen most often in *cystic fibrosis.*

Before using the term "hemoptysis," try to confirm the source of the bleeding by both history and physical examination. Blood or blood-streaked material may originate in the mouth, pharynx, or gastrointestinal tract and is easily mislabeled. When vomited, it probably originates in the gastrointestinal tract. Occasionally, however, blood from the nasopharynx or the gastrointestinal tract is aspirated and then coughed out.

Blood originating in the stomach is usually darker than blood from the respiratory tract and may be mixed with food particles.

HEALTH PROMOTION AND COUNSELING

Important Topics for Health Promotion and Counseling

- Tobacco cessation
- Immunizations

Tobacco Cessation. Despite declines in smoking over the past several decades, 23% of U.S. adults continue to smoke. Smoking rates are highest among young adults 18 to 24 years. Approximately 90% of smokers start by 18 years, with 2000 adolescents becoming regular smokers each day.[5,6] Smoking accounts for 1 in 5 U.S. deaths each year. Be familiar with the extensive risks of disease and death in smokers.

● Adverse Effects of Smoking on Health and Disease

Condition	Increased Risk Compared with Nonsmokers
● Coronary artery disease	2–3 times higher
● Stroke	2 times higher
● Peripheral vascular disease	10 times higher
● COPD mortality	10 times higher
● Lung cancer mortality	23 times higher in men
	13 times higher in women

(Source: Centers for Disease Control and Prevention, DHHS. Smoking and tobacco use. Fact sheet. Health effects of cigarette smoking. Available at: http://www.cdc.gov/tobacco/data_statistics/Factsheets/health_effects.htm. Accessed September 16, 2007.)

In addition, smoking contributes to many types of cancer and increases risk of infertility, preterm birth, low birth weight, and sudden infant death syndrome. Nonsmokers exposed to smoke also have increased risk of lung cancer, ear and respiratory infections, asthma, and residential fires.

Smoking is the leading preventable cause of death. Although a number of tests, such as helical computerized tomography, have been studied, screening for lung cancer is currently not recommended.[6] Instead, clinicians should focus on prevention and cessation, especially in teenagers and pregnant women.[7] Because 70% of smokers see a physician each year and 70% express interest in quitting, the benefits from brief counseling interventions are considerable.[8,9] Clinicians should advise smokers to quit during every visit. This advice has been shown to raise quit rates by 30%.[10] Use the "5 A's" framework or the Stages of Change model (precontemplation, contemplation, preparation, action, maintenance)[11] to assess readiness to quit.

Nicotine is highly addicting, comparable to heroin and cocaine, and quitting tobacco use is difficult. Learn to use cognitive therapy techniques to help your patients recognize signs of withdrawal such as irritability, difficulty concentrating, anxiety, and depressed mood.[8,9] Guide patients to better understand craving, triggers for smoking, and strategies for managing withdrawal, coping with stress, and preventing relapse. Combining counseling with pharmacotherapy is recommended. Three drugs have been shown to improve and sustain quit rates: nicotine replacement therapies; buproprion, a norepinephrine and dopamine reuptake inhibitor and nicotinic receptor antagonist; and

---

Assessing Readiness to Quit Smoking: The "5 A's"

1. **Ask** about tobacco use.
2. **Advise** to quit through clear, personalized messages.
3. **Assess** willingness to quit.
4. **Assist** to quit.
5. **Arrange** follow-up and support.

(Source: U.S. Preventive Services Task Force. Counseling to prevent tobacco use and tobacco-related diseases: recommendation statement. Agency for Healthcare Research and Quality, Rockville, MD. November 2003. Available at: http://www.ahrq.gov/clinic/3rduspstf/tobacccoun/tobcounrs.htm. Accessed September 11, 2007.)

---

more recently, varenicline, a nicotinic receptor partial agonist that stimulates dopamine release, thought to relieve craving.[12]

Immunizations (Adults). *Influenza* claims more than 36,000 deaths and 200,000 hospitalizations annually, especially during the late fall and winter, peaking in February.[13] The CDC Advisory Committee on Immunization Practices updates its recommendations for vaccination annually. Two types of vaccine are available: the "flu shot," an inactivated vaccine containing killed virus, and a nasal-spray vaccine containing attenuated live viruses, approved only for healthy people between 5 and 49 years. Because influenza viruses change from year to year, each vaccine contains three vaccine strains and is modified yearly. All people wishing to reduce risk of infection should be vaccinated, especially these groups:

● Adults with chronic pulmonary conditions and chronic medical illnesses, and adults who are immunosuppressed

● Residents of nursing homes and chronic care facilities

● Health care personnel

● Healthy household contacts and caregivers of children younger than 5 years and adults 50 years or older, particularly those with medical conditions placing them at higher risk for complications from influenza.

Streptococcus pneumoniae causes approximately 175,000 cases of U.S. pneumococcal pneumonia each year; 25% to 30% of these cases are accompanied by sepsis.[14] Incubation is as short as 1 to 3 days, and fatalities are 5%. There are an additional 3,000 to 6,000 cases of pneumococcal meningitis annually, many in children. The two types of *pneumococcal vaccine*, polysaccharide and conjugated, are both inactivated. The CDC recommends the pneumococcal vaccine for these groups:

● All adults 65 years and older

● People between the ages of 2 and 64 with chronic illnesses specifically associated with increased risk from pneumococcal infection, such as sickle cell anemia, cardiovascular and pulmonary disease, diabetes, cirrhosis, or leaks of cerebrospinal fluid

- Anyone with or about to receive a cochlear implant

- Persons 2 years or older who are immunocompromised, including those with HIV infection or AIDS and those receiving steroids, radiation, or chemotherapy

- Alaska natives of certain Native American groups.

TECHNIQUES OF EXAMINATION

It is helpful to examine the posterior thorax and lungs while the patient is sitting, and the anterior thorax and lungs with the patient supine. Proceed in an orderly fashion: inspect, palpate, percuss, and auscultate. Try to visualize the underlying lobes, and compare one side with the other, so that the patient serves as his or her own control. For men, arrange the patient's gown so that you can see the chest fully. For women, cover the anterior chest when you examine the back. For the anterior examination, drape the gown over each half of the chest as you examine the other half.

- *With the patient sitting,* examine the posterior thorax and lungs. The patient's arms should be folded across the chest with hands resting, if possible, on the opposite shoulders. This position moves the scapulae partly out of the way and increases your access to the lung fields. Then ask the patient to lie down.

- *With the patient supine,* examine the anterior thorax and lungs. The supine position makes it easier to examine women because the breasts can be gently displaced. Furthermore, wheezes, if present, are more likely to be heard. (Some authorities prefer to examine both the back and the front of the chest with the patient sitting. This technique is also satisfactory.)

- *For patients who cannot sit up without aid,* try to get help so that you can examine the posterior chest in the sitting position. If this is impossible, roll the patient to one side and then to the other. Percuss the upper lung, and auscultate both lungs in each position. Because ventilation is relatively greater in the dependent lung, your chances of hearing abnormal wheezes or crackles are greater on the dependent side (see p. 303).

INITIAL SURVEY OF RESPIRATION AND THE THORAX

Even though you may have already recorded the respiratory rate when you took the vital signs, it is wise to again *observe the rate, rhythm, depth, and effort of breathing.* A healthy resting adult breathes quietly and regularly about 14 to 20 times a minute. An occasional sigh is to be expected. Note whether expiration lasts longer than usual.

See Table 4-8, Abnormalities in Rate and Rhythm of Breathing, p. 134.

Always inspect the patient for any signs of respiratory difficulty.

- *Assess the patient's color* for cyanosis. Recall any relevant findings from earlier parts of your examination, such as the shape of the fingernails.

Cyanosis signals hypoxia. Clubbing of the nails (see p. 193) in *lung abscesses, malignancy, congenital heart disease*

- *Listen to the patient's breathing.* Is there any *audible wheezing*? If so, where does it fall in the respiratory cycle?

Audible *stridor,* a high-pitched wheeze, is an ominous sign of airway obstruction in the larynx or trachea.

- *Inspect the neck.* During inspiration, is there contraction of the accessory muscles, namely the sternomastoid and scalene muscles, or supraclavicular retraction? Is the trachea midline?

Inspiratory contraction of the sternomastoids and scalenes at rest signals severe difficulty in breathing. Lateral displacement of the trachea in *pneumothorax, pleural effusion,* or *atelectasis*

Also *observe the shape of the chest.* The anteroposterior (AP) diameter may increase with aging, compared with the lateral chest diameter.

The AP diameter also may increase in *chronic obstructive pulmonary disease* (COPD), although evidence is not definitive.[15]

 EXAMINATION OF THE POSTERIOR CHEST

Inspection

From a midline position behind the patient, note the *shape of the chest* and *how the chest moves,* including:

- Deformities or asymmetry

See Table 8-4, Deformities of the Thorax (p. 317).

- Abnormal retraction of the interspaces during inspiration. Retraction is most apparent in the lower interspaces.

Retraction in severe *asthma, COPD,* or upper airway obstruction

- Impaired respiratory movement on one or both sides or a unilateral lag (or delay) in movement.

Unilateral impairment or lagging of respiratory movement suggests disease of the underlying lung or pleura.

Palpation

As you palpate the chest, focus on areas of tenderness and abnormalities in the overlying skin, respiratory expansion, and fremitus.

Intercostal tenderness over inflamed pleura

- *Identify tender areas.* Carefully palpate any area where pain has been reported or where lesions or bruises are evident.

Bruises over a fractured rib

- *Assess any observed abnormalities* such as masses or sinus tracts (blind, inflammatory, tubelike structures opening onto the skin).

Although rare, sinus tracts usually indicate infection of the underlying pleura and lung (as in *tuberculosis, actinomycosis*).

- *Test chest expansion.* Place your thumbs at about the level of the 10th ribs, with your fingers loosely grasping and parallel to the lateral rib cage. As you position your hands, slide them medially just enough to raise a loose fold of skin on each side between your thumb and the spine.

  Ask the patient to inhale deeply. Watch the distance between your thumbs as they move apart during inspiration, and feel for the range and symmetry of the rib cage as it expands and contracts.

Causes of unilateral decrease or delay in chest expansion include *chronic fibrosis* of the underlying lung or pleura, *pleural effusion, lobar pneumonia,* pleural pain with associated splinting, and unilateral bronchial obstruction.

- *Feel for tactile fremitus.* Fremitus refers to the palpable vibrations transmitted through the bronchopulmonary tree to the chest wall as the patient is speaking. To detect fremitus, use either the ball (the bony part of the palm at the base of the fingers) or the ulnar surface of your hand to optimize the vibratory sensitivity of the bones in your hand. Ask the patient to repeat the words "ninety-nine" or "one-one-one." If fremitus is faint, ask the patient to speak more loudly or in a deeper voice.

  Use one hand until you have learned the feel of fremitus. Some clinicians find using one hand more accurate. The simultaneous use of both hands to compare sides, however, increases your speed and may facilitate detection of differences.

Fremitus is decreased or absent when the voice is soft or when the transmission of vibrations from the larynx to the surface of the chest is impeded. Causes include a very thick chest wall; an obstructed bronchus; *COPD*; separation of the pleural surfaces by fluid (*pleural effusion*), fibrosis (*pleural thickening*), air (*pneumothorax*), or an infiltrating tumor.

- *Palpate and compare symmetric areas* of the lungs in the pattern shown in the photograph. Identify and locate any areas of increased, decreased, or absent fremitus. Fremitus is typically more prominent in the interscapular area than in the lower lung fields and is often more prominent on the right side than on the left. It disappears below the diaphragm.

  Tactile fremitus is a somewhat imprecise assessment tool, but as

Look for *asymmetric* fremitus: asymmetric *decreased* fremitus in unilateral pleural effusion, pneumothorax, neoplasm from decreased transmission of low frequency sounds; asymmetric *increased* fremitus in unilateral pneumonia from increased transmission.[15]

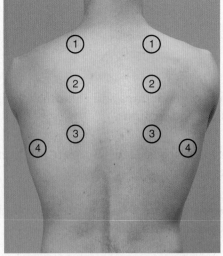

LOCATIONS FOR FEELING FREMITUS

a scouting technique, it directs your attention to possible abnormalities. Later in the examination you will check any suggested findings by listening for breath sounds, voice sounds, and whispered voice sounds. All these attributes tend to increase or decrease together.

Percussion

Percussion is one of the most important techniques of physical examination. Percussion sets the chest wall and underlying tissues in motion, producing audible sound and palpable vibrations. Percussion helps you establish whether the underlying tissues are air-filled, fluid-filled, or solid. It penetrates only 5 cm to 7 cm into the chest, however, and will not help you to detect deep-seated lesions.

How to Percuss...

The technique of percussion can be practiced on any surface. As you practice, listen for changes in percussion notes over different types of materials or different parts of the body. The key points for good technique, described for a right-handed person, are as follows:

- Hyperextend the middle finger of your left hand, known as the *pleximeter finger*. Press its distal interphalangeal joint firmly on the surface to be percussed. *Avoid surface contact by any other part of the hand, because this dampens out vibrations.* Note that the thumb and 2nd, 4th, and 5th fingers are not touching the chest.

- Position your right forearm quite close to the surface, with the hand cocked upward. The middle finger should be partially flexed, relaxed, and poised to strike.

- With a *quick, sharp but relaxed wrist motion*, strike the pleximeter finger with the right middle finger, or plexor finger. Aim at your distal interphalangeal joint. You are trying to transmit vibrations through the bones of this joint to the underlying chest wall.

- Strike using the *tip of the plexor finger,* not the finger pad. Your finger should be almost at right angles to the pleximeter. A short fingernail is recommended to avoid self-injury.

- Withdraw your striking finger quickly to avoid damping the vibrations you have created.

In summary, the movement is at the wrist. It is directed, brisk yet relaxed, and a bit bouncy.

Percussion Notes.   With your plexor or tapping finger, use the lightest percussion that produces a clear note. A thick chest wall requires stronger percussion than a thin one. However, if a *louder* note is needed, apply more pressure with the *pleximeter* finger (this is more effective for increasing percussion note volume than tapping harder with the plexor finger).

- *When percussing the lower posterior chest,* stand somewhat to the side rather than directly behind the patient. This allows you to place your pleximeter finger more firmly on the chest and your plexor is more effective, making a better percussion note.

- *When comparing two areas,* use the same percussion technique in both areas. Percuss or strike twice in each location. It is easier to detect differences in percussion notes by comparing one area with another than by striking repetitively in one place.

- *Learn to identify five percussion notes.* You can practice four of them on yourself. These notes differ in their basic qualities of sound: intensity, pitch, and duration. Train your ear to distinguish these differences by concentrating on one quality at a time as you percuss first in one location, then in another. Review the table below. Healthy lungs are *resonant.*

● **Percussion Notes and Their Characteristics**

	Relative Intensity	Relative Pitch	Relative Duration	Example of Location	Pathologic Examples
Flatness	Soft	High	Short	Thigh	Large pleural effusion
Dullness	Medium	Medium	Medium	Liver	Lobar pneumonia
Resonance	Loud	Low	Long	Healthy lung	Simple chronic bronchitis
Hyperresonance	Very loud	Lower	Longer	Usually none	COPD, pneumothorax
Tympany	Loud	High*	*	Gastric air bubble or puffed-out cheek	Large pneumothorax

* Distinguished mainly by its musical timbre.

While the patient keeps both arms crossed in front of the chest, percuss the thorax in symmetric locations on each side from the apex to the base.

● *Percuss one side of the chest and then the other at each level* in a ladder-like pattern, as shown by the numbers below. Omit the areas over the scapulae—the thickness of muscle and bone alters the percussion notes over the lungs. Identify and locate the area and quality of any abnormal percussion note.

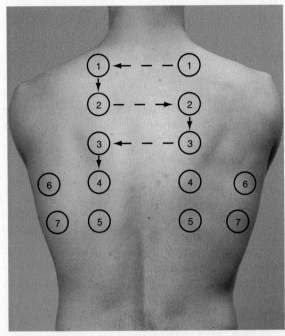

"LADDER" PATTERN FOR PERCUSSION AND AUSCULTATION

● *Identify the descent of the diaphragm,* or *diaphragmatic excursion.* First, *determine the level of diaphragmatic dullness* during quiet respiration. Holding the pleximeter finger *above and parallel* to the expected level of dullness, percuss downward in progressive steps until dullness clearly replaces resonance. Confirm this level of change by percussion near the middle of the hemothorax and also more laterally.

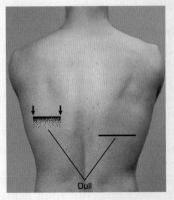

Dullness replaces resonance when fluid or solid tissue replaces air-containing lung or occupies the pleural space beneath your percussing fingers. Examples include: *lobar pneumonia,* in which the alveoli are filled with fluid and blood cells; and pleural accumulations of serous fluid (*pleural effusion*), blood (*hemothorax*), pus (*empyema*), fibrous tissue, or tumor.

Generalized hyperresonance may be heard over the hyperinflated lungs of COPD or *asthma,* but is not a reliable sign. *Unilateral hyperresonance* suggests a large pneumothorax or possibly a large air-filled bulla in the lung.

An abnormally high level suggests *pleural effusion,* or a high diaphragm as in *atelectasis* or *diaphragmatic paralysis.*

Location and sequence of percussion

Resonant

Level of diaphragm

Dull

Dull

Note that with this technique, you are identifying the boundary between the resonant lung tissue and the duller structures below the diaphragm. You are not percussing the diaphragm itself. You can infer the probable location of the diaphragm from the level of dullness.

Now, *estimate the extent of diaphragmatic excursion* by determining the distance between the level of dullness on full expiration and the level of dullness on full inspiration, normally about 5 or 6 cm.

Auscultation

Auscultation is the most important examination technique for assessing air flow through the tracheobronchial tree. Together with percussion, it also helps the clinician assess the condition of the surrounding lungs and pleural space. Auscultation involves (1) listening to the sounds generated by breathing, (2) listening for any adventitious (added) sounds, and (3) if abnormalities are suspected, listening to the sounds of the patient's spoken or whispered voice as they are transmitted through the chest wall.

Breath Sounds (Lung Sounds).   You will learn to identify patterns of breath sounds by their intensity, their pitch, and the relative duration of their inspiratory and expiratory phases. Normal breath sounds are:

- *Vesicular,* or soft and low pitched. They are heard through inspiration, continue without pause through expiration, and then fade away about one third of the way through expiration.

- *Bronchovesicular,* with inspiratory and expiratory sounds about equal in length, at times separated by a silent interval. Detecting differences in pitch and intensity is often easier during expiration.

- *Bronchial,* or louder and higher in pitch, with a short silence between inspiratory and expiratory sounds. Expiratory sounds last longer than inspiratory sounds.

The characteristics of these three kinds of breath sounds are summarized in the next table. Also shown are the *tracheal* breath sounds—very loud, harsh sounds that are heard by listening over the trachea in the neck.

Listen to the breath sounds with the diaphragm of a stethoscope after instructing the patient to breathe deeply through an open mouth. Use the pattern suggested for percussion, moving from one side to the other and comparing symmetric areas of the lungs. If you hear or suspect abnormal sounds, auscultate adjacent areas so that you can fully describe the extent of any abnormality. Listen to at least one full breath in each location. Be alert for patient discomfort resulting from hyperventilation (e.g., lightheadedness, faintness), and allow the patient to rest as needed.

Note the *intensity* of the breath sounds. Breath sounds are usually louder in the lower posterior lung fields and may also vary from area to area. If the breath sounds seem faint, ask the patient to breathe more deeply. You may then hear them easily. When patients do not breathe deeply enough or have a thick chest wall, as in obesity, breath sounds may remain diminished.

Sounds from bedclothes, paper gowns, and the chest itself can generate confusion in auscultation. Hair on the chest may cause crackling sounds. Either press harder or wet the hair. If the patient is cold or tense, you may hear muscle contraction sounds—muffled, low-pitched rumbling or roaring noises. A change in the patient's position may eliminate this noise. You can reproduce this sound on yourself by doing a Valsalva maneuver (straining down) as you listen to your own chest.

Breath sounds may be decreased when air flow is decreased (as in obstructive lung disease or muscular weakness) or when the transmission of sound is poor (as in *pleural effusion, pneumothorax,* or *COPD*).

● Characteristics of Breath Sounds[16]

	Duration of Sounds	Intensity of Expiratory Sound	Pitch of Expiratory Sound	Locations Where Heard Normally
Vesicular*	Inspiratory sounds last longer than expiratory ones.	Soft	Relatively low	Over most of both lungs
Broncho-vesicular	Inspiratory and expiratory sounds are about equal.	Intermediate	Intermediate	Often in the 1st and 2nd interspaces anteriorly and between the scapulae
Bronchial	Expiratory sounds last longer than inspiratory ones.	Loud	Relatively high	Over the manubrium, if heard at all
Tracheal	Inspiratory and expiratory sounds are about equal.	Very loud	Relatively high	Over the trachea in the neck

* The thickness of the bars indicates intensity; the steeper their incline, the higher the pitch.

If bronchovesicular or bronchial breath sounds are heard in locations distant from those listed, suspect that air-filled lung has been replaced by fluid-filled or solid lung tissue. See Table 8-5, Normal and Altered Breath and Voice Sounds (p. 318).

Is there a *silent gap* between the inspiratory and expiratory sounds?

A gap suggests bronchial breath sounds.

Listen for the *pitch, intensity, and duration of the expiratory and inspiratory sounds.* Are vesicular breath sounds distributed normally over the chest wall? Or are there bronchovesicular or bronchial breath sounds in unexpected places? If so, where are they?

Adventitious (Added) Sounds. Listen for any added, or adventitious, sounds that are superimposed on the usual breath sounds. Detection of adventitious sounds—*crackles* (sometimes called *rales*), *wheezes,* and *rhonchi*—is an important part of your examination, often leading to diagnosis of cardiac and pulmonary conditions. The most common kinds of these sounds are described on the next page.

For further discussion and other added sounds, see Table 8-6, Adventitious (Added) Lung Sounds: Causes and Qualities (p. 319).

If you hear *crackles,* especially those that do not clear after coughing, listen carefully for the following characteristics.[16–19] These are clues to the underlying condition:

● Loudness, pitch, and duration (summarized as fine or coarse crackles)

● Number (few to many)

Fine late inspiratory crackles that persist from breath to breath suggest abnormal lung tissue.

● **Adventitious or Added Breath Sounds**[16]

Crackles (or Rales)	Wheezes and Rhonchi
● **Discontinuous**	● **Continuous**
● Intermittent, nonmusical, and brief	● ≥250 msec, musical, prolonged (but not necessarily persisting throughout the respiratory cycle)
● Like dots in time	● Like dashes in time
● *Fine crackles:* soft, high-pitched, very brief (5–10 msec)	● *Wheezes:* relatively high-pitched (≥400 Hz) with hissing or shrill quality
● ● ● ● ●	WWWWW
● *Coarse crackles:* somewhat louder, lower in pitch, brief (20–30 msec)	● *Rhonchi:* relatively low-pitched (≤200 Hz) with snoring quality
● ● ● ● ●	WWW

Crackles may be from abnormalities of the lungs (*pneumonia, fibrosis, early congestive heart failure*) or of the airways (bronchitis, bronchiectasis).

Wheezes suggest narrowed airways, as in *asthma, COPD,* or *bronchitis.*

Rhonchi suggest secretions in large airways.

● Timing in the respiratory cycle

● Location on the chest wall

● Persistence of their pattern from breath to breath

● Any change after a cough or a change in the patient's position

Clearing of crackles, wheezes, or rhonchi after coughing or position change suggests inspissated secretions, as in *bronchitis* or *atelectasis.*

In some normal people, crackles may be heard at the lung bases anteriorly after maximal expiration. Crackles in dependent portions of the lungs may also occur after prolonged recumbency.

If you hear *wheezes* or *rhonchi,* note their timing and location. Do they change with deep breathing or coughing?

Findings predictive of *COPD* include combinations of symptoms and signs, especially wheezing by self-report or examination, plus history of smoking, age, and decreased breath sounds. Diagnosis requires pulmonary function tests such as spirometry.[20–25]

Transmitted Voice Sounds. If you hear abnormally located bronchovesicular or bronchial breath sounds, assess transmitted voice sounds. With a stethoscope, listen in symmetric areas over the chest wall as you:

Increased transmission of voice sounds suggests that air-filled lung has become airless. See Table 8-5, Normal and Altered Breath and Voice Sounds (p. 318).

- Ask the patient to say "ninety-nine." Normally the sounds transmitted through the chest wall are muffled and indistinct.

Louder, clearer voice sounds are called *bronchophony*.

- Ask the patient to say "ee." You will normally hear a muffled long E sound.

When "ee" is heard as "ay," an *E-to-A change (egophony)* is present, as in lobar consolidation from *pneumonia*. The quality sounds nasal.

- Ask the patient to whisper "ninety-nine" or "one-two-three." The whispered voice is normally heard faintly and indistinctly, if at all.

Louder, clearer whispered sounds are called *whispered pectoriloquy*.

EXAMINATION OF THE ANTERIOR CHEST

When examined in the supine position, the patient should lie comfortably with arms somewhat abducted. A patient who is having difficulty breathing should be examined in the sitting position or with the head of the bed elevated to a comfortable level.

Persons with severe *COPD* may prefer to sit leaning forward, with lips pursed during exhalation and arms supported on their knees or a table.

Inspection

Observe *the shape of the patient's chest* and *the movement of the chest wall*. Note:

- Deformities or asymmetry

See Table 8-4, Deformities of the Thorax (p. 317).

- Abnormal retraction of the lower interspaces during inspiration. Supraclavicular retraction is often present.

Severe *asthma, COPD,* or upper airway obstruction

- Local lag or impairment in respiratory movement

Underlying disease of lung or pleura

Palpation

Palpation has four potential uses:

- *Identification of tender areas*

Tender pectoral muscles or costal cartilages corroborate, but do not prove, that chest pain has a musculoskeletal origin.

- *Assessment of observed abnormalities*

- *Further assessment of chest expansion.* Place your thumbs along each costal margin, your hands along the lateral rib cage. As you position your hands, slide them medially a bit to raise loose skin folds between your thumbs. Ask the patient to inhale deeply. Observe how far your thumbs diverge as the thorax expands, and feel for the extent and symmetry of respiratory movement.

- *Assessment of tactile fremitus.* Compare both sides of the chest, using the ball or ulnar surface of your hand. Fremitus is usually decreased or absent over the precordium. When examining a woman, gently displace the breasts as necessary.

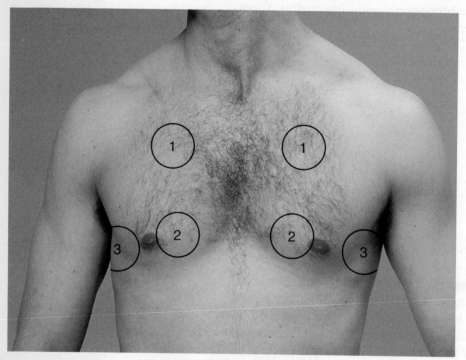

LOCATIONS FOR FEELING FREMITUS

Percussion

Percuss the anterior and lateral chest, again comparing both sides. The heart normally produces an area of dullness to the left of the sternum from the 3rd to the 5th interspaces. Percuss the left lung lateral to it.

Dullness replaces resonance when fluid or solid tissue replaces air-containing lung or occupies the pleural space. Because pleural fluid usually sinks to the lowest part of the pleural space (posteriorly in a supine patient), only a very large effusion can be detected anteriorly.

The hyperresonance of *COPD* may totally replace cardiac dullness.

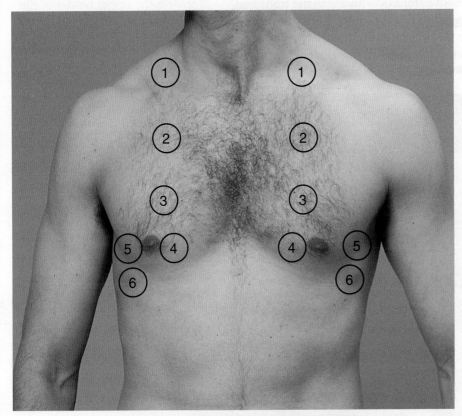

LOCATIONS FOR PERCUSSION AND AUSCULTATION

In a woman, to enhance percussion, gently displace the breast with your left hand while percussing with the right.

The dullness of right middle lobe pneumonia typically occurs behind the right breast. Unless you displace the breast, you may miss the abnormal percussion note.

Alternatively, you may ask the patient to move her breast for you.

Identify and locate any area with an abnormal percussion note.

With your pleximeter finger above and parallel to the expected upper border of liver dullness, percuss in progressive steps downward in the right midclavicular line. Identify the upper border of liver dullness. Later, during the abdominal examination, you will use this method to estimate the size of the liver. As you percuss down the chest on the left, the resonance of normal lung usually changes to the tympany of the gastric air bubble.

A lung affected by *COPD* often displaces the upper border of the liver downward. It also lowers the level of diaphragmatic dullness posteriorly.

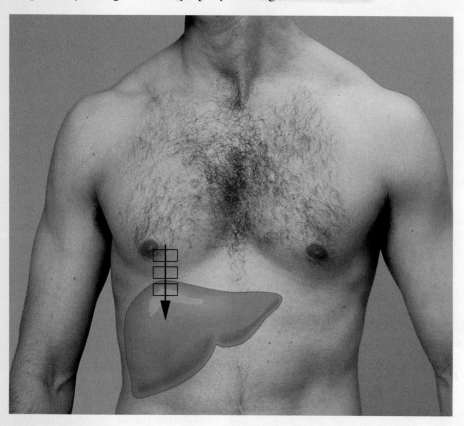

Auscultation

Listen to the chest anteriorly and laterally as the patient breathes with mouth open, somewhat more deeply than normal. Compare symmetric areas of the lungs, using the pattern suggested for percussion and extending it to adjacent areas as indicated.

Listen to the breath sounds, noting their intensity and identifying any variations from normal vesicular breathing. Breath sounds are usually louder in the upper anterior lung fields. Bronchovesicular breath sounds may be heard over the large airways, especially on the right.

Identify any adventitious sounds, time them in the respiratory cycle, and locate them on the chest wall. Do they clear with deep breathing?

If indicated, *listen for transmitted voice sounds.*

See Table 8-6, Adventitious (Added) Lung Sounds: Causes and Qualities (p. 319), and Table 8-7, Physical Findings in Selected Chest Disorders (pp. 320–321).

SPECIAL TECHNIQUES

Clinical Assessment of Pulmonary Function.   A simple but informative way to assess the pulmonary function is "the walk test." Time an 8-foot walk at the patient's normal pace. Repeat the walk and note the faster time. Also observe the rate, effort, and sound of the patient's breathing.

Nondisabled older adults taking 5.6 seconds or longer are more likely to be disabled over time than those taking 3.1 seconds or fewer. Early intervention may prevent onset of subsequent disability.[26]

Forced Expiratory Time.   This test assesses the expiratory phase of breathing, which is typically slowed in obstructive pulmonary disease. Ask the patient to take a deep breath in and then breathe out as quickly and completely as possible with mouth open. Listen over the trachea with the diaphragm of a stethoscope and time the audible expiration. Try to get three consistent readings, allowing a short rest between efforts if necessary.

Patients older than 60 years with a forced expiratory time of 6 to 8 seconds are twice as likely to have COPD.[27]

Identification of a Fractured Rib.   Local pain and tenderness of one or more ribs raise the question of fracture. By anteroposterior compression of the chest, you can help to distinguish a fracture from soft-tissue injury. With one hand on the sternum and the other on the thoracic spine, squeeze the chest. Is this painful, and where?

An increase in the local pain (distant from your hands) suggests rib fracture rather than just soft-tissue injury.

RECORDING YOUR FINDINGS

Note that initially you may use sentences to describe your findings; later you will use phrases. The style below contains phrases appropriate for most write-ups.

Recording the Physical Examination—The Thorax and Lungs

> "Thorax is symmetric with good expansion. Lungs resonant. Breath sounds vesicular; no rales, wheezes, or rhonchi. Diaphragms descend 4 cm bilaterally."
>
> **OR**
>
> "Thorax symmetric with moderate kyphosis and increased anteroposterior (AP) diameter, decreased expansion. Lungs are hyperresonant. Breath sounds distant with delayed expiratory phase and scattered expiratory wheezes. Fremitus decreased; no bronchophony, egophony, or whispered pectoriloquy. Diaphragms descend 2 cm bilaterally."

Suggests *COPD.*[20–25]

BIBLIOGRAPHY

CITATIONS

1. American Thoracic Society. Dyspnea—mechanisms, assessment, and management: a consensus statement. Am J Respir Crit Care Med 159(1):321–340, 1999.
2. Irwin RS, Madison JM. The diagnosis and treatment of cough. N Engl J Med 3432(3):1715–1721, 2000.
3. Barker A. Bronchiectasis. N Engl J Med 346(18):1383–1393, 2002.
4. Wenzel RP, Fowler AA. Acute bronchitis. N Engl J Med 355(20):2125–2130, 2006.
5. U.S. Preventive Services Task Force. Counseling to prevent tobacco use and tobacco-caused diseases: recommendation statement. Rockville, MD, Agency for Healthcare Research and Quality, November 2003. Available at: http://www.ahrq.gov/clinic/3rduspstf/tobacccoun/tobcounrs.htm. Accessed September 11, 2007.
6. U.S. Preventive Services Task Force. Lung cancer screening: recommendation statement. Rockville, MD, Agency for Healthcare Research and Quality, May 2004. Available at: http://www.ahrq.gov/clinic/3rduspstf/lungcancer/lungcanrs.htm. Accessed September 11, 2007.
7. U.S. Public Health Service. Treating tobacco use and dependence—clinician's packet. A how-to guide for implementing the Public Health Service clinical practice guideline. March 2003. Available at: http://www.surgeongeneral.gov/tobacco/clinpack.html. Accessed September 16, 2007.
8. Rigotti N. Treatment of tobacco use and dependence. N Engl J Med 346(7):506–512, 2002.
9. Centers for Disease Control and Prevention, DHHS. Fact sheet: smoking and tobacco use. Cessation. Available at: http://www.cdc.gov/tobacco/data_statistics/Factsheets/cessation2.htm. Accessed September 16, 2007.
10. Ranney L, Melvin C, Lux L, et al. Systematic review: smoking cessation intervention strategies for adults and adults in special populations. Ann Intern Med 145(11):845–856, 2006.
11. Norcross JC, Prochaska JO. Using the stages of change. Harvard Mental Health Letter May:5–7, 2002.
12. Varenicline (Chantix) for tobacco dependence. Med Lett Drugs Ther 48(1241–1242):66–68, 2006.
13. Advisory Committee on Immunization Practices (ACIP), Centers for Disease Control and Prevention. Prevention and control of influenza: recommendations of the ACIP. MMWR Morb Mortal Wkly Rep 56(RR-6):1–54, 2007.
14. Centers for Disease Control and Prevention. Vaccines and preventable diseases: pneumococcal vaccination. Available at: http://www.cdc.gov/vaccines/vpd-vac/pneumo/default.htm#recs. Accessed September 16, 2007.
15. McGee S. Evidence-Based Physical Diagnosis, 2nd ed. Philadelphia: Saunders: 314, 2007.
16. Loudon R, Murphy LH. Lungs sounds. Am Rev Respir Dis 130(4):663–673, 1994.
17. Epler GR, Carrrington CB, Gaensler EA. Crackles (rales) in the interstitial pulmonary diseases. Chest 73(3):333–339, 1978.
18. Nath AR, Capel LH. Inspiratory crackles and mechanical events of breathing. Thorax 29(6):695–698, 1974.
19. Nath AR, Capel LH. Lung crackles in bronchiectasis. Thorax 35(9):694–699, 1980.
20. Badgett RG, Tanaka DJ, Hunt DK, et al. Can moderate chronic obstructive pulmonary disease be diagnosed by historical and physical findings alone? Am J Med 94(2):188–196, 1993.
21. Holleman DR, Simel DL. Does the clinical examination predict airflow limitation? JAMA 273(4):63–68, 1995.
22. Straus SE, McAlister FA, Sackett DL, et al. The accuracy of patient history, wheezing, and laryngeal measurements in diagnosing obstructive airway disease. JAMA 283(14):1853–1857, 2000.
23. Pauwels RA, Buist AS, Calverley PM, et al. GOLD Scientific Committee. Global strategy for the diagnosis, management, and prevention of chronic obstructive pulmonary disease: NHLBI/WHO Global Initiative for Chronic Obstructive Lung Disease (GOLD) workshop summary. Am J Respir Crit Care Med 163(5):1256–1276, 2001.
24. Sin DD, McAlister FA, Man WEP, et al. Contemporary management of chronic obstructive pulmonary disease: scientific review. JAMA 290(17):2310–2312, 2003.
25. Sutherland ER, Cherniack RM. Management of chronic obstructive pulmonary disease. N Engl J Med 350(26):2689–2697, 2004.
26. Gurlanik JM, Ferrucci L, Simonsick EM, et al. Lower extremity function in persons over the age of 70 years as a predictor of subsequent disability. N Engl J Med 332(9):556–561, 1995.
27. Schapira RM, Schapira MM, Funahashi A, et al. The value of the forced expiratory time in the physical diagnosis of obstructive airway disease. JAMA 270(6):731–736, 1993.
28. Panettieri RA. In the clinic. Asthma. Ann Intern Med 146(11):ITC6-1–ITC6-14, 2007.
29. Metlay JP, Kapoor WN, Fine MJ. Does this patient have community-acquired pneumonia? Diagnosing pneumonia by history and physical examination. JAMA 378(17):1440–1445, 1997.
30. Chunilal SD, Eikelboom JW, Attia J, et al. Does this patient have pulmonary embolism? JAMA 290(21):2849–2858, 2003.
31. American Thoracic Society. Diagnostic standards/classification of TB in adults and children. Am J Respir Crit Care Med 161:1376–1395, 2000.

ADDITIONAL REFERENCES

Examination of the Lungs

Bettancourt PE, DelBono EA, Speigelman D, et al. Clinical utility of chest auscultation in common pulmonary disease. Am J Resp Crit Care Med 150:1921, 1994.

Cugell DW. Lung sound nomenclature. Am Rev Respir Dis 136:1016, 1987.

Koster MEY, Baughmann RP, Loudon RG. Continuous adventitious lung sounds. J Asthma 27:237, 1990.

Kraman SS. Lung sounds for the clinician. Arch Intern Med 146: 1411, 1986.

Lehrer S. Understanding Lung Sounds, 3rd ed. Philadelphia, WB Saunders, 2002.

Lichtenstein D, Goldstein I, Mourgeon E, et al. Comparative diagnostic performances of auscultation, chest radiography, and lung ultrasonography in acute respiratory distress syndrome. Anesthesiology 100(1):9–15, 2004.

Pulmonary Conditions

American Thoracic Society and Centers for Disease Control and Prevention. Diagnostic standards and classification of tuberculosis in adults and children. Am J Respir Crit Care Med 161(4 Pt 1): 1376–1395, 2000.

Baum GL, Crapo JD, Celli BR, et al., eds. Baum's Textbook of Pulmonary Diseases, 7th ed. Philadelphia: Lippincott Williams & Wilkins, 2004.

Chung KF, Pavord ID. Prevalence, pathogenesis, and causes of chronic cough. Lancet 371(9621):1364–1374, 2008.

Eder W, Ege MJ, Mutius E. The asthma epidemic. N Engl J Med 355(21):2226–2235, 2006.

Evans SE, Scanlon PD. Current practice in pulmonary function testing. Mayo Clin Proc 78(6):758–763, 2003.

Fiore MC, Jaén CR, Baker TB, et al. Treating Tobacco Use and Dependence: 2008 Update. Rockville, MD: U.S. Department of Health and Human Services, May 2008. Available at: http://www.ahrq.gov/path/tobacco.htm#Clinic. Accessed May 26, 2008.

Global Initiative for Chronic Obstructive Lung Disease (GOLD). Global Strategy for the Diagnosis, Management, and Prevention of Chronic Obstructive Pulmonary Disease. Bethesda, MD: Global Initiative for Chronic Obstructive Lung Disease, World Health Organization, National Heart, Lung and Blood Institute, 2007. Available at: http://www.guidelines.gov/summary/summary.aspx?doc_id=12178&nbr=006275&string=GOLD. Accessed May 26, 2008.

Qaseem A, Snow V, Shekelle P, et al. Diagnosis and management of stable chronic obstructive pulmonary disease: a clinical practice guideline from the American College of Physicians. Ann Intern Med 147(9):633–638, 2007.

Ware LB, Matthay MA. Acute pulmonary edema. N Engl J Med 353(26):2788–2796, 2005.

Weinberger SE, Cockrill BA, Mandel J. Principles of Pulmonary Medicine, 5th ed. Philadelphia: Saunders/Elsevier, 2008.

Williams SG, Schmidt DK, Redd SC, et al. Key clinical activities for quality asthma care: recommendations of the National Asthma Education and Prevention Program. MMWR Recomm Rep 52 (RR–6):1–8, 2003.

Witt TJ, Niewoehner D, Macdonald R, et al. Management of stable chronic obstructive pulmonary disease: a systematic review for a clinical practice guideline. Ann Intern Med 147(9):639–653, 2007.

The Bates' suite offers these additional resources to enhance learning and facilitate understanding of this chapter:

- Bates' Pocket Guide to Physical Examination and History Taking, 6th edition
- Bates' Nursing Online
- Bates' Visual Guide to Physical Examination, 4th edition
- thePoint online resources, http://thepoint.lww.com
- Student CD-ROM included with the book

Chest Pain

Problem	Process	Location	Quality	Severity
Cardiovascular				
Angina Pectoris	Temporary myocardial ischemia, usually secondary to coronary atherosclerosis	Retrosternal or across the anterior chest, sometimes radiating to the shoulders, arms, neck, lower jaw, or upper abdomen	Pressing, squeezing, tight, heavy, occasionally burning	Mild to moderate, sometimes perceived as discomfort rather than pain
Myocardial Infarction	Prolonged myocardial ischemia, resulting in irreversible muscle damage or necrosis	Same as in angina	Same as in angina	Often but not always a severe pain
Pericarditis	■ Irritation of parietal pleura adjacent to the pericardium	Precordial, may radiate to the tip of the shoulder and to the neck	Sharp, knifelike	Often severe
	■ Mechanism unclear	Retrosternal	Crushing	Severe
Dissecting Aortic Aneurysm	A splitting within the layers of the aortic wall, allowing passage of blood to dissect a channel	Anterior chest, radiating to the neck, back, or abdomen	Ripping, tearing	Very severe
Pulmonary				
Tracheobronchitis	Inflammation of trachea and large bronchi	Upper sternal or on either side of the sternum	Burning	Mild to moderate
Pleuritic Pain	Inflammation of the parietal pleura, as in pleurisy, pneumonia, pulmonary infarction, or neoplasm	Chest wall overlying the process	Sharp, knifelike	Often severe
Gastrointestinal and Other				
Reflex Esophagitis	Inflammation of the esophageal mucosa by reflux of gastric acid	Retrosternal, may radiate to the back	Burning, may be squeezing	Mild to severe
Diffuse Esophageal Spasm	Motor dysfunction of the esophageal muscle	Retrosternal, may radiate to the back, arms, and jaw	Usually squeezing	Mild to severe
Chest Wall Pain, Costochondritis	Variable, often unclear	Often below the left breast or along the costal cartilages; also elsewhere	Stabbing, sticking, or dull, aching	Variable
Anxiety	Unclear	Precordial, below the left breast, or across the anterior chest	Stabbing, sticking, or dull, aching	Variable

Note: Remember that chest pain may be referred from extrathoracic structures such as the neck (*arthritis*) and abdomen (*biliary colic, acute cholecystitis*). Pleural pain may be from abdominal conditions such as *subdiaphragmatic abscess*.

Timing	Factors That Aggravate	Factors That Relieve	Associated Symptoms
Usually 1–3 min but up to 10 min. Prolonged episodes up to 20 min	Exertion, especially in the cold; meals; emotional stress. May occur at rest	Rest, nitroglycerin	Sometimes dyspnea, nausea, sweating
20 min to several hours			Nausea, vomiting, sweating, weakness
Persistent	Breathing, changing position, coughing, lying down, sometimes swallowing	Sitting forward may relieve it.	Of the underlying illness
Persistent			Of the underlying illness
Abrupt onset, early peak, persistent for hours or more	Hypertension		Syncope, hemiplegia, paraplegia
Variable	Coughing	Lying on the involved side may relieve it.	Cough
Persistent	Inspiration, coughing, movements of the trunk		Of the underlying illness
Variable	Large meal; bending over, lying down	Antacids, sometimes belching	Sometimes regurgitation, dysphagia
Variable	Swallowing of food or cold liquid; emotional stress	Sometimes nitroglycerin	Dysphagia
Fleeting to hours or days	Movement of chest, trunk, arms		Often local tenderness
Fleeting to hours or days	May follow effort, emotional stress		Breathlessness, palpitations, weakness, anxiety

Dyspnea[1]

Problem	Process	Timing
Left-Sided Heart Failure (*left ventricular failure or mitral stenosis*)	Elevated pressure in pulmonary capillary bed with transudation of fluid into interstitial spaces and alveoli, decreased compliance (increased stiffness) of the lungs, increased work of breathing	Dyspnea may progress slowly, or suddenly as in acute pulmonary edema.
Chronic Bronchitis*[4]	Excessive mucus production in bronchi, followed by chronic obstruction of airways	Chronic productive cough followed by slowly progressive dyspnea
Chronic Obstructive Pulmonary Disease (COPD)*[20–25]	Overdistention of air spaces distal to terminal bronchioles, with destruction of alveolar septa and chronic obstruction of the airways	Slowly progressive dyspnea; relatively mild cough later
Asthma[28]	Bronchial hyperresponsiveness involving release of inflammatory mediators, increased airway secretions, and bronchoconstriction	Acute episodes, separated by symptom-free periods. Nocturnal episodes common
Diffuse Interstitial Lung Diseases (*such as sarcoidosis, widespread neoplasms, asbestosis, and idiopathic pulmonary fibrosis*)	Abnormal and widespread infiltration of cells, fluid, and collagen into interstitial spaces between alveoli. Many causes	Progressive dyspnea, which varies in its rate of development with the cause
Pneumonia[29]	Inflammation of lung parenchyma from the respiratory bronchioles to the alveoli	An acute illness, timing varies with the causative agent
Spontaneous Pneumothorax	Leakage of air into pleural space through blebs on visceral pleura, with resulting partial or complete collapse of the lung	Sudden onset of dyspnea
Acute Pulmonary Embolism[30]	Sudden occlusion of all or part of pulmonary arterial tree by a blood clot that usually originates in deep veins of legs or pelvis	Sudden onset of dyspnea
Anxiety With Hyperventilation	Overbreathing, with resultant respiratory alkalosis and fall in the partial pressure of carbon dioxide in the blood	Episodic, often recurrent

Chronic bronchitis and *chronic obstructive pulmonary disease (COPD)* may coexist.

Factors That Aggravate	Factors That Relieve	Associated Symptoms	Setting
Exertion, lying down	Rest, sitting up, though dyspnea may become persistent	Often cough, orthopnea, paroxysmal nocturnal dyspnea; sometimes wheezing	History of heart disease or its predisposing factors
Exertion, inhaled irritants, respiratory infections	Expectoration; rest, though dyspnea may become persistent	Chronic productive cough, recurrent respiratory infections; wheezing may develop	History of smoking, air pollutants, recurrent respiratory infections
Exertion	Rest, though dyspnea may become persistent	Cough, with scant mucoid sputum	History of smoking, air pollutants, sometimes a familial deficiency in alpha$_1$-antitrypsin
Variable, including allergens, irritants, respiratory infections, exercise, and emotion	Separation from aggravating factors	Wheezing, cough, tightness in chest	Environmental and emotional conditions
Exertion	Rest, though dyspnea may become persistent	Often weakness, fatigue. Cough less common than in other lung diseases	Varied. Exposure to one of many substances may be causative.
		Pleuritic pain, cough, sputum, fever, though not necessarily present	Varied
		Pleuritic pain, cough	Often a previously healthy young adult
		Often none. Retrosternal oppressive pain if the occlusion is massive. Pleuritic pain, cough, and hemoptysis may follow an embolism if pulmonary infarction ensues. Symptoms of anxiety (see below).	Postpartum or postoperative periods; prolonged bed rest; congestive heart failure, chronic lung disease, and fractures of hip or leg; deep venous thrombosis (often not clinically apparent)
More often occurs at rest than after exercise. An upsetting event may not be evident.	Breathing in and out of a paper or plastic bag sometimes helps the associated symptoms.	Sighing, lightheadedness, numbness or tingling of the hands and feet, palpitations, chest pain	Other manifestations of anxiety may be present.

Cough[2] and Hemoptysis*

Problem	Cough and Sputum	Associated Symptoms and Setting
Acute Inflammation		
Laryngitis	Dry cough (without sputum), may become productive of variable amounts of sputum	An acute, fairly minor illness with hoarseness. Often associated with viral nasopharyngitis
Tracheobronchitis	Dry cough, may become productive	An acute, often viral illness, with burning retrosternal discomfort
Mycoplasma and Viral Pneumonias[29]	Dry hacking cough, often becoming productive of mucoid sputum	An acute febrile illness, often with malaise, headache, and possibly dyspnea
Bacterial Pneumonias[29]	Pneumococcal: sputum mucoid or purulent; may be blood-streaked, diffusely pinkish, or rusty	An acute illness with chills, high fever, dyspnea, and chest pain. Often preceded by acute upper respiratory infection
	Klebsiella: similar; or sticky, red, and jellylike	Typically occurs in older alcoholic men
Chronic Inflammation		
Postnasal Drip	Chronic cough; sputum mucoid or mucopurulent	Repeated attempts to clear the throat. Postnasal discharge may be sensed by patient or seen in posterior pharynx. Associated with chronic rhinitis, with or without sinusitis
Chronic Bronchitis[4]	Chronic cough; sputum mucoid to purulent, may be blood-streaked or even bloody	Often long-standing cigarette smoking. Recurrent superimposed infections. Wheezing and dyspnea may develop.
Bronchiectasis[3]	Chronic cough; sputum purulent, often copious and foul-smelling; may be blood-streaked or bloody	Recurrent bronchopulmonary infections common; sinusitis may coexist.
Pulmonary Tuberculosis[31]	Cough dry or sputum that is mucoid or purulent; may be blood-streaked or bloody	Early, no symptoms. Later, anorexia, weight loss, fatigue, fever, and night sweats
Lung Abscess	Sputum purulent and foul-smelling; may be bloody	A febrile illness. Often poor dental hygiene and a prior episode of impaired consciousness
Asthma[28]	Cough, with thick mucoid sputum, especially near end of an attack	Episodic wheezing and dyspnea, but cough may occur alone. Often a history of allergy
Gastroesophageal Reflux	Chronic cough, especially at night or early in the morning	Wheezing, especially at night (often mistaken for asthma), early morning hoarseness, and repeated attempts to clear the throat. Often a history of heartburn and regurgitation
Neoplasm		
Cancer of the Lung	Cough dry to productive; sputum may be blood-streaked or bloody	Usually a long history of cigarette smoking. Associated manifestations are numerous.
Cardiovascular Disorders		
Left Ventricular Failure or Mitral Stenosis	Often dry, especially on exertion or at night; may progress to the pink frothy sputum of pulmonary edema or to frank hemoptysis	Dyspnea, orthopnea, paroxysmal nocturnal dyspnea
Pulmonary Emboli[30]	Dry to productive; may be dark, bright red, or mixed with blood	Dyspnea, anxiety, chest pain, fever; factors that predispose to deep venous thrombosis
Irritating Particles, Chemicals, or Gases	Variable. There may be a latent period between exposure and symptoms.	Exposure to irritants. Eyes, nose, and throat may be affected.

*Characteristics of hemoptysis are printed in red.

Normal Adult
The thorax in the normal adult is wider than it is deep. Its lateral diameter is larger than its anteroposterior diameter.

Funnel Chest (*Pectus Excavatum*)
Note depression in the lower portion of the sternum. Compression of the heart and great vessels may cause murmurs.

Barrel Chest
There is an increased anteroposterior diameter. This shape is normal during infancy, and often accompanies aging and chronic obstructive pulmonary disease.

Depressed costal cartilages

Anteriorly displaced sternum

Pigeon Chest (*Pectus Carinatum*)
The sternum is displaced anteriorly, increasing the anteroposterior diameter. The costal cartilages adjacent to the protruding sternum are depressed.

Expiration
Inspiration

Traumatic Flail Chest
Multiple rib fractures may result in paradoxical movements of the thorax. As descent of the diaphragm decreases intrathoracic pressure, on inspiration the injured area caves inward; on expiration, it moves outward.

Spinal convexity to the right
(patient bending forward)

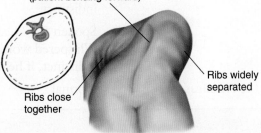

Ribs widely separated

Ribs close together

Thoracic Kyphoscoliosis
Abnormal spinal curvatures and vertebral rotation deform the chest. Distortion of the underlying lungs may make interpretation of lung findings very difficult.

TABLE 8-5

Normal and Altered Breath and Voice Sounds

The origins of breath sounds are still unclear. According to leading theories, turbulent air flow in the central airways produces the tracheal and bronchial breath sounds. As these sounds pass through the lungs to the periphery, lung tissue filters out their higher-pitched components, and only the soft and lower-pitched components reach the chest wall, where they are heard as vesicular breath sounds. Normally, tracheal and bronchial sounds may be heard over the trachea and mainstem bronchi; vesicular breath sounds predominate throughout most of the lungs.

When lung tissue loses its air, it transmits high-pitched sounds much better. If the tracheobronchial tree is open, bronchial breath sounds may replace the normal vesicular sounds over airless areas of the lung. This change is seen in lobar pneumonia when the alveoli fill with fluid, red cells, and white cells—a process called *consolidation*. Other causes include pulmonary edema or hemorrhage. Bronchial breath sounds usually correlate with an increase in tactile fremitus and transmitted voice sounds. These findings are summarized below.

	Normal Air-Filled Lung	Airless Lung, as in Lobar Pneumonia
		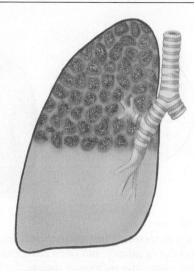
Breath Sounds	Predominantly vesicular	Bronchial or bronchovesicular over the involved area
Transmitted Voice Sounds	Spoken words muffled and indistinct	Spoken words louder, clearer (*bronchophony*)
	Spoken "ee" heard as "ee" Whispered words faint and indistinct, if heard at all	Spoken "ee" heard as "ay" (*egophony*) Whispered words louder, clearer (*whispered pectoriloquy*)
Tactile Fremitus	Normal	Increased

Adventitious (Added) Lung Sounds: Causes and Qualities[16–19]

Crackles

Crackles have two leading explanations. (1) They result from a series of tiny explosions when small airways, deflated during expiration, pop open during inspiration. This mechanism probably explains the late inspiratory crackles of interstitial lung disease and early congestive heart failure. (2) Crackles result from air bubbles flowing through secretions or lightly closed airways during respiration. This mechanism probably explains at least some coarse crackles.

Inspiration Expiration

Late inspiratory crackles may begin in the first half of inspiration but must continue into late inspiration. They are usually fine, fairly profuse, and persist from breath to breath. They appear first at the bases of the lungs, spread upward as the condition worsens, and shift to dependent regions with changes in posture. Causes include *interstitial lung disease* (such as fibrosis) and early *congestive heart failure*.

Early inspiratory crackles appear and end soon after the start of inspiration. They are often coarse and relatively few in number. Expiratory crackles are sometimes associated. Causes include *chronic bronchitis* and *asthma*.

Midinspiratory and expiratory crackles are heard in *bronchiectasis* but are not specific for this diagnosis. Wheezes and rhonchi may be associated.

Wheezes and Rhonchi

Wheezes occur when air flows rapidly through bronchi that are narrowed nearly to the point of closure. They are often audible at the mouth as well as through the chest wall. Causes of wheezes throughout the chest include *asthma, chronic bronchitis, COPD,* and *congestive heart failure* (cardiac asthma). In *asthma*, wheezes may be heard only in expiration or in both phases of the respiratory cycle. Rhonchi suggest secretions in the larger airways. In chronic bronchitis, wheezes and rhonchi often clear with coughing.

Occasionally in severe obstructive pulmonary disease, the patient is unable to force enough air through the narrowed bronchi to produce wheezing. The resulting *silent chest* is ominous and warrants immediate attention.

Persistent localized wheezing suggests partial obstruction of a bronchus, as by a tumor or foreign body. It may be inspiratory, expiratory, or both.

Stridor

A wheeze that is entirely or predominantly inspiratory is called *stridor*. It is often louder in the neck than over the chest wall. It indicates a partial obstruction of the larynx or trachea, and demands immediate attention.

Pleural Rub

Inflamed and roughened pleural surfaces grate against each other as they are momentarily and repeatedly delayed by increased friction. These movements produce creaking sounds known as a *pleural rub* (or pleural friction rub).

Pleural rubs resemble crackles acoustically, although they are produced by different pathologic processes. The sounds may be discrete, but sometimes are so numerous that they merge into a seemingly continuous sound. A rub is usually confined to a relatively small area of the chest wall, and typically is heard in both phases of respiration. When inflamed pleural surfaces are separated by fluid, the rub often disappears.

Mediastinal Crunch
(Hamman's Sign)

A *mediastinal crunch* is a series of precordial crackles synchronous with the heart beat, not with respiration. Best heard in the left lateral position, it is due to mediastinal emphysema (*pneumomediastinum*).

TABLE 8-7

Physical Findings in Selected Chest Disorders

The black boxes in this table suggest a framework for clinical assessment. Start with the three boxes under Percussion Note: resonant, dull, and hyperresonant. Then move from each of these to other boxes that emphasize some of the key differences among various conditions. The changes described vary with the extent and severity of the disorder. Abnormalities deep in the chest usually produce fewer signs than superficial ones, and may cause no signs at all. Use the table for the direction of typical changes, not for absolute distinctions.

Condition	Percussion Note	Trachea	Breath Sounds	Adventitious Sounds	Tactile Fremitus and Transmitted Voice Sounds
Normal The tracheobronchial tree and alveoli are clear; pleurae are thin and close together; mobility of the chest wall is unimpaired.	**Resonant**	Midline	Vesicular, except perhaps bronchovesicular and bronchial sounds over the large bronchi and trachea, respectively	None, except perhaps a few transient inspiratory crackles at the bases of the lungs	Normal
Chronic Bronchitis The bronchi are chronically inflamed and a productive cough is present. Airway obstruction may develop.	**Resonant**	Midline	Vesicular (normal)	None; or scattered coarse *crackles* in early inspiration and perhaps expiration; or *wheezes* or *rhonchi*	Normal
Left-Sided Heart Failure *(Early)* Increased pressure in the pulmonary veins causes congestion and interstitial edema (around the alveoli); bronchial mucosa may become edematous.	**Resonant**	Midline	Vesicular	*Late inspiratory crackles* in the dependent portions of the lungs; possibly *wheezes*	Normal
Consolidation Alveoli fill with fluid or blood cells, as in pneumonia, pulmonary edema, or pulmonary hemorrhage.	**Dull** over the airless area	Midline	*Bronchial* over the involved area	*Late inspiratory crackles* over the involved area	*Increased* over the involved area, with *bronchophony, egophony,* and *whispered pectoriloquy*
Atelectasis *(Lobar Obstruction)* When a plug in a mainstem bronchus (as from mucus or a foreign object) obstructs air flow, affected lung tissue collapses into an airless state.	**Dull** over the airless area	May be *shifted toward involved side*	*Usually absent* when bronchial plug persists. Exceptions include right upper lobe atelectasis, where adjacent tracheal sounds may be transmitted.	None	*Usually absent* when the bronchial plug persists. In exceptions (e.g., right upper lobe atelectasis) may be increased

(table continues on page 321)

Condition	Percussion Note	Trachea	Breath Sounds	Adventitious Sounds	Tactile Fremitus and Transmitted Voice Sounds
Pleural Effusion Fluid accumulates in the pleural space, separates air-filled lung from the chest wall, blocking the transmission of sound.	**Dull** to flat over the fluid	*Shifted toward opposite side* in a large effusion	*Decreased to absent,* but bronchial breath sounds may be heard near top of large effusion.	None, except a *possible pleural* rub	*Decreased to absent, but may be increased* toward the top of a large effusion
Pneumothorax When air leaks into the pleural space, usually unilaterally, the lung recoils from the chest wall. Pleural air blocks transmission of sound.	**Hyperresonant** or tympanitic over the pleural air	*Shifted toward opposite side* if much air	*Decreased to absent* over the pleural air	None, except a *possible pleural rub*	*Decreased to absent* over the pleural air
Chronic Obstructive Pulmonary Disease (COPD) Slowly progressive disorder in which the distal air spaces enlarge and lungs become hyperinflated. Chronic bronchitis is often associated.	Diffusely **hyperresonant**	Midline	*Decreased to absent*	None, or the crackles, wheezes, and rhonchi of associated chronic bronchitis	*Decreased*
Asthma Widespread narrowing of the tracheobronchial tree diminishes air flow to a fluctuating degree. During attacks, air flow decreases further, and lungs hyperinflate.	**Resonant** to diffusely **hyperresonant**	Midline	*Often obscured by wheezes*	*Wheezes, possibly crackles*	*Decreased*

The Cardiovascular System

ANATOMY AND PHYSIOLOGY

SURFACE PROJECTIONS OF THE HEART AND GREAT VESSELS

Listening to the heart has long been a symbol for the panoply of skills of bedside diagnosis. It is particularly vulnerable to evolving technology and ever more compressed time that limits opportunities for trainees to gain mastery through practice and repetition.[1,2] Many observers report the decline in clinician skills of physical examination—more amply documented for the cardiovascular system than for any other area of examination, and at

all levels of training.[3-7] As you study this chapter, combining the cognitive knowledge of anatomy and physiology with the hands-on practice of inspection, palpation, percussion, and especially auscultation will be critical. An exciting world of proven diagnostic value awaits you.

First, learn to visualize the underlying structures of the heart as you inspect the anterior chest. Note that the *right ventricle* occupies most of the anterior cardiac surface. This chamber and the pulmonary artery form a wedgelike structure behind and to the left of the sternum, outlined in black.

The inferior border of the right ventricle lies below the junction of the sternum and the xiphoid process. The right ventricle narrows superiorly and joins the pulmonary artery at the level of the sternum or *"base of the heart"*—a clinical term that refers

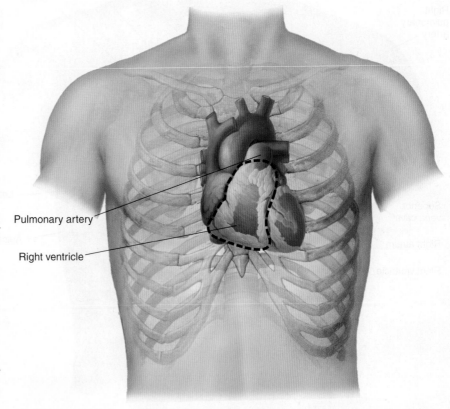

Pulmonary artery

Right ventricle

to the superior aspect of the heart at the right and left 2nd interspaces next to the sternum.

The *left ventricle*, behind the right ventricle and to the left, outlined below in black, forms the left lateral margin of the heart. Its tapered inferior tip is often termed the *cardiac "apex."* It is clinically important because it produces the apical impulse, identified during palpation of the precordium as the *point of maximal impulse*, or *PMI*. This impulse locates the left border of the heart and is normally found in the 5th interspace 7 cm to 9 cm lateral to the midsternal line, typically at or just medial to the left midclavicular line. The PMI may not be readily felt in a healthy patient with a normal heart, however.

- In supine patients the *diameter of the PMI* may be as large as a quarter, approximately 1 to 2.5 cm. A PMI greater than 2.5 cm is evidence of left ventricular hypertrophy (LVH), or enlargement.

- Similarly, *displacement of the PMI* lateral to the midclavicular line or greater than 10 cm lateral to the midsternal line also suggests LVH, or enlargement.

- Note that in some patients the most prominent precordial impulse may not be at the apex of the left ventricle. For example, in patients with chronic obstructive pulmonary disease, the most prominent palpable impulse or PMI may be in the xiphoid or epigastric area as a result of *right ventricular hypertrophy.*

Above the heart lie the *great vessels.* The *pulmonary artery,* already mentioned, bifurcates quickly into its left and right branches. The *aorta* curves upward from the left ventricle to the level of the sternal angle, where it arches backward to the left and then downward. On the medial border, the *superior* and *inferior venae cavae* channel venous blood from the upper and lower portions of the body into the right atrium.

CARDIAC CHAMBERS, VALVES, AND CIRCULATION

Circulation through the heart is shown in the diagram below, which identifies the cardiac chambers, valves, and direction of blood flow. Because of their positions, the *tricuspid* and *mitral valves* are often called *atrioventricular valves.* The *aortic* and *pulmonic valves* are called *semilunar valves* because each of their leaflets is shaped like a half moon. Although this diagram shows all valves in an open position, they do not open simultaneously in the living heart.

As the heart valves close, the heart sounds arise from vibrations emanating from the leaflets, the adjacent cardiac structures, and the flow of blood.

RA = Right atrium   ⟹ Course of oxygenated blood   LA = Left atrium
RV = Right ventricle   ⟶ Course of unoxygenated blood   LV = Left ventricle

Study carefully the positions and movements of the valves in relation to events in the cardiac cycle. This knowledge will improve your diagnostic accuracy when you auscultate the heart.

EVENTS IN THE CARDIAC CYCLE

The heart serves as a pump that generates varying pressures as its chambers contract and relax. *Systole is the period of ventricular contraction*. In the diagram below, pressure in the left ventricle rises from less than 5 mm Hg in its resting state to a normal peak of 120 mm Hg. After the ventricle ejects much of its blood into the aorta, the pressure levels off and starts to fall. *Diastole is the period of ventricular relaxation*. Ventricular pressure falls further to below 5 mm Hg, and blood flows from atrium to ventricle. Late in diastole, ventricular pressure rises slightly during inflow of blood from atrial contraction.

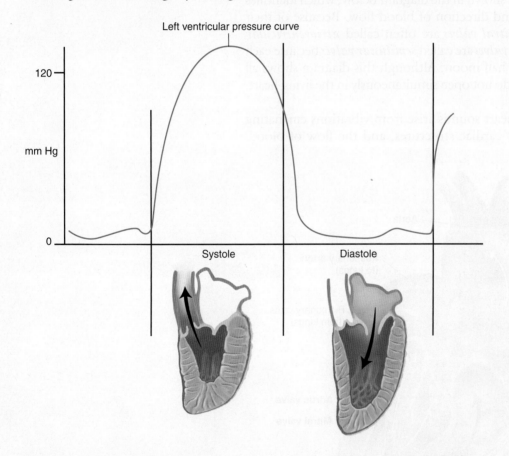

Note that during *systole* the aortic valve is open, allowing ejection of blood from the left ventricle into the aorta. The mitral valve is closed, preventing blood from regurgitating back into the left atrium. In contrast, during *diastole* the aortic valve is closed, preventing regurgitation of blood from the aorta back into the left ventricle. The mitral valve is open, allowing blood to flow from the left atrium into the relaxed left ventricle.

Understanding the interrelationships of the *pressure gradients* in these three chambers—left atrium, left ventricle, and aorta—together with the position and movement of the valves is fundamental to understanding heart sounds. Trace these changing pressures and sounds through one cardiac cycle. Note that during auscultation the first and second heart sounds define the duration of *systole* and *diastole*. An extensive literature deals with the exact causes of heart sounds. Possible explanations include actual closure of valve leaflets, tensing of related structures, leaflet positions and pressure gradients at the time of atrial and ventricular systole, and the effects of columns of blood. The explanations given here are oversimplified but retain clinical usefulness.

During *diastole,* pressure in the blood-filled left atrium slightly exceeds that in the relaxed left ventricle, and blood flows from left atrium to left ventricle across the open mitral valve. Just before the onset of ventricular systole, atrial contraction produces a slight pressure rise in both chambers.

During *systole,* the left ventricle starts to contract and ventricular pressure rapidly exceeds left atrial pressure, shutting the mitral valve. *Closure of the mitral valve produces the first heart sound, S₁.*

As left ventricular pressure continues to rise, it quickly exceeds the pressure in the aorta and forces the aortic valve open. In some pathologic conditions, an early systolic ejection sound (Ej) accompanies the opening of the aortic valve. *Normally, maximal left ventricular pressure corresponds to systolic blood pressure.*

As the left ventricle ejects most of its blood, ventricular pressure begins to fall. When left ventricular pressure drops below aortic pressure, the aortic valve shuts. *Aortic valve closure produces the second heart sound, S₂,* and another diastole begins.

In *diastole,* left ventricular pressure continues to drop and falls below left atrial pressure. The mitral valve opens. This event is usually silent, but may be audible as a pathologic opening snap (OS) if valve leaflet motion is restricted, as in mitral stenosis.

Aortic pressure

Mitral valve opens

Left atrial pressure

Left ventricular pressure

S₁ Eⱼ   S₂ OS

After the mitral valve opens, there is a period of rapid ventricular filling as blood flows early in diastole from left atrium to left ventricle. In children and young adults, a third heart sound, S₃, may arise from rapid deceleration of the column of blood against the ventricular wall. In older adults, an S₃, sometimes termed "an S₃ gallop," usually indicates a pathologic change in ventricular compliance.

Period of rapid ventricular filling

S₁ Eⱼ   S₂ OS S₃

Finally, although not often heard in normal adults, a fourth heart sound, S₄, marks atrial contraction. It immediately precedes S₁ of the next beat and also reflects a pathologic change in ventricular compliance.

Augmented ventricular filling as a result of atrial contraction

S₁ Eⱼ   S₂ OS S₃   S₄

Systole   Diastole

THE SPLITTING OF HEART SOUNDS

While these events are occurring on the left side of the heart, similar changes are occurring on the right, involving the right atrium, right ventricle, tricuspid valve, pulmonic valve, and pulmonary artery. Right ventricular and pulmonary arterial pressures are significantly lower than corresponding pressures on the left side. Furthermore, right-sided events usually occur slightly later than those on the left. Instead of a single heart sound, you may hear two discernible components, the first from left-sided aortic valve closure, or A₂, and the second from right-sided closure of the pulmonic valve, or P₂.

Consider the second heart sound, S_2, and its two components, A_2 and P_2, caused primarily by closure of the aortic and pulmonic valves, respectively. During inspiration the right heart filling time is increased, which increases right ventricular stroke volume and the duration of right ventricular ejection compared with the neighboring left ventricle. This delays the closure of the pulmonic valve, P_2, splitting S_2 into its two audible components. During expiration, these two components fuse into a single sound, S_2. Note that because walls of veins contain less smooth muscle, the venous system has more capacitance than the arterial system and lower systemic pressure. Distensibility and impedance in the pulmonary vascular bed contribute to the "hangout time" that delays P_2.[8]

Of the two components of the S_2, A_2 is normally louder, reflecting the high pressure in the aorta. It is heard throughout the precordium. P_2, in contrast, is relatively soft, reflecting the lower pressure in the pulmonary artery. It is heard best in its own area—the 2nd and 3rd left interspaces close to the sternum. It is here that you should search for splitting of the S_2.

S_1 also has two components, an earlier mitral and a later tricuspid sound. The mitral sound, its principal component, is much louder, again reflecting the high pressures on the left side of the heart. It can be heard throughout the precordium and is loudest at the cardiac apex. The softer tricuspid component is heard best at the lower left sternal border, and it is here that you may hear a split S_1. The earlier, louder mitral component may mask the tricuspid sound, however, and splitting is not always detectable. Splitting of S_1 does not vary with respiration.

HEART MURMURS

Heart murmurs are distinguishable from heart sounds by their longer duration. They are attributed to turbulent blood flow and may be "innocent," as with flow murmurs of young adults, or diagnostic of valvular heart disease. A *stenotic valve* has an abnormally narrowed valvular orifice that obstructs blood flow, as in *aortic stenosis,* and causes a characteristic murmur. So does a valve that fails to fully close, as in *aortic regurgitation* or *insufficiency.* Such a valve allows blood to leak backward in a retrograde direction and produces a *regurgitant* murmur.

To identify murmurs accurately, you must learn to assess the chest wall location where they are best heard, their timing in systole or diastole, and their qualities. In the section on Techniques of Examination, you will learn to integrate several characteristics, including murmur intensity, pitch, duration, and direction of radiation (see pp. 364–368).

RELATION OF AUSCULTATORY FINDINGS TO THE CHEST WALL

The locations on the chest wall where you hear heart sounds and murmurs help to identify the valve or chamber where they originate. Sounds and murmurs arising from the mitral valve are usually heard best at and around the cardiac apex. Those originating in the tricuspid valve are heard best at or near the lower left sternal border. Murmurs arising from the pulmonic valve are usually heard best in the 2nd and 3rd left interspaces close to the sternum but at times may also be heard at higher or lower levels. Murmurs originating in the aortic valve may be heard anywhere from the right 2nd interspace to the apex. *These areas overlap,* as illustrated below, and you will need to correlate auscultatory findings with other cardiac examination findings to identify sounds and murmurs accurately.

THE CONDUCTION SYSTEM

An electrical conduction system stimulates and coordinates the contraction of cardiac muscle.

Each normal electrical impulse is initiated in the *sinus node*, a group of specialized cardiac cells located in the right atrium near the junction of the vena cava. The sinus node acts as the cardiac pacemaker and automatically discharges an impulse about 60 to 100 times a minute. This impulse travels through both atria to the *atrioventricular node*, a specialized group of cells located low in the atrial septum. Here the impulse is delayed before passing down the bundle of His and its branches to the ventricular myocardium. Muscular contraction follows: first the atria, then the ventricles. The normal conduction pathway is diagrammed here in simplified form.

The electrocardiogram, or ECG, records these events. Contraction of cardiac smooth muscle produces electrical activity, resulting in a series of waves on the ECG. The ECG consists of *six limb leads* in the *frontal plane* and *six chest or precordial leads* in the *transverse plane*.

- Electrical vectors approaching a lead cause a *positive, or upward, deflection*.

- Electrical vectors moving away from the lead cause a *negative, or downward, deflection*.

- When positive and negative vectors balance, they are *isoelectric*, appearing as a straight line.

The components of the *normal ECG* and their duration are briefly summarized here, but you will need further instruction and practice to interpret recordings from patients. Note:

- The small *P wave* of atrial depolarization (duration up to 80 milliseconds; *PR interval* 120 to 200 milliseconds)

- The larger *QRS complex* of ventricular depolarization (up to 100 milliseconds), consisting of one or more of the following:

 –the *Q wave*, a downward deflection from septal depolarization
 –the *R wave*, an upward deflection from ventricular depolarization
 –the *S wave*, a downward deflection following an R wave

- A *T wave* of ventricular repolarization, or recovery (duration relates to QRS)

LIMB LEADS: FRONTAL PLANE

CHEST LEADS: TRANSVERSE PLANE

The electrical impulse slightly precedes the myocardial contraction that it stimulates. The relation of electrocardiographic waves to the cardiac cycle is shown below.

Electrocardiogram

Heart sounds

Systole   Diastole

THE HEART AS A PUMP

The left and right ventricles pump blood into the systemic and pulmonary arterial trees, respectively. *Cardiac output,* the volume of blood ejected from each ventricle during 1 minute, is the product of *heart rate* and *stroke volume*. Stroke volume (the volume of blood ejected with each heartbeat) depends in turn on preload, myocardial contractility, and afterload.

- *Preload* refers to the load that stretches the cardiac muscle before contraction. The volume of blood in the right ventricle at the end of diastole, then, constitutes its preload for the next beat. Right ventricular preload is increased by increasing venous return to the right heart. Physiologic causes include inspiration and the increased volume of blood flow from exercising muscles. The increased blood volume in a dilated right ventricle of congestive heart failure also increases preload. Causes of decreased right ventricular preload include exhalation, decreased left ventricular output, and pooling of blood in the capillary bed or the venous system.

- *Myocardial contractility* refers to the ability of the cardiac muscle, when given a load, to shorten. Contractility increases when stimulated by action of the sympathetic nervous system and decreases when blood flow or oxygen delivery to the myocardium is impaired.

- *Afterload* refers to the degree of vascular resistance to ventricular contraction. Sources of resistance to left ventricular contraction include the tone in the walls of the aorta, the large arteries, and the peripheral vascular tree (primarily the small arteries and arterioles), as well as the volume of blood already in the aorta.

Pathologic increases in preload and afterload, called *volume overload* and *pressure overload*, respectively, produce changes in ventricular function that may be clinically detectable. These changes include alterations in ventricular impulses, detectable by palpation, and in normal heart sounds. Pathologic heart sounds and murmurs may also develop.

The term *heart failure* is now preferred over "congestive heart failure" because not all patients have volume overload on initial presentation.[9]

ARTERIAL PULSES AND BLOOD PRESSURE

With each contraction, the left ventricle ejects a volume of blood into the aorta and on into the arterial tree. The ensuing pressure wave moves rapidly through the arterial system, where it is felt as the *arterial pulse*. Although the pressure wave travels quickly—many times faster than the blood itself—a palpable delay between ventricular contraction and peripheral pulses makes the pulses in the arms and legs unsuitable for timing events in the cardiac cycle.

Blood pressure in the arterial system varies during the cardiac cycle, peaking in systole and falling to its lowest trough in diastole. These are the levels that are measured with the blood pressure cuff, or sphygmomanometer. The difference between systolic and diastolic pressures is known as the *pulse pressure*.

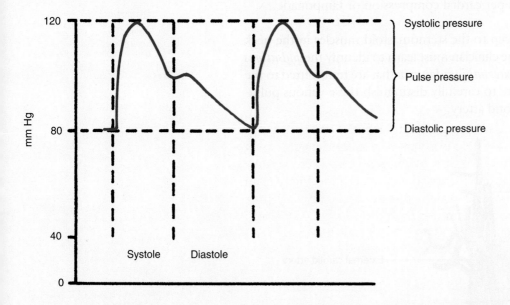

FACTORS INFLUENCING ARTERIAL PRESSURE

- Left ventricular stroke volume
- Distensibility of the aorta and the large arteries
- Peripheral vascular resistance, particularly at the arteriolar level
- Volume of blood in the arterial system.

Changes in any of these four factors alter systolic pressure, diastolic pressure, or both. Blood pressure levels fluctuate strikingly throughout any 24-hour period, varying with physical activity; emotional state; pain; noise; environmental temperature; use of coffee, tobacco, and other drugs; and even time of day.

JUGULAR VENOUS PRESSURE (JVP)

The jugular veins provide the astute clinician with an important clinical index of right heart pressures and cardiac function. *Jugular venous pressure (JVP)* reflects right atrial pressure, which in turn equals *central venous pressure (CVP)* and right ventricular end-diastolic pressure. The JVP is best estimated from the *right internal jugular vein*, which has a more direct anatomical channel into the right atrium. Contrary to widely held views, a recent study has reaffirmed inspection of the *right external jugular vein* as a useful and accurate method for estimating CVP.[10–12]

Pressure changes from right atrial filling, contraction, and emptying cause fluctuations in the JVP and its waveforms that are visible to the examiner. Careful observation of changes in these fluctuations also yields clues about volume status, right and left ventricular function, patency of the tricuspid and pulmonary valves, pressures in the pericardium, and arrhythmias such as junctional rhythms and atrioventricular blocks. For example, JVP falls with loss of blood and increases with right or left heart failure, pulmonary hypertension, tricuspid stenosis, and pericardial compression or tamponade.

The internal jugular veins lie deep to the sternomastoid muscles in the neck and are not directly visible, so the clinician must learn to identify the *pulsations* of the *internal jugular vein* or *external jugular vein* that are transmitted to the surface of the neck, making sure to carefully distinguish these venous pulsations from pulsations of the carotid artery.

To estimate the level of the JVP, you will learn to find the *highest point of oscillation in the internal jugular vein* or, if necessary, the point above which the external jugular vein appears collapsed. The JVP is usually measured in vertical distance above the *sternal angle*, the bony ridge adjacent to the second rib where the manubrium joins the body of the sternum.

Study carefully the illustrations below. Note that regardless of the patient's position, the sternal angle remains roughly 5 cm above the right atrium. In this patient, however, the pressure in the internal jugular vein is somewhat elevated.

● In *Position A*, the head of the bed is raised to the usual level, approximately 30°, but the JVP cannot be measured because the meniscus, or level of oscillation, is above the jaw and therefore not visible.

● In *Position B*, the head of the bed is raised to 60°. The "top" of the internal jugular vein is now easily visible, so the vertical distance from the sternal angle or right atrium can now be measured.

● In *Position C*, the patient is upright and the veins are barely discernible above the clavicle, making measurement untenable.

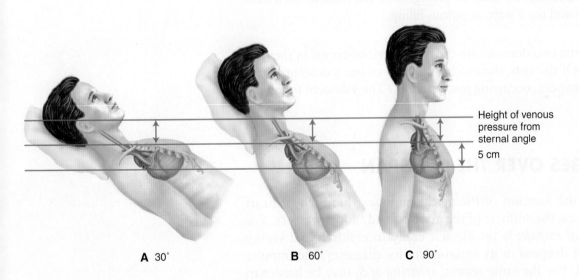

A 30°   **B** 60°   **C** 90°

Height of venous pressure from sternal angle

5 cm

Note that the height of the venous pressure as measured from the sternal angle is the *same* in all three positions, but your ability to *measure* the height of the column of venous blood, or JVP, differs according to how you position the patient. Jugular venous pressure measured at more than 4 cm above the sternal angle, or more than 9 cm above the right atrium, is considered elevated or abnormal. The techniques for measuring the JVP are fully described in Techniques of Examination on pp. 349–357.

JUGULAR VENOUS PULSATIONS

The oscillations that you see in the internal jugular veins, and often in the externals, reflect changing pressures within the right atrium. Careful observation reveals that the undulating pulsations of the internal jugular veins, and sometimes the externals, are composed of two quick peaks and two troughs.

The first elevation, the presystolic *a wave*, reflects the slight rise in atrial pressure that accompanies atrial contraction. It occurs just before S_1 and before the carotid pulse. The following trough, the *x descent*, starts with atrial relaxation. It continues as the right ventricle, contracting during systole, pulls the floor of the atrium downward. During ventricular systole, blood continues to flow into the right atrium from the venae cavae. The tricuspid valve is closed, the chamber begins to fill, and right atrial pressure begins to rise again, creating the second elevation, the *v wave*. When the tricuspid valve opens early in diastole, blood in the right atrium flows passively into the right ventricle, and right atrial pressure falls again, creating the second trough, or *y descent*. To remember these four oscillations in an oversimplified way, think of the following sequence: atrial contraction, atrial relaxation, atrial filling, and atrial emptying. (You can think of the *a* wave as <u>a</u>trial contraction and the *v* wave as <u>v</u>enous filling.)

To the naked eye, the two descents are the most obvious events in the normal jugular pulse. Of the two, the sudden collapse of the *x* descent late in systole is more prominent, occurring just before S_2. The *y* descent follows S_2 early in diastole.

CHANGES OVER THE LIFE SPAN

Aging may affect the location of the apical impulse, the pitch of heart sounds and murmurs, the stiffness of the arteries, and blood pressure. For example, the *apical impulse* is usually felt easily in children and young adults; as the chest deepens in its anteroposterior diameter, the impulse gets harder to find. For the same reason, *splitting of S_2* may be harder to hear in older people as its pulmonic component becomes less audible. Further, at some time over the life span, almost everyone has a *heart murmur*. Most murmurs occur without other evidence of cardiovascular abnormality and may therefore be considered normal variants. These common murmurs vary with age, and familiarity with their patterns helps you to distinguish normal from abnormal. Turn to pp. 780–782, Chapter 18, Assessing Children: Infancy Through Adolescence, and to p. 884, Chapter 19, The Pregnant Woman, for information on how to distinguish these innocent murmurs.

Murmurs may originate in large blood vessels as well as in the heart. The *jugular venous hum,* which is common in children, may still be heard through young adulthood (see p. 823). A second, more important example is the *cervical systolic murmur* or *bruit,* which may be innocent in children but suspicious for arterial obstruction in adults.

THE HEALTH HISTORY

Common or Concerning Symptoms

- Chest pain
- Palpitations
- Shortness of breath: dyspnea, orthopnea, or paroxysmal nocturnal dyspnea
- Swelling or edema

Assessing Cardiac Symptoms—Overview and Comparison With Baseline Activity Levels.

This section approaches chest symptoms from a *cardiac standpoint,* including chest pain, palpitations, shortness of breath from orthopnea or paroxysmal dyspnea (PND), and peripheral swelling from edema. For chest symptoms, make a habit of thinking through the range of possible cardiac, pulmonary, and extrathoracic etiologies. Review the Health History section of Chapter 8, The Thorax and Lungs, on pp. 290–292, Table 8-1, Chest Pain, on pp. 312–313, and Table 8-2, Dyspnea, on pp. 314–315. Study the various sources of *chest pain, dyspnea, wheezing, cough,* and even *hemoptysis,* because these symptoms can be cardiac as well as pulmonary in origin.

When assessing cardiac symptoms, it is important to habitually *quantify the patient's baseline level of activity.* For example, in patients with chest pain, does the pain occur with climbing stairs? How many flights? How about with walking—50 feet, one block, more? What about carrying groceries or doing housework (e.g., making beds, vacuuming)? How does this compare with these activities in the past? When did the symptoms appear or change? If the patient is short of breath, does this occur at rest, during exercise, or after climbing stairs? Sudden shortness of breath is more serious in an athlete than in a person who usually walks only from one room to another. Quantifying baseline level of activity helps establish both the severity of the patient's symptoms and their significance as the clinician considers the next steps for management.

Chest Pain.

Chest pain is one of the most serious and important symptoms you will assess as a clinician and is the second leading cause of emergency room visits, after abdominal pain. Chest pain often signals *coronary heart disease,* which currently affects 15 million people in the United States.[13] Approximately 9 million of these people have *angina pectoris,* and 8 million

Classic exertional pain, pressure, or discomfort in the chest, shoulder, back, neck, or arm in *angina pectoris,* seen in 50% of patients with acute myocardial infarction; atypihave had a *myocardial infarction*. Coronary heart disease is the leading cause of death for both men and women, and accounted for one in every five U.S. deaths in 2004. Death rates are highest in African-American men and women, compared with other ethnic groups.

cal descriptors also are common, such as cramping, grinding, pricking; rarely, tooth or jaw pain.[17,18] Annual incidence of *exertional angina* is 1 per 1000 in the population 30 years or older.

As you listen to the patient's story, always keep serious adverse events in mind, such as *angina pectoris, myocardial infarction*, or even *dissecting aortic aneurysm*.[14–16] Learn to distinguish how patients present with serious cardiovascular diseases from other possible sources, including the pericardium, trachea and bronchi, parietal pleura, esophagus, and chest wall, as well as extrathoracic structures such as the neck, gallbladder, and stomach. Inappropriate discharge from the emergency room, often because of an error in ECG interpretation, can lead to a 25% mortality rate.[14,15]

Acute coronary syndrome is increasingly used to refer to any of the clinical syndromes caused by acute myocardial ischemia, including *unstable angina, non-ST elevation myocardial infarction,* and *ST elevation infarction.*[19,20]

Your initial questions should be broad: "Do you have any pain or discomfort in your chest?" Ask the patient to point to the pain and to describe all seven of its attributes. After listening closely to the patient's description, move on to more specific questions such as "Is the pain related to exertion?" and "What kinds of activities bring on the pain?" Also "How intense is the pain, on a scale of 1 to 10?" . . . "Does it radiate into the neck, shoulder, back, or down your arm?" . . . "Are there any associated symptoms like shortness of breath, sweating, palpitations, or nausea?" . . . "Does it ever wake you up at night?" . . . "What do you do to make it better?"

Anterior chest pain, often tearing or ripping, often radiating into the back or neck, in *acute aortic dissection*[21]

Palpitations.   *Palpitations* involve an unpleasant awareness of the heartbeat. When describing palpitations, patients use terms such as skipping, racing, fluttering, pounding, or stopping of the heart. Palpitations may result from an irregular heartbeat, from rapid acceleration or slowing of the heart, or from increased forcefulness of cardiac contraction. Such perceptions also depend on how patients respond to their own body sensations. Palpitations do not necessarily mean heart disease. In contrast, the most serious dysrhythmias, such as ventricular tachycardia, often do not produce palpitations.

See Tables 9-1 and 9-2 for selected heart rates and rhythms (pp. 375–376).

Symptoms or signs of irregular heart action warrant an ECG. Only *atrial fibrillation,* which is "irregularly irregular," can be reliably identified at the bedside.

You may ask directly about palpitations, but if the patient does not understand your question, reword it. "Are you ever aware of your heartbeat? What is it like?" Ask the patient to tap out the rhythm with a hand or finger. Was it fast or slow? Regular or irregular? How long did it last? If there was an episode of rapid heartbeats, did they start and stop suddenly or gradually? (For this group of symptoms, an ECG is indicated.)

It is helpful to teach selected patients how to make serial measurements of their pulse rates in case they have further episodes.

Clues in the history include transient skips and flip-flops (possible premature contractions); rapid regular beating of sudden onset and offset (possible paroxysmal supraventricular tachycardia); a rapid regular rate of less than 120 beats per minute, especially if starting and stopping more gradually (possible sinus tachycardia).

Shortness of Breath.   *Shortness of breath* is a common patient concern and may represent *dyspnea, orthopnea,* or *paroxysmal nocturnal dyspnea. Dyspnea* is an uncomfortable awareness of breathing that is inappropriate

Sudden dyspnea in *pulmonary embolus, spontaneous pneumothorax,* anxiety to a given level of exertion. This complaint is common in patients with cardiac or pulmonary problems, as discussed in Chapter 8, The Thorax and Lungs, p. 291.

Orthopnea is dyspnea that occurs when the patient is lying down and improves when the patient sits up. Classically, it is quantified according to the number of pillows the patient uses for sleeping, or by the fact that the patient needs to sleep sitting up. Make sure, however, that the reason the patient uses extra pillows or sleeps upright is shortness of breath and not other causes.

Orthopnea in *left ventricular heart failure* or *mitral stenosis;* also in *obstructive lung disease*

Paroxysmal nocturnal dyspnea, or *PND,* describes episodes of sudden dyspnea and orthopnea that awaken the patient from sleep, usually 1 or 2 hours after going to bed, prompting the patient to sit up, stand up, or go to a window for air. There may be associated wheezing and coughing. The episode usually subsides but may recur at about the same time on subsequent nights.

PND in *left ventricular heart failure* or *mitral stenosis;* may be mimicked by *nocturnal asthma attacks.*

Edema. *Edema* refers to the accumulation of excessive fluid in the extravascular interstitial space. Interstitial tissue can absorb several liters of fluid, accommodating up to a 10% weight gain before pitting edema appears.[22] Causes vary from local to systemic. Focus your questions on the location, timing, and setting of the swelling, and on associated symptoms. "Have you had any swelling anywhere? Where? . . . Anywhere else? When does it occur? Is it worse in the morning or at night? Do your shoes get tight?"

Dependent edema appears in the lowest body parts: the feet and lower legs when sitting, or the sacrum when bedridden. Causes may be cardiac (*congestive heart failure*), nutritional (*hypoalbuminemia*), or positional.

Continue with "Are the rings tight on your fingers? Are your eyelids puffy or swollen in the morning? Have you had to let out your belt?" Also, "Have your clothes gotten too tight around the middle?" It is useful to ask patients who retain fluid to record daily morning weights, because edema may not be obvious until several liters of extra fluid have accumulated.

Edema occurs in renal and liver disease: periorbital puffiness, tight rings in *nephrotic syndrome;* enlarged waistline from *ascites* and *liver failure.*

HEALTH PROMOTION AND COUNSELING

Important Topics for Health Promotion and Counseling

- Screening for hypertension
- Screening for coronary heart disease and stroke
- Screening for dyslipidemias
- Promoting lifestyle modification and risk-factor reduction

Cardiovascular disease affects 80 million U.S. adults and includes hypertension, coronary heart disease, heart failure, stroke, and congenital cardiovascular defects. It remains the leading cause of death for both men and women, accounting for approximately one-third of all U.S. deaths.[13] Both *primary prevention,* in those without evidence of cardiovascular disease, and *secondary prevention,* in those with known cardiovascular events such as angina or myocardial infarction, remain important priorities for the office, the hospital, and the nation's public health. Education and counseling will guide your patients to maintain optimal levels of blood pressure, cholesterol, weight, and exercise and reduce risk factors for cardiovascular disease and stroke. As emerging clinicians, your task is three-fold:

● To understand important demographic data about cardiovascular disease and stroke in the population

● To identify related risk factors

● To form partnerships with patients to help reduce or control risk factors

The information presented here is designed to improve your effectiveness as you assess cardiovascular disease in your patients and engage in primary and secondary risk-factor reduction.

Screening for Hypertension. According to the U.S. Preventive Services Task Force, hypertension accounts for "35% of all myocardial infarctions and strokes, 49% of all episodes of heart failure, and 24% of all premature deaths."[23] The Task Force strongly recommends *screening all people 18 years or older for high blood pressure.* Recent long-term population-based studies have fueled a dramatic shift in national strategies to prevent and reduce blood pressure (BP). "The Seventh Report of the Joint National Committee on Prevention, Detection, Evaluation, and Treatment of High Blood Pressure," known as JNC 7, the National High Blood Pressure Education Program, and clinical investigators have issued several key messages (see box on p. 341).[24–26] These findings underlie the tougher and simpler blood pressure classification of JNC 7, reaffirmed in 2007 (see the box below).[27]

JNC 7: KEY FEATURES FOR ASSESSING BLOOD PRESSURE[24]

- There are now four categories of blood pressure. **Normal** is defined as less than 120/80 mm Hg.
- Systolic blood pressures of 120 to 139 mm Hg, diastolic blood pressures of 80 to 89 mm Hg, or both, are **pre-hypertension** (previously "high normal") and warrant lifestyle change interventions.
- **Stage 1 hypertension,** namely systolic BP 140 to 159 mm Hg, diastolic BP 90 to 99 mm Hg, or both, warrants initiation of antihypertensive drug therapy.
- The blood pressure target for patients with diabetes and chronic kidney disease is less than 130/80 mm Hg.
- Adoption of healthy lifestyles by all people is now considered "indispensable."

Important messages from recent studies that are useful for clinicians counseling patients are summarized below.

IMPORTANT MESSAGES ABOUT HYPERTENSION

- "Individuals who are normotensive at 55 years have a 90% lifetime risk for developing hypertension."[24]
- "More than 1 of every 2 adults older than 60 years of age has hypertension,"[25] and only 34% of those with hypertension have achieved blood pressure goals.[24]
- "The relationship between pressure and risk of cardiovascular disease (CVD) events is continuous, consistent, and independent of other risk factors. . . . For individuals aged 40 to 70 years, each increment of 20 mm Hg in systolic BP or 10 mm Hg in diastolic BP doubles the risk of CVD across the entire BP range from 115/75 to 185/115 mm Hg."[24,28]
- Recent large population studies of cardiovascular risk factors reveal two striking findings[29]:
  1. Only 4.8% to 9.9% of the young and middle-aged population is at low risk.
  2. The benefits of low-risk status are enormous: a 72% to 85% reduction in CVD mortality and a 40% to 58% reduction in mortality from all causes, leading to a gain of 5.8 to 9.5 years in life expectancy. This gain "holds for both African-Americans and whites, and for those of lower and higher socioeconomic status."[29]
- Identifying and treating people with risk factors are not enough. *A population-wide strategy is critical to prevent and reduce the magnitude of all the major risk factors* so that people develop favorable behaviors in childhood and *remain* at *low risk for life.*[29]

Risk factors for hypertension include physical inactivity, microalbuminuria or estimated GFR less than 60 mL/min, family history of premature CVD (younger than 55 years for men and younger than 65 years for women), excess intake of dietary sodium, insufficient intake of potassium, and excess consumption of alcohol.[24]

Screening for Coronary Heart Disease and Stroke. The American Heart Association (AHA) in its 2002 update placed the challenge for implementing risk factor reduction squarely on clinicians[30]:

- "The challenge for health care professionals is to engage greater numbers of patients, at an earlier stage of their disease, in comprehensive cardiovascular risk reduction" to expand the benefits of primary prevention.

- "The continuing message is that adoption of healthy life habits remains the cornerstone of primary prevention."

- "The imperative is to prevent the first episode of coronary disease or stroke or the development of aortic aneurysm and peripheral vascular disease because of the still-high rate of first events that are fatal or disabling."

As a first step, clinicians need to identify not only elevated blood pressure but also other well-studied risk factors for coronary heart disease (CHD). In its "Guidelines for Primary Prevention of Cardiovascular Disease and Stroke," the AHA recommends[30]:

- *Risk factor screening* for adults beginning at 20 years

- *Global absolute CHD risk estimation* for all adults 40 years and older. The goal of global risk estimates is to help patients keep their risk as low as possible. Note that diabetes, or 10-year risk of more than 20%, is considered equivalent to established CHD risk equivalents.

RISK FACTORS AND SCREENING FREQUENCY FOR ADULTS BEGINNING AT 20 YEARS

Risk Factor	Frequency
Family history of coronary heart disease (CHD)	Update regularly
Smoking status Diet Alcohol intake Physical activity	At each routine visit
Blood pressure Body mass index Waist circumference Pulse (to detect atrial fibrillation)	At each routine visit (at least every 2 years)
Fasting lipoprotein profile Fasting glucose	At least every 5 years If risk factors for hyperlipidemia or diabetes present, every 2 years

(Source: Pearson TA, Blair SN, Daniels SR, et al. AHA guidelines for primary prevention of cardiovascular disease and stroke: 2000 update. Circulation 106(3):388–391, 2002.)

ESTIMATING GLOBAL RISK FOR 10-YEAR RISK FOR CORONARY HEART DISEASE FOR ADULTS 40 YEARS OR OLDER

Establish multiple risk score for CHD based on:

- Age, gender
- Height, weight, and waist circumference, or BMI
- Smoking status

(continued)

ESTIMATING GLOBAL RISK FOR 10-YEAR RISK FOR CORONARY HEART DISEASE FOR ADULTS 40 YEARS OR OLDER (CONTINUED)

- History of cardiovascular disease or diabetes
- Systolic and diastolic blood pressure
- Total cholesterol, LDL and HDL cholesterol
- Triglycerides
- Family history of early heart disease

For calculation of global CHD risk, use the risk calculators found at either of the Web sites below (or other equations):

http://www.americanheart.org/presenter.jhtml?identifier=3003499
http://hin.nhlbi.nih.gov/atpiii/calculator.asp?usertype=prof

(Source: Pearson TA, Blair SN, Daniels SR, et al. AHA guidelines for primary prevention of cardiovascular disease and stroke: 2000 update. Circulation 106(3):388–391, 2002.)

Screening for Dyslipidemias. In 2001 the National Heart, Lung, and Blood Institute of the National Institutes of Health published the "Third Report of the National Cholesterol Education Program Expert Panel," known as ATP III.[31] Publication of the full NCEP report followed in 2002.[32] These reports provide evidence-based recommendations on the management of high cholesterol and related lipid disorders, and document that "epidemiological surveys have shown that serum cholesterol levels are continuously correlated with CHD risk over a broad range of cholesterol values," in many of the world's populations.[33] Key features of ATP III are summarized below:

ATP III: KEY RECOMMENDATIONS

- Identify LDL as the primary target of cholesterol-lowering therapy.
- Classify three 10-year risk categories:
  - *High risk (10-year risk greater than 20%):* established CHD and CHD risk equivalents
  - *Moderately high risk (10-year risk 10%–20%):* multiple, or 2+, risk factors
  - *Low risk (10-year risk less than 10%):* zero to 1 risk factor
- *Risk factors* include cigarette smoking, BP greater than 140/90 mm Hg or use of antihypertensive medication, HDL less than 40 mg/dL, family history of CHD in male first-degree relative before 55 years or female first-degree relative before 65 years, and age 45 years or older for men or 55 years or older for women.

  CHD includes history of myocardial infarction, stable or unstable angina, coronary artery procedures such as angioplasty or bypass surgery, or evidence of significant myocardial ischemia.

  (continued)

ATP III: KEY RECOMMENDATIONS (CONTINUED)

CHD risk equivalents include *noncoronary atherosclerotic disease,* such as peripheral arterial disease, abdominal aortic aneurysm, and carotid artery disease (transient ischemic attacks or stroke of carotid origin or more than 50% obstruction of the carotid artery); *diabetes;* and *2+ risk factors with 10-year risk for CHD of greater than 20%.*

- Define *high risk* as "all persons with CHD or CHD risk equivalents," with an *LDL goal for high-risk people of 100 mg/dL or less.*
- Identify secondary targets of therapy such as *metabolic syndrome* and *triglycerides greater than 150 mg/dL,* an independent risk for CHD (see table below).

ATP III defines *metabolic syndrome* as "a constellation of lipid and non-lipid risk factors of metabolic origin."[31,32] This syndrome is closely linked to the metabolic disorder of insulin resistance, seen in people who are obese, physically inactive, or genetically predisposed. Clinical criteria for metabolic syndrome are listed in the accompanying table. Note that waist circumference is correlated more closely than BMI with risk factors for metabolic syndrome.

● ATP III: Clinical Identifiers for Metabolic Syndrome

Risk Factor	Defining Level
Abdominal Obesity	Waist Circumference
Men	>102 cm (>40 in)
Women	>88 cm (>35 in)
Triglycerides	≥150 mg/dL
HDL cholesterol	
Men	<40 mg/dL
Women	<50 mg/dL
Blood Pressure	≥130/≥85 mm Hg
Fasting Glucose	≥110 mg/dL

In July 2004, NCEP updated these reports based on the findings in five major clinical trials.[33] For *high-risk people,* NCEP now recommends an LDL goal of less than 70 mg/dL and intensive lipid therapy as a *therapeutic option.*[34] The NCEP cites data showing that high-risk patients benefit from a further 30% to 40% drop in LDL even when LDL is less than 100 mg/dL.

The U.S. Preventive Services Task Force recommends routine screening of LDL for men 35 years or older and for women 45 years or older.[35] Screening should begin at 20 years for those with risk factors for CHD.[36,37]

Counsel your patients to obtain a *fasting lipid profile* to determine levels of total and LDL cholesterol. Use the risk calculators on p. 343, or consult ATP III, to *establish your patient's 10-year risk category.* Use the 2004 guidelines below, which now have four risk groups, to plan your interventions regarding lifestyle change and lipid-lowering medications.

● **Updated ATP III Guidelines: 10-Year Risk and LDL Goals**

10-year Risk Category	LDL Goal	Consider Drug Therapy if LDL:
High risk (>20%)	<100 mg/dL *Optional goal:* <70 mg/dL	≥100 mg/dL (<100 mg/dL: consider drug options, including further 30%–40% reduction in LDL)
Moderately high risk (10%–20%)	<130 mg/dL *Optional goal:* <100 mg/dL	≥130 mg/dL (100–129 mg/dL: consider drug options to achieve goal of <100 mg/dL)
Moderate risk (<10%)	<130 mg/dL	≥160 mg/dL
Lower risk (0–1 risk factor)	<160 mg/dL	≥190 mg/dL (160–189 mg/dL: drug therapy *optional*)

(Source: Adapted from Grundy SM, Cleeman JI, Merz NB, et al, for the Coordinating Committee of the National Cholesterol Education Program. Implications of recent clinical trials for the National Cholesterol Education Adult Treatment Panel III guidelines. Circulation 110(2):227–239, 2004.)

Promoting Lifestyle Modification and Risk Factor Reduction. JNC 7, the National High Blood Pressure Education Program, and the AHA encourage a series of well-studied effective lifestyle modifications and risk inter-

---

LIFESTYLE MODIFICATIONS TO PREVENT OR MANAGE HYPERTENSION

- Optimal weight, or BMI of 18.5–24.9 kg/m²
- Salt intake of less than 6 grams of sodium chloride or 2.4 grams of sodium per day
- Regular aerobic exercise such as brisk walking for at least 30 minutes per day, most days of the week
- Moderate alcohol consumption per day of 2 drinks or fewer for men and 1 drink or fewer for women (2 drinks = 1 oz ethanol, 24 oz beer, 10 oz wine, or 2–3 oz whiskey)
- Dietary intake of more than 3,500 mg of potassium
- Diet rich in fruits, vegetables, and low-fat dairy products with reduced content of saturated and total fat

(Source: Whelton PK, He J, Appel LJ, et al. Primary prevention of hypertension. Clinical and Public Health Advisory from the National High Blood Pressure Education Program. JAMA 288(15):1882–1888, 2002.)

ventions to prevent hypertension, CVD, and stroke. Lifestyle modifications for hypertension can lower systolic blood pressure from 2 to 20 mm Hg.[24] Lifestyle modifications to reduce hypertension overlap with those recommended for reducing risk for CVD and stroke, as seen below.

RISK INTERVENTIONS TO PREVENT CARDIOVASCULAR DISEASE AND STROKE

- Complete cessation of smoking
- Optimal blood pressure control—see table for JNC 7 guidelines on p. 340
- Healthy eating—see diet recommendations on previous page
- Lipid management—see table on pp. 343–344
- Regular aerobic exercise—see previous page
- Optimal weight—see previous page
- Diabetes management so that fasting glucose level is below 110 mg/dL and HgA1C is less than 7%
- Conversion of atrial fibrillation to normal sinus rhythm or, if chronic, anticoagulation

(Source: Pearson TA, Blair SN, Daniels SR, et al. AHA guidelines for primary prevention of cardiovascular disease and stroke: 2002 update. Circulation 106(3):388–391, 2002.)

Healthy Eating. Begin with a dietary history (see pp. 106–107), then target low intake of cholesterol and total fat, especially less saturated and *trans* fat. Foods with monounsaturated fats, polyunsaturated fats, and omega-3 fatty acids in fish oils help to lower blood cholesterol. Review the food sources of these healthy and unhealthy fats.[38]

FOOD SOURCES OF HEALTHY AND UNHEALTHY FATS

Healthy Fats

- *Foods high in monounsaturated fat:* nuts, such as almonds, pecans, and peanuts; sesame seeds; avocados; canola oil; olive and peanut oil; peanut butter
- *Foods high in polyunsaturated fat:* corn, safflower, cottonseed, and soybean oil; walnuts; pumpkin or sunflower seeds; soft (tub) margarine; mayonnaise; salad dressings
- *Foods high in omega-3 fatty acids:* albacore tuna, herring, mackerel, rainbow trout, salmon, sardines

Unhealthy Fats

- *Foods high in cholesterol:* dairy products, egg yolks, liver and organ meats, high-fat meat and poultry
- *Foods high in saturated fat:* high-fat dairy products—cream, cheese, ice cream, whole and 2% milk, butter, and sour cream; bacon; chocolate; coconut oil; lard and gravy from meat drippings; high-fat meats like ground beef, bologna, hot dogs, and sausage
- *Foods high in* trans *fat:* snacks and baked goods with hydrogenated or partially hydrogenated oil, stick margarines, shortening, french fries

---

Counseling About Weight and Exercise.   The January 2004 "Progress Review—Nutrition and Overweight" in *Healthy People 2010* reports that "Dietary factors are associated with 4 of the 10 leading causes of death—coronary heart disease, some types of cancer, stroke, and type 2 diabetes—as well as with high blood pressure and osteoporosis. Overall, the data on the three *Healthy People 2010* objectives for the weight status of adults and children reflect a trend for the worse."[38] More than 60% of all Americans are now obese or overweight, with a BMI equal to or greater than 25.

Counseling about weight has become a clinician imperative. Assess body mass index (BMI) as described in Chapter 4, pp. 112–114. Discuss the principles of healthy eating—patients with high fat intake are more likely to accumulate body fat than patients with high intake of protein and carbohydrate. Review the patient's eating habits and weight patterns in the family. Set realistic goals that will help the patient maintain healthy eating habits *for life*.

Regular exercise is the number one health indicator for *Healthy People 2010*. In its April 2004 "Progress Review—Physical Activity and Fitness," *Healthy People 2010* states that "in 2000, poor diet coupled with lack of exercise was the second leading actual cause of death. The gap between this risk factor and tobacco use, the leading cause, has narrowed substantially over the past decade."[39] To reduce the risk for CHD, counsel patients to pursue aerobic exercise, or exercise that increases muscle oxygen uptake, for at least 30 minutes on most days of the week. Spur motivation by emphasizing the immediate benefits to health and well-being. Deep breathing, sweating in cool temperatures, and pulse rates exceeding 60% of the maximum normal age-adjusted heart rate, or 220 minus the person's age, are markers that help patients recognize onset of aerobic metabolism. Be sure to evaluate any cardiovascular, pulmonary, or musculoskeletal conditions that present risks before selecting an exercise regimen.

TECHNIQUES OF EXAMINATION

You are now ready to learn the classic techniques for examining the cardio-vascular system. A sound knowledge of cardiac anatomy and physiology is key to understanding the hemodynamics of this closed-pump, forward-flow system. It is only through diligent and repetitive practice of the techniques of examination, however, that you will gain confidence and accuracy in your clinical findings, both normal and abnormal.[40] Examine each patient carefully and methodically. Many thorough repetitions of examining normal patients will serve you well by helping you identify important cardiac pathology.

Blood Pressure and Heart Rate.   As you begin the cardiovascular examination, review the blood pressure and heart rate recorded during the General Survey and Vital Signs at the start of the physical examination. If you need to repeat these measurements, or if they have not already been done, take the time to measure the blood pressure and heart rate using optimal technique (see Chapter 4, Beginning the Physical Examination: General Survey, Vital Signs, and Pain, especially pp. 114–119).[41–45]

In brief, for *blood pressure*, after letting the patient rest for at least 5 minutes in a quiet setting, choose a correctly sized cuff and position the patient's arm at heart level, either resting on a table if seated or supported at mid-chest level if standing. Make sure the bladder of the cuff is centered over the brachial artery. Inflate the cuff approximately 30 mm Hg above the pressure at which the brachial or radial pulse disappears. As you deflate the cuff, listen first for the sounds of at least two consecutive heartbeats—these mark the *systolic* pressure. Then listen for the disappearance point of the heartbeats, which marks the *diastolic* pressure. For *heart rate*, measure the radial pulse using the pads of your index and middle fingers, or assess the apical pulse using your stethoscope (see p. 119).

Basic Cardiac Examination Skills: Objectives for Mastery.   As you study this chapter and practice the cardiac examination, be sure you are proficient in the basic objectives listed below.

✓ Describe the chest wall anatomy and identify the key listening areas.
✓ Evaluate the jugular venous pulse, the carotid upstroke, and presence or absence of carotid bruits.
✓ Correctly identify and describe the point of maximal impulse (PMI).
✓ Correctly identify the first and second sounds (S_1 and S_2) at the base and apex.
✓ Recognize the effect of the P-R interval on the intensity of S_1.
✓ Identify physiologic and paradoxical splitting of S_2.
✓ Recognize key abnormal sounds in *early diastole,* including the third heart sound (S_3), pericardial knock, and opening snap of mitral stenosis.

✓ Recognize a fourth heart sound (S_4) *later in diastole.*

✓ Evaluate the timing of murmurs and correctly identify systolic and diastolic murmurs as well as friction rubs.

✓ Evaluate and interpret pulsus paradoxis.

✓ Correctly identify the physical findings of a normal heart examination, including rate, rhythm, and characteristics of the heart sounds.

✓ Correctly identify heart murmurs, using maneuvers when needed.

JUGULAR VENOUS PRESSURE AND PULSATIONS

Jugular Venous Pressure (JVP). Estimating the JVP is one of the most important and frequently used skills of physical examination. At first it will seem difficult, but with practice and supervision you will find that the JVP provides valuable information about the patient's volume status and cardiac function. As you have learned, the JVP reflects pressure in the right atrium, or central venous pressure, and is best assessed from pulsations in the right internal jugular vein. Note, however, that the jugular veins and pulsations are difficult to see in children younger than 12 years, so they are not useful for evaluating the cardiovascular system in this age group.

To help you learn this portion of the cardiac examination, steps for assessing the JVP are outlined on the next page. As you begin your assessment, consider the patient's volume status and how you may need to alter the elevation of the head of the bed or examining table.

● The usual starting point for assessing the JVP is to elevate the head of the bed to 30°. Identify the external jugular vein on each side, then find the internal jugular venous pulsations transmitted from deep in the neck to the overlying soft tissues. The JVP is the highest oscillation point, or meniscus, of the jugular venous pulsations that is usually evident in euvolemic patients.

● In patients who are *hypovolemic,* you may anticipate that *the JVP will be low,* causing you to subsequently *lower the head of the bed,* sometimes even to 0°, to see the point of oscillation best.

● Likewise, in volume-overloaded or *hypervolemic* patients, you may anticipate that *the JVP will be high,* causing you to subsequently *raise the head of the bed.*

A hypovolemic patient may have to lie flat before you see the neck veins. In contrast, when jugular venous pressure is increased, an elevation up to 60° or even 90° may be required. In all these positions, the sternal angle usually remains about 5 cm above the right atrium, as diagrammed on p. 335.

STEPS FOR ASSESSING THE JVP

● Make the patient comfortable. *Raise the head slightly on a pillow to relax the sternomastoid muscles.*

● *Raise the head of the bed or examining table to about 30°. Turn the patient's head slightly away from the side you are inspecting.*

(continued)

STEPS FOR ASSESSING THE JVP (continued)

- Use *tangential lighting* and examine both sides of the neck. Identify the external jugular vein on each side, then find the internal jugular venous pulsations.
- *If necessary, raise or lower the head of the bed* until you can see the oscillation point or meniscus of the internal jugular venous pulsations in the lower half of the neck.
- Focus on the *right internal jugular vein.* Look for pulsations in the suprasternal notch, between the attachments of the sternomastoid muscle on the sternum and clavicle, or just posterior to the sternomastoid. The table below helps you distinguish internal jugular pulsations from those of the carotid artery.
- *Identify the highest point of pulsation in the right internal jugular vein.* Extend a long rectangular object or card horizontally from this point and a centimeter ruler vertically from the sternal angle, making an exact right angle. Measure the vertical distance in centimeters above the sternal angle where the horizontal object crosses the ruler. *This distance, measured in centimeters above the sternal angle or the right atrium, is the JVP.*

Picture

The following features help to distinguish jugular from carotid artery pulsations:[10]

● Distinguishing Internal Jugular and Carotid Pulsations

Internal Jugular Pulsations	Carotid Pulsations
Rarely palpable	Palpable
Soft, biphasic, undulating quality, usually with two elevations and two troughs per heart beat	A more vigorous thrust with a *single outward component*
Pulsations eliminated by light pressure on the vein(s) just above the sternal end of the clavicle	Pulsations not eliminated by this pressure
Height of pulsations changes with position, dropping as the patient becomes more upright	Height of pulsations unchanged by position
Height of pulsations usually falls with inspiration	Height of pulsations not affected by inspiration

Establishing the true vertical and horizontal lines to measure the JVP is difficult, much like the problem of hanging a picture straight when you are close to it. Place your ruler on the sternal angle and line it up with something in the room that you know to be vertical. Then place a card or rectangular object at an exact right angle to the ruler. This constitutes your horizontal line. Move it up or down—still horizontal—so that the lower edge rests at the top of the

Increased pressure suggests *right-sided congestive heart failure* or, less commonly, *constrictive pericarditis, tricuspid stenosis,* or *superior vena cava obstruction.*[46–51]

jugular pulsations, and read the vertical distance on the ruler. Round your measurement off to the nearest centimeter.

In patients with obstructive lung disease, venous pressure may appear elevated on expiration only; the veins collapse on inspiration. This finding does not indicate congestive heart failure.

normal 3-5

Venous pressure measured at greater than 3 cm or possibly 4 cm above the sternal angle, or more than 8 cm or 9 cm in total distance above the right atrium, is considered elevated *above normal.*

An elevated JVP is 98% specific for an increased left ventricular end diastolic pressure and low left ventricular ejection fraction, and it increases risk of death from heart failure.[52,53]

If you cannot see pulsations in the internal jugular vein, look for them in the external jugular vein. If you see no pulsation, use *the point above which the external jugular veins appear to collapse*. Make this observation on each side of the neck. Measure the vertical distance of this point from the sternal angle.

Local kinking or obstruction is the usual cause of unilateral distention of the external jugular vein.

The highest point of venous pulsations may lie below the level of the sternal angle. Under these circumstances, venous pressure is not elevated and seldom needs to be measured.

Jugular Venous Pulsations. *Observe the amplitude and timing of the jugular venous pulsations.* To time them, feel the left carotid artery with your right thumb or listen to the heart simultaneously. The *a* wave just precedes S₁ and the carotid pulse, the *x* descent can be seen as a systolic collapse, the *v* wave almost coincides with S₂, and the *y* descent follows early in diastole. Look for absent or unusually prominent waves.

Prominent *a waves* in increased resistance to right atrial contraction, as in *tricuspid stenosis;* also in first-degree atrioventricular block, supraventricular tachycardia, junctional rhythms, *pulmonary hypertension,* and *pulmonic stenosis.*

Absent *a waves* in atrial fibrillation. Large *v waves* in *tricuspid regurgitation, constrictive pericarditis*

Jugular venous pulsations

Jugular venous pressure curves
a = atrial contraction
c = carotid transmission not visible clinically
x = descent in right atrium following *a*
v = passive venous filling of atria from the vena cavae
y = descent during atrial resting phase before contraction

Considerable practice and experience are required to master jugular venous pulsations. A beginner is well-advised to concentrate primarily on jugular venous pressure.

THE CAROTID PULSE

After you measure the JVP, move on to assessment of the *carotid pulse*. The carotid pulse provides valuable information about cardiac function and is especially useful for detecting stenosis or insufficiency of the aortic valve. Take the time to assess the quality of the carotid upstroke, its amplitude and contour, and presence or absence of any overlying *thrills* or *bruits*.

For irregular rhythms, see Table 9-1, Selected Heart Rates and Rhythms (p. 375), and Table 9-2, Selected Irregular Rhythms (p. 376).

To assess *amplitude and contour*, the patient should be lying down with the head of the bed still elevated to about 30°. When feeling for the carotid artery, first inspect the neck for carotid pulsations. These may be visible just medial to the sternomastoid muscles. Then place your index and middle fingers (or left thumb) on the right carotid artery in the lower third of the neck, press posteriorly, and feel for pulsations.

A tortuous and kinked carotid artery may produce a unilateral pulsatile bulge.

Causes of decreased pulsations include decreased stroke volume and local factors in the artery such as atherosclerotic narrowing or occlusion.

Press just inside the medial border of a well-relaxed sternomastoid muscle, roughly at the level of the cricoid cartilage. Avoid pressing on the *carotid sinus*, which lies at the level of the top of the thyroid cartilage. For the left carotid artery, use your right fingers or thumb. Never press both carotids at the same time. This may decrease blood flow to the brain and induce syncope.

Pressure on the carotid sinus may cause a reflex drop in pulse rate or blood pressure.

Slowly increase pressure until you feel a maximal pulsation, then slowly decrease pressure until you best sense the arterial pressure and contour. Try to assess:

See Table 9-3, Abnormalities of the Arterial Pulse and Pressure Waves (p. 377).

- *Normal* The *amplitude of the pulse*. This correlates reasonably well with the pulse pressure.

Small, thready, or weak pulse in *cardiogenic shock; bounding* pulse in *aortic insufficiency* (see p. 377)

- *normal* The *contour of the pulse wave,* namely the speed of the upstroke, the duration of its summit, and the speed of the downstroke. The normal upstroke is *brisk*. It is smooth, rapid, and follows S_1 almost immediately. The summit is smooth, rounded, and roughly midsystolic. The downstroke is less abrupt than the upstroke.

Delayed carotid upstroke in *aortic stenosis*

- *abnormal* Any *variations in amplitude,* either from beat to beat or with respiration.

Pulsus alternans (see p. 377), bigeminal pulse (beat-to-beat variation); paradoxical pulse (respiratory variation)

- *abnormal* The *timing of the carotid upstroke in relation to S_1 and S_2.* Note that the normal carotid upstroke follows S_1 and precedes S_2. This relationship is very helpful in correctly identifying S_1 and S_2, especially when the heart rate is increased and the duration of diastole, normally shorter than systole, is shortened and approaches the duration of systole.

Thrills and Bruits.   During palpation of the carotid artery, you may detect humming vibrations, or *thrills,* that feel like the throat of a purring cat. Routinely, but especially in the presence of a thrill, listen over both carotid arteries with the diaphragm of your stethoscope for a *bruit,* a murmur-like sound of vascular rather than cardiac origin.

Note that an aortic valve murmur may radiate to the neck and sound like a carotid bruit.

You should also listen for carotid bruits if the patient is middle-aged or elderly or if you suspect cerebrovascular disease. Ask the patient to hold breathing for a moment so that breath sounds do not obscure the vascular sound, then listen with the bell. Heart sounds alone do not constitute a bruit.

The prevalence of asymptomatic carotid bruits increases with age, reaching 8% in people 75 years or older, with a threefold increased risk of ischemic heart disease and stroke. Presence of a carotid bruit does not predict the degree of underlying stenosis, so pursue further investigation.[54]

Further examination of arterial pulses is described in Chapter 12, The Peripheral Vascular System.

The Brachial Artery. The carotid arteries reflect aortic pulsations more accurately, but in patients with carotid obstruction, kinking, or thrills, they are unsuitable. If so, assess the pulse in the *brachial artery,* applying the techniques described above for determining amplitude and contour.

Use the index and middle fingers or thumb of your opposite hand. Cup your hand under the patient's elbow and feel for the pulse just medial to the biceps tendon. The patient's arm should rest with the elbow extended, palm up. With your free hand, you may need to flex the elbow to a varying degree to get optimal muscular relaxation.

 THE HEART

For much of the cardiac examination, the patient should be *supine,* with the upper body raised by elevating the head of the bed or table to about 30°. Two other positions are also needed: (1) *turning to the left side* and (2) *sitting and leaning forward.* These positions bring the ventricular apex and left ventricular outflow tract closer to the chest wall, enhancing detection of the PMI and aortic insufficiency. *The examiner should stand at the patient's right side.*

The table below summarizes patient positions and a suggested sequence for the examination.

● Sequence of the Cardiac Examination

Patient Position	Examination	Accentuated Findings
Supine, with the head elevated 30°	Inspect and palpate the precordium: the 2nd right and left interspaces; the right ventricle; and the left ventricle, including the apical impulse (diameter, location, amplitude, duration).	
Left lateral decubitus	Palpate the apical impulse if not previously detected. Listen at the apex with the *bell* of the stethoscope.	Low-pitched extra sounds such as an S_3, opening snap, diastolic rumble of *mitral stenosis*
Supine, with the head elevated 30°	Listen at the 2nd right and left interspaces, along the left sternal border, across to the apex with the *diaphragm.* Listen at the right sternal border for tricuspid murmurs and sounds with the *bell.*	
Sitting, leaning forward, after full exhalation	Listen along the left sternal border and at the apex with the *diaphragm.*	Soft decrescendo diastolic murmur of *aortic insufficiency*

During the cardiac examination, remember to correlate your findings with the patient's jugular venous pressure and carotid pulse. It is also important to identify both the anatomical location of your findings and their timing in the cardiac cycle.

- Note the *anatomical location* of sounds in terms of interspaces and their distance from the midsternal, midclavicular, or axillary lines. The midsternal line offers the most reliable zero point for measurement, but some feel that the midclavicular line accommodates the different sizes and shapes of patients.

- Identify the *timing of impulses or sounds* in relation to the cardiac cycle. Timing of sounds is often possible through auscultation alone. In most people with normal or slow heart rates, it is easy to identify the paired heart sounds by listening through a stethoscope. S_1 is the first of these sounds, S_2 is the second, and the relatively long diastolic interval separates one pair from the next.

The relative intensity of these sounds is also helpful. *S_1 is usually louder than S_2 at the apex; S_2 is usually louder than S_1 at the base.*

Even experienced clinicians are sometimes uncertain about the timing of heart sounds, especially extra sounds and murmurs. "Inching" can then be helpful. Return to a place on the chest—most often the base—where it is easy to identify S_1 and S_2. Get their rhythm clearly in mind. Then inch your stethoscope down the chest in steps until you hear the new sound.

Auscultation alone, however, can be misleading. The intensities of S_1 and S_2, for example, may be abnormal. At rapid heart rates, moreover, diastole shortens, and at about a rate of 120, the durations of systole and diastole become indistinguishable. *Use palpation of the carotid pulse or of the apical impulse to help determine whether the sound or murmur is systolic or diastolic.* Because both the carotid upstroke and the apical impulse occur in systole, right after S_1, sounds or murmurs coinciding with them are systolic; sounds or murmurs occurring after the carotid upstroke or apical impulse are diastolic.

For example, S_1 is decreased in *first-degree heart block*, and S_2 is decreased in *aortic stenosis*.

Inspection and Palpation

Overview. Careful *inspection* of the anterior chest may reveal the location of the *apical impulse* or *point of maximal impulse (PMI)*, or less commonly, the ventricular movements of a left-sided S_3 or S_4. Tangential light is useful for making these observations. Use *palpation* to confirm the characteristics of the apical impulse.

Palpation is also valuable for detecting thrills, the timing of S_1 and S_2, and the ventricular movements of S_3 or S_4.

● Begin with general palpation of the chest wall. First palpate for *heaves*, *lifts*, or *thrills*, using your *fingerpads*. Hold them flat or obliquely on the body surface. Ventricular impulses may heave or lift your fingers.

● Check for *thrills*, formed by the turbulence of underlying murmurs, by pressing the *ball of your hand* firmly on the chest. If subsequent auscultation reveals a loud murmur, go back to that area and check for thrills again.

● Now use firm pressure for an S_1 and S_2 and lighter pressure for S_3 or S_4. When palpating for S_1 and S_2, place your right hand on the chest wall and your left index and middle fingers on the right carotid artery in the lower third of the neck. Identify S_1, which occurs just before the carotid upstroke. Now identify S_2, which occurs after the carotid upstroke. This may take some practice. At first the upstroke may seem to happen too fast. If you perform this check each time you examine a patient, you will discover that you can correctly identify S_1 and S_2 by palpation as well as by auscultation.

Thrills may accompany loud, harsh, or rumbling murmurs as in a*ortic stenosis, patent ductus arteriosus, ventricular septal defect,* and, less commonly, *mitral stenosis.* They are palpated more easily in patient positions that accentuate the murmur.

On rare occasions, a patient has *dextrocardia*—a heart situated on the right side. The apical impulse will then be found on the right. If you cannot find an apical impulse, percuss for the dullness of the heart and liver and for the tympany of the stomach. In *situs inversus,* all three of these structures are on opposite sides from normal. A right-sided heart with a normally placed liver and stomach is usually associated with congenital heart disease.

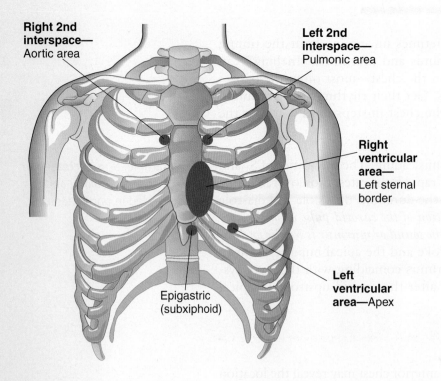

Right 2nd interspace—
Aortic area

Left 2nd interspace—
Pulmonic area

Right ventricular area—
Left sternal border

Left ventricular area—Apex

Epigastric (subxiphoid)

- Be sure to assess the *right ventricle* by palpating the right ventricular area at the lower left sternal border and in the subxiphoid area, the pulmonary artery in the left 2nd interspace, and the aortic area in the right 2nd interspace (see p. 356).

Review the diagram on the previous page, which pertains to most patients with normal anatomy of the heart and great vessels.

Left Ventricular Area—The Apical Impulse or Point of Maximal Impulse (PMI).

The apical impulse represents the brief early pulsation of the left ventricle as it moves anteriorly during contraction and touches the chest wall. Note that in most examinations the apical impulse is the point of maximal impulse, or PMI; however, some pathologic conditions may produce a pulsation that is more prominent than the apex beat, such as an enlarged right ventricle, a dilated pulmonary artery, or an aneurysm of the aorta.

If you cannot identify the apical impulse with the patient supine, ask the patient to roll partly onto the left side—this is the *left lateral decubitus* position. Palpate again, using the palmar surfaces of several fingers. If you cannot find the apical impulse, ask the patient to exhale fully and stop breathing for a few seconds. When examining a woman, it may be helpful to displace the left breast upward or laterally as necessary; alternatively, ask her to do this for you.

The apex beat is palpable in only 25% to 40% of healthy adults in the supine position and in 50% of healthy adults in the left lateral decubitus position, especially those who are thin.[55]

Once you have found the apical impulse, make finer assessments with your fingertips, and then with one finger.

With experience, you will learn to feel the apical impulse in a high percentage of patients. Obesity, a very muscular chest wall, or an increased antero-posterior diameter of the chest, however, may make it undetectable. Some apical impulses hide behind the rib cage, despite positioning.

Now assess the location, diameter, amplitude, and duration of the apical impulse. You may wish to have the patient breathe out and briefly stop breathing to check your findings.

See Table 9-4, Variations and Abnormalities of the Ventricular Impulses (p. 378).

- *Location.* Try to assess location with the patient *supine,* because the left lateral decubitus position displaces the apical impulse to the left. Locate two points: the interspaces, usually the 5th or possibly the 4th, which give the vertical location; and the distance in centimeters from the *midsternal line,* which gives the horizontal location. Some authors recommend measurement from the *midclavicular line,* because the apical impulse falls roughly at this line. Clinicians using this line should use a ruler to mark the midpoint between the sternoclavicular and acromid-clavicular joints; otherwise, use of this line is less reproducible because clinicians vary in their estimates of the midpoint of the clavicle.

Pregnancy or a high left diaphragm may displace the apical impulse upward and to the left.

Lateral displacement from cardiac enlargement in *congestive heart failure, cardiomyopathy, ischemic heart disease.* Displacement in deformities of the thorax and mediastinal shift.

Lateral displacement outside the midclavicular line increases the likelihood of cardiac enlargement and a low-left ventricular ejection fraction by 3–4 and 10, respectively.[55]

Midsternal line Midclavicular line

Apical pulse

ex/ 1 am
9th rib
7.0cm from midsternal line

- *Diameter*. Palpate the diameter of the apical impulse. In the supine patient, it usually measures less than 2.5 cm and occupies only one interspace. It may feel larger in the left lateral decubitus position.

In the left lateral decubitus position, a *diffuse* PMI with a diameter greater than 3 cm indicates left ventricular enlargement.[56]

- *Amplitude*. Estimate the amplitude of the impulse. It is usually small and feels *brisk* and *tapping*. Some young people have an increased amplitude, or hyperkinetic impulse, especially when excited or after exercise; its duration, however, is normal.

Increased amplitude may also reflect *hyperthyroidism, severe anemia,* pressure overload of the left ventricle (as in *aortic stenosis*), or volume overload of the left ventricle (as in *mitral regurgitation*).

Normal

Hyperkinetic

- *Duration*. Duration is the most useful characteristic of the apical impulse for identifying hypertrophy of the left ventricle. To assess duration, listen to the heart sounds as you feel the apical impulse, or watch the movement of your stethoscope as you listen at the apex. Estimate the proportion of systole occupied by the apical impulse. Normally it lasts through the first two-thirds of systole, and often less, but does not continue to the second heart sound.

A *sustained,* high-amplitude impulse that is normally located suggests left ventricular hypertrophy from pressure overload (as in *hypertension*). If such an impulse is displaced laterally, consider volume overload.

Normal

Sustained

A sustained low-amplitude (hypokinetic) impulse may result from *dilated cardiomyopathy*.

S₃ and S₄. By inspection and palpation, you may detect ventricular movements that are synchronous with pathologic third and fourth heart sounds. For the left ventricular impulses, feel the apical beat gently with one finger. The patient should lie partly on the left side, breathe out, and briefly stop breathing. By inking an X on the apex, you may be able to see these movements.

A brief middiastolic impulse indicates an S_3; an impulse just before the systolic apical beat itself indicates an S_4.

Right Ventricular Area—The Left Sternal Border in the 3rd, 4th, and 5th Interspaces. The patient should rest supine at 30°. Place the tips of your curved fingers in the 3rd, 4th, and 5th interspaces and try to feel the systolic impulse of the right ventricle. Again, asking the patient to breathe out and then briefly stop breathing improves your observation.

If an impulse is palpable, assess its location, amplitude, and duration. A brief systolic tap of low or slightly increased amplitude is sometimes felt in thin or shallow-chested people, especially when stroke volume is increased, as by anxiety.

A marked increase in amplitude with little or no change in duration occurs in chronic volume overload of the right ventricle, as from an *atrial septal defect.*

An impulse with increased amplitude and duration occurs with pressure overload of the right ventricle, as in *pulmonic stenosis* or *pulmonary hypertension.*

The diastolic movements of *right-sided S₃ and S₄* may be felt occasionally. Feel for them in the 4th and 5th left interspaces. Time them by auscultation or carotid palpation.

In patients with an increased anteroposterior (AP) diameter, palpation of the *right ventricle* in the *epigastric* or *subxiphoid area* is also useful. With your hand flattened, press your index finger just under the rib cage and up toward the left shoulder and try to feel right ventricular pulsations.

In obstructive pulmonary disease, hyperinflated lung may prevent palpation of an enlarged right ventricle in the left parasternal area. The impulse is felt easily, however, high in the epigastrium where heart sounds are also often heard best.

Asking the patient to inhale and briefly stop breathing is helpful. The inspiratory position moves your hand well away from the pulsations of the abdominal aorta, which might otherwise be confusing. The diastolic movements of S_3 and S_4, if present, may also be felt here.

Pulmonic Area—The Left 2nd Interspace.   This interspace overlies the *pulmonary artery*. As the patient holds expiration, look and feel for an impulse and feel for possible heart sounds. In thin or shallow-chested patients, the pulsation of a pulmonary artery may sometimes be felt here, especially after exercise or with excitement.

A prominent pulsation here often accompanies dilatation or increased flow in the pulmonary artery. A palpable S_2 suggests increased pressure in the pulmonary artery (*pulmonary hypertension*).

Aortic Area—The Right 2nd Interspace.   This interspace overlies the aortic outflow tract. Search for pulsations and palpable heart sounds.

A palpable S_2 suggests systemic *hypertension*. A pulsation here suggests a dilated or aneurysmal aorta.

Percussion

Palpation has replaced percussion in the estimation of cardiac size. When you cannot feel the apical impulse, however, percussion may be your only tool, but may not be reliable. Under these circumstances, cardiac dullness often occupies a large area. Starting well to the left on the chest, percuss from resonance toward cardiac dullness in the 3rd, 4th, 5th, and possibly 6th interspaces.

A markedly dilated failing heart may have a hypokinetic apical impulse that is displaced far to the left. A large pericardial effusion may make the impulse undetectable.

Auscultation

Overview.   Auscultation of heart sounds and murmurs is a rewarding and important skill of physical examination that leads directly to several clinical diagnoses. In this section, you will learn the techniques for identifying S_1 and S_2, extra sounds in systole and diastole, and systolic and diastolic murmurs. Review the auscultatory areas on the next page with the following caveats: (1) Many authorities discourage use of names such as "aortic area," because murmurs may be loudest in other areas; and (2) these areas may not apply to patients with cardiac enlargment, anomalies of the great vessels, or dextrocardia. It is best to use locations such as "base of the heart," apex, or parasternal border to describe your findings.

"Inching" Your Stethoscope.   In a quiet room, listen to the heart with your stethoscope, starting at either the base or apex. Either pattern is satisfactory.

● Some experts recommend *starting at the apex and inching to the base*: move the stethoscope from the PMI medially to the left sternal border, superiorly to the second interspace, then across the sternum to the second interspace at the right sternal border.

- Alternatively, you can *start at the base and inch your stethoscope to the apex*: with your stethoscope in the right 2nd interspace close to the sternum, move along the left sternal border in each interspace from the 2nd through the 5th, and then to the apex.

The Importance of Timing S₁ and S₂. Regardless of the direction you move your stethoscope, keep your left index and middle fingers on the right carotid artery in the lower third of the neck to facilitate correct identification of S_1, just before the carotid upstroke, and S_2, which follows the carotid upstroke. Be sure to compare the intensities of S_1 and S_2 as you move your stethoscope through the listening areas above.

- At the base you will note that S_2 is louder than S_1 and may split with respiration. At the apex, S_1 is usually louder than S_2 unless the PR interval is prolonged.

- By carefully noting the intensities of S_1 and S_2, you will confirm each of these sounds and thereby correctly identify *systole*, the interval between S_1 and S_2, and *diastole*, the interval between S_2 and S_1.

As you will observe when listening to the extra sounds of S_3 and S_4 and to murmurs, timing systole and diastole is an absolute prerequisite to the correct identification of these events in the cardiac cycle.

Heart sounds and murmurs that originate in the four valves range widely, as illustrated below. Use anatomical location rather than valve area to describe where murmurs and sounds are best heard.

2nd right interspace— aortic area

2nd left interspace— pulmonic area

Apex— mitral area

Lower left sternal border— tricuspid area

Aortic   Pulmonic

Tricuspid   Mitral

(Redrawn form Leatham A: Introduction to the Examination of the Cardiovascular System, 2nd ed. Oxford, Oxford University Press, 1979)

Know your stethoscope! It is important to understand the uses of both the diaphragm and the bell.

● ***The diaphragm.*** The diaphragm is better for picking up the relatively high-pitched sounds of S_1 and S_2, the murmurs of aortic and mitral regurgitation, and pericardial friction rubs. *Listen throughout the precordium* with the diaphragm, pressing it firmly against the chest.

● ***The bell.*** The bell is more sensitive to the low-pitched sounds of S_3 and S_4 and the murmur of mitral stenosis. Apply the bell lightly, with just enough pressure to produce an air seal with its full rim. *Use the bell at the apex, then move medially along the lower sternal border.* Resting the heel of your hand on the chest like a fulcrum may help you to maintain light pressure.

Pressing the bell firmly on the chest makes it function more like the diaphragm by stretching the underlying skin. Low-pitched sounds such as S_3 and S_4 may disappear with this technique—an observation that may help to identify them. In contrast, high-pitched sounds such as a midsystolic click, an ejection sound, or an opening snap will persist or get louder.

Listen to the entire precordium with the patient supine. For new patients and patients needing a complete cardiac examination, use two other important positions to listen for mitral stenosis and aortic regurgitation.

Use important maneuvers. Ask the patient to *roll partly onto the left side into the left lateral decubitus position*, bringing the left ventricle close to the chest wall. Place the bell of your stethoscope lightly on the apical impulse.

This position accentuates or brings out a left-sided S_3 and S_4 and mitral murmurs, especially *mitral stenosis*. Otherwise, you may miss these important findings.

Ask the patient to *sit up, lean forward, exhale completely, and stop breathing in expiration.* Pressing the diaphragm of your stethoscope on the chest, listen along the left sternal border and at the apex, pausing periodically so the patient may breathe.

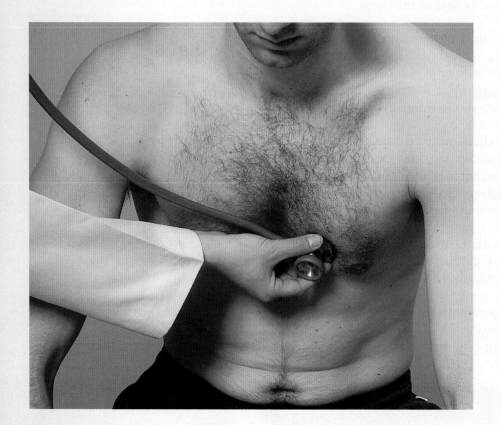

This position accentuates or brings out aortic murmurs. You may easily miss the soft diastolic murmur of *aortic regurgitation* unless you listen at this position.

Listening for Heart Sounds. Throughout your examination, take your time at each auscultatory area. Concentrate on each of the events in the cardiac cycle listed on the next page and sounds you may hear in systole and diastole.

Correctly Identifying Heart Murmurs. Correctly identifying heart murmurs is an exciting diagnostic challenge. A logical and systematic approach, a thorough understanding of cardiac anatomy and physiology, and *above all, your dedication to the study, practice, and mastery of techniques of examination and the tables in this chapter will lead to your success.* Whenever possible, compare your findings with those of an experienced clinician to improve your clinical acumen. Review the tips for identifying heart murmurs summarized in the following table, and then study the following sections carefully for more detail.

● Auscultatory Sounds

Heart Sounds	Guides to Auscultation
S_1	Note its intensity and any apparent splitting. Normal splitting is detectable along the lower left sternal border.
S_2	Note its intensity.
Split S_2	Listen for splitting of this sound in the 2nd and 3rd left interspaces. Ask the patient to breathe quietly, and then slightly more deeply than normal. Does S_2 split into its two components, as it normally does? If not, ask the patient to (1) breathe a little more deeply, or (2) sit up. Listen again. A thick chest wall may make the pulmonic component of S_1 inaudible.
	Width of split. How wide is the split? It is normally quite narrow.
	Timing of split. When in the respiratory cycle do you hear the split? It is normally heard late in inspiration.
	Does the split disappear as it should, during exhalation? If not, listen again with the patient sitting up.
	Intensity of A_2 and P_2. Compare the intensity of the two components, A_2 and P_2. A_2 is usually louder.
Extra Sounds in Systole	Such as ejection sounds or systolic clicks
	Note their location, timing, intensity, and pitch, and the effects of respiration on the sounds.
Extra Sounds in Diastole	Such as S_3, S_4, or an opening snap
	Note the location, timing, intensity, and pitch, and the effects of respiration on the sounds. (An S_3 or S_4 in athletes is a normal finding.)
Systolic and Diastolic Murmurs	Murmurs are differentiated from heart sounds by their longer duration.

See Table 9-5, Variations in the First Heart Sound—S_1 (p. 379). Note that S_1 is louder at more rapid heart rates (and PR intervals are shorter).

See Table 9-6, Variations in the Second Heart Sound—S_2 (p. 380). When either A_2 or P_2 is absent, as in disease of the respective valves, S_2 is persistently single.

Expiratory splitting suggests an abnormality (p. 380).

Persistent splitting results from delayed closure of the pulmonic valve or early closure of the aortic valve.

A loud P_2 suggests pulmonary hypertension.

The systolic click of mitral valve prolapse is the most common of these sounds. See Table 9-7, Extra Heart Sounds in Systole (p. 381).

See Table 9-8, Extra Heart Sounds in Diastole (p. 382).

See Table 9-9, Pansystolic (Holosystolic) Murmurs (p. 383), Table 9-10, Midsystolic Murmurs (pp. 384–385), and Table 9-11, Diastolic Murmurs (p. 386).

● *Timing.* First decide if you are hearing a *systolic murmur,* falling between S_1 and S_2, or a *diastolic murmur,* falling between S_2 and S_1. Palpating the carotid pulse as you listen can help you with timing. *Murmurs that coincide with the carotid upstroke are systolic.*

Systolic murmurs are usually *midsystolic* or *pansystolic.* Late systolic murmurs may also be heard.

Diastolic murmurs usually indicate valvular heart disease. Systolic murmurs may indicate valvular disease but often occur when the heart valves are normal.

TIPS FOR IDENTIFYING HEART MURMURS

- Time the murmur—is it in systole or diastole?
- Locate where the murmur is loudest on the precordium—at the base, along the sternal border, at the apex?
- Conduct any necessary maneuvers, such as having the patient lean forward and exhale or turn to the left lateral decubitus position.
- Determine the shape of the murmur—for example, is it crescendo or decrescendo, is it holosystolic?
- Grade the intensity of the murmur from 1 to 6.
- Identify associated features such as the quality of S_1 and S_2, the presence of extra sounds such as S_3, S_4, or an opening snap, or the presence of additional murmurs.
- Be sure you are listening in a quiet room!

A *midsystolic murmur* begins after S_1 and stops before S_2. Brief gaps are audible between the murmur and the heart sounds. Listen carefully for the gap just before S_2. It is heard more easily and, if present, usually confirms the murmur as midsystolic, not pansystolic.

Midsystolic murmurs typically arise from blood flow across the semilunar (aortic and pulmonic) valves. See Table 9-10, Midsystolic Murmurs (pp. 384–385).

A *pansystolic (holosystolic) murmur* starts with S_1 and stops at S_2, without a gap between murmur and heart sounds.

Pansystolic murmurs often occur with regurgitant (backward) flow across the atrioventricular valves. See Table 9-9, Pansystolic (Holosystolic) Murmurs (p. 383).

A *late systolic murmur* usually starts in mid- or late systole and persists up to S_2.

This is the murmur of mitral valve prolapse and is often, but not always, preceded by a systolic click (see p. 383).

Diastolic murmurs may be *early diastolic, middiastolic,* or *late diastolic.*

An *early diastolic murmur* starts immediately after S_2, without a discernible gap, and then usually fades into silence before the next S_1.

Early diastolic murmurs typically accompany regurgitant flow across incompetent semilunar valves.

A *middiastolic murmur* starts a short time after S_2. It may fade away, as illustrated, or merge into a late diastolic murmur.

Middiastolic and presystolic murmurs reflect turbulent flow across the atrioventricular valves. See Table 9-11, Diastolic Murmurs (p. 386).

A *late diastolic (presystolic) murmur* starts late in diastole and typically continues up to S_1.

An occasional murmur, such as the murmur of a patent ductus arteriosus, starts in systole and continues without pause through S_2, into but not necessarily throughout diastole. It is then called a *continuous murmur*. Other cardiovascular sounds, such as pericardial friction rubs or venous hums, have *both systolic and diastolic components*. Observe and describe these sounds according to the characteristics used for systolic and diastolic murmurs.

See Table 9-12, Cardiovascular Sounds With Both Systolic and Diastolic Components (p. 387).

- *Shape.* The shape or configuration of a murmur is determined by its intensity over time.

 A *crescendo murmur* grows louder.

The presystolic murmur of *mitral stenosis* in normal sinus rhythm

 A *decrescendo murmur* grows softer.

The early diastolic murmur of *aortic regurgitation*

 A *crescendo–decrescendo murmur* first rises in intensity, then falls.

The midsystolic murmur of *aortic stenosis* and *innocent flow murmurs*

 A *plateau murmur* has the same intensity throughout.

The pansystolic murmur of *mitral regurgitation*

- *Location of Maximal Intensity.* This is determined by the site where the murmur originates. Find the location by exploring the area where you hear the murmur. Describe where you hear it best in terms of the interspace and its relation to the sternum, the apex, or the midsternal, the midclavicular, or one of the axillary lines.

For example, a murmur best heard in the 2nd right interspace often originates at or near the aortic valve.

- *Radiation or Transmission From the Point of Maximal Intensity.* This reflects not only the site of origin but also the intensity of the murmur and the direction of blood flow. Explore the area around a murmur and determine where else you can hear it.

A loud murmur of *aortic stenosis* often radiates into the neck (in the direction of arterial flow), especially on the right side.

- *Intensity.* This is usually graded on a 6-point scale and expressed as a fraction. The numerator describes the intensity of the murmur wherever it is loudest; the denominator indicates the scale you are using. Intensity is influenced by the thickness of the chest wall and the presence of intervening tissue.

An identical degree of turbulence would cause a louder murmur in a thin person than in a very muscular or obese person. Emphysematous lungs may diminish the intensity of murmurs.

Learn to grade murmurs using the 6-point scale below. Note that grades 4 through 6 require the added presence of a palpable thrill.

● Gradations of Murmurs

Grade	Description
Grade 1	Very faint, heard only after listener has "tuned in"; may not be heard in all positions
Grade 2	Quiet, but heard immediately after placing the stethoscope on the chest
Grade 3	Moderately loud
Grade 4	Loud, with palpable thrill
Grade 5	Very loud, with thrill. May be heard when the stethoscope is partly off the chest
Grade 6	Very loud, with thrill. May be heard with stethoscope entirely off the chest

● *Pitch.* This is categorized as high, medium, or low.

● *Quality.* This is described in terms such as blowing, harsh, rumbling, and musical.

A fully described murmur might be: a "medium-pitched, grade 2/6, blowing decrescendo diastolic murmur, heard best in the 4th left interspace, with radiation to the apex" (*aortic regurgitation*).

Other useful characteristics of murmurs—and heart sounds too—include variation with respiration, with the position of the patient, or with other special maneuvers.

Murmurs originating in the right side of the heart tend to vary with respiration more than left-sided murmurs.

 ## INTEGRATING CARDIOVASCULAR ASSESSMENT

A good cardiovascular examination requires more than observation. You need to think about the possible meanings of your individual observations, fit them together in a logical pattern, and correlate your cardiac findings with the patient's blood pressure, arterial pulses, venous pulsations, jugular venous pressure, the remainder of your physical examination findings, and the patient's history.

Evaluating the common systolic murmur illustrates this point. In examining an asymptomatic teenager, for example, you might hear a grade 2/6 mid-systolic murmur in the 2nd and 3rd left interspaces. Because this suggests a murmur of pulmonic origin, you should assess the size of the right ventricle by carefully palpating the left parasternal area. Because pulmonic stenosis and atrial septal defects can occasionally cause such murmurs, listen carefully to the splitting of the second heart sound and try to hear any ejection sounds. Listen to the murmur after the patient sits up. Look for evidence of anemia, hyperthyroidism, or pregnancy that could produce such a murmur

In a 60-year-old person with angina, you might hear a harsh 3/6 mid-systolic crescendo–decrescendo murmur in the right 2nd interspace radiating to the neck. These findings suggest *aortic stenosis* but could arise from *aortic sclerosis* (leaflets sclerotic but not stenotic), a dilated aorta, or increased flow across a normal valve. Assess any delay in the carotid upstroke and the intensity of A_2 for evidence of *aortic stenosis.* Check the apical impulse for left ventricular hypertrophy. Listen for *aortic regurgitation* as the patient leans forward and exhales.

by increasing the flow across the aortic or the pulmonic valve. If all your findings are normal, your patient probably has an *innocent* or *functional murmur*—one with no pathologic significance.

Functional murmurs are short, early, midsystolic murmurs that decrease in intensity with maneuvers that reduce left ventricular volume, such as standing, sitting up, and straining during the Valsalva maneuver.

Put all this information together to make a hypothesis about the origin of the murmur.

 SPECIAL TECHNIQUES

Aids to Identify Systolic Murmurs. Elsewhere in this chapter you have learned how to improve your auscultation of heart sounds and murmurs by placing the patient in different positions. Two additional techniques help you distinguish the murmurs of mitral valve prolapse and hypertrophic cardiomyopathy from aortic stenosis.

(1) Standing and Squatting. When a person stands, venous return to the heart decreases, as does peripheral vascular resistance. Arterial blood pressure, stroke volume, and the volume of blood in the left ventricle all decline. When squatting, changes occur in the opposite direction. These changes help (1) to identify a prolapsed mitral valve and (2) to distinguish hypertrophic cardiomyopathy from aortic stenosis.

Secure the patient's gown so that it will not interfere with your examination, and ready yourself for prompt auscultation. Instruct the patient to squat next to the examining table and hold on to it for balance. Listen to the heart with the patient in the squatting position and again in the standing position.

● Maneuvers to Identify Systolic Murmurs

Maneuver	Cardiovascular Effect	Effect on Systolic Sounds and Murmurs		
		Mitral Valve Prolapse	Hypertrophic Cardiomyopathy	Aortic Stenosis
Standing; Strain Phase of Valsalva	**Decreased left ventricular volume** from ↓ venous return to heart	↑ prolapse of mitral valve	↑ outflow obstruction	↓ blood volume ejected into aorta
	Decreased vascular tone: ↓ arterial blood pressure	*Click moves earlier in systole* and *murmur lengthens*	↑ **intensity of murmur**	↓ **intensity of murmur**
Squatting; Release of Valsalva	**Increased left ventricular volume** from ↑ venous return to heart	↓ prolapse of mitral valve	↓ outflow obstruction	↑ blood volume ejected into aorta
	Increased vascular tone: ↑ arterial blood pressure; ↑ peripheral vascular resistance	*Delay of click* and *murmur shortens*	↓ **intensity of murmur**	↑ **intensity of murmur**

(2) Valsalva Maneuver.   When a person strains down against a closed glottis, venous return to the right heart is decreased, and after a few seconds, left ventricular volume and arterial blood pressure both fall. Release of the effort has the opposite effects. These changes help to distinguish prolapse of the mitral valve and hypertrophic cardiomyopathy from aortic stenosis.

The patient should be lying down. Ask the patient to "bear down," or place one hand on the midabdomen and instruct the patient to strain against it. By adjusting the pressure of your hand you can alter the patient's effort to the desired level. Use your other hand to place your stethoscope on the patient's chest.

The murmur of hypertrophic cardiomyopathy is the only systolic murmur that increases in intensity during the Valsalva maneuver (strain phase).[57]

Pulsus Alternans.   In *pulsus alternans,* the rhythm of the pulse remains regular, but the *force* of the arterial pulse alternates because of alternating strong and weak ventricular contractions. *Pulsus alternans* almost always indicates severe left-sided heart failure and is usually best felt by applying light pressure on the radial or femoral arteries.[58] Use a blood pressure cuff to confirm your finding. After raising the cuff pressure, lower it slowly to the systolic level—the initial Korotkoff sounds are the strong beats. As you lower the cuff, you will hear the softer sounds of the alternating weak beats.

Alternately loud and soft Korotkoff sounds or a sudden doubling of the apparent heart rate as the cuff pressure declines indicates a *pulsus alternans* (see p. 377).

The upright position may accentuate the alternation.

Paradoxical Pulse.   If you have noted that the pulse varies in amplitude with respiration or if you suspect pericardial tamponade (because of increased jugular venous pressure, a rapid and diminished pulse, and dyspnea, for example), use a blood-pressure cuff to check for a *paradoxical pulse.* This is a greater than normal drop in systolic pressure during inspiration. As the patient breathes, quietly if possible, lower the cuff pressure slowly to the systolic level. Note the pressure level at which the first sounds can be heard. Then drop the pressure very slowly until sounds can be heard throughout the respiratory cycle. Again note the pressure level. The difference between these two levels is normally no greater than 3 or 4 mm Hg.

The level identified by first hearing Korotkoff sounds is the highest systolic pressure during the respiratory cycle. The level identified by hearing sounds throughout the cycle is the lowest systolic pressure. A difference between these levels of more than 10 mm Hg indicates a paradoxical pulse and suggests *pericardial tamponade,* possible *constrictive pericarditis,* but most commonly *obstructive airway disease* (see p. 377).

RECORDING YOUR FINDINGS

Note that initially you may use sentences to describe your findings; later you will use phrases. The style below contains phrases appropriate for most write-ups.

Recording the Physical Examination—
The Cardiovascular Examination

> "The jugular venous pulse (JVP) is 3 cm above the sternal angle with the head of bed elevated to 30°. Carotid upstrokes are brisk, without bruits. The point of maximal impulse (PMI) is tapping, 7 cm lateral to the mid-sternal line in the 5th intercostal space. Crisp S_1 and S_2. At the base S_2 is greater than S_1 and physiologically split, with $A_2 > P_2$. At the apex S_1 is greater than S_2 and constant. No murmurs or extra sounds."
>
> **OR**
>
> "The JVP is 5 cm above the sternal angle with the head of bed elevated to 50°. Carotid upstrokes are brisk; a bruit is heard over the left carotid artery. The PMI is diffuse, 3 cm in diameter, palpated at the anterior axillary line in the 5th and 6th intercostal spaces. S_1 and S_2 are soft. S_3 present at the apex. High-pitched harsh 2/6 holosystolic murmur best heard at the apex, radiating to the axilla."

Suggests congestive heart failure with volume overload with possible left carotid occlusion and mitral regurgitation.[59–61]

BIBLIOGRAPHY

CITATIONS

1. Markel H. The stethoscope and the art of listening. N Engl J Med 354(6):551–552, 2006.
2. Simel DS. Time, now, to recover the fun in the physical examination rather than abandon it. Arch Intern Med 166(6): 603–604, 2006.
3. Mangione S. Cardiac auscultatory skills of physicians-in-training: a comparison of three English-speaking countries. Am J Med 110(3):210–216, 2001.
4. Mangione S. Cardiac auscultatory skills of internal medicine and family practice trainees: a comparison of diagnostic proficiency. JAMA 278(9):717–722, 1997.
5. Mangione S. The teaching and practice of cardiac auscultation during internal medicine and cardiology training. Ann Intern Med 119(1):47–54, 1993.
6. Marcus G, Vessey J, Jordan MV, et al. Relationship between accurate auscultation of a clinically useful third heart sound and level of experience. Arch Intern Med 166(6):617–622, 2006.
7. Vukanovic-Criley JM, Criley S, Warde CM, et al. Competency in cardiac examination skills in medical students, trainees, physicians, and faculty: a multicenter study. Arch Intern Med 166(6):610–616, 2006.
8. O'Rourke RA, Braunwald E. Physical examination of the cardiovascular system. In: Kasper DL, Braunwald E, Hauser S, et al., eds. Harrison's Principles of Internal Medicine, 16th ed. New York: McGraw-Hill, 2005:1307.
9. Hunt SA, Abraham WT, Chin MH, et al. ACC/AHA 2005 guideline update for the diagnosis and management of chronic heart failure in the adult—summary article. Circulation 112(12): 154–235, 2005.
10. Cook DJ, Simel DL. Does this patient have abnormal central venous pressure? JAMA 275(8):630–654, 1996.
11. Vinayak AG, Levitt J, Gehlbach B, et al. Usefulness of the external jugular vein examination in detecting abnormal central venous pressure in critically ill patients. Arch Intern Med 166(19):2132–2137, 2006.
12. Davison R, Cannon R. Estimation of central venous pressure by examination of jugular veins. Am Heart J 87(3):279–282, 1974.
13. American Heart Association–American Stroke Association. Heart Disease and Stroke Statistics, 2007. Available at: http://www.americanheart.org/downloadable/heart/1166712318459HS_StatsInsideText.pdf; Cardiovascular Disease Statistics. Available at: http://www.americanheart.org/presenter.jhtml?

identifier=4478; National Center for Health Statistics, Fast Stats A to Z. Available at: http://www.cdc.gov/nchs/fastats/heart.htm. Accessed December 2, 2007.

14. Lee TH, Goldman L. Evaluation of the patient with acute chest pain. N Engl J Med 342(16):1187–1195, 2000.

15. Goldman L, Kirtane AJ. Triage of patient with acute chest syndrome and possible cardiac ischemia: the elusive search for diagnostic perfection. Ann Intern Med 139(12):987–995, 2003.

16. Snow V, Barry P, Fihn SD, et al. Evaluation of primary care patients with chronic stable angina: guidelines from the American College of Physicians. Ann Intern Med 141(1):57–64, 2004.

17. Hofgren C, Karlson BW, Gaston-Johansson F, et al. Word descriptors in suspected acute myocardial infarction: a comparison between patients with and without confirmed myocardial infarction. Heart Lung 23(5):397–403, 1994.

18. Abrams J. Chronic stable angina. N Engl J Med 352(24): 2524–2533, 2005.

19. Gibbons RJ, Abrams J, Chatterjee K, et al. ACC/AHA 2002 ACC/AHA 2002 guideline update for the management of patients with chronic stable angina—summary article. Circulation 107(1):149–158, 2003.

20. Fraker TD, Fihn SD, Gibbons RJ, et al. 2007 Chronic angina focused update of the ACC/AHA 2002 guideline update for the management of patients with chronic stable angina. Circulation. Published on-line November 12, 2007, at http://content.onlinejacc.org/cgi/content/citation/j.jacc.2007.08.002v1. Accessed November 25, 2007.

21. Klompas M. Does this patient have an acute thoracic aortic dissection? JAMA 287(17):2262–2272, 2002.

22. Cho S, Atwood JE. Peripheral edema. Am J Med 113(7): 580–586, 2002.

23. U.S. Preventive Services Task Force. Screening for high blood pressure: recommendations and rationale. Rockville, MD, Agency for Healthcare Research and Quality, July 2003. Available at: http://www.ahrq.gov/clinic/3rduspstf/hibloodrr.htm. Accessed November 25, 2007.

24. Chobanion AV, Bakris GL, Black HR, et al. The Seventh Report of the Joint National Committee on Preventions, Detection, Evaluation, and Treatment of High Blood Pressure—The JNC 7 Report. JAMA 289(19):2560–2572, 2003. Available at: www.nhlbi.nih.gov/guidelines/hypertension/jncintro.htm. Accessed December 2, 2007.

25. Whelton PK, He J, Appel LJ, et al. Primary prevention of hypertension. Clinical and Public Health Advisory from the National High Blood Pressure Education Program. JAMA 288(15):1882–1888, 2002.

26. U.S. Preventive Services Task Force. Screening for high blood pressure: U.S. Preventive Services Task Force reaffirmation recommendation statement. Ann Intern Med 147(11):783–786, 2007; See also: Woolff T, Miller T. Evidence for the reaffirmation of the U.S. Preventive Services Task Force recommendation on screening for high blood pressure. Ann Intern Med 147(11):787–791, 2007.

27. Vidt DG, Borazanian RA. Treat high blood pressure sooner: tougher, simpler JNC 7 guidelines. Cleve Clin J Med 70(8): 721–728, 2003.

28. Vasan RS, Larson MG, Leip EP, et al. Impact of high-normal blood pressure on the risk of cardiovascular disease. N Engl J Med 345(18):1291–1297, 2001.

29. Stamler J, Stamler R, Neaton JD, et al. Low risk-factor profile and long-term cardiovascular and noncardiovascular mortality and life expectancy—findings for 5 large cohorts of young adult and middle-aged men and women. JAMA 282(21): 2012–2018, 1999.

30. Pearson TA, Blair SN, Daniels SR, et al. AHA guidelines for primary prevention of cardiovascular disease and stroke: 2002 update. Circulation 106(3):388–391, 2002.

31. Third Report of the National Cholesterol Education Program (NCEP) Expert Panel. Detection, evaluation, and treatment of high blood cholesterol in adults: executive summary. National Cholesterol Education Program, National Heart, Lung, and Blood Institute, National Institutes of Health. NIH Publication No. 01-3670. May 2001. Available at: www.nhlbi.nih.gov/guidelines/cholesterol/index.htm. Accessed November 26, 2007.

32. National Cholesterol Education Panel. Third report of the National Cholesterol Education Program (NCEP) Expert Panel on detection, evaluation, and treatment of high blood cholesterol in adults (Adult Treatment Panel III) final report. Circulation 106(25):3143–3421, 2002.

33. Grundy SM, Cleeman JI, Merz NB, et al, for the Coordinating Committee of the National Cholesterol Education Program. Implications of recent clinical trials for the National Cholesterol Education Program Adult Treatment Panel III guidelines. Circulation 110(2):227–239, 2004.

34. Heart Protection Study Collaborative Group. MRC/BHF Heart Protection Study of cholesterol lowering with simvastatin in 20,356 high risk individuals: a randomized placebo-controlled trial. Lancet 360(9326):7–22, 2002.

35. U.S. Preventive Services Task Force. Screening for lipid disorders: recommendations and rationale. Am J Prev Med 20(3S):73–76, 2001. Agency for Healthcare Research and Quality, Rockville MD. Available at: http://www.ahrq.gov/clinic/ajpmsuppl/lipidrr.htm. Accessed November 16, 2007.

36. Pignone MP, Phillips CJ, Atkins D, et al. Summary of the evidence. Screening and treating adults for lipid disorders. Agency for Healthcare Research and Quality, Rockville, MD. Available at: http://www.ahrq.gov/clinic/ajpmsuppl/pignone1.htm. Accessed December 2, 2007.

37. Walsh JME, Pignone M. Drug treatment of hyperlipidemia in women. JAMA 291(18):2243–2252, 2004; American Diabetes Association. Toolkit No. 7. Protect your heart: choose fats wisely. March 2004. Available at: http://www.diabetes.org/type-1-diabetes/well-being/Choose-Fats.jsp. Accessed November 27, 2007.

38. Healthy People 2010. Progress review: nutrition and overweight. U.S. Department of Health and Human Services—Public Health Service. January 21, 2004. Available at: http://www.healthypeople.gov/data/2010prog/focus19/default.htm. Accessed November 27, 2007.

39. Healthy People 2010. Progress review: physical activity and fitness. U.S. Department of Health and Human Services—Public Health Service. April 14, 2004. Available at: http://www.healthypeople.gov/data/2010prog/focus22/. Accessed November 27, 2007.

40. Barrett MJ, Kuzma MA, Seto TC, et al. The power of repetition in mastering cardiac auscultation. Am J Med 119(1): 73–75, 2006.

41. Beevers G, Lip GY, O'Brien E. ABC of hypertension: blood pressure measurement. Part I. Sphygmomanometry: factors common in all techniques. BMJ 322(7292):981–985, 2001.

42. Beevers G, Lip GY, O'Brien E. ABC of hypertension: blood pressure measurement. Part II Conventional sphygmomanometry: technique of auscultatory blood pressure measurement. BMJ 322(7293):1043–1047, 2001.

43. McAlister FA, Straus SE. Evidence-based treatment of hypertension. Measurement of blood pressure: an evidence based review. BMJ 322(7292):908–911, 2001.

44. Tholl U, Forstner K, Anlauf M. Measuring blood pressure: pitfalls and recommendations. Nephrol Dial Transplant 19(4): 766–770, 2004.

45. Edmonds ZV, Mower WR, Lovato LM, et al. The reliability of vital sign measurements. Ann Emerg Med 39(3):233–237, 2002.

46. Lange RA, Hillis LD. Acute pericarditis. N Engl J Med 351(21): 2195–2202, 2004.

47. Spodick D. Acute pericarditis: current concepts and practice. JAMA 289(9):1150–1153, 2003.

48. Khot UN. Prognostic importance of physical examination of heart failure in non-ST elevation acute coronary syndromes: the enduring value of Killip classification. JAMA 290(16): 2174–2181, 2003.

49. Jessup M, Brozena S. Medical progress: heart failure. N Engl J Med 348(20):2007–2017, 2003.

50. Aurigemma GP, Gasach WH. Diastolic heart failure. N Engl J Med 351(11):1097–1104, 2004.

51. Badgett RG, Lucey CR, Muirow CD. Can the clinical examination diagnose left-sided heart failure in adults? JAMA 277(21): 1712–1719, 1997.

52. McGee S. Inspection of the neck veins. In: Evidence-Based Physical Diagnosis, 2nd ed. St. Louis, Saunders, 2007:378.

53. Drazner MH, Rame E, Stevenson LW, et al. Prognostic importance of elevated jugular venous pressure and a third heart sound in patients with heart failure. N Engl J Med 345(8):574–581, 2001.

54. Sauve JS, Laupacis A, Feagan B, et al. Does this patient have a clinically important carotid bruit? JAMA 270(23):2843–2845, 1993.

55. McGee S. Palpation of the heart. In: Evidence-Based Physical Diagnosis, 2nd ed. St. Louis, Saunders, 2007:400–404.

56. Dans AL, Bossone EF, Guyatt GH, et al. Evaluation of the reproducibility and accuracy of apex beat measurement in the detection of echocardiographic left ventricular dilation. Can J Cardiol 11(6):493–407, 1995.

57. Lembo NJ, Dell'Italia LJ, Crawford MH, et al. Bedside diagnosis of systolic murmurs. N Engl J Med 318(24):1572–1578, 1988.

58. Cha K, Falk RH. Images in clinical medicine: pulsus alternans. N Engl J Med 334(13):834, 1996.

59. Halder AW, Larson MG, Franklin SS, et al. Systolic blood pressure, diastolic blood pressure, and pulse pressure as predictors of risk for congestive heart failure in the Framingham Heart Study. Ann Intern Med 138(1):10–16, 2003.

60. Thomas JT, Kelly RF, Thomas SJ, et al. Utility of history, physical examination, electrocardiogram, and chest radiograph for differentiating normal from decreased systolic function in patients with heart failure. Am J Med 112(6):437–445, 2002.

61. Fonarow GC, Adams KF, Abraham WT, et al. Risk stratification for in-hospital mortality in acutely decompensated heart failure: classification and regression tree analysis. JAMA 293(5): 572–580, 2005.

62. Kono T, Rosman H, Alam M, et al. Hemodynamic correlates of the third heart sound during the evolution of chronic heart failure. J Am Coll Cardiol 21(2):419–423, 1993.

63. Homma S, Bhattacharjee D, Gopal A, et al. Relationship of auscultatory fourth heart sound to the quantitated left atrial filling fraction. Clin Cardiol 14(8):671–674, 1991.

64. Pierard LA, Lancellotti P. The role of ischemic mitral regurgitation in the pathogenesis of acute pulmonary edema. N Engl J Med 351(16):1627–1634, 2004.

65. Otto CM. Evaluation and management of chronic mitral regurgitation. N Engl J Med 345(10):740–746, 2001.

66. Etchells E, Bell C, Robb K. Does this patient have an abnormal systolic murmur? JAMA 277(7):564–571, 1997.

67. Etchells E, Glenns, Shadowitz S, et al. A bedside clinical prediction rule for detecting moderate or severe aortic stenosis. J Gen Intern Med 13(10):699–704, 1998.

68. Carabello BA. Aortic stenosis. N Engl J Med 356(9):677–682, 2001.

69. Enriquez-Serano M, Tajik AJ. Aortic regurgitation. N Engl J Med 351(15):1539–1546, 2004.

ADDITIONAL REFERENCES

Beckman JA, Creager MA, Libby P. Diabetes and atherosclerosis: epidemiology, pathophysiology, and management. JAMA 287(19):2570–2581, 2002.

Bossone E, Rampoldi, Nienaber CA, et al. Usefulness of pulse deficit to predict in-hospital complications and mortality in patients with acute type A aortic dissection. Am J Cardiol 89(7):851–855, 2002.

Capuzzi DM, Freeman JS. C-reactive protein and cardiovascular risk in the metabolic syndrome and type 2 diabetes: controversy and challenge. Clin Diabetes 25(1):16–22, 2007.

Carnici PG, Crea F. Coronary microvascular dysfunction. N Engl J Med 356(8):830–840, 2007.

Cohn JN, Hoke L, Whitwam W, et al. Screening for early detection of cardiovascular disease in asymptomatic individuals. Am Heart J 146(4):679–685, 2003.

Criley JM. The Physiological Origins of Heart Sounds and Murmurs: The Unique Interactive Guide to Cardiac Diagnosis. English/Spanish (CD-ROM). Palo Alto, CA: Blaufuss Multimedia, 1997.

Devereux RB, Wachtell K, Gerdts E, et al. Prognostic significance of left ventricular mass change during treatment of hypertension. JAMA 292(19):2350–2356, 2004.

Fuster V, Alexander RW, O'Rourke RA, et al. Hurst's The Heart, 11th ed. New York: McGraw-Hill, Medical Publishing Division, 2004.

Hansson GK. Inflammation, atherosclerosis, and coronary artery disease. N Engl J Med 352(16):1685–1695, 2005.

Klein LW. Atherosclerosis regression, vascular remodeling, and plaque stabilization. J Am Coll Cardiol 49:271–273, 2007.

Kuperstein R, Feinberg MS, Eldar M, et al. Physical determinants of systolic murmur intensity in aortic stenosis. Am J Cardiol 95(6):774–776, 2005.

Libby P, ed. Braunwald's Heart Disease: A Textbook of Cardiovascular Medicine, 8th ed. Philadelphia: Elsevier–Saunders, 2008.

Maron BJ, Thompson PD, Ackerman MJ, et al. Recommendations and considerations related to preparticipation screening for cardiovascular abnormalities in competitive athletes: 2007 update. A scientific statement from the American Heart Association Council on Nutrition, Physical Activity, and Metabolism, endorsed by the American College of Cardiology Foundation. Circulation 115(12):1643–1655, 2007.

National Cholesterol Education Program. Risk Assessment Tool for Estimating 10-year Risk of Developing Hard CHD (Myocardial Infarction and Coronary Death). Available at: http://hp2010.nhlbihin.net/atpiii/calculator.asp?usertype= prof. Accessed May 30, 2008.

Neubauer S. The failing heart: an engine out of fuel. N Engl J Med 356(11):1140–1151, 2007.

Perloff JK. Physical Examination of the Heart and Circulation, 3rd ed. Philadelphia: Saunders, 2000.

Pryor DB, Shaw L, McCants CB. Value of the history and physical in identifying patients at increased risk for coronary artery disease. Ann Intern Med 118(2):81–90, 1993.

Sebastian TP, Kostis JB, Cassazza L, et al. Heart rate and blood pressure response in adult men and women during exercise and sexual activity. Am J Cardiol 100(12):1795–1801, 2007.

Selvanayagam J, De Pasquale C, Arnolda L. Usefulness of clinical assessment of the carotid pulse in the diagnosis of aortic stenosis. Am J Cardiol 93(4):493–495, 2004.

Sharma UC, Barenbrug P, Pokharel S, et al. Systematic review of the outcome of aortic valve replacement in patients with aortic stenosis. Ann Thorac Surg 78(1):90–95, 2004.

Sinisalo J, Rapola J, Rossinen J, et al. Simplifying the estimation of jugular venous pressure. Am J Cardiol 100(12):1779–1781, 2007.

Sipahi I, Tuzcu EM, Schoenhagen P, et al. Effects of normal, prehypertensive, and hypertensive blood pressure levels on progression of coronary atherosclerosis. J Am Coll Cardiol 48(4):833–838, 2006.

The Bates' suite offers these additional resources to enhance learning and facilitate understanding of this chapter:

- Bates' Pocket Guide to Physical Examination and History Taking, 6th edition
- Bates' Nursing Online
- Bates' Visual Guide to Physical Examination, 4th edition
- thePoint online resources, http://thepoint.lww.com
- Student CD-ROM included with the book

TABLE	
9-1	**Selected Heart Rates and Rhythms**

Cardiac rhythms may be classified as *regular or irregular*. When rhythms are irregular or rates are fast or slow, obtain an ECG to identify the origin of the beats (sinus node, AV node, atrium, or ventricle) and the pattern of conduction. Note that with AV (atrioventricular) block, arrhythmias may have a fast, normal, or slow ventricular rate. Some authors consider 90 beats/minute the upper limit of normal.

	ECG Pattern	Usual Resting Rate
	Sinus tachycardia	100–180
FAST (>100)	Supraventricular (atrial or nodal) tachycardia	150–250
	Atrial flutter with a regular ventricular response	100–175
	Ventricular tachycardia	110–250
NORMAL (60–100)	Normal sinus rhythm	60–90
	Second-degree AV block	60–100
	Atrial flutter with a regular ventricular response	75–100
SLOW (<60)	Sinus bradycardia	<60
	Second-degree AV block	30–60
	Complete heart block	<40
RHYTHMIC OR SPORADIC	With early beats, atrial or nodal (supraventricular) premature contraction OR ventricular premature contractions	See Table 9-2
	Sinus arrhythmia	
TOTAL	Atrial fibrillation	
	Atrial flutter with varying block	

WHAT IS THE RATE?

REGULAR

IS THE RHYTHM REGULAR OR IRREGULAR?

IRREGULAR

WHAT IS THE PATTERN OF IRREGULARITY?

Selected Irregular Rhythms

Type of Rhythm	ECG Waves and Heart Sounds	

Atrial or Nodal Premature Contractions (*Supraventricular*)

Aberrant P wave   Normal QRS and T

QRS
P   T

S₁ S₂

Early beat   Pause

Rhythm. A beat of atrial or nodal origin comes earlier than the next expected normal beat. A pause follows, and then the rhythm resumes.

Heart Sounds. S_1 may differ in intensity from the S_1 of normal beats, and S_2 may be decreased.

Ventricular Premature Contractions

No P wave   Aberrant QRS and T

S₁ S₂

Early beat with split sounds   Pause

Rhythm. A beat of ventricular origin comes earlier than the next expected normal beat. A pause follows, and the rhythm resumes.

Heart Sounds. S_1 may differ in intensity from the S_1 of the normal beats, and S_2 may be decreased. Both sounds are likely to be split.

Sinus Arrhythmia

S₁ S₂   S₁ S₂ S₁ S₂   S₁ S₂   S₁ S₂

INSPIRATION   EXPIRATION

Rhythm. The heart varies cyclically, usually speeding up with inspiration and slowing down with expiration.

Heart Sounds. Normal, although S_1 may vary with the heart rate.

Atrial Fibrillation and Atrial Flutter With Varying AV Block

No P waves   Fibrillation waves

S₁ S₂   S₁ S₂ S₁ S₂   S₁ S₂

Rhythm. The ventricular rhythm is totally irregular, although short runs of the irregular ventricular rhythm may seem regular.

Heart Sounds. S_1 varies in intensity.

TABLE
9-3

Abnormalities of the Arterial Pulse and Pressure Waves

Normal

mm Hg

The pulse pressure is approximately 30–40 mm Hg. The pulse contour is smooth and rounded. (The notch on the descending slope of the pulse wave is not palpable.)

Small, Weak Pulses

The pulse pressure is diminished, and the pulse feels weak and small. The upstroke may feel slowed, the peak prolonged. Causes include (1) decreased stroke volume, as in heart failure, hypovolemia, and severe aortic stenosis, and (2) increased peripheral resistance, as in exposure to cold and severe congestive heart failure.

Large, Bounding Pulses

The pulse pressure is increased, and the pulse feels strong and bounding. The rise and fall may feel rapid, the peak brief. Causes include (1) increased stroke volume, decreased peripheral resistance, or both, as in fever, anemia, hyperthyroidism, aortic regurgitation, arteriovenous fistulas, and patent ductus arteriosus; (2) increased stroke volume because of slow heart rates, as in bradycardia and complete heart block; and (3) decreased compliance (increased stiffness) of the aortic walls, as in aging or atherosclerosis.

Bisferiens Pulse

A bisferiens pulse is an increased arterial pulse with a double systolic peak. Causes include pure aortic regurgitation, combined aortic stenosis and regurgitation, and, though less commonly palpable, hypertrophic cardiomyopathy.

Pulsus Alternans

The pulse alternates in amplitude from beat to beat even though the rhythm is basically regular (and must be for you to make this judgment). When the difference between stronger and weaker beats is slight, it can be detected only by sphygmomanometry. Pulsus alternans indicates left ventricular failure and is usually accompanied by a left-sided S_3.

Bigeminal Pulse

Premature contractions

This disorder of rhythm may mimic pulsus alternans. A bigeminal pulse is caused by a normal beat alternating with a premature contraction. The stroke volume of the premature beat is diminished in relation to that of the normal beats, and the pulse varies in amplitude accordingly.

Paradoxical Pulse

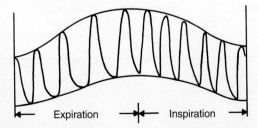

Expiration   Inspiration

A paradoxical pulse may be detected by a palpable decrease in the pulse's amplitude on quiet inspiration. If the sign is less pronounced, a blood pressure cuff is needed. Systolic pressure decreases by more than 10 mm Hg during inspiration. A paradoxical pulse is found in pericardial tamponade, constrictive pericarditis (though less commonly), and obstructive lung disease.

TABLE 9-4

Variations and Abnormalities of the Ventricular Impulses

In the healthy heart, the *left ventricular impulse* is usually the *point of maximal impulse,* or *PMI.* This brief impulse is generated by the movement of the ventricular apex against the chest wall during contraction. The *right ventricular impulse* is normally not palpable beyond infancy, and its characteristics are indeterminate. In contrast, learn the classical descriptors of the left ventricular PMI:

- *Location:* in the 4th or 5th interspace, ~7–10 cm lateral to the midsternal line, depending on the diameter of the chest
- *Diameter: discrete,* or ≤2 cm
- *Amplitude: brisk* and *tapping*
- *Duration:* ≤2/3 of systole

Careful examination of the ventricular impulse gives you important clues about underlying cardiovascular hemodynamics. The quality of the ventricular impulse changes as the left and right ventricles adapt to high-output states (anxiety, hyperthyroidism, and severe anemia) and to the more pathologic conditions of chronic pressure or volume overload. Note below the distinguishing features of three types of ventricular impulses: the *hyperkinetic ventricular impulse* from transiently increased stroke volume—this change does not necessarily indicate heart disease; the *sustained* ventricular impulse of ventricular hypertrophy from chronic pressure load, known as *increased afterload* (see p. 359); and the *diffuse* ventricular impulse of ventricular dilation from chronic volume overload, or *increased preload.*

	Left Ventricular Impulse			Right Ventricular Impulse		
	Hyperkinetic	Pressure Overload	Volume Overload	Hyperkinetic	Pressure Overload	Volume Overload
Examples of Causes	Anxiety, hyperthyroidism, severe anemia	Aortic stenosis, hypertension	Aortic or mitral regurgitation	Anxiety, hyperthyroidism, severe anemia	Pulmonic stenosis, pulmonary hypertension	Atrial septal defect
Location	Normal	Normal	Displaced to the left and possibly downward	3rd, 4th, or 5th left interspaces	3rd, 4th, or 5th left interspaces, also subxiphoid	Left sternal border, extending toward the left cardiac border, also subxiphoid
Diameter	~2 cm, though increased amplitude may make it seem larger	>2 cm	>2 cm	Not useful	Not useful	Not useful
Amplitude	More forceful tapping	More forceful tapping	*Diffuse*	Slightly more forceful	More forceful	Slightly to markedly more forceful
Duration	<2/3 systole	*Sustained* (up to S_2)	Often slightly sustained	Normal	Sustained	Normal to slightly sustained

TABLE 9-5

Variations in the First Heart Sound—S_1

Normal Variations	S_1 S_2	S_1 is softer than S_2 at the *base* (right and left 2nd interspaces).
	S_1 S_2	S_1 is often but not always louder than S_2 at the *apex*.
Accentuated S_1	S_1 S_2	S_1 is accentuated in (1) tachycardia, rhythms with a short PR interval, and high cardiac output states (e.g., exercise, anemia, hyperthyroidism) and (2) mitral stenosis. In these conditions, the mitral valve is still open wide at the onset of ventricular systole and then closes quickly.
Diminished S_1	S_1 S_2	S_1 is diminished in first-degree heart block (delayed conduction from atria to ventricles). Here the mitral valve has had time after atrial contraction to float back into an almost closed position before ventricular contraction shuts it. It closes more quietly. S_1 is also diminished (1) when the mitral valve is calcified and relatively immobile, as in mitral regurgitation and (2) when left ventricular contractility is markedly reduced, as in congestive heart failure or coronary heart disease.
Varying S_1	S_1 S_2 S_1 S_2	S_1 varies in intensity (1) in complete heart block, when atria and ventricles are beating independently of each other and (2) in any totally irregular rhythm (e.g., atrial fibrillation). In these situations, the mitral valve is in varying positions before being shut by ventricular contraction. Its closure sound, therefore, varies in loudness.
Split S_1	S_1 S_2	S_1 may be split normally along the lower left sternal border where the tricuspid component, often too faint to be heard, becomes audible. This split may sometimes be heard at the apex, but consider also an S_4, an aortic ejection sound, and an early systolic click. Abnormal splitting of both heart sounds may be heard in right bundle branch block and in premature ventricular contractions.

Variations in the Second Heart Sound—S_2

	Inspiration	Expiration	

Physiologic Splitting

Listen for *physiologic splitting* of S_2 in the *2nd or 3rd left interspace*. The pulmonic component of S_2 is usually too faint to be heard at the apex or aortic area, where S_2 is a single sound derived from aortic valve closure alone. Normal splitting is *accentuated by inspiration* and usually *disappears on expiration*. In some patients, especially younger ones, S_2 may not become single on expiration. It may merge when the patient sits up.

Pathologic Splitting
(involves splitting during expiration and suggests heart disease)

Wide splitting of S_2 refers to an increase in the usual splitting that persists throughout the respiratory cycle. Wide splitting can be caused by delayed closure of the pulmonic valve (as in pulmonic stenosis or right bundle branch block). As illustrated here, right bundle branch block also causes splitting of S_1 into its mitral and tricuspid components. Wide splitting can also be caused by early closure of the aortic valve, as in mitral regurgitation.

Fixed splitting refers to wide splitting that does not vary with respiration. It occurs in atrial septal defect and right ventricular failure.

Paradoxical or reversed splitting refers to splitting that appears on expiration and disappears on inspiration. Closure of the aortic valve is abnormally delayed so that A_2 follows P_2 in expiration. Normal inspiratory delay of P_2 makes the split disappear. The most common cause of paradoxical splitting is left bundle branch block.

Increased Intensity of A_2 in the Right Second Interspace (where only A_2 can usually be heard) occurs in systemic hypertension because of the increased pressure load. It also occurs when the aortic root is dilated, probably because the aortic valve is then closer to the chest wall.

Decreased or Absent A_2 in the Right Second Interspace is noted in calcific aortic stenosis because of valve immobility. If A_2 is inaudible, no splitting is heard.

Increased Intensity of P_2. When P_2 is equal to or louder than A_2, suspect pulmonary hypertension. Other causes include a dilated pulmonary artery and an atrial septal defect. When a split S_2 is heard widely, even at the apex and the right base, P_2 is accentuated.

Decreased or Absent P_2 is usually from the increased anteroposterior diameter of the chest associated with aging. It can also result from pulmonic stenosis. If P_2 is inaudible, no splitting is heard.

TABLE
9-7

Extra Heart Sounds in Systole

There are two kinds of extra heart sounds in systole: (1) early ejection sounds and (2) clicks, commonly heard in mid- and late systole.

Early Systolic Ejection Sounds

S_1 E_j S_2

Early systolic ejection sounds occur shortly after S_1, coincident with opening of the aortic and pulmonic valves. They are relatively high in pitch, have a sharp, clicking quality, and are heard better with the diaphragm of the stethoscope. An ejection sound indicates cardiovascular disease.

Listen for an *aortic ejection sound* at both the base and apex. It may be louder at the apex and usually does not vary with respiration. An aortic ejection sound may accompany a dilated aorta, or aortic valve disease from congenital stenosis or a bicuspid valve.

A *pulmonic ejection sound* is heard best in the 2nd and 3rd left interspaces. When S_1, usually relatively soft in this area, appears to be loud, you may be hearing a pulmonic ejection sound. Its intensity often *decreases with inspiration*. Causes include dilatation of the pulmonary artery, pulmonary hypertension, and pulmonic stenosis.

Systolic Clicks

S_1 C_1 S_2

Systolic clicks are usually caused by *mitral valve prolapse*—an abnormal systolic ballooning of part of the mitral valve into the left atrium. The clicks are usually mid- or late systolic. Prolapse of the mitral valve is a common cardiac condition, affecting about 5% of the general population. There is equal prevalence in men and women.

The click is usually single, but you may hear more than one, usually *at or medial to the apex*, but also *at the lower left sternal border*. It is high-pitched, so listen with the diaphragm. The click is often followed by a late systolic murmur from mitral regurgitation—a flow of blood from left ventricle to left atrium. The murmur usually crescendos up to S_2. Auscultatory findings are notably variable. Most patients have only a click, some have only a murmur, and some have both. Systolic clicks may also be of extracardial or mediastinal origin.

Squatting

S_1 C_1 S_2

Standing

S_1 C_1 S_2

Findings vary from time to time and often change with body position. Several positions are recommended to identify the syndrome: supine, seated, squatting, and standing. *Squatting delays the click and murmur; standing moves them closer to S_1.*

Extra Heart Sounds in Diastole

Opening Snap

S_1 S_2 OS S_1

The *opening snap* is a very early diastolic sound usually produced by the opening of a *stenotic mitral valve*. It is heard best just medial to the apex and along the lower left sternal border. When it is loud, an opening snap radiates to the apex and to the pulmonic area, where it may be mistaken for the pulmonic component of a split S_2. Its high pitch and snapping quality help to distinguish it from an S_2. It is heard better with the *diaphragm*.

S_3

S_1 S_2 S_3 S_1

You will detect *physiologic* S_3 frequently in children and in young adults to the age of 35 or 40. It is common during the last trimester of pregnancy. Occurring early in diastole during rapid ventricular filling, it is later than an opening snap, dull and low in pitch, and heard best at the apex in the left lateral decubitus position. The *bell* of the stethoscope should be used with very light pressure.

A *pathologic* S_3 or *ventricular gallop* sounds just like a physiologic S_3. An S_3 in a person over age 40 (possibly a little older in women) is almost certainly pathologic, arising from altered left ventricular compliance at the end of the rapid filling phase of diastole.[62] Causes include decreased myocardial contractility, congestive heart failure, and volume overloading of a ventricle, as in mitral or tricuspid regurgitation. A *left-sided* S_3 is heard typically at the apex in the left lateral decubitus position. A *right-sided* S_3 is usually heard along the lower left sternal border or below the xiphoid with the patient supine, and is louder on inspiration. The term *gallop* comes from the cadence of three heart sounds, especially at rapid heart rates, and sounds like "Kentucky."

S_4

S_1 S_2 S_4 S_1

An S_4 (*atrial sound* or *atrial gallop*) occurs just before S_1. It is dull, low in pitch, and heard better with the bell. An S_4 is heard occasionally in an apparently normal person, especially in trained athletes and older age groups. More commonly, it is due to increased resistance to ventricular filling following atrial contraction. This increased resistance is related to decreased compliance (increased stiffness) of the ventricular myocardium.[63]

Causes of a left-sided S_4 include hypertensive heart disease, coronary artery disease, aortic stenosis, and cardiomyopathy. A *left-sided* S_4 is heard best at the apex in the left lateral position; it may sound like "Tennessee." The less common *right-sided* S_4 is heard along the lower left sternal border or below the xiphoid. It often gets louder with inspiration. Causes of a right-sided S_4 include pulmonary hypertension and pulmonic stenosis.

An S_4 may also be associated with delayed conduction between the atria and ventricles. This delay separates the normally faint atrial sound from the louder S_1 and makes it audible. An S_4 is never heard in the absence of atrial contraction, which occurs with atrial fibrillation.

Occasionally, a patient has both an S_3 and an S_4, producing a *quadruple rhythm* of four heart sounds. At rapid heart rates, the S_3 and S_4 may merge into one loud extra heart sound, called a *summation gallop*.

TABLE
9-9

Pansystolic (Holosystolic) Murmurs

Pansystolic (holosystolic) murmurs are pathologic, arising from blood flow from a chamber with high pressure to one of lower pressure, through a valve or other structure that should be closed. The murmur begins immediately with S_1 and continues up to S_2.

	Mitral Regurgitation[64,65]	Tricuspid Regurgitation	Ventricular Septal Defect
	Decreased ↓ S_1 ‖‖‖ S_2 S_3	S_1 ‖‖‖ S_2 S_3	S_1 ‖‖‖ S_2
Murmur	*Location.* Apex	*Location.* Lower left sternal border	*Location.* 3rd, 4th, and 5th left interspaces
	Radiation. To the left axilla, less often to the left sternal border	*Radiation.* To the right of the sternum, to the xiphoid area, and perhaps to the left midclavicular line, but not into the axilla	*Radiation.* Often wide
	Intensity. Soft to loud; if loud, associated with an apical thrill	*Intensity.* Variable	*Intensity.* Often very loud, with a thrill
	Pitch. Medium to high	*Pitch.* Medium	*Pitch.* High, holosystolic
	Quality. Harsh, holosystolic	*Quality.* Blowing, holosystolic	*Quality.* Often harsh
	Aids. Unlike tricuspid regurgitation, it does not become louder in inspiration.	*Aids.* Unlike mitral regurgitation, the intensity may increase slightly with inspiration.	
Associated Findings	S_1 normal (75%), loud (12%), soft (12%) An apical S_3 reflects volume overload of the left ventricle. The apical impulse is increased in amplitude (diffuse), laterally displaced, and may be sustained.	The right ventricular impulse is increased in amplitude and may be sustained. An S_3 may be audible along the lower left sternal border. The jugular venous pressure is often elevated, with large *v* waves in the jugular veins.	S_2 may be obscured by the loud murmur. Findings vary with the severity of the defect and with associated lesions.
Mechanism	When the *mitral valve fails to close fully in systole,* blood regurgitates from left ventricle to left atrium, causing a murmur. This leakage creates volume overload on the left ventricle, with subsequent dilatation. Several structural abnormalities cause this condition, and findings may vary accordingly.	When the *tricuspid valve fails to close fully in systole,* blood regurgitates from right ventricle to right atrium, producing a murmur. The most common cause is right ventricular failure and dilatation, with resulting enlargement of the tricuspid orifice. Either pulmonary hypertension or left ventricular failure is the usual initiating cause.	A ventricular septal defect is a congenital abnormality in which *blood flows from the relatively high-pressure left ventricle into the low-pressure right ventricle through a hole.* The defect may be accompanied by other abnormalities, but an uncomplicated lesion is described here.

TABLE
9-10

Midsystolic Murmurs

Midsystolic ejection murmurs are the most common kind of heart murmur. They may be (1) *innocent*—without any detectable physiologic or structural abnormality; (2) *physiologic*—from physiologic changes in body metabolism; or (3) *pathologic*—arising from a structural abnormality in the heart or great vessels.[57,66] Midsystolic murmurs tend to peak near midsystole and usually stop before S_2. The crescendo–decrescendo or "diamond" shape is not always audible, but the gap between the murmur and S_2 helps to distinguish midsystolic from pansystolic murmurs.

	Innocent Murmurs	**Physiologic Murmurs**
Murmur	*Location.* 2nd to 4th left interspaces between the left sternal border and the apex *Radiation.* Little *Intensity.* Grade 1 to 2, possibly 3 *Pitch.* Soft to medium *Quality.* Variable *Aids.* Usually decreases or disappears on sitting	Similar to innocent murmurs
Associated Findings	None: normal splitting, no ejection sounds, no diastolic murmurs, and no palpable evidence of ventricular enlargement. Occasionally, both an innocent murmur and another kind of murmur are present.	Possible signs of a likely cause
Mechanism	Innocent murmurs result from turbulent blood flow, probably generated by ventricular ejection of blood into the aorta from the left and occasionally the right ventricle. Very common in children and young adults—may also be heard in older people. There is no underlying cardiovascular disease.	Turbulence due to a temporary increase in blood flow in predisposing conditions such as anemia, pregnancy, fever, and hyperthyroidism.

Pathologic Murmurs

Aortic Stenosis[67,68]	Hypertrophic Cardiomyopathy	Pulmonic Stenosis

Location. Right 2nd interspace

Radiation. Often to the carotids, down the left sternal border, even to the apex

Intensity. Sometimes soft but often loud, with a thrill

Pitch. Medium, harsh; crescendo–decrescendo may be higher at the apex

Quality. Often harsh; may be more musical at the apex

Aids. Heard best with the patient sitting and leaning forward

A$_2$ decreases as aortic stenosis worsens. A$_2$ may be delayed and merge with P$_2$ → single S$_2$ on expiration or paradoxical S$_2$ split. Carotid upstroke may be *delayed,* with slow rise and small amplitude. Hypertrophied left ventricle may → *sustained* apical impulse and an S$_4$ from decreased compliance.

Significant aortic valve stenosis impairs blood flow across the valve, causing turbulence, and increases left ventricular afterload. Causes are congenital, rheumatic, and degenerative; findings may differ with each cause. Other conditions mimic aortic stenosis without obstructing flow: *aortic sclerosis,* a stiffening of aortic valve leaflets associated with aging; a *bicuspid aortic valve,* a congenital condition that may not be recognized until adulthood; *a dilated aorta,* as in arteriosclerosis, syphilis, or Marfan's syndrome; *pathologically increased flow across the aortic valve* during systole can accompany aortic regurgitation.

Location. 3rd and 4th left interspaces

Radiation. Down the left sternal border to the apex, possibly to the base, but not to the neck

Intensity. Variable

Pitch. Medium

Quality. Harsh

Aids. Decreases with squatting, increases with straining down from Valsalva and standing

S$_3$ may be present. An S$_4$ is often present at the apex (unlike mitral regurgitation). The apical impulse may be *sustained* and have two palpable components. The carotid pulse rises *quickly,* unlike the pulse in aortic stenosis.

Massive ventricular hypertrophy is associated with unusually rapid ejection of blood from the left ventricle during systole. Outflow tract obstruction of flow may coexist. Accompanying distortion of the mitral valve may cause mitral regurgitation.

Location. 2nd and 3rd left interspaces

Radiation. If loud, toward the left shoulder and neck

Intensity. Soft to loud; if loud, associated with a thrill

Pitch. Medium; crescendo–decrescendo

Quality. Often harsh

In severe stenosis, S$_2$ is widely split, and P$_2$ is diminished or inaudible. An early pulmonic ejection sound is common. May hear a right-sided S$_4$. Right ventricular impulse often increased in amplitude and *sustained.*

Pulmonic valve stenosis impairs flow across the valve, increasing right ventricular afterload. Congenital and usually found in children. In an *atrial septal defect,* the systolic murmur from pathologically increased flow across the pulmonic valve may mimic pulmonic stenosis.

TABLE
9-11

Diastolic Murmurs

Diastolic murmurs almost always indicate heart disease. There are two basic types. *Early decrescendo diastolic murmurs* signify regurgitant flow through an incompetent semilunar valve, more commonly the aortic. *Rumbling diastolic murmurs in mid- or late diastole* suggest stenosis of an atrioventricular valve, usually the mitral.

	Aortic Regurgitation[69]	**Mitral Stenosis**

Murmur

Aortic Regurgitation[69]	**Mitral Stenosis**
Location. 2nd to 4th left interspaces	*Location.* Usually limited to the apex
Radiation. If loud, to the apex, perhaps to the right sternal border	*Radiation.* Little or none
Intensity. Grade 1 to 3	*Intensity.* Grade 1 to 4
Pitch. High. *Use the diaphragm.*	*Pitch.* Decrescendo low-pitched rumble. *Use the bell.*
Quality. Blowing decrescendo; may be mistaken for breath sounds	
Aids. The murmur is heard best with the *patient sitting, leaning forward*, with breath held after exhalation.	*Aids.* Placing the bell exactly on the apical impulse, turning the patient into a *left lateral position*, and mild exercise all help to make the murmur audible. It is heard better in exhalation.

Associated Findings

An ejection sound may be present.	S_1 is accentuated and may be palpable at the apex.
An S_3 or S_4, if present, suggests severe regurgitation.	An opening snap (OS) often follows S_2 and initiates the murmur.
Progressive changes in the apical impulse include increased amplitude, displacement laterally and downward, widened diameter, and increased duration.	If pulmonary hypertension develops, P_2 is accentuated, and the right ventricular impulse becomes palpable.
The pulse pressure increases, and *arterial pulses are often large and bounding.* A midsystolic flow murmur or an Austin Flint murmur suggests large regurgitant flow.	Mitral regurgitation and aortic valve disease may be associated with mitral stenosis.

Mechanism

The leaflets of the aortic valve fail to close completely during diastole, and blood regurgitates from the aorta back into the left ventricle. Volume overload on the left ventricle results. Two other murmurs may be associated: (1) a midsystolic murmur from the resulting increased forward flow across the aortic valve and (2) a mitral diastolic (*Austin Flint*) murmur, attributed to diastolic impingement of the regurgitant flow on the anterior leaflet of the mitral valve.	When the leaflets of the mitral valve thicken, stiffen, and become distorted from the effects of rheumatic fever, the *mitral valve fails to open sufficiently in diastole.* The resulting murmur has two components: (1) middiastolic (during rapid ventricular filling) and (2) presystolic (during atrial contraction). The latter disappears if atrial fibrillation develops, leaving only a middiastolic rumble.

Cardiovascular Sounds With Both Systolic and Diastolic Components

Some cardiovascular sounds extend beyond one phase of the cardiac cycle. Three examples, further described below, are: (1) a *venous hum*, a benign sound produced by turbulence of blood in the jugular veins—common in children; (2) a *pericardial friction rub*, produced by inflammation of the pericardial sac; and (3) *patent ductus arteriosus*, a congenital abnormality in which an open channel persists between the aorta and pulmonary artery. *Continuous murmurs* begin in systole and extend through S_2 into all or part of diastole, as in *patent ductus arteriosus*.

	Venous Hum	**Pericardial Friction Rub**	**Patent Ductus Arteriosus**
Timing	Continuous murmur without a silent interval. Loudest in diastole	May have three short components, each associated with friction from cardiac movement in the pericardial sac: (1) atrial systole, (2) ventricular systole, and (3) ventricular diastole. Usually the first two components are present; all three make diagnosis easy; only one (usually the systolic) invites confusion with a murmur.	Continuous murmur in both systole and diastole, often with a silent interval late in diastole. Loudest in late systole, obscures S_2, and fades in diastole
Location	Above the medial third of the clavicles, especially on the right	Variable, but usually heard best in the 3rd interspace to the left of the sternum	Left 2nd interspace
Radiation	1st and 2nd interspaces	Little	Toward the left clavicle
Intensity	Soft to moderate. Can be obliterated by pressure on the jugular veins	Variable. May increase when the patient leans forward, exhales, and holds breath (in contrast to pleural rub)	Usually loud, sometimes associated with a thrill
Quality	Humming, roaring	Scratchy, scraping	Harsh, machinery-like
Pitch	Low (heard better with the *bell*)	High (heard better with the *diaphragm*)	Medium

The Breasts and Axillae

THE FEMALE BREAST

The female breast lies against the anterior thoracic wall, extending from the clavicle and 2nd rib down to the 6th rib, and from the sternum across to the midaxillary line. Its surface area is generally rectangular rather than round.

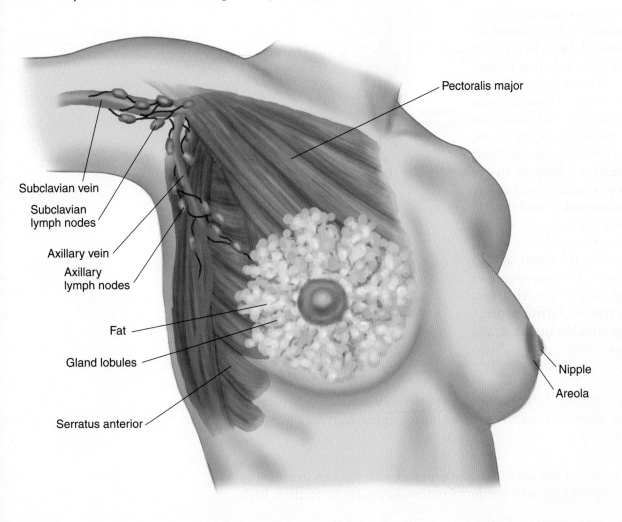

Pectoralis major

Subclavian vein

Subclavian
lymph nodes

Axillary vein

Axillary
lymph nodes

Fat

Gland lobules

Serratus anterior

Nipple

Areola

The breast overlies the pectoralis major and, at its inferior margin, the serratus anterior.

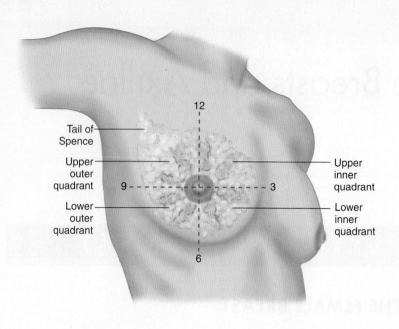

To describe clinical findings, the breast is often divided into four quadrants based on horizontal and vertical lines crossing at the nipple. An axillary tail of breast tissue, sometimes termed the "tail of Spence," extends laterally across the anterior axillary fold. Alternatively, findings can be localized as the time on the face of a clock (e.g., 3 o'clock) and the distance in centimeters from the nipple.

The breast is hormonally sensitive tissue, responsive to the changes of monthly cycling and aging. *Glandular tissue*, namely secretory tubuloalveolar glands and ducts, forms 15 to 20 septated *lobes* radiating around the nipple. Within each lobe are many smaller *lobules*. These drain into milk-producing ducts and sinuses that open onto the surface of the *areola*, or nipple. *Fibrous connective tissue* provides structural support in the form of fibrous bands or suspensory ligaments connected to both the skin and the underlying fascia. *Adipose tissue*, or fat, surrounds the breast, predominantly in the superficial and peripheral areas. The proportions of these components vary with age, the general state of nutrition, pregnancy, exogenous hormone use, and other factors.

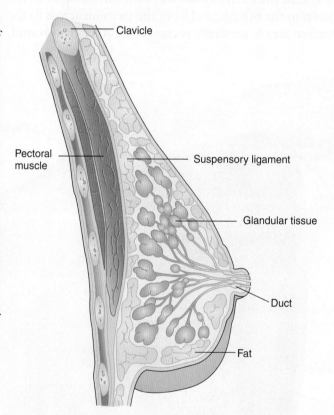

The surface of the areola has small, rounded elevations formed by sebaceous glands, sweat glands, and accessory areolar glands. A few hairs are often seen on the areola.

Both the nipple and the areola are well supplied with smooth muscle that contracts to express milk from the ductal system during breast-feeding. Rich sensory innervation, especially in the nipple, triggers "milk letdown" following neurohormonal stimulation from infant sucking. Tactile stimulation of the area, including the breast examination, makes the nipple smaller, firmer, and more erect, whereas the areola puckers and wrinkles. These smooth muscle reflexes are normal and should not be mistaken for signs of breast disease.

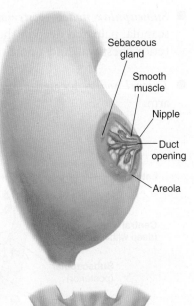

The adult breast may be soft, but it often feels granular, nodular, or lumpy. This uneven texture is normal and may be termed *physiologic nodularity*. It is often bilateral. It may be evident throughout the breast or only in parts of it. The nodularity may increase before menses—a time when breasts often enlarge and become tender or even painful. For breast changes during adolescence and pregnancy, see pp. 841–842 and p. 882.

Occasionally, one or more extra or supernumerary nipples are located along the "milk line," illustrated on the right. Only a small nipple and areola are usually present, often mistaken for a common mole. There may be underlying glandular tissue. An extra nipple has no pathologic significance.

 ## THE MALE BREAST

The male breast consists chiefly of a small nipple and areola. These overlie a thin disc of undeveloped breast tissue consisting primarily of ducts. Lacking estrogen and progesterone stimulation, ductal branching and development of lobules are minimal.[1] It may be difficult to distinguish male breast tissue from the surrounding muscles of the chest wall. A firm button of breast tissue 2 cm or more in diameter has been described in roughly one of three adult men.

 ## LYMPHATICS

Lymphatics from most of the breast drain toward the axilla. Of the axillary lymph nodes, the *central nodes* are palpable most frequently. They lie along the chest wall, usually high in the axilla and midway between the anterior and posterior axillary folds. Into them drain channels from three other groups of lymph nodes, which are seldom palpable:

- *Pectoral nodes—anterior,* located along the lower border of the pectoralis major inside the anterior axillary fold. These nodes drain the anterior chest wall and much of the breast.

- *Subscapular nodes—posterior,* located along the lateral border of the scapula; palpated deep in the posterior axillary fold. They drain the posterior chest wall and a portion of the arm.

- *Lateral nodes—*located *along the upper humerus.* They drain most of the arm.

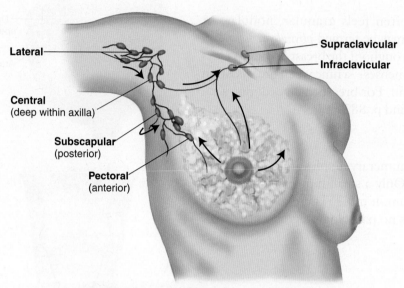

Lateral

Supraclavicular

Infraclavicular

Central
(deep within axilla)

Subscapular
(posterior)

Pectoral
(anterior)

ARROWS INDICATE DIRECTION OF LYMPH FLOW

Lymph drains from the central axillary nodes to the *infraclavicular* and *supraclavicular* nodes.

Not all the lymphatics of the breast drain into the axilla. Malignant cells from a breast cancer may spread directly to the infraclavicular nodes or into deep channels within the chest.

THE HEALTH HISTORY

Common or Concerning Symptoms

- Breast lump or mass
- Breast pain or discomfort
- Nipple discharge

Questions about a woman's breasts may be included in the history or deferred to the physical examination. Ask "Do you examine your breasts?" . . . "How often?" For a menstruating woman, ask when she examines her breast during her monthly cycle: self-examination is best done when estrogen stimulation is lowest, approximately 5 to 7 days after onset of menses. Ask whether she has any *discomfort, pain,* or *lumps* in her breasts. About 50% of women have palpable lumps or nodularity, and premenstrual enlargement and ten-

Lumps may be physiologic or pathologic, ranging from cysts and fibroadenomas to breast cancer. See Table 10-1, Common Breast Masses (p. 413), and Table 10-2, Visible Signs of Breast Cancer (p. 414).

derness are common.[2] If your patient reports a lump or mass, ask about the precise location, how long it has been present, and any change in size or variation with the menstrual cycle. Ask about any change in breast contour, dimpling, swelling, or puckering of the skin over the breasts.

Ask about any *discharge from the nipples* and when it occurs. Does the discharge appear only after compression of the nipple, or is it spontaneous? Physiologic hypersecretion is seen in pregnancy, lactation, chest wall stimulation, sleep, and stress. If spontaneous, what is the color, consistency, and quantity? Is the color milky, brown or greenish, or bloody? Ask if the discharge is unilateral or bilateral.

Galactorrhea, or the inappropriate discharge of milk-containing fluid, is abnormal if it occurs 6 or more months after childbirth or cessation of breast-feeding.

HEALTH PROMOTION AND COUNSELING

Important Topics for Health Promotion and Counseling

- Palpable masses of the breast
- Assessing risk of breast cancer
- Breast cancer screening

Overview

Women may experience a wide range of changes in breast tissue and sensation, from cyclic swelling and nodularity to a distinct lump or mass. The examination of the breast provides a meaningful opportunity for the clinician to explore concerns important to women's health—what to do if a lump or mass is detected, risk factors for breast cancer, and screening measures such as breast self-examination, the clinical breast examination (CBE) by a skilled clinician, and mammography. Women will frequently seek information during the clinical encounter.

Palpable Masses of the Breast and Breast Symptoms. Breast cancer occurs in up to 4% of women with breast complaints, in approximately 5% of women reporting a nipple discharge, and in up to 11% of women specifically complaining of a breast lump or mass.[1,2] Breast masses show marked variation in etiology, from fibroadenomas and cysts seen in younger women, to abscess or mastitis, to primary breast cancer. On initial assessment, the woman's age and physical characteristics of the mass provide clues about its etiology, as shown in the next table on Palpable Masses of the Breast, but definitive diagnosis should be pursued. All breast masses require careful assessment.

Assessing Risk of Breast Cancer. Women are increasingly interested in information about breast cancer. Clinicians are urged to be familiar with the literature detailing the epidemiology of and risk factors for breast cancer that supports recommendations for screening. Key facts and figures are presented here, but further reading will enhance your counseling of female patients.

● Palpable Masses of the Breast

Age	Common Lesion	Characteristics
15–25	Fibroadenoma	Usually fine, round, mobile, nontender
25–50	Cysts	Usually soft to firm, round, mobile; often tender
	Fibrocystic changes	Nodular, ropelike
	Cancer	Irregular, stellate, firm, not clearly delineated from surrounding tissue
Over 50	Cancer until proven otherwise	As above
Pregnancy/lactation	Lactating adenomas, cysts, mastitis, and cancer	As above

Adapted from Schultz MZ, Ward BA, Reiss M. Breast diseases. In Noble J, Greene HL, Levinson W, et al. (eds). Primary Care Medicine, 2nd ed. St. Louis, Mosby, 1996. See also Venet L, Strax P, Venet W, et al. Adequacies and inadequacies of breast examinations by physicians in mass screenings. Cancer 28(6):1546–1551, 1971.

Breast Cancer Facts and Figures.   Breast cancer is the most common cause of cancer in women worldwide, accounting for more than 10% of cancers in women. In the United States a woman born now has a 12%, or 1 in 8, lifetime risk of developing breast cancer.[3] The probability of diagnosis over the next 10 years increases by decade.[4]

● Age-Specific Probabilities of Developing Invasive Breast Cancer*

If Current Age is:	The Probability of Developing Breast Cancer in the Next 10 Years is:	or 1 in:
20	0.05%	1,837
30	0.43%	234
40	1.43%	70
50	2.51%	40
60	3.51%	28
70	3.88%	26
Lifetime risk	12.28%	8

*Among those free of cancer at beginning of age interval. Based on cases diagnosed 2002–2004. Percentages and "1 in" numbers may not be numerically equivalent due to rounding.

(Source: American Cancer Society. Breast Cancer Facts and Figures 2007–2008, p. 11. Available at: http://www.cancer.org/downloads/STT/BCFF-Final.pdf. Accessed October 20, 2007.)

Breast cancer is the second leading cause of cancer death in women, with highest mortality rates in women 35 years or younger and older than 75 years. There are several trends of note.[3]

- *Declines in new cases of invasive breast cancer.* The number of new cases of invasive breast cancer has been falling since 2000, explained by two main factors: decreased mammography screening, which leads to under-diagnosis or delayed diagnosis rather than a true decrease in disease incidence; and decreased use of hormone replacement therapy (HRT).[5]

- *Earlier and more advanced breast cancer in African-American women.* African-American women have a higher incidence of breast cancer before 40 years, are more likely to be diagnosed with larger tumors, and are more likely to die from breast cancer at every age. The disparity between death rates for white and African-American women has been increasing since 1980. In 2004 the breast cancer death rate was 36% higher for African-American women compared with white women. Analysis of stage-specific survival rates controlling for estrogen-receptor status shows that African-American women have less early-stage disease in every age group except those older than 65 years, suggesting that Medicare may level access to care and treatment. Clinicians should consider offering pertinent information and screening mammograms to African-American women at earlier ages. Insurance coverage should address costs of earlier care and screening.[6] Offering African-American women mammograms beginning at 40 years risks detection of only 83.6% of breast cancers, compared with 93.3% for white women.[7]

Assessing Risk Factors for Breast Cancer. Both *modifiable* and *non-modifiable risk factors* for breast cancer have been identified, as listed in the table on p. 396. Many risk factors cannot be readily altered, such as age, family history, age at first full-term pregnancy, early menarche, late menopause, and breast density.[3] Others can be modified, although these tend to confer lower relative risk: postmenopausal obesity, use of HRT, alcohol use, and physical inactivity. Of note, breast-feeding decreases risk, especially with longer duration. Use of contraceptives slightly increases risk. A stronger risk factor is use of estrogen-progesterone combination HRT. The table on the next page from the American Cancer Society report "Breast Cancer Facts and Figures 2007–2008,"[3] summarizes the strengths of current risk factors. Readers are encouraged to review the excellent discussions of individual risk factors presented in this report.

Establishing Patient Risk of Breast Cancer. After taking a detailed history and thoroughly examining the breast, clinicians should assess breast cancer risk by looking at probability by decade (see p. 394), and/or using the computerized Breast Cancer Risk Assessment Tool (often called the Gail model)[8,9] (see http://brca.nci.nih./gov/brc/start/htm).

This tool incorporates risk factors of age, first-degree relatives with breast cancer, previous breast biopsies and presence of hyperplasia (see p. 397), age

● Breast Cancer in Women: Factors that Increase Relative Risk

Relative Risk	Factor
>4.0	<ul><li>Female</li><li>Age (65+ versus <65 years, although risk increases across all ages until age 80)</li><li>Certain inherited genetic mutations for breast cancer (BRCA1 and/or BRCA2)</li><li>Two or more first-degree relatives with breast cancer diagnosed at an early age</li><li>Personal history of breast cancer</li><li>High breast tissue density</li><li>Biopsy-confirmed atypical hyperplasia</li></ul>
2.1–4.0	<ul><li>One first-degree relative with breast cancer</li><li>High-dose radiation to chest</li><li>High bone density (postmenopausal)</li></ul>
1.1–2.0 Factors that affect circulating hormones	<ul><li>Late age at first full-term pregnancy (>30 years)</li><li>Early menarche (<12 years)</li><li>Late menopause (>55 years)</li><li>No full-term pregnancies</li><li>Never breast-fed a child</li><li>Recent oral contraceptive use</li><li>Recent and long-term use of hormone replacement therapy</li><li>Obesity (postmenopausal)</li></ul>
Other factors	<ul><li>Personal history of endometrium, ovary, or colon cancer</li><li>Alcohol consumption</li><li>Height (tall)</li><li>High socioeconomic status</li><li>Jewish heritage</li></ul>

Adapted with permission from Hulka et al. 2001.

(Source: American Cancer Society. Breast Cancer Facts and Figures 2007–2008, p. 10. Available at: http://www.cancer.org/downloads/STT/BCFF-Final.pdf. Accessed October 20, 2007.)

at menarche, and age at first delivery. It assumes annual screening and no patient history of breast cancer. For women with a family history of second-degree maternal or paternal relatives with breast cancer, the Claus model can be used.[10] Neither the Gail or Claus models include such risk factors as breast density, plasma levels of free estradiol, bone density, post-menopausal weight gain, or waist-to-hip ratio. The Gail model accurately predicts the number of breast cancer cases expected in a given population, but it is less accurate in predicting whether an individual woman will be affected (see http://astor.jhmi.edu/brcapro).[11, 12]

Selected Risk Factors that Affect Screening Decisions

BRCA1 and 2 Mutations. It is important to begin evaluating a woman's risk for breast cancer even in her 20s. Women of all ages should be asked if there is a family history of breast or ovarian cancer, or both, on both the maternal and paternal sides. Approximately 5% to 10% of women have genetic risk of BRCA1 or BRCA2 gene mutation. These genes are autosomal dominant. Women with BRCA1 mutations and BRCA2 mutations have an estimated 65% and 45% risk of developing breast cancer by age 70 respectively.[3] To identify women who should be referred for possible genetic testing, two strategies are recommended, detailed in the table below.[13]

CRITERIA FOR IDENTIFYING WOMEN AT RISK FOR BRCA1 OR 2 MUTATION

- Using the risk calculator at http://astor.som.jhmi.edu/brcapro/, determine that the risk for a BRCA1 or 2 mutation is at least 10%

- Establish one of the following risk factors:

  - First-degree relative with a known BRCA1 or 2 mutation

  - ≥2 relatives with a diagnosis of breast cancer before age 50, and ≥1 is a first-degree relative

  - ≥3 relatives with a diagnosis of breast cancer, and ≥1 occurred before age 50

  - ≥2 relatives with a diagnosis of ovarian cancer

  - ≥1 relative with a diagnosis of breast cancer, and ≥1 relative has a diagnosis of ovarian cancer

(Source: Fletcher SW, Elmore JG. Mammographic screening for breast cancer. N Engl J Med 348[14]:1672–1680, 2003.)

Benign Breast Disorders. Mammograms are resulting in increasing numbers of breast biopsies, and clinicians should now understand the effects of benign breast disease on risk for later breast cancer.[1,14] Within a decade of starting annual screening, 20% of women have had a breast biopsy.[15] Breast lesions are believed to evolve in somewhat linear fashion from usual ductal hyperplasia, or unfolded lobules, to atypical hyperplasia, to the pathologic stages of ductal carcinoma in situ (DCIS) and invasive cancer. These disorders are now classified by degree of cellular proliferation on biopsy and degree of risk for breast cancer. Women with atypia are more likely to have strong family history of breast cancer (approximately 28% vs 20%). Their risk increases when atypia is diagnosed at younger ages. Currently studies show no increased risk for women with nonproliferative findings and no family history of breast cancer.

● Risk of Breast Cancer and Histology of Benign Breast Lesions[1,14]

- *No increased risk,* relative risk approx. 1.3

  Nonproliferative changes: including cysts and ductal ectasia, mild hyperplasia, simple fibroadenoma, mastitis, granuloma, diabetic mastopathy

- *Small increased risk,* or relative risk 1.5–2.0

  Proliferative without atypia: including usual ductal hyperplasia, complex fibroadenoma, papilloma

- *Moderate increased risk,* or relative risk >2.0 to approx. 4.2

  Proliferative with atypia: including atypical ductal hyperplasia and atypical lobular hyperplasia

Breast Density. Mammographic breast density has been identified as "the most undervalued and underused risk factor" in studies of breast cancer.[16] It is a strong independent risk factor even after adjusting for the effects of other risk factors, and it has the important attribute of "being present in the tissue from which the cancer arises."[17] Stromal and epithelial tissues appear radiologically light and dense, reflecting higher proportions of stromal and glandular tissue and increased ductal and atypical ductal hyperplasia. A proposed mechanism is proliferation of breast epithelial cells and stromal fibrosis in response to growth factors induced by circulating sex hormones.

An analysis of studies quantifying breast density found that women with radiologic density in more than 60% to 75% of the breast are at 4 to 6 times greater risk of breast cancer than women with no breast density.[16] Breast density may account for up to 30% of the risk for breast cancer and has a strong inherited component.[18] It is not yet known if breast density is associated with the increased risk of breast cancer seen in women with elevated blood levels of estrogen, free estradiol, and testosterone, which metabolizes to estrone and estradiol.[1,19]

Breast density affects the sensitivity and specificity of mammograms, dropping from 88% and 96% in women with predominantly fatty breast tissue to 62% and 89% in women with breasts that are extremely dense.[16] Sensitivity and specificity appear lowest in younger women taking HRT, leading authors to recommend that mammography reports include statements about breast density that might influence decisions about use of HRT.

Recommendations for Breast Cancer Screening and Chemoprevention

Individualized and BRCA1 and BRCA2 Screening. Discussions about risk factors for breast cancer can begin at any age. Screen all women regardless of age for general risk of breast cancer and risk of BRCA1 and 2 inheritance, using methods noted above. Also assess family history of ovarian cancer.

Mammography

Women 40 to 50 Years. Use of *mammography* in asymptomatic women in this age group has been controversial because of lower sensitivity and specificity, possibly related to breast density; increasing risk of false positives and subsequent biopsy; difficulty individualizing risks and benefits; and variation in individual values and preferences. Most professional groups, including the American Cancer Society and the U.S. Preventive Health Services Task Force, have endorsed mammography every 1 to 2 years for women in their 40s. Current evidence suggests a 15% reduction in breast cancer mortality after 14 years of follow-up, although there are wide confidence intervals around the 15% figure.[20] A recent review for the American College of Physicians supports individualized discussion of risks and benefits in this age group. *Shared decision making* is especially important for this age group given the varying risks and benefits, which can range from 0.4% for women with no risk factors to 6% if several risk factors exist.[13,20]

Women 50 Years or Older. Screening mammography reduces breast cancer mortality in women 50 to 70 years by 15% to 35%.[3] All groups recommend annual screening mammograms in this age group. Mammography detects 80% to 90% of breast cancers in asymptomatic women and has a specificity of 90%. Screening should continue for women older than 70 years, taking life expectancy and health status into account. (See Chapter 20, The Older Adult, pp. 909–921). Inform women of the increased likelihood of recall for return examinations because of unclear findings and that abnormal findings may lead to biopsy.[21] Digital mammography shows promise for even greater accuracy, especially for younger women and women with dense breasts.[22]

Clinical Breast Examination (CBE). The American Cancer Society recommends performing the *clinical breast examination* every 3 years in women 20 to 40 years, and annually after 40 years. Other professional groups find evidence of benefit insufficient to support a definitive recommendation.[3] CBE sensitivity and specificity are 54% and 94% and depend on the technique of the examiner.[2] CBE has not been clearly shown to decrease mortality and should be performed in conjunction with mammography.

Breast Self-Examination (BSE). The American Cancer Society no longer recommends monthly BSE. Although BSE does not improve detection of breast cancer, it does promote patient self-awareness, and a clinician should instruct women interested in using BSE in proper technique. Monthly BSE 5 to 7 days after the onset of menses can be taught to women as early as their 20s. (See Patient Instructions for the BSE, on p. 410.)

Magnetic Resonance Imaging (MRI). Some recent studies have investigated use of *breast MRI* in women at high risk for breast cancer, younger women, women with dense breasts, and the contralateral breast of women with newly diagnosed breast cancer. In these groups, breast MRI has helped improve detection of multicentric or contralateral breast cancer prior to management decisions about breast-conserving strategies or initiation of treatment regimens.[23-25] However, cost is high and specificity is 70% to 90%, resulting in more false positives, recalls, and biopsies.[3,13,21] Expertise in reading MRIs and MRI-guided biopsy, an important adjunct to use of breast MRI, is not widely available. Finally, breast MRI has not been evaluated for screening in the general population. Currently the American Cancer Society recommends breast MRI for women at high lifetime risk, or risk of 20% or more.[3] Women at moderately increased lifetime risk, or risk of 15% to 20%, are encouraged to discuss benefits and drawbacks with their providers. Criteria for classifying risk are given next.

● Criteria for Classifying Breast Cancer Risk and Referrals for Breast MRI

High Risk, or 20%–25%	Moderate Risk, or 15%–20%
• Known BRCA1 or 2 mutation • Known first-degree relative, including father, brother, with BRCA1 or 2 mutation, but woman not tested • Lifetime risk 20%–25% using assessment tools • History of chest radiation between ages 10 and 30 • Has high-risk genetic syndrome or first-degree relative with high-risk syndrome	• History of breast cancer, ductal or lobular carcinoma in situ, atypical ductal or lobular hyperplasia • Extremely dense breasts or unevenly dense breasts on mammograms

(Source: American Cancer Society. Breast Cancer Facts and Figures 2007–2008. pp 13–14. Available at: http://www.cancer.org/downloads/STT/BCFF-Final.pdf. Accessed October 20, 2007.)

Chemoprevention. As of 2002 the U.S. Preventive Services Task Force recommends discussion of chemoprevention with estrogen-receptor modulators in women at high risk for breast cancer and at low risk for adverse effects, but it recommends against routine use for primary prevention in women at low or average risk. The Task Force found substantial evidence that these modulators reduce the incidence of estrogen-receptor-positive breast cancer.[3,26-28] Clinicians are urged to review the literature on risks and benefits of these agents for women at high risk for developing breast cancer within 5 years. The Task Force notes that the balance of benefit and harm is more favorable for women in their 40s or 50s at increased risk and without predisposition to thromboembolic events, and for women in their 50s without a uterus. Further, key studies use the Gail model cutoff of 1.66 as high risk; however, the revised Gail model addresses prevention of invasive and noninvasive cancers, but it does not discriminate between risks of estrogen-receptor-positive versus estrogen-receptor-negative cancers.[29,30] *Prophylactic bilateral mastectomy* is also advised in women at very high genetic risk.

Counseling Women about Breast Cancer

The Challenges of Communicating Risks and Benefits. As breast cancer screening and prevention options become more complex, clinicians should consider how best to express statistics on risks and benefits in terms that patients can easily understand. Framing, or the effect of presenting the same information in terms of either increased benefit or decreased harm, is one of several ways of presenting data that can compromise informed consent. Elmore recommends, for example, that instead of reporting a Gail model risk of diagnosis of breast cancer in 5 years as 1.1%, explaining that only 11 out of 1000 women would get such a diagnosis is easier for patients to grasp.[15] Likewise, for patients absolute risk might be preferable to relative risk. Instead of stating that 379 of 6061 women with nonproliferative breast disease developed breast cancer, compared with an expected number of 298, giving a relative risk of 1.27, it is clearer to use absolute risk. In 100 women followed for 15 years, 6 in 100 with nonproliferative disease developed breast cancer, compared with 5 in the general population.

Web Sites for Breast Cancer Information. Encourage female patients to pursue breast cancer–related information from recommended sources to help them make informed choices during shared decision making.[21]

BREAST CANCER WEB SITES

Calculation of the risk of a breast cancer diagnosis and death at the level of individual women:

http://bcra.nci.nih.gov/brc/start.htm (Gail model)

http://astor.som.jhmi.edu/brcapro (Gail Model, Claus Model, and a model that predicts the probability of carrying a *BRCA1* or *BRCA2* mutation)

http://yourcancerrisk.harvard.edu/
    Breast Self-Examination Tutorials

http://www.komen.org/bse

http://www.breastselfexam.ca
    National Guidelines for Breast Cancer Screening

http://www.guidelines.gov
    Randomized Clinical Trials of New Modalities in Breast Cancer Screening

http://www.clinicaltrials.gov

http://www.acrin.org/current_protocols.html

(Source: Elmore JG, Armstrong K, Lehman CD et al. Screening for breast cancer. JAMA 293[10]:1245–1256, 2005, p 1252.)

TECHNIQUES OF EXAMINATION

 ## THE FEMALE BREAST

The clinical breast examination is an important component of women's health care: it enhances detection of breast cancers that mammography may miss and provides an opportunity to demonstrate techniques for self-examination to the patient. Clinical investigation has shown, however, that variations in examiner experience and technique affect the value of the clinical breast examination. Clinicians are advised to adopt a more standardized approach, especially for palpation, and to use a systemic and thorough search pattern, varying palpation pressure, and a circular motion with the fingerpads.[2] These techniques will be discussed in more detail in the following pages. Inspection is routinely recommended, but its value in breast cancer detection is less well studied.

As you begin the examination of the breasts, be aware that women and girls may feel apprehensive. Be reassuring and adopt a courteous and gentle approach. Before you begin, let the patient know that you are about to examine her breasts. This may be a good time to ask if she has noticed any lumps or other problems and if she performs a monthly breast self-examination. If she does not, teach her good technique and watch as she repeats the steps of examination after you, giving helpful correction as needed.

An adequate inspection initially requires full exposure of the chest, but later in the examination, cover one breast while you are palpating the other. Because breasts tend to swell and become more nodular before menses as a result of increasing estrogen stimulation, the best time for examination is 5 to 7 days *after* the onset of menstruation. Nodules appearing during the premenstrual phase should be reevaluated at this later time.

Inspection

Inspect the breasts and nipples with the patient in the sitting position and disrobed to the waist. A thorough examination of the breast includes careful inspection for skin changes, symmetry, contours, and retraction in four views—arms at sides, arms over head, arms pressed against hips, and leaning forward. When examining an adolescent girl, assess her breast development according to Tanner's sex maturity ratings described on page 842.

Arms at Sides. Note the clinical features listed below.

- The *appearance of the skin,* including:

  - Color

  - Thickening of the skin and unusually prominent pores, which may accompany lymphatic obstruction

Risk factors for breast cancer include previous breast cancer, an affected mother or sister, biopsy showing atypical hyperplasia, increasing age, early menarche, late menopause, late or no pregnancies, and previous radiation to the chest wall. See table on Breast Cancer in Women: Factors that Increase Relative Risk, p. 396.

See Patient Instructions for the Breast Self-Examination, p. 410.

Redness may be from local infection or inflammatory carcinoma.

Thickening and prominent pores suggest breast cancer.

● The *size and symmetry of the breasts*. Some difference in the size of the breasts, including the areolae, is common and is usually normal, as shown in the photograph below.

● The *contour of the breasts*. Look for changes such as masses, dimpling, or flattening. Compare one side with the other.

Flattening of the normally convex breast suggests cancer. See Table 10-2, Visible Signs of Breast Cancer (p. 414).

ARMS AT SIDES

● The *characteristics of the nipples*, including *size and shape*, *direction* in which they point, any *rashes* or *ulceration*, or any *discharge*.

Asymmetry of directions in which nipples point suggests an underlying cancer. Rash or ulceration in Paget's disease of the breast[31] (see p. 414).

Occasionally, the shape of the nipple is *inverted*, or depressed below the areolar surface. It may be enveloped by folds of areolar skin, as illustrated. Long-standing inversion is usually a normal variant of no clinical consequence, except for possible difficulty when breast-feeding.

Recent or fixed flattening or depression of the nipple suggests nipple retraction. A retracted nipple may also be broadened and thickened, suggesting an underlying cancer.

Arms Over Head; Hands Pressed Against Hips; Leaning Forward. To bring out dimpling or retraction that may otherwise be invisible, ask the patient to raise her arms over her head, then press her hands against her hips to contract the pectoral muscles. Inspect the breast contours carefully in each position. If the breasts are large or pendulous, it may be useful to have the patient stand and lean forward, supported by the back of the chair or the examiner's hands.

ARMS OVER HEAD

Dimpling or retraction of the breasts in these positions suggests an underlying cancer. When a cancer or its associated fibrous strands are attached to both the skin and the fascia overlying the pectoral muscles, pectoral contraction can draw the skin inward, causing dimpling.

HANDS PRESSED AGAINST HIPS

Occasionally, these signs may be associated with benign lesions such as posttraumatic fat necrosis or mammary duct ectasia, but they must always be further evaluated.

LEANING FORWARD

This position may reveal an asymmetry of the breast or nipple not otherwise visible. Retraction of the nipple and areola suggests an underlying cancer. See Table 10-2, Visible Signs of Breast Cancer (p. 414).

Palpation

The Breast. Palpation is best performed when the breast tissue is flattened. The patient should be supine. Plan to palpate a rectangular area extending from the clavicle to the inframammary fold or bra line, and from the midsternal line to the posterior axillary line and well into the axilla for the tail of the breast.

A thorough examination will take 3 minutes for each breast. Use the *finger-pads* of the 2nd, 3rd, and 4th fingers, keeping the fingers slightly flexed. It is important to be *systematic*. Although a circular or wedge pattern can be used, the *vertical strip pattern* is currently the best validated technique for detecting breast masses.[2] Palpate in *small, concentric circles* at each examining point, if possible applying light, medium, and deep pressure. You will need to press more firmly to reach the deeper tissues of a large breast. Your examination should cover the entire breast, including the periphery, tail, and axilla.

When pressing deeply on the breast, you may mistake a normal rib for a hard breast mass.

- To examine *the lateral portion of the breast,* ask the patient to roll onto the opposite hip, placing her hand on her forehead but keeping the shoulders pressed against the bed or examining table. This flattens the lateral breast tissue. Begin palpation in the axilla, moving in a straight line down to the bra line, then move the fingers medially and palpate in a vertical strip up the chest to the clavicle. Continue in vertical overlapping strips until you reach the nipple, then reposition the patient to flatten the medial portion of the breast.

Nodules in the tail of the breast in the axilla (the tail of Spence) are sometimes mistaken for enlarged axillary lymph nodes.

- To examine *the medial portion of the breast,* ask the patient to lie with her shoulders flat against the bed or examining table, placing her hand at her neck and lifting up her elbow until it is even with her shoulder. Palpate in a straight line down from the nipple to the bra line, then back to the clavicle, continuing in vertical overlapping strips to the midsternum.

Examine the breast tissue carefully for:

- *Consistency* of the tissues. Normal consistency varies widely, depending in part on the relative proportions of firmer glandular tissue and soft fat. Physiologic nodularity may be present, increasing before menses. There may be a firm transverse ridge of compressed tissue along the lower margin of the breast, especially in large breasts. This is the normal inframammary ridge, not a tumor.

- *Tenderness,* as in premenstrual fullness

- *Nodules.* Palpate carefully for any lump or mass that is qualitatively different from or larger than the rest of the breast tissue. This is sometimes called a dominant mass and may reflect a pathologic change that requires evaluation by mammogram, aspiration, or biopsy. Assess and describe the characteristics of any nodule:

  Location—by quadrant or clock, with centimeters from the nipple

  Size—in centimeters

  Shape—round or cystic, disclike, or irregular in contour

  Consistency—soft, firm, or hard

  Delimitation—well circumscribed or not

  Tenderness

  Mobility—in relation to the skin, pectoral fascia, and chest wall. Gently move the breast near the mass and watch for dimpling.

Tender cords suggest *mammary duct ectasia,* a benign but sometimes painful condition of dilated ducts with surrounding inflammation, sometimes with associated masses.

See Table 10-1, Common Breast Masses (p. 413).

Hard, irregular, poorly circumscribed nodules, fixed to the skin or underlying tissues, strongly suggest breast cancer.

Cysts, inflamed areas; some cancers may be tender.

- Next, try to move the mass itself while the patient relaxes her arm and then while she presses her hand against her hip.

A mobile mass that becomes fixed when the arm relaxes is attached to the ribs and intercostal muscles; if fixed when the hand is pressed against the hip, it is attached to the pectoral fascia.

The Nipple.   Palpate each nipple, noting its elasticity.

Thickening of the nipple and loss of elasticity suggest an underlying breast cancer.

 ## THE MALE BREAST

Examination of the male breast may be brief but is important. *Inspect the nipple and areola* for nodules, swelling, or ulceration. *Palpate the areola and breast tissue* for nodules. If the breast appears enlarged, distinguish between the soft fatty enlargement of obesity and the firm disc of glandular enlargement, called *gynecomastia*.

Gynecomastia arises from an imbalance of estrogens and androgens, sometimes drug related. A hard, irregular, eccentric, or ulcerating nodule suggests breast cancer.

Male breast cancer constitutes only 1% of breast cancer cases, peaking in frequency around age 71.[3, 32] Risk factors are BRCA2 mutations, obesity, family history of male or female breast cancer, testicular disorders, and work exposure to high temperatures and exhaust emission.

 ## THE AXILLAE

Although the axillae may be examined with the patient lying down, a sitting position is preferable.

Inspection

Inspect the skin of each axilla, noting evidence of:

- Rash

- Infection

- Unusual pigmentation

Deodorant and other rashes

Sweat gland infection (*hidradenitis suppurativa*)

Deeply pigmented, velvety axillary skin suggests *acanthosis nigricans*—one form is associated with internal malignancy.

Palpation

To examine the left axilla, ask the patient to relax with the left arm down. Help by supporting the left wrist or hand with your left hand. Cup together the fingers of your right hand and reach as high as you can toward the apex of the axilla. Warn the patient that this may feel uncomfortable. Your fingers should lie directly behind the pectoral muscles, pointing toward the midclavicle. Now press your fingers in toward the chest wall and slide them downward, trying to feel the central nodes against the chest wall. Of the axillary nodes, these are the most often palpable. One or more soft, small (<1 cm), nontender nodes are frequently felt.

Enlarged axillary nodes from infection of the hand or arm, recent immunizations or skin tests in the arm, or part of a generalized lymphadenopathy. Check the epitrochlear nodes and other groups of lymph nodes.

Nodes that are large (≥1 cm) and firm or hard, matted together, or fixed to the skin or to underlying tissues suggest malignant involvement.

Use your left hand to examine the right axilla.

If the central nodes feel large, hard, or tender, or if there is a suspicious lesion in the drainage areas for the axillary nodes, feel for the other groups of axillary lymph nodes:

- *Pectoral nodes*—grasp the anterior axillary fold between your thumb and fingers, and with your fingers, palpate inside the border of the pectoral muscle.

- *Lateral nodes*—from high in the axilla, feel along the upper humerus.

- *Subscapular nodes*—step behind the patient and, with your fingers, feel inside the muscle of the posterior axillary fold.

Also, feel for infraclavicular nodes and re-examine the supraclavicular nodes.

SPECIAL TECHNIQUES

Assessment of Spontaneous Nipple Discharge. If there is a history of spontaneous nipple discharge, try to determine its origin by compressing the areola with your index finger, placed in radial positions around the nipple. Watch for discharge appearing through one of the duct openings on the nipple's surface. Note the color, consistency, and quantity of any discharge and the exact location where it appears.

Milky discharge unrelated to a prior pregnancy and lactation is *nonpuerperal galactorrhea.* Causes include *hypothyroidism,* pituitary *prolactinoma,* and drugs that are dopamine agonists, including many psychotropic agents and phenothiazines.

Papilloma

Spontaneous unilateral bloody discharge from one or two ducts warrants further evaluation for intraductal *papilloma,* shown above, ductal carcinoma in situ, or Paget's disease of the breast. Clear, serous, green, black, or nonbloody discharges that are multiductal usually require only reassurance.[1]

Examination of the Mastectomy or Breast Augmentation Patient.
The woman with a mastectomy warrants special care on examination. Inspect the mastectomy scar and axilla carefully for any masses or unusual nodularity. Note any change in color or signs of inflammation. Lymphedema may be present in the axilla and upper arm from impaired lymph drainage after surgery. Palpate gently along the scar—these tissues may be unusually sensitive. Use a circular motion with two or three fingers. Pay special attention to the upper outer quadrant and axilla. Note any enlargement of the lymph nodes or signs of inflammation or infection.

Masses, nodularity, and change in color or inflammation, especially in the incision line, suggest recurrence of breast cancer.

It is especially important to carefully palpate the breast tissue and incision lines of women with breast augmentation or reconstruction.

Instructions for the Breast Self-Examination. The office or hospital visit is an important time to teach your patient how to perform the breast self-examination (BSE). A high proportion of breast masses are detected by women examining their own breasts. Although BSE has not been shown to reduce breast cancer mortality, monthly BSE is inexpensive and may promote stronger health awareness and more active self-care. For early detection of breast cancer, the BSE is most useful when coupled with regular breast examination by an experienced clinician and mammography. The BSE is best timed just after menses, when hormonal stimulation of breast tissue is low.

PATIENT INSTRUCTIONS FOR THE BREAST SELF-EXAMINATION (BSE)

Lying Supine

1. Lie down with a pillow under your right shoulder. Place your right arm behind your head.
2. Use the finger pads of the three middle fingers on your left hand to feel for lumps in the right breast. The finger pads are the top third of each finger.
3. Press firmly enough to know how your breast feels. A firm ridge in the lower curve of each breast is normal. If you're not sure how hard to press, talk with your health care provider, or try to copy the way the doctor or nurse does it.

4. Press firmly on the breast in an up-and-down or "strip" pattern. You can also use a circular or wedge pattern, but be sure to use the same pattern every time. Check the entire breast area, and remember how your breast feels from month to month.
5. Repeat the examination on your left breast, using the finger pads of the right hand.
6. If you find any masses, lumps, or skin changes, see your doctor right away.

Standing

1. Repeat the examination of both breasts while standing, with one arm behind your head. The upright position makes it easier to check the upper outer part of the breasts (toward your armpit). This is where about half of breast cancers are found. You may want to do the upright part of the BSE while you are in the shower. Your soapy hands will make it easy to check how your breasts feel as they glide over the wet skin.

2. For added safety, you might want to check your breasts by standing in front of a mirror right after your BSE each month. See if there are any changes in the way your breasts look, such as dimpling of the skin, changes in the nipple, redness, or swelling.
3. If you find any masses, lumps, or skin changes, see your doctor right away.

Adapted from the American Cancer Society. Available at: www.cancer.org. Accessed October 24, 2007.

RECORDING YOUR FINDINGS

Note that initially you may use sentences to describe your findings; later you will use phrases. The style below contains phrases appropriate for most write-ups.

Recording the Physical Examination—Breasts and Axillae

"Breasts symmetric and smooth without masses. Nipples without discharge." (Axillary adenopathy usually included after Neck in section on Lymph Nodes; see p. 245.)

OR

"Breasts pendulous with diffuse fibrocystic changes. Single firm 1 × 1 cm mass, mobile and nontender, with overlying peau d'orange appearance in right breast, upper outer quadrant at 11 o'clock, 2 cm from the nipple."

Suggests possible breast cancer

BIBLIOGRAPHY

CITATIONS

1. Santen RJ, Mansel R. Benign breast disorders. N Engl J Med 353(3):275–285, 2005.
2. Barton MB, Harris R, Fletcher SW. Does this patient have breast cancer? The screening clinical breast examination: should it be done? How? JAMA 282(13):1270–1280, 1999.
3. American Cancer Society. Breast Cancer Facts and Figures 2007–2008. Available at: http://www.cancer.org/downloads/STT/BCFF-Final.pdf. Accessed October 20, 2007.
4. U.S. Preventive Services Task Force. Screening for Breast Cancer: Recommendations and Rationale. February 2002. Rockville, MD, Agency for Healthcare Research and Quality. Available at: http://www.ahrq.gov/clinic/3rduspstf/breastcancer/brcanrr.htm. Accessed October 20, 2007.
5. Ravdin PM, Cronin KA, Howlader N, et al. The decrease in breast-cancer incidence in 2003 in the United States. N Engl J Med 356(16):1670–1674, 2007.
6. Chu KC, Lamar CA, Freeman HP. Racial disparities in breast carcinoma survival rates: separating factors that affect diagnosis from factors that affect treatment. Cancer 97(11): 2859–2863, 2003.
7. del Carmen MG, Hughes KS, Halpern E, et al. Racial differences in mammographic breast density. Cancer 98(3):590–596, 2003.
8. Gail MH, Brinton LA, Byar DP, et al. Projecting individualized probabilities of developing breast cancer for white females who are being examined annually. J Natl Cancer Inst 81(24): 1879–1886, 1989.
9. Gail MH, Benichou J. Validations studies on a model for breast cancer risk (editorial). J Natl Cancer Inst 86:73–87, 1996.
10. Claus EB, Risch N, Thompson WD. Autosomal dominant inheritance of early-onset breast cancer: implications for risk prediction. Cancer 73(3):643–651, 1994.
11. National Cancer Institute. Genetics of breast and ovarian cancer: models for prediction of breast cancer risk. Available at: http://www.cancer.gov/cancertopics/pdq/genetics/breast-and-ovarian. Accessed October 21, 2007.
12. Armstrong K, Moye E, Sankey W, et al. Screening mammography in women 40 to 49 years of age: a systematic review for the American College of Physicians. Ann Intern Med 146(7): 516–526, 2007.
13. Fletcher SW, Elmore JG. Mammographic screening for breast cancer. N Engl J Med 348(14):1672–1680, 2003.
14. Hartmann LC, Sellers TA, Frost MH, et al. Benign breast disease and the risk of breast cancer. N Engl J Med 353(3): 229–237, 2005.
15. Elmore JG, Gigerenzer G. Benign breast disease: the risks of communicating risk (editorial). N Engl J Med 353(3): 297–298, 2005.
16. Carney PA, Migloiretti DL, Yankaskas, et al. Individual and combined effects of age, breast density, and hormone replacement therapy use on the accuracy of screening mammography. Ann Intern Med 138(3):168–175, 2003.

17. Boyd NF, Lockwood GA, Byng JW, et al. Mammographic densities and breast cancer risk. Cancer Epidemiol Biomarkers Prevent 7(12):1133–1144, 1998.

18. Vachon CM, Sellers TA, Carlson EE, et al. Strong evidence of a genetic determinant for mammographic density, a major risk factor for breast cancer. Cancer Res 67(17):8412–8418, 2007.

19. Yager JD, Davidson. Estrogen carcinogenesis in breast cancer. N Engl J Med 354(3):270–282, 2006.

20. Qaseem A, Snow V, Sherif K, et al. Screening mammography in women 40 to 49 years of age: a clinical practice guideline from the American College of Physicians. Ann Intern Med 146(7):511–515, 2007.

21. Elmore JG, Armstrong K, Lehman CD, et al. Screening for breast cancer. JAMA 293(10):1245–1256, 2005.

22. Pisano ED, Gatsonis C, Hendrick E, et al. Diagnostic performance of digital versus film mammography for breast-cancer screening. N Engl J Med 353(17):1773–1783, 2005.

23. Kreige M, Brekelmans CTM, Boetes C, et al. Efficacy of MRI and mammography for breast-cancer screening in women with a familial or genetic predisposition. N Engl J Med 351(5):427–437, 2004.

24. Lehman CD, Gatsonis C, Kuhl CK, et al. MRI evaluation of the contralateral breast in women with recently diagnosed breast cancer. N Engl J Med 356(13):1295–1303, 2007.

25. Smith RA. The evolving role of MRI in the detection and evaluation of breast cancer. N Engl J Med 356(13):1362–1363, 2007.

26. U.S. Preventive Services Task Force. Chemoprevention of breast cancer: summary of the evidence. Rockville, MD, Agency for Healthcare Research and Quality. Available at: http://www.ahrq.gov/clinic/3rduspstf/breastchemo/brstchemosum1.htm. Accessed October 22, 2007.

27. U.S. Preventive Services Task Force. Chemoprevention of breast cancer: recommendations and rationale. Rockville, MD, Agency for Healthcare Research and Quality, July 2002. Available at: http://www.ahrq.gov/clinic/3rduspstf/breastchemo/breastchemorr.htm. Accessed October 22, 2007.

28. Vogel VG, Constantino JP, Wickerham DL, et al. Effects of tamoxifen vs raloxifene on the risk of developing invasive breast cancer and other disease outcomes. The NSABP study of tamoxifen and raloxifene (STAR) P-2 trial. JAMA 295(23):2727–2741, 2006.

29. Gail MH, Costantino JP. Validating and improving models for projecting the absolute risk of breast cancer. J Natl Cancer Inst 93(5)334–335, 2001.

30. Gail MH, Costantino JH, Bryant J, et al. Weighing the risks and benefits of tamoxifen treatment for preventing breast cancer. J Natl Cancer Inst 91(21):1829–1846, 1999.

31. Chen CY, Sun LM, Anderson BO. Paget disease of the breast: changing patterns of incidence, clinical presentation, and treatment in the U.S. Cancer 197(7):1448–1458, 2006.

32. Fentiman IS. Male breast cancer. Lancet 367(9510):595–604, 2006.

ADDITIONAL REFERENCES

American Geriatrics Society Clinical Practice Committee. Position Statement: breast cancer screening in older women. Available at: http://www.americangeriatrics.org/products/positionpapers/brstcncr.shtml. Accessed May 26, 2008.

Bland KI, Beenken SW, Copeland EM. The Breast. In: Brunicardi FC, Andersen DK, Billiar TM, et al., eds. Schwartz's Principles of Surgery, 8th ed. New York: McGraw-Hill Medical, 2005.

Chlebowski RT, Hentrix SL, Langer RD, et al. Influence of estrogen plus progestin on breast cancer and mammography in healthy postmenopausal women: The Women's Health Initiative randomized trial. JAMA 289(24):3243–3253, 2003.

Giordano SH, Cohen DS, Buzdar AU. Breast carcinoma in men: a population-based study. Cancer 101(1):51–57, 2004.

Harris JR, Morrow M, Bonadonna G. Cancer of the breast. In: DeVita VT, Lawrence TS, Rosenberg SA. DeVita, Hellman, and Rosenberg's Cancer: Principles & Practice of Oncology, 8th ed. Philadelphia: Lippincott Williams & Wilkins, 2008.

Jones BA, Patterson EA, Calvocoressi L. Mammography screening in African American women: evaluating the research. Cancer 97(Suppl.1):258–272, 2003.

Kudva YC, Reynolds CA, O'Brien T, et al. Mastopathy and diabetes. Curr Diab Rep 3(1):56–59, 2003.

Mandalblatt J, Saha S, Teusch S, et al. The cost-effectiveness of screening mammography beyond age 65 years: a systematic review for the U.S. Preventive Services Task Force. Ann Intern Med 139(10):835–842, 2003.

Robson M, Offit K. Clinical practice: management of an inherited predisposition to breast cancer. N Engl J Med 357(2):154–162, 2007.

> **The Bates' suite offers these additional resources to enhance learning and facilitate understanding of this chapter:**
>
> - *Bates' Pocket Guide to Physical Examination and History Taking,* 6th edition
> - *Bates' Nursing Online*
> - *Bates' Visual Guide to Physical Examination,* 4th edition
> - thePoint online resources, http://thepoint.lww.com
> - Student CD-ROM included with the book

Common Breast Masses

The three most common kinds of breast masses are *fibroadenoma* (a benign tumor), *cysts*, and *breast cancer*. The clinical characteristics of these masses are listed below. However, any breast mass should be carefully evaluated and usually warrants further investigation by ultrasound, aspiration, mammography, or biopsy. The masses depicted below are large for purposes of illustration. Ideally, breast cancer should be identified early, when the mass is small. *Fibrocystic changes,* not illustrated, are also commonly palpable as nodular, ropelike densities in women ages 25–50. They may be tender or painful. They are considered benign and are not viewed as a risk factor for breast cancer.

	Fibroadenoma	Cysts	Cancer
Usual Age	15–25, usually puberty and young adulthood, but up to age 55	30–50, regress after menopause except with estrogen therapy	30–90, most common over age 50
Number	Usually single, may be multiple	Single or multiple	Usually single, although may coexist with other nodules
Shape	Round, disclike, or lobular	Round	Irregular or stellate
Consistency	May be soft, usually firm	Soft to firm, usually elastic	Firm or hard
Delimitation	Well delineated	Well delineated	Not clearly delineated from surrounding tissues
Mobility	Very mobile	Mobile	May be fixed to skin or underlying tissues
Tenderness	Usually nontender	Often tender	Usually nontender
Retraction Signs	Absent	Absent	May be present

TABLE 10-2

Visible Signs of Breast Cancer

- Cancer
- Dimpling
- Retracted nipple

Retraction Signs

As breast cancer advances, it causes fibrosis (scar tissue). Shortening of this tissue produces *dimpling, changes in contour,* and *retraction or deviation of the nipple.* Other causes of retraction include fat necrosis and mammary duct ectasia.

Abnormal Contours

Look for any variation in the normal convexity of each breast, and compare one side with the other. Special positioning may again be useful. Shown here is marked flattening of the lower outer quadrant of the left breast.

Skin Dimpling

Look for this sign with the patient's arm at rest, during special positioning, and on moving or compressing the breast, as illustrated here.

Nipple Retraction and Deviation

A retracted nipple is flattened or pulled inward, as illustrated here. It may also be broadened, and feels thickened. When involvement is radially asymmetric, the nipple may deviate or point in a different direction from its normal counterpart, typically toward the underlying cancer.

- Dermatitis of areola
- Erosion of nipple

Paget's Disease of the Nipple

This uncommon form of breast cancer usually starts as a scaly, eczemalike lesion that may weep, crust, or erode. A breast mass may be present. Suspect Paget's disease in any persisting dermatitis of the nipple and areola. Can present with invasive breast cancer or ductal carcinoma in situ.[31]

Edema of the Skin

Edema of the skin is produced by lymphatic blockade. It appears as thickened skin with enlarged pores—the so-called *peau d'orange* (orange peel) *sign.* It is often seen first in the lower portion of the breast or areola.

11

The Abdomen

ANATOMY AND PHYSIOLOGY

Visualize or palpate the landmarks of the abdominal wall and pelvis, as illustrated. The rectus abdominis muscles become more prominent when the patient raises the head and shoulders from the supine position.

Rectus abdominis muscle

Xiphoid process

Costal margin

Midline, overlying linea alba

Umbilicus

Iliac crest

Anterior superior iliac spine

Inguinal ligament

Pubic tubercle

Symphysis pubis

For descriptive purposes, the abdomen is often divided by imaginary lines crossing at the umbilicus, forming the right upper, right lower, left upper, and left lower quadrants. Another system divides the abdomen into nine sections. Terms for three of them are commonly used: epigastric, umbilical, and hypogastric or suprapubic.

When examining the abdomen and moving in a clockwise rotation, several organs are often palpable. Exceptions are the stomach and much of the liver and spleen. The abdominal cavity extends up under the rib cage to the dome of the diaphragm, placing these organs in a protected location, beyond the reach of the palpating hand.

In the *right upper quadrant,* the soft consistency of the *liver* makes it difficult to feel through the abdominal wall. The lower margin of the liver, the liver edge, is often palpable at the right costal margin. The *gallbladder,* which rests against the inferior surface of the liver, and the more deeply lying *duodenum* are generally not palpable. At a deeper level, the *lower pole of the right kidney* may be felt, especially in thin people with relaxed abdominal muscles. Moving medially, the examiner encounters the rib cage, which protects the stomach; occasionally patients misidentify the stony hard *xiphoid process* lying in the midline as a tumor. The *abdominal aorta* often has visible pulsations and is usually palpable in the upper abdomen.

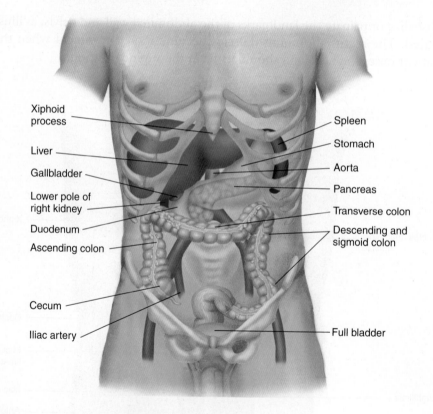

In the *left upper quadrant,* the *spleen* is lateral to and behind the stomach, just above the left kidney in the left midaxillary line. Its upper margin rests against the dome of the diaphragm. The 9th, 10th, and 11th ribs protect most of the spleen. The tip of the spleen may be palpable below the left costal margin in a small percentage of adults. The *pancreas* in healthy people escapes detection.

In the *left lower quadrant* you can often feel the firm, narrow, tubular sigmoid *colon.* Portions of the transverse and descending colon may also be palpable. In the lower midline are the *bladder*, the *sacral promontory*, the bony anterior edge of the S1 vertebra sometimes mistaken for a tumor, and in women, the *uterus* and *ovaries*.

In the *right lower quadrant* are bowel loops and the *appendix* at the tail of the cecum near the junction of the small and large intestines. In healthy people, there will be no palpable findings.

A distended *bladder* may be palpable above the symphysis pubis. The bladder accommodates roughly 300 ml of urine filtered by the kidneys into the renal pelvis and the ureters. Bladder expansion stimulates contraction of bladder smooth muscle, the *detrusor muscle,* at relatively low pressures. Rising pressure in the bladder triggers the conscious urge to void.

Increased intraurethral pressure can overcome rising pressures in the bladder and prevent incontinence. Intraurethral pressure is related to factors such as smooth muscle tone in the internal urethral sphincter, the thickness of the urethral mucosa, and in women, sufficient support to the bladder and proximal urethra from pelvic muscles and ligaments to maintain proper anatomical relationships. Striated muscle around the urethra can also contract voluntarily to interrupt voiding.

Neuroregulatory control of the bladder functions at several levels. In infants, the bladder empties by reflex mechanisms in the sacral spinal cord. Voluntary control of the bladder depends on higher centers in the brain and on motor and sensory pathways between the brain and the reflex arcs of the sacral spinal cord. When voiding is inconvenient, higher centers in the brain can inhibit detrusor contractions until the capacity of the bladder, approximately 400 to 500 ml, is exceeded. The integrity of the sacral nerves that innervate the bladder can be tested by assessing perirectal and perineal sensation in the S2, S3, and S4 dermatomes (see p. 702).

The *kidneys* are posterior organs. The ribs protect their upper portions. The *costovertebral angle*—the angle formed by the lower border of the 12th rib and the transverse processes of the upper lumbar vertebrae—defines the region to assess for kidney tenderness.

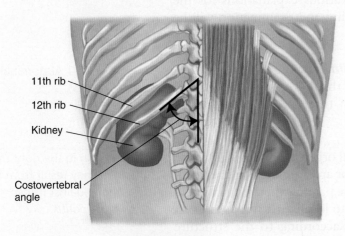

11th rib
12th rib
Kidney
Costovertebral angle

POSTERIOR VIEW

THE HEALTH HISTORY

Common or Concerning Symptoms

Gastrointestinal Disorders	Urinary and Renal Disorders
• Abdominal pain, acute and chronic • Indigestion, nausea, vomiting including blood, loss of appetite, early satiety • Dysphagia and/or odynophagia • Change in bowel function • Diarrhea, constipation • Jaundice	• Suprapubic pain • Dysuria, urgency, or frequency • Hesitancy, decreased stream in males • Polyuria or nocturia • Urinary incontinence • Hematuria • Kidney or flank pain • Ureteral colic

Gastrointestinal complaints rank high among reasons for office and emergency-room visits. You will encounter a wide variety of upper gastrointestinal symptoms, including abdominal pain, heartburn, nausea and vomiting, difficulty or pain with swallowing, vomiting of stomach contents or blood, loss of appetite, and jaundice. Abdominal pain alone accounted for more than 13 million office visits in 2004[1] and 7 million emergency-room visits in 2003.[2] Lower gastrointestinal complaints are also common: diarrhea, constipation, change in bowel habits, and blood in the stool, often described as either bright red or dark and tarry.

Numerous symptoms also originate in the *genitourinary tract:* difficulty urinating, urgency and frequency, hesitancy and decreased stream in men, high urine volume, urinating at night, incontinence, blood in the urine, and flank pain and colic from renal stones or infection.

Often you will need to cluster several findings from both the patient's story and your examination as you sort through various explanations for the patient's symptoms. Your skills in history-taking and examination will be needed for sound clinical reasoning.

Patterns and Mechanisms of Abdominal Pain.

Before exploring gastrointestinal and genitourinary symptoms, review the mechanisms and clinical patterns of abdominal pain. Be familiar with three broad categories of abdominal pain:

See Table 11-1 Abdominal Pain (pp. 454–455)

• *Visceral pain* occurs when hollow abdominal organs such as the intestine or biliary tree contract unusually forcefully or are distended or stretched. Solid organs such as the liver can also become painful when their capsules are stretched. Visceral pain may be difficult to localize. It is typically palpable near the midline at levels that vary according to the structure involved, as illustrated on the next page.

Visceral pain in the right upper quadrant may result from liver distention against its capsule in *alcoholic hepatitis.*

Visceral pain varies in quality and may be gnawing, burning, cramping, or aching. When it becomes severe, it may be associated with sweating, pallor, nausea, vomiting, and restlessness.

Visceral periumbilical pain may signify early *acute appendicitis* from distention of an inflamed appendix. It gradually changes to parietal pain in the right lower quadrant from inflammation of the adjacent parietal peritoneum.

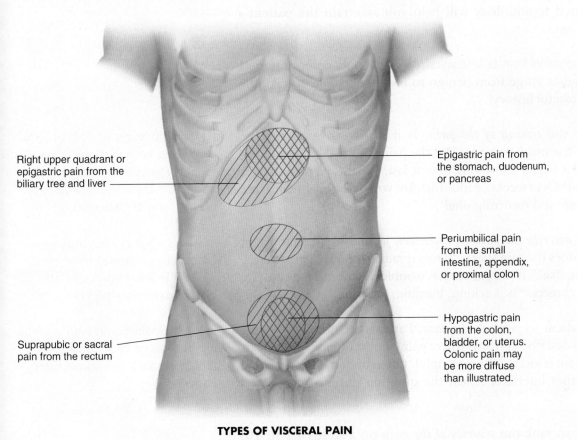

Right upper quadrant or epigastric pain from the biliary tree and liver

Epigastric pain from the stomach, duodenum, or pancreas

Periumbilical pain from the small intestine, appendix, or proximal colon

Hypogastric pain from the colon, bladder, or uterus. Colonic pain may be more diffuse than illustrated.

Suprapubic or sacral pain from the rectum

TYPES OF VISCERAL PAIN

- *Parietal pain* originates from inflammation in the parietal peritoneum. It is a steady, aching pain that is usually more severe than visceral pain and more precisely localized over the involved structure. It is typically aggravated by movement or coughing. Patients with this type of pain usually prefer to lie still.

- *Referred pain* is felt in more distant sites, which are innervated at approximately the same spinal levels as the disordered structures. Referred pain often develops as the initial pain becomes more intense and thus seems to radiate or travel from the initial site. It may be felt superficially or deeply but is usually well localized.

Pain may also be referred to the abdomen from the chest, spine, or pelvis, thus complicating the assessment of abdominal pain.

Pain of duodenal or pancreatic origin may be referred to the back; pain from the biliary tree, to the right shoulder or the right posterior chest.

Pain from *pleurisy* or *acute myocardial infarction* may be referred to the epigastric area.

THE GASTROINTESTINAL TRACT

Upper Abdominal Pain, Discomfort, and Heartburn. The prevalence of recurrent upper abdominal discomfort or pain in the United States and other Western countries is approximately 25%.[3] In recent years consensus statements from expert societies have clarified the definitions and classification of numerous abdominal symptoms, particularly the Rome III criteria for functional gastrointestinal disorders.[4] Understanding carefully defined terminology will help you ascertain the patient's underlying condition.

Studies suggest that neuropeptides like 5-hydroxytryptophan and substance P mediate interconnected symptoms of pain, bowel dysfunction, and stress.[4]

Acute Upper Abdominal Pain or Discomfort. For patients complaining of abdominal pain, causes range from benign to life-threatening, so take the time to conduct a careful history.

● First determine the *timing of the pain*. Is it *acute or chronic?* Acute abdominal pain has many patterns. Did the pain start suddenly or gradually? When did it begin? How long does it last? What is its pattern over a 24-hour period? Over weeks or months? Are you dealing with an acute illness or a chronic and recurring one?

In emergency rooms 40% to 45% of patients have nonspecific pain, but 15% to 30% need surgery, usually for appendicitis, intestinal obstruction, or cholecystitis.[5]

● Ask patients to *describe the pain in their own words*. Pursue important details: "Where does the pain start?" "Does it radiate or travel anywhere?" "What is the pain like?" If the patient has trouble describing the pain, try offering several choices: "Is it aching, burning, gnawing . . . ?"

Doubling over with cramping colicky pain indicates *renal stone*. Sudden knifelike epigastric pain occurs in *gallstone pancreatitis*.[6]

● Then ask the patient to *point to the pain*. Patients are not always clear when they try to describe in words where pain is most intense. The quadrant where the pain is located can be helpful. Often underlying organs are involved. If clothes interfere, repeat the question during the physical examination.

Epigastric pain occurs with *gastritis* or *GERD*. Right upper quadrant and upper abdominal pain signify *cholecystitis*.[7]

● Ask the patient to rank the *severity of the pain* on a scale of 1 to 10. Note that severity does not always help you to identify the cause. Sensitivity to abdominal pain varies widely and tends to diminish in older patients, masking acute abdominal conditions. Pain threshold and how patients accommodate to pain during daily activities also affect ratings of severity.

● As you probe *factors that aggravate or relieve the pain*, pay special attention to any association with meals, alcohol, medications (including aspirin and aspirin-like drugs and any over-the-counter medications), stress, body position, and use of antacids. Ask if indigestion or discomfort is related to exertion and relieved by rest.

Note that angina from inferior wall coronary artery disease may present as "indigestion," but is precipitated by exertion and relieved by rest. See Table 9-1, Chest Pain, p. 375.

Chronic Upper Abdominal Discomfort or Pain. For more chronic symptoms, *dyspepsia* is defined as chronic or recurrent discomfort or pain centered in the upper abdomen.[8] *Discomfort* is defined as a subjective negative feeling that is nonpainful. It can include various symptoms such as bloating, nausea, upper abdominal fullness, and heartburn.

● Note that bloating, nausea, or belching can occur alone and is seen in other disorders. When they occur alone they do not meet the criteria for dyspepsia.

Bloating may occur with *inflammatory bowel disease,* belching from *aerophagia,* or swallowing air.

● Many patients with upper abdominal discomfort or pain will have *functional, or nonulcer, dyspepsia,* defined as a 3-month history of nonspecific upper abdominal discomfort or nausea not attributable to structural abnormalities or peptic ulcer disease. Symptoms are usually recurring and typically present for more than 6 months.[3]

Multifactorial causes include delayed gastric emptying (20%–40%), gastritis from *H. pylori* (20%–60%), peptic ulcer disease (up to 15% if *H. pylori* is present), and psychosocial factors.[3]

Many patients with chronic upper abdominal discomfort or pain complain primarily of *heartburn, acid reflux,* or *regurgitation.* If patients report these symptoms more than once a week, they are likely to have *gastroesophageal reflux disease (GERD)* until proven otherwise.[8,9]

These symptoms or mucosal damage on endoscopy are the diagnostic criteria for GERD. Risk factors include reduced salivary flow, which prolongs acid clearance by damping action of the bicarbonate buffer; delayed gastric emptying; selected medications; and hiatal hernia.

● *Heartburn* is a rising retrosternal burning pain or discomfort occurring weekly or more often.[3] It is typically aggravated by food such as alcohol, chocolate, citrus fruits, coffee, onions, and peppermint; or positions like bending over, exercising, lifting, or lying supine.

Note that angina from inferior wall coronary ischemia along the diaphragm may present as heartburn. See Table 9-1, Chest Pain, p. 375.

● Some patients with GERD have *atypical respiratory symptoms* such as cough, wheezing, and aspiration pneumonia. Others complain of *pharyngeal symptoms,* such as hoarseness and chronic sore throat.[10]

● Some patients may have "*alarm symptoms,*" such as difficulty swallowing (dysphagia), pain with swallowing (odyophagia), recurrent vomiting, evidence of gastrointestinal bleeding, weight loss, anemia, or risk factors for gastric cancer.

Patients with uncomplicated GERD who do not respond to empiric therapy, patients older than 55 years, and those with "alarm symptoms" warrant endoscopy to detect esophagitis, peptic strictures, or Barrett's esophagus (in this condition the squamocolumnar junction is displaced proximally and replaced by intestinal metaplasia, increasing the risk of esophageal cancer 30-fold).[9,11,12] Approximately 50% of patients with GERD will have no disease on endoscopy.[13]

Lower Abdominal Pain and Discomfort—Acute and Chronic. Lower abdominal pain and discomfort may be acute or chronic. Asking the patient to point to the pain and characterize all its features, combined with findings on physical examination, will help you identify possible causes. Some acute pain, especially in the suprapubic area or radiating from the flank, originates in the genitourinary tract (see p. 428).

Acute Lower Abdominal Pain.   Patients may complain of *acute pain* localized to the *right lower quadrant*. Find out if it is sharp and continuous or intermittent and cramping, causing them to double over.

| Right lower quadrant pain or pain that migrates from the periumbilical region, combined with abdominal wall rigidity on palpation, is most likely to predict *appendicitis*. In women other causes include *pelvic inflammatory disease, ruptured ovarian follicle,* and *ectopic pregnancy.*[14]

Cramping pain radiating to the right or left lower quadrant may be a renal stone.

When patients report acute pain in the *left lower quadrant* or *diffuse abdominal pain,* investigate associated symptoms such as fever and loss of appetite.

Left lower quadrant pain with a palpable mass may be *diverticulitis.* Diffuse abdominal pain with absent bowel sounds and firmness, guarding, or rebound on palpation indicates *small or large bowel obstruction* (see p. 454).

Chronic Lower Abdominal Pain.   If there is *chronic pain* in the quadrants of the lower abdomen, ask about change in bowel habits and alternating diarrhea and constipation.

Change in bowel habits with mass lesion indicates *colon cancer.* Intermittent pain for 12 weeks of the preceding 12 months with relief from defecation, change in frequency of bowel movements, or change in form of stool (loose, watery, pellet-like), without structural or biochemical abnormalities are symptoms of *irritable bowel syndrome.*[15]

Gastrointestinal Symptoms Associated With Abdominal Pain. Patients often experience abdominal pain in conjunction with other symptoms. "How is your appetite?" is a good starting question that may lead to other concerns like *indigestion, nausea, vomiting,* and *anorexia. Indigestion* is a general term for distress associated with eating that can have many meanings. Urge your patient to be more specific.

Anorexia, nausea, and vomiting accompany many gastrointestinal disorders; these are all seen in pregnancy, *diabetic ketoacidosis, adrenal insufficiency, hypercalcemia, uremia,* liver disease, emotional states, adverse drug reactions, and other conditions. Induced vomiting without nausea is more indicative of *anorexia/bulimia.*

● *Nausea,* often described as "feeling sick to my stomach," may progress to retching and vomiting. *Retching* describes involuntary spasm of the stomach, diaphragm, and esophagus that precedes and culminates in *vomiting,* the forceful expulsion of gastric contents out of the mouth.

Some patients may not actually vomit but raise esophageal or gastric contents without nausea or retching, called *regurgitation*.

Regurgitation occurs in *GERD, esophageal stricture,* and *esophageal cancer.*

Ask about any vomitus or regurgitated material and inspect it if possible. What color is it? What does the vomitus smell like? How much has there been? You may have to help the patient with the amount: a teaspoon? Two teaspoons? A cupful?

Vomiting and pain indicate *small bowel obstruction.* Fecal odor occurs with *small bowel obstruction* or *gastrocolic fistula.*

Ask specifically if the vomitus contains any blood, and quantify the amount. Gastric juice is clear and mucoid. Small amounts of yellowish or greenish bile are common and have no special significance. Brownish or blackish vomitus with a "coffee grounds" appearance suggests blood altered by gastric acid. Coffee-grounds emesis or red blood is termed *hematemesis.*

Hematemesis may accompany *esophageal* or *gastric varices, gastritis,* or *peptic ulcer disease.*

Is there any dehydration or electrolyte imbalance from prolonged vomiting, or significant blood loss? Do the patient's symptoms suggest any complications of vomiting, such as aspiration into the lungs, seen in debilitated, obtunded, or elderly patients?

Symptoms of blood loss such as lightheadedness or syncope depend on the rate and volume of bleeding and are rare until blood loss exceeds 500 ml.

● *Anorexia* is loss or lack of appetite. Find out if it arises from intolerance to certain foods or reluctance to eat because of anticipated discomfort. Check for associated symptoms of nausea and vomiting.

Patients may complain of unpleasant *abdominal fullness* after light or moderate meals, or *early satiety,* the inability to eat a full meal. A dietary assessment or recall may be warranted (see Chapter 4, General Survey, Vital Signs, and Pain, pp. 106–107).

Consider *diabetic gastroparesis,* anticholinergic medications, *gastric outlet obstruction, gastric cancer;* early satiety in *hepatitis.*

Other Gastrointestinal Symptoms

Dysphagia and/or Odynophagia.   Less commonly, patients may report difficulty swallowing from impaired passage of solid foods or liquids from the mouth to the stomach, or *dysphagia.* Food seems to stick, hesitate, or "not go down right," suggesting motility disorders or structural anomalies. The sensation of a lump in the throat or the retrosternal area unassociated with swallowing is not true dysphagia.

For types of dysphagia, see Table 11-2, Dysphagia, p. 456.

Indicators of *oropharyngeal dysphagia* include drooling, nasopharyngeal regurgitation, and cough from aspiration in muscular or neurologic disorders affecting motility; gurgling or regurgitation of undigested food occur in structural conditions like *Zenker's diverticulum.*

Ask the patient to point to where the dysphagia occurs.

Pointing to below the sterno-clavicular notch indicates *esophageal dysphagia.*

Pursue which types of foods provoke symptoms: solid foods, or solids and liquids? Establish the timing. When does the dysphagia start? Is it intermittent or persistent? Is it progressing? If so, over what time period? Are there associated symptoms and medical conditions?

If solid foods, consider structural esophageal conditions like esophageal stricture, web or Schatzki's ring, neoplasm; if solids and liquids, a motility disorder is more likely.

Is there *odynophagia*, or pain on swallowing?

Consider esophageal ulceration from radiation, caustic ingestion, or infection from *Candida, cytomegalovirus, herpes simplex,* or *HIV.* Can be pill-induced (aspirin, nonsteroidal anti-inflammatory agents).

Change in Bowel Function. You will frequently need to assess *bowel function*. Start with open-ended questions: "How are your bowel movements?" "How frequent are they?" "Do you have any difficulties?" "Have you noticed any change?" The range of normal is broad. Current parameters suggest a minimum may be as low as two bowel movements per week.

Some patients may complain of passing excessive gas, or *flatus*, normally about 600 ml per day.

Consider aerophagia, legumes or other gas-producing foods, *intestinal lactase deficiency, irritable bowel syndrome.*

Diarrhea and Constipation. Patients vary widely in their views of diarrhea and constipation. Increased water content of the stool results in *diarrhea*, or stool volume greater than 200 grams in 24 hours. Patients, however, usually focus on the change to loose watery stools or increased frequency.

See Table 11-3, Constipation (p. 457) and Table 11-4, Diarrhea (pp. 458–459).

Ask about the duration. *Acute diarrhea* lasts 2 weeks or fewer. *Chronic diarrhea* is defined as lasting 4 weeks or more.

Acute diarrhea is usually caused by infection;[16] chronic diarrhea is typically noninfectious in origin, as in *Crohn's disease* and *ulcerative colitis.*

Query the characteristics of the diarrhea, including volume, frequency, and consistency.

High-volume, frequent watery stools usually are from the small intestine; small-volume stools with tenesmus, or diarrhea with mucus, pus, or blood occur in rectal inflammatory conditions.

Is there mucus, pus, or blood? Is there associated *tenesmus*, a constant urge to defecate, accompanied by pain, cramping, and involuntary straining?

Does diarrhea occur at night?

Nocturnal diarrhea usually has pathologic significance.

Are the stools greasy or oily? Frothy? Foul-smelling? Floating on the surface because of excessive gas?

Oily residue, sometimes frothy or floating, occurs with *steatorrhea,* or fatty diarrheal stools, from malabsorption in *celiac sprue, pancreatic insufficiency,* and *small bowel bacterial overgrowth.*

Associated features are important in identifying possible causes. Pursue current medications, including alternative medicines and especially antibiotics, recent travel, diet patterns, baseline bowel habits, and risk factors for immunocompromise.

Diarrhea is common with use of penicillins and macrolides, magnesium-based antacids, metformin, and herbal and alternative medicines.

Another common symptom is *constipation*. Recent definitions stipulate that constipation should be present for at least 12 weeks of the prior 6 months with at least two of the following conditions: fewer than 3 bowel movements per week; 25% or more defecations with either straining or sensation of incomplete evacuation; lumpy or hard stools; or manual facilitation.[17]

Ask about frequency of bowel movements, passage of hard or painful stools, straining, and a sense of incomplete rectal emptying or pressure.

Check if the patient actually looks at the stool and can describe its color and bulk.

Thin, pencil-like stool occurs in an obstructing "apple-core" lesion of the sigmoid colon.

What remedies has the patient tried? Do medications or stress play a role? Are there associated systemic disorders?

Consider medications such as anticholinergic agents, calcium-channel blockers, iron supplements, and opiates. Constipation also occurs with *diabetes, hypothyroidism, hypercalcemia, multiple sclerosis, Parkinson's disease,* and *systemic sclerosis.*

Occasionally there is no passage of either feces or gas, or *obstipation*.

Obstipation signifies *intestinal obstruction.*

Inquire about the color of stools. Is there *melena,* or black tarry stools, or *hematochezia,* stools that are red or maroon-colored? Pursue such important details as quantity and frequency of any blood.

See Table 11-5, Black and Bloody Stools, p. 460.

Melena may appear with as little as 100 ml of *upper gastrointestinal bleeding,* hematochezia if more than 1000 ml of blood, usually from *lower gastrointestinal bleeding.*

Is it mixed in with stool or on the surface? Is it streaks on the toilet paper or more copious?

Blood on the surface or toilet paper may occur with *hemorrhoids.*

Jaundice.   In some patients, you will be struck by jaundice or icterus, the yellowish discoloration of the skin and sclerae from increased levels of bilirubin, a bile pigment derived chiefly from the breakdown of hemoglobin. Normally the hepatocytes conjugate, or combine, unconjugated bilirubin with other substances, making the bile water soluble, and then excrete it into the bile. The bile passes through the cystic duct into the common bile duct, which also drains the extrahepatic ducts from the liver. More distally the common bile duct and the pancreatic ducts empty into the duodenum at the ampulla of Vater. Mechanisms of jaundice include the following:

● Increased production of bilirubin

● Decreased uptake of bilirubin by the hepatocytes

● Decreased ability of the liver to conjugate bilirubin

● Decreased excretion of bilirubin into the bile, resulting in absorption of *conjugated* bilirubin back into the blood.

> Predominantly unconjugated bilirubin occurs from the first three mechanisms, as in *hemolytic anemia* (increased production) and *Gilbert's syndrome.*

> Impaired excretion of conjugated bilirubin occurs with *viral hepatitis, cirrhosis, primary biliary cirrhosis,* and drug-induced cholestasis, as from oral contraceptives, methyl testosterone, and chlorpromazine.

Intrahepatic jaundice can be *hepatocellular,* from damage to the hepatocytes, or *cholestatic,* from impaired excretion as a result of damaged hepatocytes or intrahepatic bile ducts. *Extrahepatic* jaundice arises from obstruction of the extrahepatic bile ducts, most commonly the cystic and common bile ducts.

> Gallstones or *pancreatic carcinoma* may obstruct the common bile duct.

As you assess the patient with jaundice, pay special attention to the associated symptoms and the setting in which the illness occurred. What was the *color of the urine* as the patient became ill? When the level of conjugated bilirubin increases in the blood, it may be excreted into the urine, turning the urine a dark yellowish brown or tea color. Unconjugated bilirubin is not water-soluble, so it is not excreted into urine.

> Dark urine from bilirubin indicates impaired excretion of bilirubin into the gastrointestinal tract.

Ask also about the *color of the stools.* When excretion of bile into the intestine is completely obstructed, the stools become gray or light colored, or *acholic,* without bile.

> Acholic stools may occur briefly in *viral hepatitis;* they are common in obstructive jaundice.

Does the skin itch without other obvious explanation? Is there associated pain? What is its pattern? Has it been recurrent in the past?

> Itching indicates cholestatic or obstructive jaundice; pain may signify a distended liver capsule, *biliary cholic,* or *pancreatic cancer.*

Ask about risk factors for liver diseases, such as:

● *Hepatitis:* Travel or meals in areas of poor sanitation, ingestion of contaminated water or foodstuffs (hepatitis A); parenteral or mucous membrane exposure to infectious body fluids such as blood, serum, semen, and saliva, especially through sexual contact with an infected partner or use of shared needles for injection drug use (hepatitis B); intravenous illicit drug use; or blood transfusion (hepatitis C)

● *Alcoholic hepatitis* or *alcoholic cirrhosis* (interview the patient carefully about alcohol use)

● *Toxic liver damage* from medications, industrial solvents, or environmental toxins

● *Gallbladder disease* or *surgery* that may result in extrahepatic biliary obstruction

● *Hereditary disorders* in the Family History

THE URINARY TRACT

General questions for a urinary history include: "Do you have any difficulty passing your urine?" "How often do you go?" "Do you have to get up at night? How often?" "How much urine do you pass at a time?" "Is there any pain or burning?" "Do you ever have trouble getting to the toilet in time?" "Do you ever leak any urine? Or wet yourself involuntarily?" Does the patient sense when the bladder is full and when voiding occurs?

Ask women if sudden coughing, sneezing, or laughing makes them lose urine. Roughly half of young women report this experience even before bearing children. Occasional leakage is not necessarily significant. Ask older men, "Do you have trouble starting your stream?" "Do you have to stand close to the toilet to void?" "Is there a change in the force or size of your stream, or straining to void?" "Do you hesitate or stop in the middle of voiding?" "Is there dribbling when you're through?"

Suprapubic Pain.   Disorders in the urinary tract may cause pain in either the abdomen or the back. Bladder disorders may cause *suprapubic pain*. In *bladder infection*, pain in the lower abdomen is typically dull and pressure-like. In sudden overdistention of the bladder, pain is often agonizing; in contrast, chronic bladder distention is usually painless.

Dysuria, Urgency, or Frequency.   Infection or irritation of either the bladder or urethra often provokes several symptoms. Frequently there is *pain on urination*, usually felt as a burning sensation. Some clinicians refer to this as *dysuria*, whereas others reserve the term *dysuria* for difficulty voiding. Women may report internal urethral discomfort, sometimes described as a pressure or an external burning from the flow of urine across irritated or inflamed labia. Men typically feel a burning sensation proximal to the glans penis. In contrast, *prostatic pain* is felt in the perineum and occasionally in the rectum.

Other associated symptoms are common. Urinary *urgency* is an unusually intense and immediate desire to void, sometimes leading to involuntary voiding or *urge incontinence*. Urinary *frequency*, or abnormally frequent voiding, may occur. Ask about any related fever or chills, blood in the urine, or any pain in the abdomen, flank, or back (see illustration on next page). Men with partial obstruction to urinary outflow often report *hesitancy* in starting the urine stream, *straining to void, reduced caliber and force of the urinary stream*, or *dribbling* as voiding is completed.

See Table 11-6, Frequency, Nocturia, and Polyuria (p. 461).

Involuntary voiding or lack of awareness suggests cognitive or neurosensory deficits.

Stress incontinence arises from decreased intraurethral pressure (see pp. 462–463).

These problems are common in men with partial bladder outlet obstruction from *benign prostatic hyperplasia*; also seen with *urethral stricture.*

Pain of sudden overdistention accompanies acute urinary retention.

Painful urination accompanies *cystitis* or *urethritis.*

If dysuria, consider bladder stones, foreign bodies, tumors; also *acute prostatitis.* In women, internal burning occurs in *urethritis,* and external burning in *vulvovaginitis.*

Urgency suggests bladder infection or irritation. In men, painful urination without frequency or urgency suggests *urethritis.*

See Table 15-2, Abnormalities of the Prostate (pp. 568–569).

Polyuria or Nocturia.   Three additional terms describe important alterations in the pattern of urination. *Polyuria* refers to a significant increase in 24-hour urine volume, roughly defined as exceeding 3 liters. It should be distinguished from urinary frequency, which can involve voiding in high amounts, seen in polyuria, or in small amounts, as in infection. *Nocturia* refers to urinary frequency at night, sometimes defined as awakening the patient more than once; urine volumes may be large or small. Clarify the patient's daily fluid intake. Note any change in nocturnal voiding patterns and the number of trips to the bathroom.

Abnormally high renal production of urine suggests polyuria. Frequency without polyuria during the day or night suggests bladder disorder or impairment to flow at or below the bladder neck.

Urinary Incontinence.   Up to 30% of older patients are concerned about *urinary incontinence*, an involuntary loss of urine that may become socially embarrassing or cause problems with hygiene. If the patient reports incontinence, ask when it happens and how often. Find out if the patient is leaking small amounts of urine with increased intra-abdominal pressure from coughing, sneezing, laughing, or lifting. Or is it difficult for the patient to hold the urine once there is an urge to void, and loss of large amounts of urine? Is there a sensation of bladder fullness, frequent leakage, or voiding of small amounts but difficulty emptying the bladder?

See Table 11-7, Urinary Incontinence (pp. 462–463).

Stress incontinence with increased intra-abdominal pressure suggests decreased contractility of urethral sphincter or poor support of bladder neck; *urge incontinence,* if unable to hold the urine, suggests detrusor overactivity; *overflow incontinence,* when the bladder cannot be emptied until bladder pressure exceeds urethral pressure, indicates anatomical obstruction by prostatic hypertrophy or stricture, or neurogenic abnormalities.

As described earlier, bladder control involves complex neuroregulatory and motor mechanisms (see p. 417). Several central or peripheral nerve lesions may affect normal voiding. Can the patient sense when the bladder is full? And when voiding occurs? Although there are four broad categories of incontinence, a patient may have a combination of causes.

In addition, the patient's functional status may significantly affect voiding behaviors even when the urinary tract is intact. Is the patient mobile? Alert? Able to respond to voiding cues and reach the bathroom? Is alertness or voiding affected by medications?

Functional incontinence may arise from impaired cognition, musculo-skeletal problems, or immobility.

Hematuria.   Blood in the urine, or *hematuria*, is an important cause for concern. When visible to the naked eye, it is called *gross hematuria*. The urine may appear frankly bloody. Blood may be detected only during microscopic urinalysis, known as *microscopic hematuria*. Smaller amounts of blood may tinge the urine with a pinkish or brownish cast. In women, be sure to distinguish menstrual blood from hematuria. If the urine is reddish, ask about ingestion of beets or medications that might discolor the urine. Test the urine with a dipstick and microscopic examination before you settle on the term *hematuria*.

Kidney or Flank Pain; Ureteral Colic.   Disorders of the urinary tract may also cause *kidney pain*, often reported as *flank pain* at or below the posterior costal margin near the costovertebral angle. It may radiate anteriorly toward the umbilicus. Kidney pain is a visceral pain usually produced by distention of the renal capsule and typically dull, aching, and steady. *Ureteral pain* is dramatically different. It is usually severe and colicky, originating at the costovertebral angle and radiating around the trunk into the lower quadrant of the abdomen, or possibly into the upper thigh and testicle or labium. Ureteral pain results from sudden distention of the ureter and associated distention of the renal pelvis. Ask about any associated fever, chills, or hematuria.

Kidney pain, fever, and chills occur in *acute pyelonephritis*.

Renal or ureteral colic is caused by sudden obstruction of a ureter, for example, from urinary stones or blood clots.

Kidney pain

Ureteral pain

HEALTH PROMOTION AND COUNSELING

Important Topics for Health Promotion and Counseling

- Screening for alcohol abuse
- Risk factors for hepatitis A, B, and C
- Screening for colon cancer

Screening for Alcohol Abuse. Alert clinicians often notice clues of unhealthy alcohol use from social patterns and behavioral problems that emerge during the history. The patient may report past episodes of pancreatitis, family history of alcoholism, or arrest for driving under the influence of alcohol. Examination of the abdomen may reveal such classic findings as hepatosplenomegaly, ascites, or even *caput medusa,* a collateral pathway of recanalized umbilical veins radiating up the abdomen that decompresses portal vein hypertension.

Other classic findings include spider angiomas, palmar erythema, and peripheral edema.

Alcohol abuse or dependence is on the rise, affecting 8.5% of the U.S. population, or 17.6 million people.[18] Lifetime prevalence is approximately 13.5%, and in emergency rooms and trauma admissions, prevalence reaches 30% to 40% and 50% respectively.[19,20] The addictions are increasingly viewed as chronic relapsing behavioral disorders with substance-induced rearrangements of brain neurotransmitters resulting in tolerance, physical dependence, sensitization, craving, and relapse (see p. 144). Alcohol addiction has numerous sequelae and is highly correlated with fatal car accidents, suicide and other mental health disorders, family disruption, violence, hypertension, cirrhosis, and malignancies of the upper gastrointestinal tract and liver.

See Chapter 5, Behavior and Mental Status, pp. 143–144.

Because early at-risk behaviors may be hard to identify, knowledge of basic alcohol screening criteria is critical. The U.S. Preventive Services Task Force recommends screening and behavioral counseling interventions for all adults in primary care settings, including pregnant women.[21] If your patient drinks alcoholic beverages, choose one of three well-validated screening tools: the CAGE questionnaire, the Alcohol Use Disorders Identification Test (AUDIT), or the screening question about heavy drinking days, "How many times in the past year have you had 4 or more drinks a day (women) or 5 or more drinks a day (men)?" Cutoffs for risky or hazardous drinking are:

See the four CAGE questions, Chapter 3, Interviewing and the Health History, p. 84.

● Women: ≥3 drinks per occasion and ≥7 drinks per week

● Men: ≥4 drinks per occasion and ≥14 drinks per week

Tailor your recommendations for treatment to the severity of the problem, ranging from brief interventions to inpatient detoxification to long-term rehabilitation (see Chapter 5, Behavior and Mental Status, p. 144).

Risk Factors for Hepatitis A, B, and C. The mainstay for protecting adults against viral hepatitis is adherence to vaccination guidelines for hepatitis A and hepatitis B, the most effective method for preventing infection and transmission. Educating patients about how the hepatitis viruses spread and the benefits of vaccination for groups at risk is also important.

Hepatitis A.   Transmission of hepatitis A is fecal:oral: fecal shedding by those handling food causes contamination of water and foods, leading to infection for those in close contact in households and extended family settings. Infected children are often asymptomatic and play a key role in spreading infection. In 2006 the CDC recommended hepatitis A vaccination for children and for persons at increased risk for infection, such as travelers to endemic areas, male–male partners, injection and illicit drug users, and persons with chronic liver disease. For immediate protection and prophylaxis for household contacts and travelers, immune serum globulin can be administered before and within 2 weeks of contact with hepatitis A. Advise handwashing with soap and water before bathroom use, changing diapers, and preparing and eating food.[22,23]

Hepatitis B.   Hepatitis B poses more serious threats to patient health. Approximately 95% of infections in healthy adults are self-limited, with elimination of the virus from blood and development of immunity.[24] Chronic infection occurs in 5% of those older than 5 years, and approximately 15% of those infected after childhood die prematurely from cirrhosis or liver cancer. Most (approximately 70%) are asymptomatic until they develop advanced liver disease. The Centers for Disease Control and Prevention has identified three risk categories:

● *Sexual contacts,* including sex partners for those already infected, people with more than one sex partner in the prior 6 months, people seeking evaluation and treatment for sexually transmitted diseases, and men having sex with men

● *People with percutaneous or mucosal exposure to blood,* including injection drug users, household contacts of antigen-positive persons, residents and staff of facilities for the developmentally disabled, health-care workers, and people on dialysis

● *Other,* including travelers to endemic areas, people with chronic liver disease and HIV infection, and people seeking protection from hepatitis B infection

The Centers for Disease Control and Prevention issued new recommendations for expanded hepatitis B immunization in 2006.[24] The following groups should receive vaccination:

● All adults in high-risk settings, such as STD clinics, HIV testing and treatment programs, drug-abuse treatment programs and programs for injection drug users, correctional facilities, programs for men having sex with men, chronic hemodialysis facilities and end-stage renal disease programs, and facilities for people with developmental disabilities

● In primary care and specialty settings, adults in at-risk groups or requesting the hepatitis B vaccine even without acknowledging a specific risk factor

● Adults in occupations involving exposure to blood or other potentially infectious body fluids

The U.S. Preventive Services Task Force recommends screening for all pregnant women at their first prenatal visit.[22]

Hepatitis C.   Hepatitis C is transmitted by repeated percutaneous exposure to blood and is present in approximately 2% of U.S. adults. However, prevalence reaches 50% to 90% in groups at high risk.[22] The strongest risk factors are injection drug use and transfusion with clotting factors before 1987. Additional risk factors include hemodialysis, sex partners using injection drugs, blood transfusion or organ transplant before 1992, undiagnosed liver disease, infants born to infected mothers, occupational exposure, and multiple sex partners or an infected sex partner. Sexual transmission is rare. Chronic infection occurs in 55% to 85% of those infected; chronic liver disease occurs in 70% of those with chronic infections.[25] There is no vaccine for prevention, so screening for risk factors and referral of those infected, plus counseling to avoid risk factors, including tattoos, are critical.

Screening for Colorectal Cancer.   Colorectal cancer is the third most common cancer in both men and women and accounts for almost 10% of all cancer deaths.[26] More than 90% of cases occur after age 50, primarily from neoplastic changes in adenomatous polyps. Mortality rates are declining, reflecting improvements in early detection and treatment. Recent evidence has prompted revision of screening guidelines by multi-society task forces, including the American Cancer Society in both 2003 and 2006, placing new emphasis on risk stratification, use of colonoscopy, and post-polypectomy management.[27,28]

- *Assessing risk status.* Clinicians should assess risk status when patients are around age 20 by asking the questions below. If 50 years or older, patients answering no to these three questions are at *average risk;* if younger than 50 years, no screening is indicated. A positive response warrants screening for increased or high colorectal cancer risk and referral for more complex patient management.[27,28]

  - Has the patient had colorectal cancer or an adenomatous polyp?

  - Does the patient have an illness such as inflammatory bowel disease that increases risk for colorectal cancer?

  - Has a family member had colorectal cancer or an adenomatous polyp? If so, how many, at what age, and was it a first-degree relative (parent, sibling, or child)?

- *Screening for people at average risk.* Because no one screening option is clearly superior, beginning at age 50 average-risk patients should be offered one of the following five options:

  - Fecal occult blood test (FOBT) annually, using six samples and tested without rehydration. Single samples have a sensitivity for detecting advanced neoplasia of approximately 5%, compared with approximately 24% using six samples, so a single-sample office test is not sufficient.[29,30] Aggressive follow-up with colonoscopy is recommended for a positive test on any specimen.

  - Flexible sigmoidoscopy every 5 years

  - Combined FOBT and flexible sigmoidoscopy

  - Colonoscopy every 10 years

  - Double-contrast barium enema every 5 years

- *Screening for people at increased risk.* Colonoscopy at the intervals noted below is indicated for the following increased risk factors:

  - Single small adenoma (<1 cm): 3 to 6 years after initial polypectomy

  - Single large adenoma (>1 cm), multiple adenomas, adenoma with high-grade dysplasia or villous change: within 3 years of initial polypectomy

  - History of resection of colorectal cancer: within 1 year after resection

  - Any first-degree relative younger than 60 years, two or more first-degree relatives with either colorectal cancer or adenomatous polyps: at age 40 or 10 years before youngest case in immediate family, whichever is earlier. Approximately 15% of those with colorectal cancer have familial disease.[31]

- *Screening for people at high risk.* High-risk factors include family history of familial adenomatous polyposis (found in ~1% of colorectal cancers);

family history of hereditary nonpolyposis colon cancer (in approximately 3% to 4%); and history of inflammatory bowel disease, chronic ulcerative colitis, or Crohn's disease. Referral, genetic testing, and early surveillance are recommended in these groups.[28,31,32]

Other Risk Factors for Colorectal Cancer.   Some studies show possible increased risk from diabetes (approximately 30% increase), alcohol use, obesity, smoking, and high-fat diet. Some evidence suggests that several factors may be protective: diet high in fruits and vegetables; diet high in fiber; regular physical activity; and use of aspirin or nonsteroidal anti-inflammatory agents (NSAIDs). Study findings remain conflicting about the benefits of high-fiber and low-fat high fruit and vegetable diets.[33,34] The U.S. Preventive Services Task Force recommends *against* routine use of aspirin and NSAIDs to prevent colorectal cancer in average-risk people because of poor-quality evidence that these agents lead to a reduction in colorectal cancer mortality and good evidence of increased incidence of gastrointestinal bleeding and renal impairment.[35]

TECHNIQUES OF EXAMINATION

For a skilled abdominal examination, you need good light and a relaxed and well-draped patient, with exposure of the abdomen from just above the xiphoid process to the symphysis pubis. The groin should be visible. The genitalia should remain draped. The abdominal muscles should be relaxed to enhance all aspects of the examination, but especially palpation.

Tips for Enhancing Examination of the Abdomen

- Check that the patient has an empty bladder.
- Make the patient comfortable in the supine position, with a pillow under the head and perhaps another under the knees. Slide your hand under the low back to see if the patient is relaxed and lying flat on the table.
- Ask the patient to keep the arms at the sides or folded across the chest. If the arms are above the head, the abdominal wall stretches and tightens, making palpation difficult. Move the gown to below the nipple line, and the drape to the level of the symphysis pubis.
- Before you begin palpation, ask the patient to point to any areas of pain so you can examine these areas last.
- Warm your hands and stethoscope. To warm your hands, rub them together or place them under hot water. You can also palpate through the patient's gown to absorb warmth from the patient's body before exposing the abdomen.
- Approach the patient calmly and avoid quick, unexpected movements. *Watch the patient's face for any signs of pain or discomfort.* Make sure you avoid long fingernails.
- Distract the patient if necessary with conversation or questions. If the patient is frightened or ticklish, begin palpation with the patient's hand under yours. After a few moments, slip your hand underneath to palpate directly.

An arched back thrusts the abdomen forward and tightens the abdominal muscles.

Visualize each organ in the region you are examining. Stand at the patient's right side and proceed in an orderly fashion with inspection, auscultation, percussion, and palpation. Assess the liver, spleen, kidneys, and aorta.

THE ABDOMEN

Inspection

Starting from your usual standing position at the right side of the bed, inspect the abdomen. As you look at the contour of the abdomen, watch for peristalsis. It is helpful to sit or bend down so that you can view the abdomen tangentially.

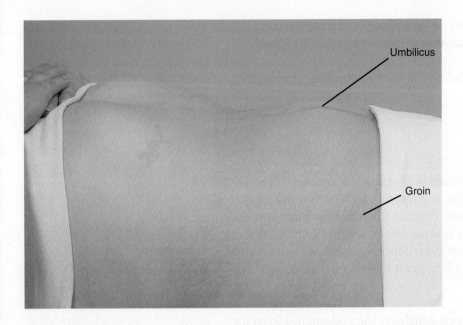

Inspect the surface, contours, and movements of the abdomen, including the following:

- *The skin.* Note:

    Scars. Describe or diagram their location.

    Striae. Old silver striae or stretch marks are normal.

    Pink–purple striae of *Cushing's syndrome*

    Dilated veins. A few small veins may be visible normally.

    Dilated veins of *hepatic cirrhosis* or of *inferior vena cava obstruction*

    Rashes and lesions

- *The umbilicus.* Observe its contour and location and any inflammation or bulges suggesting a hernia.

    See Table 11-8, Localized Bulges in the Abdominal Wall (p. 464).

- *The contour of the abdomen*

    Is it flat, rounded, protuberant, or scaphoid (markedly concave or hollowed)?

    See Table 11-9, Protuberant Abdomens (p. 465).

    Do the flanks bulge, or are there any local bulges? Also survey the inguinal and femoral areas.

    Bulging flanks of *ascites*; suprapubic bulge of a distended bladder or pregnant uterus; hernias

    Is the abdomen symmetric?

    Asymmetry from an enlarged organ or mass

    Are there visible organs or masses? Look for an enlarged liver or spleen that has descended below the rib cage.

    Lower abdominal mass of an ovarian or a uterine tumor

- *Peristalsis.* Observe for several minutes if you suspect intestinal obstruction. Peristalsis may be visible normally in very thin people.

Increased peristaltic waves of *intestinal obstruction*

- *Pulsations.* The normal aortic pulsation is frequently visible in the epigastrium.

Increased pulsation of an *aortic aneurysm* or of *increased pulse pressure*

Auscultation

Auscultation provides important information about bowel motility. *Listen to the abdomen before performing percussion or palpation because these maneuvers may alter the frequency of bowel sounds.* Practice auscultation until you are thoroughly familiar with variations in normal bowel sounds and can detect changes suggestive of inflammation or obstruction. Auscultation may also reveal *bruits,* or vascular sounds resembling heart murmurs, over the aorta or other arteries in the abdomen.

See Table 11-10, Sounds in the Abdomen (p. 466).
Bruits suggest vascular occlusive disease.

Place the diaphragm of your stethoscope gently on the abdomen. Listen for bowel sounds and note their frequency and character. Normal sounds consist of clicks and gurgles, occurring at an estimated frequency of 5 to 34 per minute. Occasionally you may hear *borborygmi*—prolonged gurgles of hyperperistalsis—the familiar "stomach growling." Because bowel sounds are widely transmitted through the abdomen, listening in one spot, such as the right lower quadrant, is usually sufficient.

Bowel sounds may be altered in diarrhea, intestinal obstruction, *paralytic ileus,* and *peritonitis.*

Abdominal Bruits and Friction Rub. If the patient has high blood pressure, listen in the epigastrium and in each upper quadrant for *bruits.* Later in the examination, when the patient sits up, listen also in the costovertebral angles. Epigastric bruits confined to systole may be heard normally.

A bruit in one of these areas that has both systolic and diastolic components strongly suggests *renal artery stenosis* as the cause of hypertension.

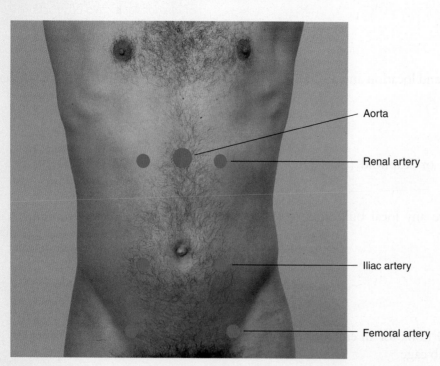

Aorta

Renal artery

Iliac artery

Femoral artery

Listen for bruits over the aorta, the iliac arteries, and the femoral arteries. Bruits confined to systole are relatively common, however, and do not necessarily signify occlusive disease.

Listening points for bruits in these vessels are illustrated on the previous page.

Listen over the liver and spleen for *friction rubs*.

Bruits with both systolic and diastolic components suggest the turbulent blood flow of *partial arterial occlusion* or *arterial insufficiency*.

Friction rubs in liver tumor, gonococcal infection around the liver, splenic infarction

Percussion

Percussion helps you to assess the amount and distribution of gas in the abdomen and to identify possible masses that are solid or fluid-filled. Its use in estimating the size of the liver and spleen will be described in later sections.

Percuss the abdomen lightly in all four quadrants to assess the distribution of *tympany* and *dullness*. Tympany usually predominates because of gas in the gastrointestinal tract, but scattered areas of dullness from fluid and feces are also typical.

A protuberant abdomen that is tympanitic throughout suggests *intestinal obstruction*. See Table 11-9, Protuberant Abdomens (p. 465).

- Note any large dull areas that might indicate an underlying mass or enlarged organ. This observation will guide your palpation.

Pregnant uterus, ovarian tumor, distended bladder, large liver or spleen

- On each side of a protuberant abdomen, note where abdominal tympany changes to the dullness of solid posterior structures.

Dullness in both flanks prompts further assessment for ascites (see pp. 448–449).

Briefly percuss the lower anterior chest, between the lungs above and costal margins below. On the right, you will usually find the dullness of the liver; on the left, the tympany that overlies the gastric air bubble and the splenic flexure of the colon.

In *situs inversus* (rare), organs are reversed: air bubble on the right, liver dullness on the left.

Palpation

Light Palpation. Feeling the abdomen gently is especially helpful for identifying abdominal tenderness, muscular resistance, and some superficial organs and masses. It also serves to reassure and relax the patient.

Keeping your hand and forearm on a horizontal plane, with fingers together and flat on the abdominal surface, palpate the abdomen with a light, gentle, dipping motion. When moving your hand from place to place, raise it just off the skin. Moving smoothly, feel in all quadrants.

Identify any superficial organs or masses and any area of tenderness or increased resistance to your hand. If resistance is present, try to distinguish voluntary guarding from involuntary muscular spasm. To do this:

● Try all the relaxing methods you know (see p. 434).

(see p. 434)

Involuntary rigidity (muscular spasm) typically persists despite these maneuvers. It indicates *peritoneal inflammation.*

● Feel for the relaxation of abdominal muscles that normally accompanies exhalation.

● Ask the patient to mouth-breathe with the jaw dropped open.

Voluntary guarding usually decreases with these maneuvers.

Deep Palpation.   This is usually required to delineate abdominal masses. Again using the palmar surfaces of your fingers, feel in all four quadrants. Identify any masses and note their location, size, shape, consistency, tenderness, pulsations, and any mobility with respiration or with the examining hand. Correlate your palpable findings with their percussion notes.

Abdominal masses may be categorized in several ways: physiologic (pregnant uterus), inflammatory (*diverticulitis* of the colon), vascular (an abdominal aortic aneurysm), neoplastic (carcinoma of the colon), or obstructive (a distended bladder or dilated loop of bowel).

Assessment for Peritoneal Inflammation.   Abdominal pain and tenderness, especially when associated with muscular spasm, suggest inflammation of the parietal peritoneum. Localize the pain as accurately as possible. First, even before palpation, *ask the patient to cough* and determine where the cough produces pain. Then, *palpate gently with one finger* to map the tender area. Pain produced by light percussion has similar localizing value. These gentle maneuvers may be all you need to establish an area of peritoneal inflammation.

Abdominal pain with coughing or light percussion suggests peritoneal inflammation. See Table 11-11, Tender Abdomens (pp. 467–468).

TWO-HANDED DEEP PALPATION

If not, look for *rebound tenderness*. Press down with your fingers firmly and slowly, then withdraw them quickly. Watch and listen to the patient for signs of pain. Ask the patient "Which hurts more, when I press or let go?" Have the patient locate the pain exactly. Pain induced or increased by quick withdrawal constitutes *rebound tenderness* caused by rapid movement of an inflamed peritoneum.

Rebound tenderness suggests peritoneal inflammation. If tenderness is felt elsewhere than where you were trying to elicit rebound, that area may be the real source of the problem.

 ## THE LIVER

Because the rib cage shelters most of the liver, assessment is difficult. Liver size and shape can be estimated by percussion and perhaps palpation, however, and the palpating hand helps you to evaluate its surface, consistency, and tenderness.

Percussion

Measure the vertical span of liver dullness in the right midclavicular line. Locate the midclavicular line carefully to avoid inaccurate measurement from use of a "wandering landmark." Use a light to moderate percussion stroke, because examiners with a heavier stroke underestimate liver size.[36] Starting at a level below the umbilicus (in an area of tympany, not dullness), percuss upward toward the liver. Identify the *lower border of dullness* in the midclavicular line.

Next, identify the *upper border of liver dullness* in the midclavicular line. Starting at the nipple line, lightly percuss from lung resonance down toward liver dullness. Gently displace a woman's breast as necessary to be sure that you start in a resonant area. The course of percussion is shown next.

The span of liver dullness is *increased* when the liver is enlarged.

PERCUSSING LIVER SPAN

The span of liver dullness is *decreased* when the liver is small, or when free air is present below the diaphragm, as from a *perforated hollow viscus*. Serial observations may show a decreasing span of dullness with resolution of *hepatitis* or *congestive heart failure* or, less commonly, with progression of *fulminant hepatitis*.

Liver dullness may be displaced downward by the low diaphragm of *chronic obstructive pulmonary disease*. Span, however, remains normal.

Now measure in centimeters the distance between your two points—the vertical span of liver dullness. Normal liver spans, shown below, are generally greater in men than in women and greater in tall people than in short people. If the liver seems to be enlarged, outline the lower edge by percussing in other areas.

4–8 cm in midsternal line

6–12 cm in right midclavicular line

NORMAL LIVER SPANS

Dullness of a right pleural effusion or consolidated lung, if adjacent to liver dullness, may falsely *increase* the estimate of liver size.

Gas in the colon may produce tympany in the right upper quadrant, obscure liver dullness, and falsely *decrease* the estimate of liver size.

Measurements of liver span by percussion are more accurate when the liver is enlarged with a palpable edge.[37]

Only about half of livers with an edge below the right costal margin are palpable, but when the edge is palpable, the likelihood of hepatomegaly roughly doubles.[36]

Palpation

Place your left hand behind the patient, parallel to and supporting the right 11th and 12th ribs and adjacent soft tissues below. Remind the patient to relax on your hand if necessary. By pressing your left hand forward, the patient's liver may be felt more easily by your other hand.

Place your right hand on the patient's right abdomen lateral to the rectus muscle, with your fingertips well below the lower border of liver dullness. Some examiners like to point their fingers up toward the patient's head, whereas others prefer a somewhat more oblique position, as shown on the next page. In either case, press gently in and up.

Ask the patient to take a deep breath. Try to feel the liver edge as it comes down to meet your fingertips. If you feel it, lighten the pressure of your palpating hand slightly so that the liver can slip under your finger pads and you can feel its anterior surface. Note any tenderness. If palpable at all, the normal liver edge is soft, sharp, and regular, with a smooth surface. The normal liver may be slightly tender.

Firmness or hardness of the liver, bluntness or rounding of its edge, and irregularity of its contour suggest an abnormality of the liver.

On inspiration, the liver is palpable about 3 cm below the right costal margin in the midclavicular line. Some people breathe more with the chest than with the diaphragm. It may be helpful to train such a patient to "breathe with the abdomen," thus bringing the liver, as well as the spleen and kidneys, into a palpable position during inspiration.

An obstructed, distended gallbladder may form an oval mass below the edge of the liver and merge with it. It is dull to percussion.

In order to feel the liver, you may have to alter your pressure according to the thickness and resistance of the abdominal wall. If you cannot feel it, move your palpating hand closer to the costal margin and try again.

Try to trace the liver edge both laterally and medially. Palpation through the rectus muscles, however, is especially difficult. Describe or sketch the liver edge, and measure its distance from the right costal margin in the midclavicular line.

The "hooking technique" may be helpful, especially when the patient is obese. Stand to the right of the patient's chest. Place both hands, side by side, on the right abdomen below the border of liver dullness. Press in with your fingers and up toward the costal margin. Ask the patient to take a deep breath. The liver edge shown below is palpable with the fingerpads of both hands.

The edge of an enlarged liver may be missed by starting palpation too high in the abdomen, as shown above.

See Table 11-12, Liver Enlargement: Apparent and Real (p. 469).

Assessing Percussion Tenderness of a Nonpalpable Liver. Place your left hand flat on the lower right rib cage and then gently strike your hand with the ulnar surface of your right fist. Ask the patient to compare the sensation with that produced by a similar strike on the left side.

Tenderness over the liver suggests inflammation, as in *hepatitis*, or congestion, as in *heart failure*.

 THE SPLEEN

When a spleen enlarges, it expands anteriorly, downward, and medially, often replacing the tympany of stomach and colon with the dullness of a solid organ. It then becomes palpable below the costal margin. Percussion suggests but does not confirm splenic enlargement. Palpation can confirm the enlargement but often misses large spleens that do not descend below the costal margin.

Percussion

Two techniques may help you to detect *splenomegaly,* an enlarged spleen:

- *Percuss the left lower anterior chest wall* between lung resonance above and the costal margin, an area termed *Traube's space.* As you percuss along the routes suggested by the arrows in the following figures, note the lateral extent of tympany. Percussion is moderately accurate in detecting splenomegaly (sensitivity, 60%–80%; specificity, 72%–94%).[38]

If percussion dullness is present, palpation correctly detects presence or absence of splenomegaly more than 80% of the time.[38]

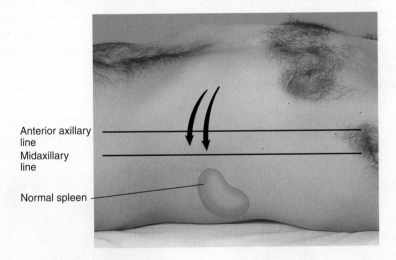

Anterior axillary line
Midaxillary line
Normal spleen

If tympany is prominent, especially laterally, splenomegaly is not likely. The dullness of a normal spleen is usually hidden within the dullness of other posterior tissues.

Fluid or solids in the stomach or colon may also cause dullness in Traube's space.

- *Check for a splenic percussion sign.* Percuss the lowest interspace in the left anterior axillary line, as shown next. This area is usually tympanitic. Then ask the patient to take a deep breath, and percuss again. When spleen size is normal, the percussion note usually remains tympanitic.

A change in percussion note from tympany to dullness on inspiration suggests splenic enlargement. This is a *positive splenic percussion sign.*

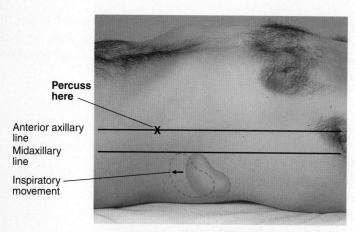

Percuss here

Anterior axillary line

Midaxillary line

Inspiratory movement

NEGATIVE SPLENIC PERCUSSION SIGN

POSITIVE SPLENIC PERCUSSION SIGN

If either or both of these tests is positive, pay extra attention to palpation of the spleen.

The splenic percussion sign may also be positive when spleen size is normal.

Palpation

With your left hand, reach over and around the patient to support and press forward the lower left rib cage and adjacent soft tissue. With your right hand below the left costal margin, press in toward the spleen. Begin palpation low enough so that you are below a possibly enlarged spleen. (If your hand is close to the costal margin, moreover, it is not sufficiently mobile to reach up under the rib cage.) Ask the patient to take a deep breath. Try to feel the tip or edge of the spleen as it comes down to meet your fingertips. Note any tenderness, assess the splenic contour, and measure the distance between the spleen's lowest point and the left costal margin. In approximately 5% of normal adults, the tip of the spleen is palpable. Causes include a low, flat diaphragm, as in chronic obstructive pulmonary disease, and a deep inspiratory descent of the diaphragm.

An enlarged spleen may be missed if the examiner starts too high in the abdomen to feel the lower edge.

Splenomegaly is eight times more likely when the spleen is palpable.[36] Causes include portal hypertension, hematologic malignancies, HIV infection, and splenic infarct or hematoma.

The spleen tip below is just palpable deep to the left costal margin.

Repeat with the patient lying on the right side with legs somewhat flexed at hips and knees. In this position, gravity may bring the spleen forward and to the right into a palpable location.

The enlarged spleen is palpable about 2 cm below the left costal margin on deep inspiration.

Umbilicus

PALPATING THE SPLEEN—PATIENT LYING ON RIGHT SIDE

THE KIDNEYS

Palpation

Although kidneys are not usually palpable, you should learn and practice the techniques for examination. Detecting an enlarged kidney may prove to be very important.

Palpation of the Left Kidney. Move to the patient's left side. Place your right hand behind the patient, just below and parallel to the 12th rib, with your fingertips just reaching the costovertebral angle. Lift, trying to displace the kidney anteriorly. Place your left hand gently in the left upper quadrant, lateral and parallel to the rectus muscle. Ask the patient to take a deep breath. At the peak of inspiration, press your left hand firmly and deeply into the left upper quadrant, just below the costal margin, and try to "capture" the kidney between your two hands. Ask the patient to breathe out and then to stop breathing briefly. Slowly release the pressure of your left hand, feeling at the same time for the kidney to slide back into its expiratory position. If the kidney is palpable, describe its size, contour, and any tenderness.

Alternatively, try to feel for the left kidney by a method similar to feeling for the spleen. With your left hand, reach over and around the patient to lift the left loin, and with your right hand feel deep in the left upper quadrant. Ask the patient to take a deep breath, and feel for a mass. A normal left kidney is rarely palpable.

A left flank mass may represent marked *splenomegaly* or an enlarged left kidney. Suspect *splenomegaly* if a notch is palpated on medial border, the edge extends beyond the midline, percussion is dull, and your fingers can probe deep to the medial and lateral borders but *not* between the mass and the costal margin. Confirm findings with further evaluation.

Attributes favoring an *enlarged kidney* over an enlarged spleen include preservation of normal tympany in the left upper quadrant and the ability to probe with your fingers between the mass and the costal margin, but not deep to its medial and lower borders.

Palpation of the Right Kidney. To capture the right kidney, return to the patient's right side. Use your left hand to lift from in back, and your right hand to feel deep in the left upper quadrant. Proceed as before.

A normal right kidney may be palpable, especially in thin, well-relaxed women. It may or may not be slightly tender. The patient is usually aware of a capture and release. Occasionally, a right kidney is located more anteriorly than usual and then must be distinguished from the liver. The edge of the liver, if palpable, tends to be sharper and to extend farther medially and laterally. It cannot be captured. The lower pole of the kidney is rounded.

Causes of kidney enlargement include hydronephrosis, cysts, and tumors. Bilateral enlargement suggests *polycystic kidney disease.*

Assessing Percussion Tenderness of the Kidneys. You may note tenderness when examining the abdomen, but also search for it at each costovertebral angle. Pressure from your fingertips may be enough to elicit tenderness, but if not, use fist percussion. Place the ball of one hand in the costovertebral angle and strike it with the ulnar surface of your fist. Use enough force to cause a perceptible but painless jar or thud in a normal person.

To save the patient needless exertion, integrate this assessment with your examination of the back (see p. 20).

Pain with pressure or fist percussion suggests *pyelonephritis* but may also have a musculoskeletal cause.

ASSESSING COSTOVERTEBRAL ANGLE TENDERNESS

THE BLADDER

The bladder normally cannot be examined unless it is distended above the symphysis pubis. On palpation, the dome of the distended bladder feels smooth and round. Check for tenderness. Use percussion to check for dullness and to determine how high the bladder rises above the symphysis pubis.

Bladder distention from outlet obstruction due to *urethral stricture, prostatic hyperplasia;* also from medications and neurologic disorders such as *stroke, multiple sclerosis.*

Suprapubic tenderness in *bladder infection*

THE AORTA

Press firmly deep in the upper abdomen, slightly to the left of the midline, and identify the aortic pulsations. In people older than age 50, assess the width of the aorta by pressing deeply in the upper abdomen with one hand on each side of the aorta, as illustrated. In this age group, a normal aorta is not more than 3.0 cm wide (average, 2.5 cm). This measurement does not include the thickness of the abdominal wall. The ease of feeling aortic pulsations varies greatly with the thickness of the abdominal wall and with the anteroposterior diameter of the abdomen.

Risk factors for abdominal aortic aneurysm (AAA) are age 65 years or older, history of smoking, male gender, and a first-degree relative with a history of AAA repair.[39,40]

A periumbilical or upper abdominal mass with expansile pulsations that is 3 cm or more wide suggests an AAA. Sensitivity of palpation increases as AAAs enlarge: for widths of 3.0–3.9 cm, 29%; 4.0–4.9 cm, 50%; ≥5.0 cm, 76%.[41]

Screening by palpation followed by ultrasound decreases mortality, especially in male smokers 65 years or older. Pain may signal rupture. Rupture is 15 times more likely in AAAs >4 cm than in smaller aneurysms.[41]

SPECIAL TECHNIQUES

Assessment Techniques for:

- Ascites
- Appendicitis
- Acute cholecystitis
- Ventral hernia
- Mass in abdominal wall

Assessing Possible Ascites

A protuberant abdomen with bulging flanks suggests the possibility of ascitic fluid. Because ascitic fluid characteristically sinks with gravity, whereas gas-filled loops of bowel float to the top, percussion gives a dull note in dependent areas of the abdomen. Look for such a pattern by percussing outward in several directions from the central area of tympany. Map the border between tympany and dullness.

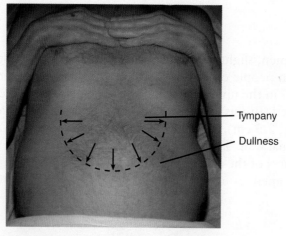

Ascites from increased hydrostatic pressure in cirrhosis, congestive heart failure, constrictive pericarditis, or inferior vena cava or hepatic vein obstruction; from decreased osmotic pressure in nephrotic syndrome, malnutrition. Also in ovarian cancer.

Two additional techniques help to confirm ascites, although both signs may be misleading.

- *Test for shifting dullness.* After mapping the borders of tympany and dullness, ask the patient to turn onto one side. Percuss and mark the borders again. In a person without ascites, the borders between tympany and dullness usually stay relatively constant.

In ascites, dullness shifts to the more dependent side, whereas tympany shifts to the top.

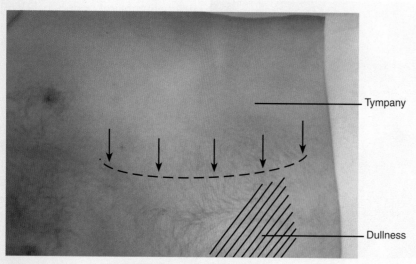

PATIENT LYING ON RIGHT SIDE

● *Test for a fluid wave.* Ask the patient or an assistant to press the edges of both hands firmly down the midline of the abdomen. This pressure helps to stop the transmission of a wave through fat. While you tap one flank sharply with your fingertips, feel on the opposite flank for an impulse transmitted through the fluid. Unfortunately, this sign is often negative until ascites is obvious, and it is sometimes positive in people without ascites.

An easily palpable impulse suggests ascites. A positive fluid wave, shifting dullness, and peripheral edema make the diagnosis of ascites highly likely (likelihood ratios of 3.0–6.0).[42]

Identifying an Organ or a Mass in an Ascitic Abdomen.
Try to *ballotte* the organ or mass, exemplified here by an enlarged liver. Straighten and stiffen the fingers of one hand together, place them on the abdominal surface, and make a brief jabbing movement directly toward the anticipated structure. This quick movement often displaces the fluid so that your fingertips can briefly touch the surface of the structure through the abdominal wall.

Assessing Possible Appendicitis

● Ask the patient to point to where the pain began and where it is now. Ask the patient to cough. Determine whether and where pain results.

The pain of *appendicitis* classically begins near the umbilicus, then shifts to the right lower quadrant, where coughing increases it. Older patients report this pattern less frequently than younger ones.[14]

● Search carefully for an area of local tenderness.

Localized tenderness anywhere in the right lower quadrant, even in the right flank, may indicate *appendicitis*.

● Feel for muscular rigidity.

Early voluntary guarding may be replaced by involuntary muscular rigidity.

● *Perform a rectal examination and, in women, a pelvic examination.* These maneuvers may not help you to discriminate between a normal and an inflamed appendix, but they may help to identify an inflamed appendix atypically located within the pelvic cavity. They may also suggest other causes of the abdominal pain.

Right-sided rectal tenderness may also be caused by an inflamed adnexa or an inflamed seminal vesicle.

Additional techniques are sometimes helpful:

● Check the tender area for rebound tenderness. (If other signs are typically positive, you can save the patient unnecessary pain by omitting this test.)

Rebound tenderness suggests peritoneal inflammation, if *appendicitis*.

● Check for *Rovsing's sign* and for referred rebound tenderness. Press deeply and evenly in the *left* lower quadrant. Then quickly withdraw your fingers.

Pain in the *right* lower quadrant during *left*-sided pressure suggests *appendicitis* (a positive Rovsing's sign). So does right lower quadrant pain on quick withdrawal (*referred rebound tenderness*).

● Look for a *psoas sign*. Place your hand just above the patient's right knee and ask the patient to raise that thigh against your hand. Alternatively, ask the patient to turn onto the left side. Then extend the patient's right leg at the hip. Flexion of the leg at the hip makes the psoas muscle contract; extension stretches it.

Increased abdominal pain on either maneuver constitutes a *positive psoas sign,* suggesting irritation of the psoas muscle by an inflamed appendix.

● Look for an *obturator sign*. Flex the patient's right thigh at the hip, with the knee bent, and rotate the leg internally at the hip. This maneuver stretches the internal obturator muscle. (Internal rotation of the hip is described on p. 624.)

Right hypogastric pain constitutes a *positive obturator sign,* suggesting irritation of the obturator muscle by an inflamed appendix.

● Test for *cutaneous hyperesthesia*. At a series of points down the abdominal wall, gently pick up a fold of skin between your thumb and index finger, without pinching it. This maneuver should not normally be painful.

Localized pain with this maneuver, in all or part of the right lower quadrant, may accompany *appendicitis*.

Assessing Possible Acute Cholecystitis

When right upper quadrant pain and tenderness suggest acute cholecystitis, look for *Murphy's sign*. Hook your left thumb or the fingers of your right hand under the costal margin at the point where the lateral border of the rectus muscle intersects with the costal margin. Alternatively, if the liver is enlarged, hook your thumb or fingers under the liver edge at a comparable point below. Ask the patient to take a deep breath. Watch the patient's breathing and note the degree of tenderness.

A sharp increase in tenderness with a sudden stop in inspiratory effort constitutes a *positive Murphy's sign* of *acute cholecystitis.* Hepatic tenderness may also increase with this maneuver but is usually less well localized.

Assessing Ventral Hernias

Ventral hernias are hernias in the abdominal wall exclusive of groin hernias. If you suspect but do not see an umbilical or incisional hernia, ask the patient to raise both head and shoulders off the table.

The bulge of a hernia will usually appear with this action (see p. 511).

Inguinal and femoral hernias are discussed in Chapter 13, Male Genitalia and Hernias. They can give rise to important abdominal problems and must not be overlooked.

The cause of intestinal obstruction or peritonitis may be missed by overlooking a strangulated femoral hernia.

Mass in the Abdominal Wall

Distinguishing an Abdominal Mass From a Mass in the Abdominal Wall.
An occasional mass is in the abdominal wall rather than inside the abdominal cavity. Ask the patient either to raise the head and shoulders or to strain down, thus tightening the abdominal muscles. Feel for the mass again.

A mass in the abdominal wall remains palpable; an intra-abdominal mass is obscured by muscular contraction.

RECORDING YOUR FINDINGS

Note that initially you may use sentences to describe your findings; later you will use phrases. The style below contains phrases appropriate for most write-ups.

Recording the Physical Examination—The Abdomen

"Abdomen is protuberant with active bowel sounds. It is soft and non-tender; no palpable masses or hepatosplenomegaly. Liver span is 7 cm in the right midclavicular line; edge is smooth and palpable 1 cm below the right costal margin. Spleen and kidneys not felt. No costovertebral angle (CVA) tenderness."

OR

"Abdomen is flat. No bowel sounds heard. It is firm and boardlike, with increased tenderness, guarding, and rebound in the right midquadrant. Liver percusses to 7 cm in the midclavicular line; edge not felt. Spleen and kidneys not felt. No palpable masses. No CVA tenderness.

Suggests peritonitis from possible *appendicitis* (see p. 450 and pp. 450–458)

BIBLIOGRAPHY

CITATIONS

1. Hing E, Cherry DK, Woodwell DA. National ambulatory medical care survey: 2004 summary. Advance Data from Vital and Health Statistics 374. June 23, 2006. Centers for Disease Control and Prevention. Available at: http://www.cdc.gov/nchs/data/ad/ad374.pdf. Accessed September 23, 2007.

2. McCaig LF, Burt CW. National hospital ambulatory medical care survey: 2003 emergency department summary. Advance Data from Vital and Health Statistics 358. May 26, 2005. Centers for Disease Control and Prevention. Available at: http://www.cdc.gov/nchs/data/ad/ad358.pdf. Accessed September 23, 2007.

3. Talley NJ, Vakil NB, Moayyedi P, et al. American Gastroenterological Association technical review on the evaluation of dyspepsia. Gastroenterology 129(5):1756–1780, 2005.

4. Drossman DA. The functional gastrointestinal disorders and the Rome III process. Gastroenterology 130(5):1377–1390, 2007.

5. Ranji SR, Goldman LE, Simel DL, et al. Do opiates affect the clinical evaluation of patients with acute abdominal pain? JAMA 296(14):1764–1774, 2006.

6. Whitcomb DC. Acute pancreatitis. N Engl J Med 354(20):2142–2150, 2006.

7. Trowbridge RL, Rutkowshi NK, Shojania KG. Does this patient have acute cholecystitis? JAMA 289(1):80–86, 2003.

8. Talley NJ, Vakil N. Practice guidelines: guidelines for management of dyspepsia. Am J Gastroenterol 100(10):2324–2337, 2005.

9. DeVault KR, Castell DO. Updated guidelines for the diagnosis and treatment of gastroesophageal reflux disease. Am J Gastroenterol 100(1):190–200, 2005.

10. Vaezi MF, Hicks DM, Abelson TI, et al. Laryngeal signs and symptoms and gastroesophageal reflux disease (GERD): a critical assessment of cause and effect association. Gastroenterol Hepatol 1(5):333–344, 2003.

11. Talley NJ. American Gastroenterological Association medical position statement: evaluation of dyspepsia. Gastroenterology 129(5):1753–1755, 2005.

12. Shaheen N, Ransohoff DF. Gastroesophageal reflux, Barrett esophagus, and esophageal cancer. Scientific review. JAMA 287(15):1972–1981, 2002.

13. Moayyedi P, Talley NJ, Fennerty MB, et al. Can the clinical history distinguish between organic and functional dyspepsia? JAMA 295(13):1566–1576, 2006.

14. Paulson EK, Kalady MF, Pappas TN. Suspected appendicitis. N Engl J Med 348(3):236–242, 2003.

15. Horwitz BJ, Fisher RS. The irritable bowel syndrome. N Engl J Med 344(24):1846–1850, 2001.

16. Theilman NM, Guerrant RL. Acute infectious diarrhea. N Engl J Med 350(1):38–46, 2004.

17. Longstreth GF, Thompson WG, Chey WD, et al. Functional bowel disorders. Gastroenterology 130(5):1480–1491, 2006. Available at: http://www.romecriteria.org/pdfs/p1480FBDs.pdf. Accessed October 5, 2007.

18. Grant BF, Dawson DA, Stinson FS, et al. The 12-month prevalence and trends in DSM-IV alcohol abuse and dependence: United States, 1991–1992 and 2001–2002. Drug and Alcohol Dependence 74(3):223–234, 2004.

19. Regier DA, Farmer ME, Rae DS, et al. Comorbidity of mental disorders with alcohol and other drug abuse: results from the Epidemiologic Catchment Study. JAMA 264(19):2511–2518, 1990.

20. Saitz R. Unhealthy alcohol use. N Engl J Med 352(6):596–607, 2005.

21. U.S. Preventive Services Task Force. Screening and Behavioral Counseling Interventions in Primary Care to Reduce Alcohol Misuse: Recommendation Statement. Rockville, MD, Agency for Healthcare Research and Quality, April 2004. Updated in Guide to Clinical Preventive Services, 2006. Available at: http://www.ahrq.gov/clinic/pocketgd/gcps2c.htm#Alcohol. Accessed September 6, 2007.

22. U.S. Preventive Services Task Force. Screening for hepatitis B infection; Screening for hepatitis C in adults. Guide to Clinical Preventive Services, 2006. Available at: http://www.ahrq.gov/clinic/pocketgd/gcps2b.htm#HepB. Accessed October 14, 2007.

23. Fiore AF, Wasley A, Bell BP. Recommendations of the Advisory Committee on Immunization Practices: prevention of hepatitis A through active or passive immunization. MMWR Morb Mortal Wkly Rep 55(RR07):1–23, 2006. Available at: http://www.cdc.gov/mmwr/preview/mmwrhtml/rr5507a1.htm. Accessed October 14, 2007.

24. Mast E, Weinbaum CM, Fiore AE, et al. Recommendations of the Advisory Committee on Immunization Practices. Part II: Immunization of adults. A comprehensive immunization strategy to eliminate transmission of hepatitis B virus infection in the United States. MMWR Morb Mortal Wkly Rep 55(RR16):1–25, 2006. Available at: http://www.cdc.gov/mmwr/preview/mmwrhtml/rr5516a1.htm?s_cid=rr5516a1_e. Accessed October 14, 2007.

25. Centers for Disease Control and Prevention. National Center for HIV/AIDS, Viral Hepatitis, STD, and TB Prevention. Hepatitis C Fact Sheet. May 24, 2005. Available at: http://www.cdc.gov/ncidod/diseases/hepatitis/c/fact.htm. Accessed October 14, 2007.

26. American Cancer Society. Cancer Facts and Figures 2007. Atlanta, National Home Office. Available at: http://www.cancer.org/downloads/STT/CAFF2007PWSecured.pdf. Accessed October 14, 2007.

27. Winawer S, Fletcher R, Rex D, et al. Gastrointestinal Consortium Panel. Colorectal cancer screening and surveillance: clinical guidelines and rationale. Update based on new evidence. Gastroenterology 124(2):544–560, 2003.

28. Winawer S, Zauber A, Fletcher RH, et al. Guidelines for colonoscopy surveillance after polypectomy: a consensus update by the US Multi-Society Task Force on Colorectal Cancer and the American Cancer Society. Gastroenterology 130(6):1872–1885, 2006.

29. Collins JF, Leiberman DA, Dirbom TE, et al. Accuracy of screening for fecal occult blood on a single stool sample obtained by digital rectal examination: a comparison with

recommended sampling practice. Ann Intern Med 142(2): 81–85, 2005.

30. Boolchand V, Olds G, Singh J, et al. Colorectal screening after polypectomy: a national survey study of primary care physicians. Ann Intern Med 145(9):654–659, 2006.

31. American Cancer Society. What are the risk factors for colorectal cancer? Available at: http://www.cancer.org/docroot/CRI/content/CRI_2_4_2X_What_are_the_risk_factors_for_colon_and_rectum_cancer.asp?sitearea=CRI&viewmode=print&. Accessed October 14, 2007.

32. American Cancer Society. Can colorectal polyps and cancer be found early? Available at: http://www.cancer.org/docroot/CRI/content/CRI_2_4_3X_Can_colon_and_rectum_cancer_be_found_early.asp. Accessed October 14, 2007.

33. Schatzkin A, Lanza E, Corle D, et al. Lack of effect of a low-fat, high-fiber diet on the recurrence of colorectal adenomas. N Engl J Med 342(16):1149–1155, 2000.

34. Alberts DS, Martinez ME, Roe DJ, et al. Lack of effect of a high-fiber cereal supplement on the recurrence of colorectal adenomas. N Engl J Med 342(16):1156–1162, 2000.

35. U.S. Preventive Services Task Force. Routine aspirin or non-steroidal anti-inflammatory drugs for the primary prevention of colorectal cancer: U.S. Preventive Services Task Force Recommendation Statement. Ann Intern Med 146(5):361–364, 2007.

36. McGee S. Chapter 47, Palpation and percussion of the abdomen; Chapter 48, Abdominal pain and tenderness. In Evidence-Based Physical Diagnosis. St. Louis, Saunders, 2007, pp. 553–555, 572–582.

37. Naylor CD. Physical examination of the liver. JAMA 271(23): 1857–1859, 1994.

38. Grover SA, Barkun AN, Sackett DL. Does this patient have splenomegaly? JAMA 270(18):2218–2221, 1993.

39. U.S. Preventive Services Task Force. Screening for abdominal aortic aneurysm: recommendation statement. Ann Intern Med 142(3):198–202, 2005.

40. Birkmeyer JD, Upchurch GR. Evidence-based screening and management of abdominal aortic aneurysm (editorial). Ann Intern Med 146(10): 749–750, 2007.

41. Lederle FA, Simel DL. Does this patient have abdominal aortic aneurysm? JAMA 281(1):77–82, 1999.

42. Williams JW, Simel DL. Does this patient have ascites? How to divine fluid in the abdomen. JAMA 267(19):2645–2648, 1992.

ADDITIONAL REFERENCES

Examination of the Abdomen

Fink HA, Lederle FA, Rptj CS. The accuracy of physical examination to detect abdominal aortic aneurysm. Arch Intern Med 160(6):833–836, 2000.

Kim LG, Scott AP, Ashton HA, et al. A sustained mortality benefit from screening for abdominal aortic aneurysm. Ann Intern Med 146(10): 696–706, 2007.

McGee SR. Percussion and physical diagnosis: separating myth from science. Dis Mon 41(10):641–688, 1995.

Silen W, Cope Z. Cope's Early Diagnosis of the Acute Abdomen, 21st ed. Oxford, UK, and New York, Oxford University Press, 2005.

Sleisenger MH, Feldman M, Griedman LS, et al (eds). Sleisenger and Fortran's Gastrointestinal and Liver Disease: Pathophysiology, Diagnosis, Management, 8th ed. Philadelphia, WB Saunders, 2006.

Turnbull JM. Is listening for abdominal bruits useful in the evaluation of hypertension? JAMA 274(16):1299–1301, 1995.

Yamamoto W, Kono H, Maekawa H, et al. The relationship between abdominal pain regions and specific diseases: an epidemiologic approach to clinical practice. J Epidemiol 7(1):27–32, 1997.

Examination of the Liver

Meidl EJ, Ende J. Evaluation of liver size by physical examination. J Gen Intern Med 8(11):635–637, 1993.

Zoli M, Magliotti D, Drimaldi M, et al. Physical examination of the liver: is it still worth it? Am J Gastroenterol 90(9):1428–1432, 1995.

Examination of the Spleen

Barkun ANB, Camus M, Green L, et al. The bedside assessment of splenic enlargement. Am J Med 91(5):512–518, 1991.

Barkun AN, Camus M, Meagher T, et al. Splenic enlargement and Traube's space: how useful is percussion? Am J Med 87(5): 562–566, 1989.

Tamayo SG, Rickman LS, Matthews WC, et al. Examiner dependence on physical diagnostic tests of splenomegaly: a prospective study with multiple observers. J Gen Intern Med 8(2):69–75, 1993.

Gastrointestinal Conditions

American Gastroenterological Association. American Gastroenterological Association Medical Position Statement: guidelines on constipation. Gastroenterology 119(6):1761–1778, 2000.

Bak E, Raman G, Chung M, et al. Effectiveness of management strategies for renal artery stenosis: a systematic review. Ann Intern Med 145(12):901–912, 2006.

Craig AS, Schaffner W. Prevention of hepatitis A with the hepatitis A vaccine. N Engl J Med 350(5):476–480, 2004.

Lembo A, Camilleri M. Chronic constipation. N Engl J Med 349(14):1360–1368, 2003.

Mertz HR. Irritable bowel syndrome. N Engl J Med 349(22): 2136–2146, 2003.

Ouslander JG. Management of the overactive bladder. N Engl J Med 350(8):786–799, 2004.

Shaheen N, Ransohoff DF. Gastroesophageal reflux, Barrett esophagus, and esophageal cancer: clinical applications. JAMA 287(15): 1982–1986, 2002.

Thielman NM, Guerrant RL. Acute infectious diarrhea. N Engl J Med 350(1):38–47, 2004.

> **The Bates' suite offers these additional resources to enhance learning and facilitate understanding of this chapter:**
>
> - Bates' Pocket Guide to Physical Examination and History Taking, 6th edition
> - Bates' Nursing Online
> - Bates' Visual Guide to Physical Examination, 4th edition
> - thePoint online resources, http://thepoint.lww.com
> - Student CD-ROM included with the book

Abdominal Pain

Problem	Process	Location	Quality
Peptic Ulcer and Dyspepsia[3,4]	Peptic ulcer refers to a demonstrable ulcer, usually in the duodenum or stomach. Dyspepsia causes similar symptoms but no ulceration. Infection by *Helicobacter pylori* is often present.	Epigastric, may radiate to the back	Variable: gnawing burning, boring, aching, pressing, or hungerlike
Cancer of the Stomach	Predominantly adenocarcinoma (90%–95%)	Increasingly in 'cardia' and GE junction; also in distal stomach	Variable
Acute Pancreatitis[6]	An acute inflammation of the pancreas	Epigastric, may radiate to the back or other parts of the abdomen; may be poorly localized	Usually steady
Chronic Pancreatitis	Fibrosis of the pancreas secondary to recurrent inflammation	Epigastric, radiating through to the back	Steady, deep
Cancer of the Pancreas	Predominantly adenocarcinoma (95%)	Epigastric and in either upper quadrant; often radiates to the back	Steady, deep
Biliary Colic	Sudden obstruction of the cystic duct or common bile duct by a gallstone	Epigastric or right upper quadrant; may radiate to the right scapula and shoulder	Steady, aching; *not* colicky
Acute Cholecystitis[7]	Inflammation of the gallbladder, usually from obstruction of the cystic duct by a gallstone	Right upper quadrant or upper abdominal; may radiate to the right scapular area	Steady, aching
Acute Diverticulitis	Acute inflammation of a colonic diverticulum, a saclike mucosal outpouching through the colonic muscle	Left lower quadrant	May be cramping at first, but becomes steady
Acute Appendicitis[14]	Acute inflammation of the appendix with distention or obstruction	• Poorly localized *periumbilical pain*, followed usually by • *Right lower quadrant pain*	• Mild but increasing, possibly cramping • Steady and more severe
Acute Mechanical Intestinal Obstruction	Obstruction of the bowel lumen, most commonly caused by (1) adhesions or hernias (small bowel), or (2) cancer or diverticulitis (colon)	• *Small bowel:* periumbilical or upper abdominal • *Colon:* lower abdominal or generalized	• Cramping • Cramping
Mesenteric Ischemia	Blood supply to the bowel and mesentery blocked from thrombosis or embolus (acute arterial occlusion), or reduced from hypoperfusion	May be periumbilical at first, then diffuse	Cramping at first, then steady

Timing	Factors That May Aggravate	Factors That May Relieve	Associated Symptoms and Setting
Intermittent. Duodenal ulcer is more likely than gastric ulcer or dyspepsia to cause pain that (1) wakes the patient at night, and (2) occurs intermittently over a few weeks, then disappears for months, and then recurs.	Variable	Food and antacids may bring relief, but not necessarily in any of these disorders and least commonly in gastric ulcer.	Nausea, vomiting, belching, bloating; heartburn (more common in duodenal ulcer); weight loss (more common in gastric ulcer). Dyspepsia is more common in the young (20–29 yrs), gastric ulcer in those over 50 yrs, and duodenal ulcer in those 30–60 yrs.
The history of pain is typically shorter than in peptic ulcer. The pain is persistent and slowly progressive.	Often food	*Not* relieved by food or antacids	Anorexia, nausea, early satiety, weight loss, and sometimes bleeding. Most common in ages 50–70
Acute onset, persistent pain	Lying supine	Leaning forward with trunk flexed	Nausea, vomiting, abdominal distention, fever. Often a history of previous attacks and alcohol abuse or gallstones
Chronic or recurrent course	Alcohol, heavy or fatty meals	Possibly leaning forward with trunk flexed; often intractable	Symptoms of decreased pancreatic function may appear: diarrhea with fatty stools (steatorrhea) and diabetes mellitus.
Persistent pain; relentlessly progressive illness		Possibly leaning forward with trunk flexed; often intractable	Anorexia, nausea, vomiting, weight loss, and jaundice; depression
Rapid onset over a few minutes, lasts one to several hours and subsides gradually. Often recurrent			Anorexia, nausea, vomiting, restlessness
Gradual onset; course longer than in biliary colic	Jarring, deep breathing		Anorexia, nausea, vomiting, fever
Often a gradual onset			Fever, constipation. There may be initial brief diarrhea.
• Lasts roughly 4–6 hours			Anorexia, nausea, possibly vomiting, which typically follow the onset of pain; low fever
• Depends on intervention	• Movement or cough	• If it subsides temporarily, suspect perforation of the appendix.	
• Paroxysmal; may decrease as bowel mobility is impaired			• Vomiting of bile and mucus (high obstruction) or fecal material (low obstruction). Obstipation develops.
• Paroxysmal, though typically milder			• Obstipation early. Vomiting late if at all. Prior symptoms of underlying cause.
Usually abrupt in onset, then persistent			Vomiting, diarrhea (sometimes bloody), constipation, shock

Process and Problem	Timing	Factors That Aggravate	Factors That Relieve	Associated Symptoms and Conditions
Oropharyngeal Dysphagia, *due to motor disorders affecting the pharyngeal muscles*	Acute or gradual onset and a variable course, depending on the underlying disorder	Attempts to start the swallowing process		Aspiration into the lungs or regurgitation into the nose with attempts to swallow. Neurologic evidence of stroke, bulbar palsy, or other neuromuscular conditions
Esophageal Dysphagia *Mechanical Narrowing*				
• Mucosal rings and webs	Intermittent	Solid foods	Regurgitation of the bolus of food	Usually none
• Esophageal stricture	Intermittent; may become slowly progressive	Solid foods	Regurgitation of the bolus of food	A long history of heartburn and regurgitation
• Esophageal cancer	May be intermittent at first; progressive over months	Solid foods, with progression to liquids	Regurgitation of the bolus of food	Pain in the chest and back and weight loss, especially late in the course of illness
Motor Disorders				
• Diffuse esophageal spasm	Intermittent	Solids or liquids	Maneuvers described below; sometimes nitroglycerin	Chest pain that mimics angina pectoris or myocardial infarction and lasts minutes to hours; possibly heartburn
• Scleroderma	Intermittent; may progress slowly	Solids or liquids	Repeated swallowing; movements such as straightening the back, raising the arms, or a Valsalva maneuver (straining down against a closed glottis)	Heartburn; other manifestations of scleroderma
• Achalasia	Intermittent; may progress	Solids or liquids		Regurgitation, often at night when lying down, with nocturnal cough; possibly chest pain precipitated by eating

TABLE
11-3

Constipation

Problem	Process	Associated Symptoms and Setting
Life Activities and Habits *Inadequate Time or Setting for the Defecation Reflex*	Ignoring the sensation of a full rectum inhibits the defecation reflex.	Hectic schedules, unfamiliar surroundings, bed rest
False Expectations of Bowel Habits	Expectations of "regularity" or more frequent stools than a person's norm	Beliefs, treatments, and advertisements that promote the use of laxatives
Diet Deficient in Fiber	Decreased fecal bulk	Other factors such as debilitation and constipating drugs may contribute.
Irritable Bowel Syndrome[15]	Change in frequency or form of bowel movement without structural or chemical abnormality	Small, hard stools, often with mucus; periods of diarrhea; intermittent pain for 12 weeks of preceding 12 months, relieved by defecation; stress may aggravate.
Mechanical Obstruction *Cancer of the Rectum or Sigmoid Colon*	Progressive narrowing of the bowel lumen	Change in bowel habits; often diarrhea, abdominal pain, and bleeding. In rectal cancer, tenesmus and pencil-shaped stools
Fecal Impaction	A large, firm, immovable fecal mass, most often in the rectum	Rectal fullness, abdominal pain, and diarrhea around the impaction; common in debilitated, bedridden, and often elderly patients
Other Obstructing Lesions (such as diverticulitis, volvulus, intussusception, or hernia)	Narrowing or complete obstruction of the bowel	Colicky abdominal pain, abdominal distention, and in intussusception, often "currant jelly" stools (red blood and mucus)
Painful Anal Lesions	Pain may cause spasm of the external sphincter and voluntary inhibition of the defecation reflex.	Anal fissures, painful hemorrhoids, perirectal abscesses
Drugs	A variety of mechanisms	Opiates, anticholinergics, antacids containing calcium or aluminum, and many others
Depression	A disorder of mood. See Table 5-2, Disorders of Mood.	Fatigue, anhedonia, sleep disturbance, weight loss
Neurologic Disorders	Interference with the autonomic innervation of the bowel	Spinal cord injuries, multiple sclerosis, Hirschsprung's disease, and other conditions
Metabolic Conditions	Interference with bowel motility	Pregnancy, hypothyroidism, hypercalcemia

Problem	Process	Characteristics of Stool
Acute Diarrhea[16]		
Secretory Infection	Infection by viruses, preformed bacterial toxins (such as *Staphylococcus aureus, Clostridium perfringens,* toxigenic *Escherichia coli, Vibrio cholerae*), cryptosporidium, *Giardia lamblia*	Watery, without blood, pus, or mucus
Inflammatory Infection	Colonization or invasion of intestinal mucosa (nontyphoid *Salmonella, Shigella, Yersinia, Campylobacter,* enteropathic *E. coli, Entamoeba histolytica*)	Loose to watery, often with blood, pus, or mucus
Drug-Induced Diarrhea	Action of many drugs, such as magnesium-containing antacids, antibiotics, antineoplastic agents, and laxatives	Loose to watery
Chronic Diarrhea		
Diarrheal Syndrome		
• Irritable bowel syndrome[15]	Change in frequency and form of bowel movements without chemical or structural abnormality	Loose; may show mucus but no blood. Small, hard stools with constipation
• Cancer of the sigmoid colon	Partial obstruction by a malignant neoplasm	May be blood-streaked
Inflammatory Bowel Disease		
• Ulcerative colitis	Inflammation of the mucosa and submucosa of the rectum and colon with ulceration; typically extends proximally from the rectum	Soft to watery, often containing blood
• Crohn's disease of the small bowel (regional enteritis) or colon (granulomatous colitis)	Chronic transmural inflammation of the bowel wall, in a skip pattern typically involving the terminal ileum and/or proximal colon	Small, soft to loose or watery, usually free of gross blood (enteritis) or with less bleeding than ulcerative colitis (colitis)
Voluminous Diarrhea		
• Malabsorption syndrome	Defective absorption of fat, including fat-soluble vitamins, with steatorrhea (excessive excretion of fat) as in pancreatic insufficiency, bile salt deficiency, bacterial overgrowth	Typically bulky, soft, light yellow to gray, mushy, greasy or oily, and sometimes frothy; particularly foul-smelling; usually floats in the toilet
• Osmotic diarrhea		
Lactose intolerance	Deficiency in intestinal lactase	Watery diarrhea of large volume
Abuse of osmotic purgatives	Laxative habit, often surreptitious	Watery diarrhea of large volume
• Secretory diarrhea from bacterial infection, secreting villous adenoma, fat or bile salt malabsorption, hormone-mediated conditions (gastrin in Zollinger–Ellison syndrome, vasoactive intestinal peptide)	Variable	Watery diarrhea of large volume

Timing	Associated Symptoms	Setting, Persons at Risk
Duration of a few days, possibly longer. Lactase deficiency may lead to a longer course.	Nausea, vomiting, periumbilical cramping pain. Temperature normal or slightly elevated	Often travel, a common food source, or an epidemic
An acute illness of varying duration	Lower abdominal cramping pain and often rectal urgency, tenesmus; fever	Travel, contaminated food or water. Men and women who have had frequent anal intercourse
Acute, recurrent, or chronic	Possibly nausea; usually little if any pain	Prescribed or over-the-counter medications
Often worse in the morning Diarrhea rarely wakes the patient at night.	Crampy lower abdominal pain, abdominal distention, flatulence, nausea, constipation	Young and middle-aged adults, especially women
Variable	Change in usual bowel habits, crampy lower abdominal pain, constipation	Middle-aged and older adults, especially older than 55 yrs
Onset ranges from insidious to acute. Typically recurrent; may be persistent. Diarrhea may wake the patient at night.	Crampy lower or generalized abdominal pain, anorexia, weakness; fever if severe. May include episcleritis, uveitis, arthritis, erythema nodosum.	Often young people. Increases risk of colon cancer.
Insidious onset; chronic or recurrent. Diarrhea may wake the patient at night.	Crampy periumbilical or right lower quadrant (enteritis) or diffuse (colitis) pain, with anorexia, low fever, and/or weight loss. Perianal or perirectal abscesses and fistulas. May cause small or large bowel obstruction	Often young people, especially in late teens, but also in middle age. More common in people of Jewish descent. Increases risk of colon cancer
Onset of illness typically insidious	Anorexia, weight loss, fatigue, abdominal distention, often crampy lower abdominal pain. Symptoms of nutritional deficiencies such as bleeding (vitamin K), bone pain and fractures (vitamin D), glossitis (vitamin B), and edema (protein)	Variable, depending on cause
Follows the ingestion of milk and milk products; relieved by fasting	Crampy abdominal pain, abdominal distention, flatulence	In >50% of African-Americans, Asians, Native Americans, Hispanics; in 5%–20% of Caucasians
Variable	Often none	Persons with anorexia nervosa or bulimia nervosa
Variable	Weight loss, dehydration, nausea, vomiting, and cramping abdominal pain	Variable depending on cause

| TABLE
11-5

Black and Bloody Stools

Problem	Selected Causes	Associated Symptoms and Setting
Melena Refers to passage of black, tarry (sticky and shiny) stools. Tests for occult blood are positive. Involves loss of at least 60 ml of blood into the gastrointestinal tract (less in infants and children), usually from the esophagus, stomach, or duodenum. Less commonly, when intestinal transit is slow, blood may originate in the jejunum, ileum, or ascending colon. In infants, melena may result from swallowing blood during the birth process.	Peptic ulcer	Often, but not necessarily, a history of epigastric pain
	Gastritis or stress ulcers	Recent ingestion of alcohol, aspirin, or other anti-inflammatory drugs; recent bodily trauma, severe burns, surgery, or increased intracranial pressure
	Esophageal or gastric varices	Cirrhosis of the liver or other cause of portal hypertension
	Reflux esophagitis	History of heartburn
	Mallory-Weiss tear, a mucosal tear in the esophagus due to retching and vomiting	Retching, vomiting, often recent ingestion of alcohol
Black, Nonsticky Stools May result from other causes, then give negative results when tested for occult blood. (Ingestion of iron or other substances, however, may cause a positive test result in the absence of blood.) These stools have no pathologic significance.	Ingestion of iron, bismuth salts as in Pepto-Bismol, licorice, or even commercial chocolate cookies	
Red Blood in the Stools Usually originates in the colon, rectum, or anus, and much less frequently in the jejunum or ileum. Upper gastrointestinal hemorrhage may also cause red stools. The amount of blood lost is then usually large (more than a liter). Rapid transit time through the intestinal tract leaves insufficient time for the blood to turn black.	Cancer of the colon	Often a change in bowel habits
	Benign polyps of the colon	Often no other symptoms
	Diverticula of the colon	Often no other symptoms
	Inflammatory conditions of the colon and rectum	
	• Ulcerative colitis, Crohn's disease	See Table 11-4, Diarrhea.
	• Infectious diarrhea	See Table 11-4, Diarrhea.
	• Proctitis (various causes) from frequent anal intercourse	Rectal urgency, tenesmus
	Ischemic colitis	Lower abdominal pain, sometimes fever or shock in older adults. Abdomen typically soft to palpation
	Hemorrhoids	Blood on the toilet paper, on the surface of the stool, or dripping into the toilet
	Anal fissure	Blood on the toilet paper or on the surface of the stool; anal pain
Reddish but Nonbloody Stools	Ingestion of beets	Pink urine, which usually precedes the reddish stool

TABLE
11-6

Frequency, Nocturia, and Polyuria

Problem	Mechanisms	Selected Causes	Associated Symptoms
Frequency	Decreased capacity of the bladder		
	• Increased bladder sensitivity to stretch because of inflammation	*Infection*, stones, tumor, or foreign body in the bladder	Burning on urination, urinary urgency, sometimes gross hematuria
	• Decreased elasticity of the bladder wall	Infiltration by scar tissue or tumor	Symptoms of associated inflammation (see above) are common.
	• Decreased cortical inhibition of bladder contractions	Motor disorders of the central nervous system, such as a stroke	Urinary urgency; neurologic symptoms such as weakness and paralysis
	Impaired emptying of the bladder, with residual urine in the bladder		
	• Partial mechanical obstruction of the bladder neck or proximal urethra	Most commonly, benign prostatic hyperplasia; also urethral stricture and other obstructive lesions of the bladder or prostate	Prior obstructive symptoms: hesitancy in starting the urinary stream, straining to void, reduced size and force of the stream, and dribbling during or at the end of urination
	• Loss of peripheral nerve supply to the bladder	Neurologic disease affecting the sacral nerves or nerve roots, e.g., diabetic neuropathy	Weakness or sensory defects
Nocturia			
With High Volumes	Most types of polyuria (see p. 428)		
	Decreased concentrating ability of the kidney with loss of the normal decrease in nocturnal urinary output	Chronic renal insufficiency due to a number of diseases	Possibly other symptoms of renal insufficiency
	Excessive fluid intake before bedtime	Habit, especially involving alcohol and coffee	
	Fluid-retaining, edematous states Dependent edema accumulates during the day and is excreted when the patient lies down at night.	Congestive heart failure, nephrotic syndrome, hepatic cirrhosis with ascites, chronic venous insufficiency	Edema and other symptoms of the underlying disorder. Urinary output during the day may be reduced as fluid reaccumulates in the body. See Table 12-5, Peripheral Causes of Edema.
With Low Volumes	Frequency Voiding while up at night without a real urge, a "pseudo-frequency"	Insomnia	Variable
Polyuria	Deficiency of antidiuretic hormone (diabetes insipidus)	A disorder of the posterior pituitary and hypothalamus	Thirst and polydipsia, often severe and persistent; nocturia
	Renal unresponsiveness to antidiuretic hormone (nephrogenic diabetes insipidus)	A number of kidney diseases, including hypercalcemic and hypokalemic nephropathy; drug toxicity, e.g., from lithium	Thirst and polydipsia, often severe and persistent; nocturia
	Solute diuresis		
	• Electrolytes, such as sodium salts	Large saline infusions, potent diuretics, certain kidney diseases	Variable
	• Nonelectrolytes, such as glucose	Uncontrolled diabetes mellitus	Thirst, polydipsia, and nocturia
	Excessive water intake	Primary polydipsia	Polydipsia tends to be episodic. Thirst may not be present. Nocturia is usually absent.

TABLE
11-7

Urinary Incontinence*

Problem	Mechanisms
Stress Incontinence The urethral sphincter is weakened so that transient increases in intra-abdominal pressure raise the bladder pressure to levels that exceed urethral resistance.	In women, often a weakness of the pelvic floor with inadequate muscular support of the bladder and proximal urethra and a change in the angle between the bladder and the urethra. Causes include childbirth and surgery. Local conditions affecting the internal urethral sphincter, such as postmenopausal atrophy of the mucosa and urethral infection, may also contribute. In men, stress incontinence may follow prostatic surgery.
Urge Incontinence Detrusor contractions are stronger than normal and overcome the normal urethral resistance. The bladder is typically *small*.	• Decreased cortical inhibition of detrusor contractions from strokes, brain tumors, dementia, and lesions of the spinal cord above the sacral level • Hyperexcitability of sensory pathways, as in bladder infections, tumors, and fecal impaction • Deconditioning of voiding reflexes, as in frequent voluntary voiding at low bladder volumes
Overflow Incontinence Detrusor contractions are insufficient to overcome urethral resistance. The bladder is typically *large*, even after an effort to void.	• Obstruction of the bladder outlet, as in benign prostatic hyperplasia or tumor • Weakness of the detrusor muscle associated with peripheral nerve disease at the sacral level • Impaired bladder sensation that interrupts the reflex arc, as from diabetic neuropathy
Functional Incontinence This is a functional inability to get to the toilet in time because of impaired health or environmental conditions.	Problems in mobility resulting from weakness, arthritis, poor vision, or other conditions. Environmental factors such as an unfamiliar setting, distant bathroom facilities, bed rails, or physical restraints
Incontinence Secondary to Medications Drugs may contribute to any type of incontinence listed.	Sedatives, tranquilizers, anticholinergics, sympathetic blockers, and potent diuretics

*Patients may have more than one kind of incontinence.

Symptoms	Physical Signs
Momentary leakage of small amounts of urine with coughing, laughing, and sneezing while the person is in an upright position. A desire to urinate is not associated with pure stress incontinence.	The bladder is not detected on abdominal examination. Stress incontinence may be demonstrable, especially if the patient is examined before voiding and in a standing position. Atrophic vaginitis may be evident.
Incontinence preceded by an urge to void. The volume tends to be moderate. Urgency Frequency and nocturia with small to moderate volumes If acute inflammation is present, pain on urination Possibly "pseudo-stress incontinence"—voiding 10–20 sec after stresses such as a change of position, going up or down stairs, and possibly coughing, laughing, or sneezing	The bladder is not detectable on abdominal examination. When cortical inhibition is decreased, mental deficits or motor signs of central nervous system disease are often, though not necessarily, present. When sensory pathways are hyperexcitable, signs of local pelvic problems or a fecal impaction may be present.
A continuous dripping or dribbling incontinence Decreased force of the urinary stream Prior symptoms of partial urinary obstruction or other symptoms of peripheral nerve disease may be present.	An enlarged bladder is often found on abdominal examination and may be tender. Other signs include prostatic enlargement, motor signs of peripheral nerve disease, a decrease in sensation (including perineal sensation), and diminished to absent reflexes.
Incontinence on the way to the toilet or only in the early morning	The bladder is not detectable on physical examination. Look for physical or environmental clues to the likely cause.
Variable. A careful history and chart review are important.	Variable

Localized bulges in the abdominal wall include *ventral hernias* (defects in the wall through which tissue protrudes) and subcutaneous tumors such as *lipomas*. The more common ventral hernias are umbilical, incisional, and epigastric. Hernias and a rectus diastasis usually become more evident when the patient raises head and shoulders from a supine position.

INFANT

Umbilical Hernia

A protrusion through a defective umbilical ring is most common in infants but also occurs in adults. In infants, but not in adults, it usually closes spontaneously within 1 to 2 years.

Diastasis Recti

Separation of the two rectus abdominis muscles, through which abdominal contents form a midline ridge when the patient raises head and shoulders. Often seen in repeated pregnancies, obesity, and chronic lung disease. It has no clinical consequences.

Ridge

Incisional Hernia

This is a protrusion through an operative scar. Palpate to detect the length and width of the defect in the abdominal wall. A small defect, through which a large hernia has passed, has a greater risk for complications than a large defect.

Epigastric Hernia

A small midline protrusion through a defect in the linea alba occurs between the xiphoid process and the umbilicus. With the patient's head and shoulders raised (or with the patient standing), run your fingerpad down the linea alba to feel it.

Lipoma

Common, benign, fatty tumors usually in the subcutaneous tissues almost anywhere in the body, including the abdominal wall. Small or large, they are usually soft and often lobulated. Press your finger down on the edge of a lipoma. The tumor typically slips out from under it.

TABLE
11-9

Protuberant Abdomens

Fat

Fat is the most common cause of a protuberant abdomen. Fat thickens the abdominal wall, the mesentery, and omentum. The umbilicus may appear sunken. A *pannus*, or apron of fatty tissue, may extend below the inguinal ligaments. Lift it to look for inflammation in the skin folds or even for a hidden hernia.

Gas

Gaseous distention may be localized or generalized. It causes a tympanitic percussion note. Increased intestinal gas production from certain foods may cause mild distention. More serious are intestinal obstruction and adynamic (paralytic) ileus. Note the location of the distention. Distention becomes more marked in colonic than in small bowel obstruction.

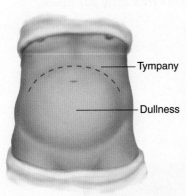

Tympany

Dullness

Tumor

A large, solid tumor, usually rising out of the pelvis, is dull to percussion. Air-filled bowel is displaced to the periphery. Causes include ovarian tumors and uterine myomata. Occasionally a markedly distended bladder may be mistaken for such a tumor.

Tympany

Dullness

Pregnancy

Pregnancy is a common cause of a pelvic "mass." Listen for the fetal heart (see pp. 885–886).

Tympany

Dullness

Umbilicus may be protuberant

Bulging flank

Tympany

Dullness

Ascitic Fluid[42]

Ascitic fluid seeks the lowest point in the abdomen, producing bulging flanks that are dull to percussion. The umbilicus may protrude. Turn the patient onto one side to detect the shift in position of the fluid level (shifting dullness). (See pp. 448–449 for the assessment of ascites.)

TABLE

11-10

Sounds in the Abdomen

Bowel Sounds

Bowel sounds may be:

- *Increased*, as in diarrhea or *early intestinal obstruction*

- *Decreased*, then absent, as in *adynamic ileus* and *peritonitis*. Before deciding that bowel sounds are absent, sit down and listen where shown for 2 min or even longer.

High-pitched tinkling sounds suggest intestinal fluid and air under tension in a dilated bowel. *Rushes of high-pitched sounds* coinciding with an abdominal cramp indicate intestinal obstruction.

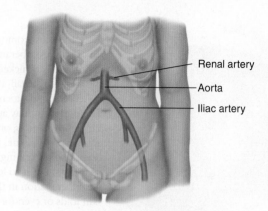

Bruits

A *hepatic bruit* suggests carcinoma of the liver or alcoholic hepatitis. *Arterial bruits* with both systolic and diastolic components suggest partial occlusion of the aorta or large arteries. Partial occlusion of a renal artery may explain hypertension.

Venous Hum

A venous hum is rare. It is a soft humming noise with both systolic and diastolic components. It indicates increased collateral circulation between portal and systemic venous systems, as in hepatic cirrhosis.

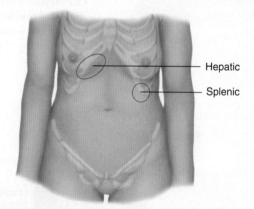

Friction Rubs

Friction rubs are rare. They are grating sounds with respiratory variation. They indicate inflammation of the peritoneal surface of an organ, as in liver cancer, chlamydial or gonococcal perihepatitis, recent liver biopsy, or splenic infarct. When a systolic bruit accompanies a hepatic friction rub, suspect carcinoma of the liver.

TABLE 11-11

Tender Abdomens

Abdominal Wall Tenderness

Superficial tender area

Deep tender area

Tenderness may originate in the abdominal wall. When the patient raises the head and shoulders, this tenderness persists, whereas tenderness from a deeper lesion (protected by the tightened muscles) decreases.

Visceral Tenderness

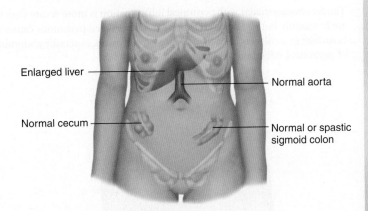

Enlarged liver

Normal aorta

Normal cecum

Normal or spastic sigmoid colon

The structures shown may be tender to deep palpation. Usually the discomfort is dull with no muscular rigidity or rebound tenderness. A reassuring explanation to the patient may prove quite helpful.

Tenderness From Disease in the Chest and Pelvis

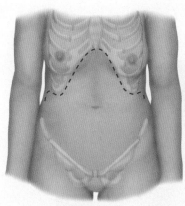

Unilateral or bilateral, upper or lower abdomen

Acute Pleurisy

Abdominal pain and tenderness may result from acute pleural inflammation. When unilateral, it may mimic acute cholecystitis or appendicitis. Rebound tenderness and rigidity are less common; chest signs are usually present.

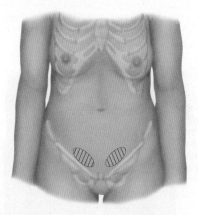

Acute Salpingitis

Frequently bilateral, the tenderness of acute salpingitis (inflammation of the fallopian tubes) is usually maximal just above the inguinal ligaments. Rebound tenderness and rigidity may be present. On pelvic examination, motion of the uterus causes pain.

(table continues on page 468)

TABLE
11-11

Tender Abdomens (continued)

Tenderness of Peritoneal Inflammation

Tenderness associated with peritoneal inflammation is more severe than visceral tenderness. Muscular rigidity and rebound tenderness are frequently but not necessarily present. Generalized peritonitis causes exquisite tenderness throughout the abdomen, together with boardlike muscular rigidity. These signs on palpation, especially abdominal rigidity, double the likelihood of peritonitis.[36] Local causes of peritoneal inflammation include:

Acute Cholecystitis[7]

Signs are maximal in the right upper quadrant. Check for Murphy's sign (see p. 451).

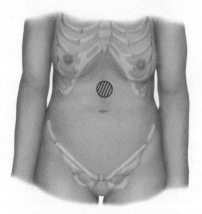

Acute Pancreatitis[6]

In acute pancreatitis, epigastric tenderness and rebound tenderness are usually present, but the abdominal wall may be soft.

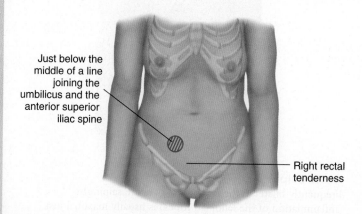

Just below the middle of a line joining the umbilicus and the anterior superior iliac spine

Right rectal tenderness

Acute Appendicitis[14]

Right lower quadrant signs are typical of acute appendicitis but may be absent early in the course. The typical area of tenderness is illustrated. Explore other portions of the right lower quadrant as well as the right flank.

Acute Diverticulitis

Acute diverticulitis most often involves the sigmoid colon and then resembles a left-sided appendicitis.

Liver Enlargement: Apparent and Real

A palpable liver does not necessarily indicate hepatomegaly (an enlarged liver), but more often results from a change in consistency—from the normal softness to an abnormal firmness or hardness, as in cirrhosis. Clinical estimates of liver size should be based on both percussion and palpation, although even these techniques are far from perfect.[36]

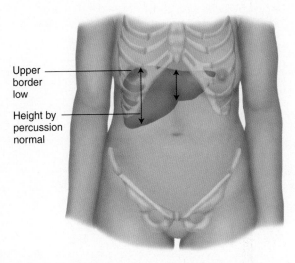

Upper
border
low

Height by
percussion
normal

Elongated
right lobe

Downward Displacement of the Liver by a Low Diaphragm

This finding is common when the diaphragm is low (e.g., in COPD). The liver edge may be readily palpable well below the costal margin. Percussion, however, reveals a low upper edge also, and the vertical span of the liver is normal.

Normal Variations in Liver Shape

In some people, especially those with a lanky build, the liver tends to be elongated so that its right lobe is easily palpable as it projects downward toward the iliac crest. Such an elongation, sometimes called *Riedel's lobe*, represents a variation in shape, not an increase in liver volume or size. Examiners can only estimate the upper and lower borders of an organ with three dimensions and differing shapes. Some error is unavoidable.

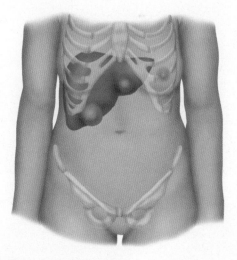

Smooth Large Liver

Cirrhosis may produce an enlarged liver with a firm, *nontender* edge. The liver is not always enlarged in this condition, however, and many other diseases may produce similar findings. An enlarged liver with a smooth, *tender* edge suggests inflammation, as in hepatitis, or venous congestion, as in right-sided heart failure.

Irregular Large Liver

An enlarged liver that is firm or hard and has an irregular edge or surface suggests malignancy. There may be one or more nodules. The liver may or may not be tender.

The Peripheral Vascular System

ANATOMY AND PHYSIOLOGY

Careful assessment of the peripheral vascular system is essential for detection of *peripheral arterial disease,* found in approximately 30% of the adult population, but "silent" in roughly half of those affected.[1] Thromboembolic disorders of the *peripheral venous system* are also common, seen in an estimated 1% of adults older than 60 years, and early detection is critical to minimizing risk of fatal pulmonary embolism.[2]

This chapter reviews the anatomy and physiology of the arteries, veins, and lymphatic system in the arms and legs, and updates health history taking, health promotion and counseling, and techniques of examination according to the *American College of Cardiology and American Heart Association 2005 Practice Guidelines for the Management of Patients with Peripheral Arterial Disease.*[3]

 ARTERIES

Arteries contain three concentric layers of tissue: the *intima,* the *media,* and the *adventitia.*

Injury to vascular endothelial cells can provoke thrombus formation, atheromas, and the vascular lesions of hypertension.[4]

Smooth muscle

Internal elastic membrane

External elastic membrane

Endothelium

Artery

Tunica externa

Tunica media

Tunica intima

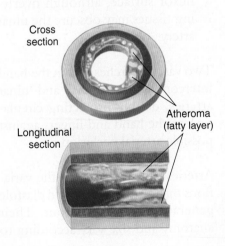

Cross section

Atheroma (fatty layer)

Longitudinal section

Surrounding the lumen of all blood vessels is the *intima,* a single continuous lining of endothelial cells with remarkable metabolic properties.[4] Intact endothelium synthesizes regulators of thrombosis like prostacyclin, plasminogen activator, and heparin-like molecules. It produces prothrombotic molecules such as Von Willebrand factor and plasminogen activator inhibitor. It modulates blood flow and vascular reactivity through synthesis of vasoconstrictors like endothelin and angiotensin-converting enzyme and vasodilators such as nitric oxide and prostacyclin. The intimal endothelium also regulates immune and inflammatory reactions through elaboration of interleukins, adhesion molecules, and histocompatibility antigens.

An *atheroma* begins in the intima as lipid-filled foam cells, then fatty streaks. *Complex atheromas* are thickened asymmetric plaques that narrow the lumen, reducing blood flow, and weaken the underlying media. They have a soft lipid core and a fibrous cap of smooth muscle cells and a collagen-rich matrix. Plaque rupture may precede thrombosis.[4,5]

The *media* is composed of smooth muscle cells that dilate and constrict to accommodate blood pressure and flow. Its inner and outer boundaries are membranes of elastic fibers, or *elastin,* called *internal and external elastic laminae.* Small arterioles called the *vasa vasorum* perfuse the media. The outer layer of the artery is the *adventitia,* connective tissue containing nerve fibers and the vasa vasorum.

Arterial pulses are palpable in arteries lying close to the body surface. In the arms, note pulsations in:

- The *brachial artery* at the bend of the elbow just medial to the biceps tendon

- The *radial artery* on the lateral flexor surface, and

- The *ulnar artery* on the medial flexor surface, although overlying tissues may obscure the ulnar artery

Two vascular arches within the hand interconnect the radial and ulnar arteries, doubly protecting circulation to the hand and fingers against possible arterial occlusion.

Arteries must respond to the variations that cardiac systole and diastole generate in cardiac output. Their anatomy and size vary according to

Brachial artery

Radial artery

Ulnar artery

Arterial arches

their distance from the heart. The aorta and its immediate branches are *large or highly elastic arteries* such as the pulmonary, common carotid, and iliac arteries. These arteries course into *medium-sized or muscular arteries* like the coronary and renal arteries. The elastic recoil and smooth muscle contraction and relaxation in the media of large and medium-sized arteries propagate arterial pulsatile flow. Medium-sized arteries divide into *small arteries* less than 2 mm in diameter and even smaller *arterioles* with diameters from 20 to 100 mm. Resistance to blood flow occurs primarily in the arterioles. (Recall that resistance is inversely proportional to the fourth power of the vessel diameter, known as the law of LaPlace.[4] From the arterioles blood flows into the vast network of *capillaries,* each the diameter of a single red blood cell, only 7 to 8 microns (µm) across. Capillaries have an endothelial cell lining but no media, facilitating rapid diffusion of oxygen and carbon dioxide.

In the legs, find pulsations in:

Anterior superior
iliac spine —————

Inguinal ligament —————

Femoral artery —————

Symphysis pubis —————

Popliteal artery —————

Posterior tibial artery —————

Dorsalis pedis artery —————

Arterial arch —————

- The *femoral artery* just below the inguinal ligament, midway between the anterior superior iliac spine and the symphysis pubis

- The *popliteal artery,* an extension of the femoral artery that passes medially behind the femur, palpable just behind the knee. The popliteal artery divides into the two arteries perfusing the lower leg and foot, namely . . .

- The *dorsalis pedis artery* on the dorsum of the foot just lateral to the extensor tendon of the big toe, and

- The *posterior tibial artery* behind the medial malleolus of the ankle. An interconnecting arch between its two chief arterial branches protects circulation to the foot.

 # VEINS

Unlike arteries, veins are thin-walled and highly distensible, with a capacity for up to two-thirds of circulating blood flow. The *venous intima* consists of nonthrombogenic endothelium. Protruding into the lumen are valves that promote unidirectional venous return to the heart. The *media* contains circumferential rings of elastic tissue and smooth muscle that change vein caliber in response to even minor changes in venous pressure.[4,6]

Veins from the arms, upper trunk, and head and neck drain into the *superior vena cava,* which empties into the right atrium. Veins from the legs and lower trunk drain upward into the *inferior vena cava.* Because of their weaker wall structure, the leg veins are susceptible to irregular dilatation, compression, ulceration, and invasion by tumors and warrant special attention.

Deep and Superficial Venous System (Legs).
The *deep veins* of the legs carry approximately 90% of venous return from the lower extremities. They are well supported by surrounding tissues.

In contrast, the *superficial veins* are subcutaneous, with relatively poor tissue support. They include:

- The *great saphenous vein*, which originates on the dorsum of the foot, passes just anterior to the medial malleolus, continues up the medial aspect of the leg, and joins the femoral vein of the deep venous system below the inguinal ligament

- The *small saphenous vein*, which begins at the side of the foot, passes upward along the posterior calf, and joins the deep venous system in the popliteal fossa

Anastomotic veins connect the two saphenous veins that are readily visible when dilated. Bridging or *perforating veins* connect the superficial system with the deep system.

When competent, the one-way valves of the deep, superficial, and perforating veins propel blood toward the heart, preventing pooling, venous stasis, and backward flow. Contraction of the calf muscles during walking also serves as a venous pump, squeezing blood upward against gravity.

THE LYMPHATIC SYSTEM AND LYMPH NODES

The lymphatic system is an extensive vascular network that drains lymph fluid from body tissues and returns it to the venous circulation. The system starts peripherally as blind lymphatic capillaries, continues centrally as thin vascular channels, then collecting ducts, and empties into the major veins at the neck. Lymph fluid transported through these channels is filtered through lymph nodes interposed along the way.

Lymph nodes are round, oval, or bean-shaped structures that vary in size according to their location. Some lymph nodes, such as the preauriculars, if palpable at all, are typically very small. The inguinal nodes, in contrast, are relatively larger—often 1 cm in diameter and occasionally even 2 cm in an adult.

In addition to its vascular functions, the lymphatic system plays an important role in the body's immune system. Cells within the lymph nodes engulf cellular debris and bacteria and produce antibodies.

Only the superficial lymph nodes are accessible to physical examination. These include the cervical nodes (p. 238), the axillary nodes (p. 391), and nodes in the arms and legs.

Recall that the axillary lymph nodes drain most of the arm. Lymphatics from the ulnar surface of the forearm and hand, the little and ring fingers, and the adjacent surface of the middle finger, however, drain first into the *epitrochlear nodes*. These are located on the medial surface of the arm approximately 3 cm above the elbow. Lymphatics from the rest of the arm drain mostly into the axillary nodes. A few may go directly to the infraclaviculars.

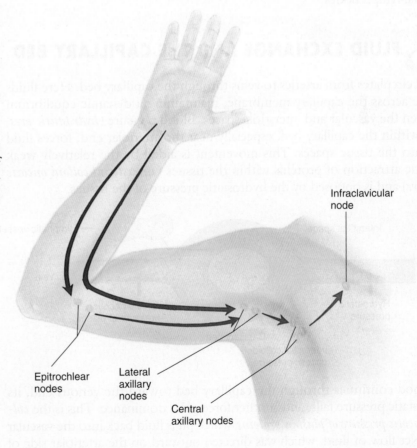

Infraclavicular node

Epitrochlear nodes

Lateral axillary nodes

Central axillary nodes

The lymphatics of the lower limb, following the venous supply, consist of both deep and superficial systems. Only the superficial nodes are palpable. The *superficial inguinal nodes* include two groups. The *horizontal group* lies in a chain high in the anterior thigh below the inguinal ligament. It drains the superficial portions of the lower abdomen and buttock, the external genitalia (but not the testes), the anal canal and perianal area, and the lower vagina.

The *vertical group* clusters near the upper part of the saphenous vein and drains a corresponding region of the leg. In contrast, lymphatics from the portion of leg drained by the small saphenous vein (the heel and outer aspect of the foot) join the deep system at the level of the popliteal space. Lesions in this area, therefore, are not usually associated with palpable inguinal lymph nodes.

Horizontal group

Femoral artery

Vertical group

Femoral vein

Great saphenous vein

 ## FLUID EXCHANGE AND THE CAPILLARY BED

Blood circulates from arteries to veins through the capillary bed. Here fluids diffuse across the capillary membrane, maintaining a dynamic equilibrium between the vascular and interstitial spaces. Blood pressure (*hydrostatic pressure*) within the capillary bed, especially near the arteriolar end, forces fluid out into the tissue spaces. This movement is aided by the relatively weak osmotic attraction of proteins within the tissues (*interstitial colloid oncotic pressure*) and is opposed by the hydrostatic pressure of the tissues.

Interstitial space

Lymphatic vessel

Artery

Vein

Hydrostatic pressure

Colloid oncotic pressure of plasma protein

Capillary bed

Interstitial colloid oncotic pressure

As blood continues through the capillary bed toward the venous end, its hydrostatic pressure falls, and another force gains dominance. This is the *colloid oncotic pressure of plasma proteins,* which pulls fluid back into the vascular tree. Net flow of fluid, which was directed outward on the arteriolar side of the capillary bed, reverses and turns inward on the venous side. Lymphatic capillaries, which also play an important role in this equilibrium, remove excessive fluid, including protein, from the interstitial space.

Lymphatic dysfunction or disturbances in hydrostatic or osmotic forces can all disrupt this equilibrium. The most common clinical result is the increased interstitial fluid known as edema (see Table 12-5, Peripheral Causes of Edema, p. 499).

THE HEALTH HISTORY

Common or Concerning Symptoms

- Pain in the arms or legs
- Intermittent claudication
- Cold, numbness, pallor in the legs; hair loss
- Swelling in calves, legs, or feet
- Color change in fingertips or toes in cold weather
- Swelling with redness or tenderness

As defined by recent guidelines from the American College of Cardiology and the American Heart Association, *peripheral arterial disease* (PAD) refers to stenotic, occlusive, and aneurysmal disease of the aorta, its visceral arterial branches, and the arteries of the lower extremities, exclusive of the coronary arteries.[3] Be aware that pain in the extremities may arise from the skin, peripheral vascular system, musculoskeletal system, or nervous system. It also may be referred, like the pain of myocardial infarction that radiates to the left arm.

See Table 12-1, Painful Peripheral Vascular Disorders and Their Mimics, pp. 494–495.

Ask about any pain or cramping in the legs during exertion that is relieved by rest within 10 minutes, termed *intermittent claudication.*

Atherosclerosis can cause symptomatic limb ischemia with exertion; distinguish this from *spinal stenosis,* which produces leg pain with exertion that may be reduced by leaning forward (stretching the spinal cord in the narrowed vertebral canal) and less readily relieved by rest.

Ask also about *coldness, numbness,* or *pallor* in the legs or *feet* or *loss of hair* over the anterior tibial surfaces.

Hair loss over the anterior tibiae occurs with decreased arterial perfusion. "Dry" or brown-black ulcers from *gangrene* may ensue.

Because most patients with PAD report minimal symptoms, asking specifically about the symptoms that follow is recommended, especially in patients older than 50 years and those with risk factors, especially smoking but also diabetes, hypertension, elevated cholesterol, or coronary artery disease (see

Only about 10% of patients have the classic triad of leg pain with exertion that stops with rest.[1] The low symptom rate may reflect

p. 342).[3] When symptoms (see below) or risk factors are present, careful examination and testing of the ankle–brachial index are warranted (see p. 479 and p. 496).

functional declines in walking, even though PAD is present or progressing.[7]

- Fatigue, aching, numbness, or pain that limits walking or exertion in the legs; if present, identify the location. Ask also about erectile dysfunction.

Symptom location suggests the site of arterial ischemia:

- buttock, hip: aortoiliac

- erectile dysfunction: iliac–pudendal

- thigh: common femoral or aortoiliac

- upper calf: superficial femoral

- lower calf: popliteal

- foot: tibial or peroneal

- Any poorly healing or nonhealing wounds of the legs or feet

- Any pain at rest in the lower leg or foot and changes when standing or supine

- Abdominal pain after meals and associated "food fear" and weight loss

Abdominal pain, "food fear," and weight loss suggest intestinal ischemia of the celiac or superior or inferior mesenteric arteries.

- Any first-degree relatives with an abdominal aortic aneurysm

Prevalence of abdominal aortic aneurysms in first-degree relatives is 15% to 28%.[3]

HEALTH PROMOTION AND COUNSELING

Important Topics for Health Promotion and Counseling

- Screening for peripheral arterial disease (PAD); the ankle–brachial index (ABI)
- Screening for renal artery disease
- Screening for abdominal aortic aneurysms

Screening for Peripheral Arterial Disease: The Ankle–Brachial Index.
PAD is a common manifestation of atherosclerosis, affecting from 12% to 29% of community populations.[1,8] Prevalence of PAD increases with age and the

presence of cardiovascular risk factors. Prevalence by age group rises from 2.5% in patients 60 years or older, to 8% in those 60–69 years, and 19% in those 70 years or older.[9] PAD and cardiovascular disease overlap in 16% of patients.[1] Despite widespread prevalence, PAD is underdiagnosed in office practices.[1,3,10] Although the U.S. Preventive Services Task Force does not advocate screening, the American College of Cardiology/American Heart Association guidelines support "case-finding" in those at risk, as detailed below.[3]

RISK FACTORS FOR LOWER-EXTREMITY PERIPHERAL ARTERIAL DISEASE

- Age younger than 50 years with diabetes or atherosclerosis risk factor of smoking, dyslipidemia, hypertension, or hyperhomocysteinemia

- Age 50 to 69 years and history of smoking or diabetes

- Age 70 years or older

- Leg symptoms with exertion or ischemic rest pain

- Abnormal lower extremity pulses

- Known atherosclerotic coronary, carotid, or renal artery disease

(Source: Hirsch AT, Haskal ZJ, Hertzer NR, et al. ACC/AHA 2005 guidelines for the management of patients with peripheral arterial disease.)

Learn to assess for PAD by using the ankle–brachial index (ABI). The ABI is reliable, reproducible, and easy to perform in the office, with a sensitivity and specificity of 90% and 95%, respectively.[10] Clinicians or office staff can readily measure systolic blood pressure in the arms and in the pedal pulses, using Doppler ultrasound. These values can be entered into calculators readily available at selected Web sites (see American College of Physicians, at http://cpsc.acponline.org/enhancements/232abiCalc.html).

See Table 12-2, Using the Ankle–Brachial Index, p. 496.

A wide range of interventions is available to reduce both onset and progression of PAD, including meticulous foot care and well-fitting shoes, tobacco cessation, treatment of hyperlipidemia, optimal control and treatment of diabetes and hypertension, use of antiplatelet agents, graded exercise, and, if needed, surgical revascularization.[11] Patients with ABIs in the lowest category have a 20% to 25% annual risk for death.[1]

Screening for Renal Artery Disease.   Atherosclerotic renal artery disease affects 7% of adults older than 65 years, rising to 22% to 55% of those with PAD and 30% of patients with documented coronary artery disease.[3,12] The American College of Cardiology and the American Heart Association recommend diagnostic studies for renal artery disease, usually beginning with ultrasound, in patients with the following conditions: hypertension before 30 years; severe hypertension (see p. 118) after 55 years; accelerated, resistant, or malignant hypertension; new worsening of renal function or worsening after use of an angiotensin-converting enzyme inhibitor or an angiotensin-receptor blocking agent; an unexplained small kidney; or sudden unexplained pulmonary edema, especially in the setting of worsening renal function.[3] Symptoms arise from these conditions rather than directly from atherosclerotic changes in the renal artery.

Screening for Abdominal Aortic Aneurysm. Recent evidence documents the benefit of early detection of abdominal aortic aneurysm (AAA), the 14th leading cause of death in the United States.[13] An AAA is present when the infrarenal aortic diameter exceeds 3.0 cm. Rupture and mortality rates dramatically increase for AAAs exceeding 5.5 cm in diameter. The strongest risk factor for rupture is excess aortic diameter. Additional risk factors are smoking, age older than 65 years, family history, coronary artery disease, PAD, hypertension, and elevated cholesterol level. Because symptoms are rare, and screening is now shown to reduce mortality by 40%, the U.S. Preventive Services Task Force recommends one-time screening by ultrasound in men between 65 and 75 years with a history of "ever smoking," defined as more than 100 cigarettes in a lifetime.[14] Due to lower prevalence, data on benefits of screening nonsmokers and women are inconclusive. Ultrasound in asymptomatic individuals is 95% sensitive and nearly 100% specific for AAA.

TECHNIQUES OF EXAMINATION

Important Areas of Examination

THE ARMS	THE LEGS
• Size, symmetry, skin color	• Size, symmetry, skin color
• Radial pulse, brachial pulse	• Femoral pulse and inguinal lymph nodes
• Epitrochlear lymph nodes	• Popliteal, dorsalis pedis, and posterior tibial pulses
	• Peripheral edema

The American College of Cardiology and the American Heart Association have urged clinicians to intensify their focus when examining the peripheral vascular system.[3] Recall that peripheral arterial disease is often asymptomatic and underdiagnosed, leading to significant morbidity and mortality. As you learn and practice the techniques of the vascular examination, observe the 2005 recommendations for examining the peripheral arterial system. Review the techniques for assessing blood pressure, the carotid artery, the aorta, and the renal and femoral arteries on the pages indicated below.

Summary: Key Components of the Peripheral Arterial Examination

• Measure blood pressure in both arms (see Ch. 4, pp. 116–117).
• Palpate carotid upstroke, auscultate for bruits (see Ch. 9, p. 353).
• Auscultate for aortic, renal, and femoral bruits; palpate aorta and determine maximal diameter (see Ch. 11, pp. 436–437).
• Palpate brachial, radial, ulnar, femoral, popliteal, dorsalis pedis, and posterior arteries.
• Inspect ankles and feet for color, temperature, skin integrity; note any ulcerations; check for hair loss, trophic skin changes, hypertrophic nails.
(Source: Hirsch AT, Haskal ZJ, Hertzer NR, et al. ACC/AHA 2005 guidelines for the management of patients with peripheral arterial disease.)

Asymmetric blood pressures seen in *coarctation of the aorta* and *dissecting aortic aneurysm*

ARMS

Inspect both arms from the fingertips to the shoulders. Note:

● Their size, symmetry, and any swelling

Lymphedema of the arm and hand may follow axillary node dissection and radiation therapy.

● The venous pattern

Prominent veins in an edematous arm suggest venous obstruction.

● The color of the skin and nail beds and the texture of the skin

Palpate the radial pulse with the pads of your fingers on the flexor surface of the wrist laterally. Partially flexing the patient's wrist may help you feel this pulse. Compare the pulses in both arms.

(*Source: Marks R: Skin Disease in Old Age. Philadelphia, JB Lippincott, 1987*)

In *Raynaud's disease,* wrist pulses are typically normal, but spasm of more distal arteries causes episodes of sharply demarcated pallor of the fingers (see Table 12-1, Painful Peripheral Vascular Disorders and Their Mimics, pp. 494–495).

There are several systems for grading the amplitude of the arterial pulses. One system uses a scale of 0 to 3, as below.[3] You should check to see what scale your institution uses.

Note that if an artery is widely dilated, it is *aneurysmal.*

Recommended Grading of Pulses[3]

3+   Bounding
2+   Brisk, expected (normal)
1+   Diminished, weaker than expected
0   Absent, unable to palpate

Bounding carotid, radial, and femoral pulses in *aortic insufficiency*; asymmetric diminished pulses in *arterial occlusion* from atherosclerosis or embolism

If you suspect arterial insufficiency, feel for the *brachial pulse.* Flex the patient's elbow slightly, and palpate the artery just medial to the biceps tendon at the antecubital crease. The brachial artery can also be felt higher in the arm in the groove between the biceps and triceps muscles.

Feel for one or more *epitrochlear nodes.* With the patient's elbow flexed to about 90° and the forearm supported by your hand, reach around behind the arm and feel in the groove between the biceps and triceps muscles, about 3 cm above the medial epicondyle. If a node is present, note its size, consistency, and tenderness.

Epitrochlear nodes are difficult or impossible to identify in most normal people.

Right hand of examiner
Medial epicondyle of humerus

MEDIAL ASPECT, LEFT ARM

An enlarged epitrochlear node may arise from local or distal infection or may be associated with generalized lymphadenopathy.

 LEGS

The patient should be lying down and draped so that the external genitalia are covered and the legs fully exposed. A good examination is impossible through stockings or socks!

Inspect both legs from the groin and buttocks to the feet. Note:

- Their size, symmetry, and any swelling

- The venous pattern and any venous enlargement

- Any pigmentation, rashes, scars, or ulcers

- The color and texture of the skin, the color of the nail beds, and the distribution of hair on the lower legs, feet, and toes.

Palpate the *superficial inguinal nodes,* including both the horizontal and the vertical groups. Note their size, consistency, and discreteness, and note any tenderness. Nontender, discrete inguinal nodes up to 1 cm or even 2 cm in diameter are frequently palpable in normal people.

Horizontal group
Femoral artery
Femoral vein
Vertical group
Great saphenous vein

See Table 12-3, Chronic Insufficiency of Arteries and Veins (p. 497).

See Table 12-4, Common Ulcers of the Ankles and Feet (p. 498).

Lymphadenopathy refers to enlargement of the nodes, with or without tenderness. Try to distinguish between local and generalized lymphadenopathy, respectively, by finding either (1) a causative lesion in the drainage area or (2) enlarged nodes in at least two other noncontiguous lymph node regions.

Palpate the pulses to assess the arterial circulation.

- *The femoral pulse.* Press deeply, below the inguinal ligament and about midway between the anterior superior iliac spine and the symphysis pubis. As in deep abdominal palpation, the use of two hands, one on top of the other, may facilitate this examination, especially in obese patients.

A diminished or absent pulse indicates partial or complete occlusion proximally; for example, at the aortic or iliac level, all pulses distal to the occlusion are typically affected. Chronic arterial occlusion, usually from atherosclerosis, causes *intermittent claudication* (p. 494), postural color changes (p. 490), and trophic changes in the skin (p. 490).

An exaggerated, widened femoral pulse suggests a *femoral aneurysm*, a pathologic dilatation of the artery.

- *The popliteal pulse.* The patient's knee should be somewhat flexed, with the leg relaxed. Place the fingertips of both hands so that they just meet in the midline behind the knee and press them deeply into the popliteal fossa. The popliteal pulse is often more difficult to find than other pulses. It is deeper and feels more diffuse.

An exaggerated, widened popliteal pulse suggests an aneurysm of the popliteal artery. Popliteal and femoral aneurysms are not common. They are usually caused by atherosclerosis and occur primarily in men older than 50 years.

If you cannot feel the popliteal pulse with this approach, try with the patient prone. Flex the patient's knee to about 90°, let the lower leg relax against your shoulder or upper arm, and press your two thumbs deeply into the popliteal fossa.

Atherosclerosis (arteriosclerosis obliterans) most commonly obstructs arterial circulation in the thigh. The femoral pulse is then normal, the popliteal decreased or absent.

- *The dorsalis pedis pulse.* Feel the dorsum of the foot (not the ankle) just lateral to the extensor tendon of the great toe. If you cannot feel a pulse, explore the dorsum of the foot more laterally.

The dorsalis pedis artery may be congenitally absent or may branch higher in the ankle. Search for a pulse more laterally.

Decreased or absent pedal pulses (assuming a warm environment) with normal femoral and popliteal pulses suggest occlusive disease in the lower popliteal artery or its branches—often seen in *diabetes mellitus.*

- *The posterior tibial pulse.* Curve your fingers behind and slightly below the medial malleolus of the ankle. (This pulse may be hard to feel in a fat or edematous ankle.)

Sudden arterial occlusion from embolism or thrombosis causes pain and numbness or tingling. The limb distal to the occlusion becomes cold, pale, and pulseless. Emergency treatment is required. If collateral circulation is good, only numbness and coolness may result.

TIPS FOR FEELING DIFFICULT PULSES

1. Position your body and examining hand comfortably; awkward positions decrease your tactile sensitivity.

2. Place your hand properly and linger there, varying the pressure of your fingers to pick up a weak pulsation. If unsuccessful, then explore the area deliberately.

3. Do not confuse the patient's pulse with your own pulsating fingertips. If you are unsure, count your own heart rate and compare it with the patient's. The rates are usually different. Your carotid pulse is convenient for this comparison.

Note the temperature of the feet and legs with the backs of your fingers. Compare one side with the other. Bilateral coldness is most often caused by a cold environment or anxiety.

Coldness, especially when unilateral or associated with other signs, suggests arterial insufficiency from inadequate arterial circulation.

Look for edema. Compare one foot and leg with the other, noting their relative size and the prominence of veins, tendons, and bones.

Edema causes swelling that may obscure the veins, tendons, and bony prominences.

Check for pitting edema. Press firmly but gently with your thumb for at least 5 seconds (1) over the dorsum of each foot, (2) behind each medial malleolus, and (3) over the shins. Look for *pitting*—a depression caused by pressure from your thumb. Normally there is none. The severity of edema is graded on a four-point scale, from slight to very marked.

See Table 12-5, Some Peripheral Causes of Edema (p. 499).

Shown below is 3+ pitting edema.

If you suspect edema, *measure the legs* to identify the edema and to follow its course. With a flexible tape, measure (1) the forefoot, (2) the smallest possible circumference above the ankle, (3) the largest circumference at the calf, and (4) the midthigh, a measured distance above the patella with the knee extended. Compare one side with the other. A difference of more than 1 cm just above the ankle or 2 cm at the calf is unusual in normal people and suggests edema.

Conditions such as muscular atrophy can also cause different circumferences in the legs.

If edema is present, look for possible causes in the peripheral vascular system. These include (1) recent deep venous thrombosis, (2) chronic venous insufficiency from previous deep venous thrombosis or incompetence of the venous valves, and (3) lymphedema. Note the extent of the swelling. How far up the leg does it go?

In *deep venous thrombosis,* the extent of edema suggests the location of the occlusion: the popliteal vein when the lower leg or the ankle is swollen; the iliofemoral veins when the entire leg is swollen.

Is the swelling unilateral or bilateral? Are the veins unusually prominent?

Venous distention suggests a venous cause of edema.

Try to identify any venous tenderness that may accompany deep venous thrombosis. Palpate the groin just medial to the femoral pulse for tenderness of the femoral vein. Next, with the patient's leg flexed at the knee and relaxed, palpate the calf. With your fingerpads, gently compress the calf muscles against the tibia, and search for any tenderness or cords. Deep venous thrombosis, however, may have no demonstrable signs, and diagnosis often depends on high clinical suspicion and other testing.

A painful, pale swollen leg, together with tenderness in the groin over the femoral vein, suggests deep *iliofemoral thrombosis.* Only half of patients with *deep venous thrombosis* in the calf have tenderness and cords deep in the calf. Calf tenderness is nonspecific and may be present without thrombosis.

Note the *color of the skin.*

- Is there a local area of redness? If so, note its temperature, and gently try to feel the firm cord of a thrombosed vein in the area. The calf is most often involved.

Local swelling, redness, warmth, and a subcutaneous cord suggest *superficial thrombophlebitis.*

- Are there brownish areas near the ankles?

Brownish discoloration or ulcers just above the malleolus suggest *chronic venous insufficiency.*

- Note any ulcers in the skin. Where are they?

- Feel the thickness of the skin.

Thickened brawny skin suggests lymphedema and advanced venous insufficiency.

Ask the patient to stand, and *inspect the saphenous system for varicosities.* The standing posture allows any varicosities to fill with blood and makes them visible. You can easily miss them when the patient is in a supine position. Feel for any varicosities, noting any signs of thrombophlebitis.

Varicose veins are dilated and tortuous. Their walls may feel somewhat thickened. Many varicose veins can be seen in the leg on p. 491.

SPECIAL TECHNIQUES

Evaluating the Arterial Supply to the Hand.   If you suspect arterial insufficiency in the arm or hand, try to feel the *ulnar pulse* as well as the radial and brachial pulses. Feel for it deeply on the flexor surface of the wrist medially. Partially flexing the patient's wrist may help you. The pulse of a normal ulnar artery, however, may not be palpable.

Arterial occlusive disease is much less common in the arms than in the legs. Absent or diminished pulses at the wrist are found in acute embolic occlusion and in *Buerger's disease,* or *thromboangiitis obliterans.*

The *Allen test* gives further information. This test is also useful to ensure the patency of the ulnar artery before puncturing the radial artery for blood samples. The patient should rest with hands in lap, palms up.

Ask the patient to make a tight fist with one hand; then compress both radial and ulnar arteries firmly between your thumbs and fingers.

Next, ask the patient to open the hand into a relaxed, slightly flexed position. The palm is pale.

Extending the hand fully may cause pallor and a falsely positive test.

Release your pressure over the ulnar artery. If the ulnar artery is patent, the palm flushes within about 3 to 5 seconds.

Persisting pallor indicates occlusion of the ulnar artery or its distal branches.

Patency of the radial artery may be tested by releasing the radial artery while still compressing the ulnar artery.

Postural Color Changes of Chronic Arterial Insufficiency. If pain or diminished pulses suggest arterial insufficiency, look for postural color changes. Raise both legs, as shown at the right, to about 60° until maximal pallor of the feet develops—usually within a minute. In light-skinned persons, either maintenance of normal color, as seen in this right foot, or slight pallor is normal.

Marked pallor on elevation suggests *arterial insufficiency.*

Then ask the patient to sit up with legs dangling down. Compare both feet, noting the time required for:

● Return of pinkness to the skin, normally about 10 seconds or less

● Filling of the veins of the feet and ankles, normally about 15 seconds

This right foot has normal color and the veins on the foot have filled. These normal responses suggest an adequate circulation.

The foot above is still pale, and the veins are just starting to fill—signs of arterial insufficiency.

Look for any unusual *rubor* (dusky redness) to replace the pallor of the dependent foot. Rubor may take a minute or more to appear.

Normal responses accompanied by diminished arterial pulses suggest that a good collateral circulation has developed around an arterial occlusion.

Color changes may be difficult to see in darker-skinned persons. Inspect the soles of the feet for these changes, and use tangential lighting to see the veins.

Persisting rubor on dependency suggests arterial insufficiency (see p. 498). When veins are incompetent, dependent rubor and the timing of color return and venous filling are not reliable tests of arterial insufficiency.

(Source of foot photos: Kappert A, Winsor T: Diagnosis of Peripheral Vascular Disease. Philadelphia, FA Davis, 1972.)

Mapping Varicose Veins. You can map out the course and connections of varicose veins by transmitting pressure waves along the blood-filled veins. With the patient standing, place your palpating fingers gently on a vein and, with your other hand below it, compress the vein sharply. Feel for a pressure wave transmitted to the fingers of your upper hand. A palpable pressure wave indicates that the two parts of the vein are connected.

A wave may also be transmitted downward, but not as easily.

Feel for a
pressure wave

Compress sharply

Evaluating the Competency of Venous Valves. By the *retrograde filling (Trendelenburg) test,* you can assess the valvular competency in both the communicating veins and the saphenous system. Start with the patient supine. Elevate one leg to about 90° to empty it of venous blood.

Next, occlude the great saphenous vein in the upper thigh by manual compression, using enough pressure to occlude this vein but not the deeper vessels. Ask the patient to stand. While you keep the vein occluded, watch for venous filling in the leg. Normally the saphenous vein fills from below, taking about 35 seconds as blood flows through the capillary bed into the venous system.

Rapid filling of the superficial veins while the saphenous vein is occluded indicates incompetent valves in the communicating veins. Blood flows quickly in a retrograde direction from the deep to the saphenous system.

After the patient stands for 20 seconds, release the compression and look for sudden additional venous filling. Normally there is none; competent valves in the saphenous vein block retrograde flow. Slow venous filling continues.

Sudden additional filling of superficial veins after release of compression indicates incompetent valves in the saphenous vein.

When both steps of this test are normal, the response is termed negative–negative. Negative–positive and positive–negative responses may also occur.

When both steps are abnormal, the test is positive–positive.

RECORDING YOUR FINDINGS

Note that initially you may use sentences to describe your findings; later you will use phrases. The style below contains phrases appropriate for most write-ups. Recall that the written description of lymph nodes appears in Chapter 7, The Head and Neck (see p. 245). Likewise, assessment of the carotid pulse is recorded in Chapter 9, The Cardiovascular System (see p. 371).

Recording the Physical Examination—
The Peripheral Vascular System

"Extremities are warm and without edema. No varicosities or stasis changes. Calves are supple and nontender. No femoral or abdominal bruits. Brachial, radial, femoral, popliteal, dorsalis pedis (DP), and posterior tibial (PT) pulses are 2+ and symmetric."

OR

"Extremities are pale below the midcalf, with notable hair loss. Rubor noted when legs dependent but no edema or ulceration. Bilateral femoral bruits; no abdominal bruits heard. Brachial and radial pulses 2+; femoral, popliteal, DP and PT pulses 1+." (Alternatively, pulses can be recorded as below.)

Suggests atherosclerotic *peripheral arterial disease*

	Radial	Brachial	Femoral	Popliteal	Dorsalis Pedis	Posterior Tibial
RT	2+	2+	1+	1+	1+	1+
LT	2+	2+	1+	1+	1+	1+

BIBLIOGRAPHY

CITATIONS

1. Hirsch AT, Criqui MH, Treat-Jacobsen D, et al. Peripheral arterial disease detection, awareness, and treatment in primary care. JAMA 286(11):1317–1324, 2001.
2. Bates SM, Ginsberg JS. Treatment of deep-vein thrombosis. N Engl J Med 351(3):268–277, 2004.
3. Hirsch AT, Haskal ZJ, Hertzer NR, et al. ACC/AHA 2005 guidelines for the management of patients with peripheral arterial disease (lower extremity, renal, mesenteric, and abdominal aortic): a collaborative report from the American Association for Vascular Surgery/Society for Vascular Surgery, Society for Cardiovascular Angiography and Interventions, Society for Vascular Medicine and Biology, Society of Interventional Radiology, and the ACC/AHA Task Force on Practice Guidelines (Writing Committee to Develop Guidelines for the Management of Patients With Peripheral Arterial Disease). Available at: http://circ.ahajournals.org/cgi/reprint/113/11/e463. Accessed June 24, 2007.
4. Schoen FJ. Blood vessels. In Kumar VK, Fausto N, & Abbas AK (eds). Robbins and Cotran Pathologic Basis of Disease, 7th ed. Philadelphia, Elsevier, 2005.
5. Hansson GK. Inflammation, atherosclerosis, and coronary artery disease. N Engl J Med 352(16):1685–1689, 2005.
6. Lam EY, Giswold ME, Moneta GL. Venous and lymphatic disease. In Brunicardi C, Anderson DA, Billiar TR, et al. (eds). Schwartz's Principles of Surgery, 8th ed. New York, McGraw Hill, 2005.
7. McDermott MM, Liu K, Greenland P, et al. Functional decline in peripheral arterial disease—associations with the ankle brachial index and leg symptoms. JAMA 292(4):453–461, 2004.
8. Newman AB. Peripheral arterial disease: insights from population studies of older adults. J Am Ger Soc 48(9):1157–1162, 2000.
9. Kanel WB. The demographics of claudication and the aging of the American population. Vasc Med 1:60–64, 1986.

10. Laine C, Goldman D, Wilson JF. In the clinic: peripheral arterial disease. Ann Intern Med 146(5):ITC 3–1, 2007.

11. McDermott MM, Liu K, Ferrucci, et al. Physical performance in peripheral arterial disease: a slower rate of decline in patients who walk more. Ann Intern Med 144(1):10–20, 2006.

12. Balk E, Raman G, Chung M, et al. Effectiveness of management strategies for renal artery stenosis: a systematic review. Ann Intern Med 145(12):901–912, 2006.

13. Kim LG, Scott AP, Ashton HA, et al. A sustained mortality benefit from screening for abdominal aortic aneurysm. Ann Intern Med 146(10):699–706, 2007.

14. U.S. Preventive Services Task Force. Screening for abdominal aortic aneurysm: recommendation statement. Ann Intern Med 142(3):198–202, 2005.

15. Falagas ME, Paschalis IV. Narrative review: diseases that masquerade as infectious cellulitis. Ann Intern Med 142(1):47–55, 2005.

16. De Araujo T, Valencia I, Federman D, et al. Managing the patient with venous ulcers. Ann Intern Med 138(4):326–334, 2003.

ADDITIONAL REFERENCES

Anand SS, Wells PS, Hunt D, et al. Does this patient have a deep vein thrombosis? JAMA 279(14):1094–1099, 1998.

Boulton AJM, Kirsner RS, Vileikyte L. Neuropathic diabetic foot ulcers. N Engl J Med 51(1):48–55, 2004.

Colman RW, Marder VJ, Clowes AW, et al., eds. Hemostasis and Thrombosis: Basic Principles and Clinical Practice, 4th ed. Philadelphia: Lippincott Williams & Wilkins, 2005.

Creager MA, Loscalzo J, Dzau VJ, eds. Vascular Medicine: A Companion to Braunwald's Heart Disease. Philadelphia: WB Saunders, 2006.

Douketis JD. Use of a clinical prediction score in patients with suspected deep venous thrombosis: two steps forward, one step back? Ann Intern Med 143(2):140–141, 2005.

Klein LW. Atherosclerosis regression, vascular remodeling, and plaque stabilization. J Am Coll Cardiol 49(2):271–273, 2007.

Qaseem A, Snow V, Barry P, et al. Current diagnosis of venous thromboembolism in primary care: a clinical practice guideline from the American Academy of Family Physicians and the American College of Physicians. Ann Intern Med 146(6):454–458, 2007.

Tiwari A, Cheng KS, Button M, et al. Differential diagnosis, investigation, and current treatment of lower limb lymphedema. Arch Surg 138(2):152–161, 2003.

Wigley FM. Raynaud's phenomenon. N Engl J Med 347(13):1001–1008, 2002.

⚭ **The Bates' suite offers these additional resources to enhance learning and facilitate understanding of this chapter:**

- Bates' Pocket Guide to Physical Examination and History Taking, 6th edition
- Bates' Nursing Online
- Bates' Visual Guide to Physical Examination, 4th edition
- thePoint online resources, http://thepoint.lww.com
- Student CD-ROM included with the book

Painful Peripheral Vascular Disorders and Their Mimics[3,16]

Problem	Process	Location of Pain
Arterial Disorders *Atherosclerosis* *(arteriosclerosis obliterans)*		
• Intermittent claudication	Episodic muscular ischemia induced by exercise, due to atherosclerosis of large or medium-sized arteries	Usually calf muscles, but also may be in the buttock, hip, thigh, or foot, depending on the level of obstruction
• Rest pain	Ischemia even at rest	Distal pain, in the toes or forefoot
Acute Arterial Occlusion	Embolism or thrombosis, possibly superimposed on arteriosclerosis obliterans	Distal pain, usually involving the foot and leg
Raynaud's Disease and Phenomenon	*Raynaud's disease:* Episodic spasm of the small arteries and arterioles; no vascular occlusion *Raynaud's phenomenon:* Syndrome secondary to other conditions such as collagen vascular disease, arterial occlusion, trauma, drugs	Distal portions of one or more fingers. Pain is usually not prominent unless fingertip ulcers develop. Numbness and tingling are common.
Venous Disorders *Superficial Thrombophlebitis*	Clot formation and acute inflammation in a superficial vein	Pain in a local area along the course of a superficial vein, most often in the saphenous system
Deep Venous Thrombosis (DVT)	Clot formation in a deep vein	Tight, bursting pain, if present, usually in the calf; may be painless.
Chronic Venous Insufficiency (deep)	Chronic venous engorgement secondary to venous occlusion or incompetency of venous valves	Diffuse aching of the leg(s)
Thromboangiitis Obliterans (Buerger's disease)	Inflammatory and thrombotic occlusions of small arteries and also of veins, occurring in smokers	• Intermittent claudication, particularly in the arch of the foot • Rest pain in the fingers or toes
Compartment Syndrome	Pressure builds from trauma or bleeding into one of the four major muscle compartments between the knee and ankle. Each compartment is enclosed by fascia and thus cannot expand to accommodate increasing pressure.	Tight, bursting pain in calf muscles, usually in the anterior tibial compartment, sometimes with overlying dusky red skin.
Acute Lymphangitis	Acute bacterial infection (usually streptococcal) spreading up the lymphatic channels from a portal of entry such as an injured area or an ulcer	An arm or a leg
Mimics* *Acute Cellulitis*	Acute bacterial infection of the skin and subcutaneous tissues	Arms, legs, or elsewhere
Erythema Nodosum	Raised tender bilateral subcutaneous lesions seen in systemic conditions such as pregnancy, sarcoidosis, tuberculosis, streptococcal infections, inflammatory bowel disease	Anterior surfaces of both lower legs

---

* Mistaken primarily for acute superficial thrombophlebitis.

Timing	Factors That Aggravate	Factors That Relieve	Associated Manifestations
Fairly brief; pain usually forces the patient to rest.	Exercise such as walking	Rest usually stops the pain in 1–3 min.	Local fatigue, numbness, diminished pulses, often signs of arterial insufficiency (see p. 498)
Persistent, often worse at night	Elevation of the feet, as in bed	Sitting with legs dependent	Numbness, tingling, trophic signs and color changes of arterial insufficiency (see p. 498)
Sudden onset; associated symptoms may occur without pain.			Coldness, numbness, weakness, absent distal pulses
Relatively brief (minutes) but recurrent	Exposure to cold, emotional upset	Warm environment	Color changes in the distal fingers: severe pallor (essential for the diagnosis) followed by cyanosis and then redness
An acute episode lasting days or longer			Local redness, swelling, tenderness, a palpable cord, possibly fever
Often hard to determine because of lack of symptoms	Walking	Elevation speeds relief	Possible swelling of the foot and calf, local calf tenderness. Prior history of DVT
Chronic, increasing as the day wears on	Prolonged standing	Elevation of the leg(s)	Chronic edema, pigmentation, possibly ulceration (see p. 498)
• Fairly brief but recurrent • Chronic, persistent, may be worse at night	• Exercise	• Rest • Permanent cessation of smoking helps both kinds of pain (but patients seldom stop)	Distal coldness, sweating, numbness, and cyanosis; ulceration and gangrene at the tips of fingers or toes; migratory thrombophlebitis
Several hours if *acute* (pressure must be relieved to overt necrosis). During exercise if *chronic*.	*Acute:* anabolic steroids; surgical complication; crush injury. *Chronic:* occurs with exercise	*Acute:* surgical incision to relieve pressure *Chronic:* avoiding exercise; ice elevation	Tingling, burning sensations in calf; muscles may feel tight, full, numbness, paralysis if unrelieved
An acute episode lasting days or longer			Red streak(s) on the skin, with tenderness, enlarged, tender lymph nodes, and fever
An acute episode lasting days or longer			A local area of diffuse swelling, redness, and tenderness with enlarged, tender lymph nodes and fever; no palpable cord
Pain associated with a series of lesions over several weeks			Lesions recur in crops; often malaise, joint pains, and fever

TABLE

12-2

Using the Ankle–Brachial Index

Instructions for Measuring the Ankle–Brachial Index (ABI)

1. Patient should rest supine in a warm room for at least 10 minutes before testing.

2. Place blood pressure cuffs on both arms and ankles as illustrated, then apply ultrasound gel over brachial, dorsalis pedis, and posterior tibial arteries.

3. Measure systolic pressures in the arms
   - Use Doppler to locate brachial pulse
   - Inflate cuff 20 mm Hg above last audible pulse
   - Deflate cuff slowly and record pressure at which pulse becomes audible
   - Obtain 2 measures in each arm and record the average as the brachial pressure in that arm

4. Measure systolic pressures in ankles
   - Use Doppler to locate dorsalis pedis pulse
   - Inflate cuff 20 mm Hg above last audible pulse
   - Deflate cuff slowly and record pressure at which pulse becomes audible
   - Obtain 2 measures in each ankle and record the average as the dorsalis pedis pressure in that leg
   - Repeat above steps for posterior tibial arteries

5. Calculate ABI

$$\text{Right ABI} = \frac{\text{highest right average ankle pressure (DP or PT)}}{\text{highest average arm pressure (right or left)}}$$

$$\text{Left ABI} = \frac{\text{highest left average ankle pressure (DP or PT)}}{\text{highest average arm pressure (right or left)}}$$

Site	1st reading	2nd reading	Average	Site	1st reading	2nd reading	Average
Left brachial				Right brachial			
Left dorsalis pedis				Right dorsalis pedis			
Left posterior tibial				Right posterior tibial			

Ankle–Brachial Index Calculator

$$A - BI = S_A \div S_B$$

Enter values for systolic pressure at:

The ankle: ☐ *mm/Hg*

The brachial artery: ☐ *mm/Hg*

Ankle–brachial index: ☐

Interpretation of Ankle–Brachial Index

>0.90 (with a range of 0.90 to 1.30) = Normal lower extremity blood flow
<0.89 to >0.60 = Mild PAD
<0.59 to >0.40 = Moderate PAD
<0.39 = Severe PAD

(Sources: *Ankle–Brachial Calculator*—American College of Physicians. Available at: http//cpsc.acponline.org/enhancements/232abiCalc.html. Accessed July 3, 2007. Laine C, Goldman D, Wilson JF. In the clinic: peripheral arterial disease. Ann Int Med 146(5):ITC 3-1, 2007.)

TABLE
12-3

Chronic Insufficiency of Arteries and Veins

Chronic Arterial Insufficiency (Advanced)	Chronic Venous Insufficiency (Advanced)

Rubor

Ischemic ulcer

	Chronic Arterial Insufficiency (Advanced)	Chronic Venous Insufficiency (Advanced)
Pain	Intermittent claudication, progressing to pain at rest	Often painful[16]
Mechanism	Tissue ischemia	Venous hypertension
Pulses	Decreased or absent	Normal, though may be difficult to feel through edema
Color	Pale, especially on elevation; dusky red on dependency	Normal, or cyanotic on dependency. Petechiae and then brown pigmentation appear with chronicity.
Temperature	Cool	Normal
Edema	Absent or mild; may develop as the patient tries to relieve rest pain by lowering the leg	Present, often marked
Skin Changes	Trophic changes: thin, shiny, atrophic skin; loss of hair over the foot and toes; nails thickened and ridged	Often brown pigmentation around the ankle, stasis dermatitis, and possible thickening of the skin and narrowing of the leg as scarring develops
Ulceration	If present, involves toes or points of trauma on feet	If present, develops at sides of ankle, especially medially
Gangrene	May develop	Does not develop

(Sources of photos: *Arterial Insufficiency*—Kappert A, Winsor T. Diagnosis of Peripheral Vascular Disease. Philadelphia, FA Davis, 1972; *Venous Insufficiency*—Marks R: Skin Disease in Old Age. Philadelphia, JB Lippincott, 1987.)

Chronic Venous Insufficiency

This condition usually appears over the medial and sometimes the lateral malleolus. The ulcer contains small, painful granulation tissue and fibrin; necrosis or exposed tendons are rare. Borders are irregular, flat, or slightly steep. Pain affects quality of life in 75% of patients. Associated findings include edema, reddish pigmentation and purpura, venous varicosities, the eczematous changes of stasis dermatitis (redness, scaling, and pruritus), and at times cyanosis of the foot when dependent. Gangrene is rare.[16]

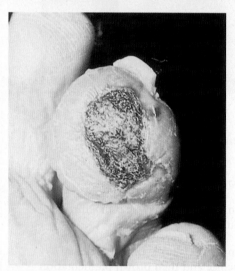

Arterial Insufficiency

This condition occurs in the toes, feet, or possibly areas of trauma (e.g., the shins). Surrounding skin shows no callus or excess pigment, although it may be atrophic. Pain often is severe unless neuropathy masks it. Gangrene may be associated, along with decreased pulses, trophic changes, foot pallor on elevation, and dusky rubor on dependency.

Neuropathic Ulcer

This condition develops in pressure points of areas with diminished sensation; seen in diabetic neuropathy, neurologic disorders, and Hansen disease. Surrounding skin is calloused. There is no pain, so the ulcer may go unnoticed. In uncomplicated cases, there is no gangrene. Associated signs include decreased sensation and absent ankle jerks.

(Source of photos: Marks R: Skin Disease in Old Age. Philadelphia, JB Lippincott, 1987.)

TABLE
12-5

Some Peripheral Causes of Edema

Approximately one third of total body water is extracellular, or outside the body's cells. Approximately 25% of extracellular fluid is plasma; the remainder is interstitial fluid. At the arteriolar end of the capillaries, *hydrostatic pressure* in the blood vessels and *colloid oncotic pressure* in the interstitium cause fluid to move into the tissues; at the venous end of the capillaries and in the lymphatics, hydrostatic pressure in the interstitium and the colloid oncotic pressure of plasma proteins cause fluid to return to the vascular compartment. Several clinical conditions disrupt this balance, resulting in *edema,* or a clinically evident accumulation of interstitial fluid. Not depicted below is *capillary leak syndrome,* in which protein leaks into the interstitial space, seen in burns, angioedema, snake bites, and allergic reactions.

Pitting

Swollen foot

Pitting Edema

Edema is soft, bilateral, with pitting on pressure, on the anterior tibiae and feet. There is no skin thickening, ulceration, or pigmentation. Pitting edema results from several conditions: when legs are dependent from prolonged standing or sitting, which leads to increased hydrostatic pressure in the veins and capillaries; congestive heart failure leading to decreased cardiac output; nephrotic syndrome, cirrhosis, or malnutrition leading to low albumin and decreased intravascular colloid oncotic pressure; and drug use.

Pitting

Pigment

Ulcer

Advanced

Chronic Venous Insufficiency

Edema is soft, with pitting on pressure, and occasionally bilateral. Look for brawny changes and skin thickening, especially near the ankle. Ulceration, brownish pigmentation, and edema in the feet are common. Arises from chronic obstruction and from incompetent valves in the deep venous system.

No pitting

Skin thick

Foot swollen

Lymphedema

Edema is soft in the early stages, then becomes indurated, hard, and nonpitting. Skin is markedly thickened; ulceration is rare. There is no pigmentation. Edema is found in the feet and toes, often bilaterally. Lymphedema develops when lymph channels are obstructed by tumor, fibrosis, or inflammation, and in cases of axillary node dissection and radiation.

Male Genitalia and Hernias

ANATOMY AND PHYSIOLOGY

Review the anatomy of the male genitalia.

The *shaft of the penis* is formed by three columns of vascular erectile tissue: the *corpus spongiosum*, containing the urethra, and two *corpora cavernosa*. The corpus spongiosum forms the bulb of the penis, ending in the cone-shaped *glans* with its expanded base, or *corona*. In uncircumcized men, the glans is covered

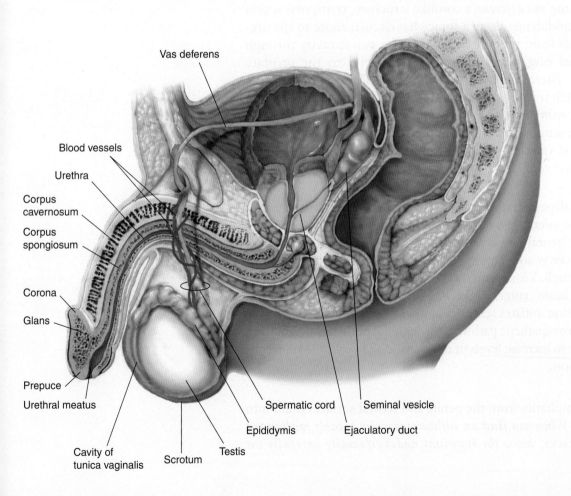

Vas deferens

Blood vessels

Urethra

Corpus cavernosum

Corpus spongiosum

Corona

Glans

Prepuce

Urethral meatus

Spermatic cord

Seminal vesicle

Ejaculatory duct

Epididymis

Testis

Cavity of tunica vaginalis

Scrotum

by a loose, hoodlike fold of skin called the *prepuce* or *foreskin* where *smegma,* or secretions of the glans, may collect. The urethra is located ventrally in the shaft of the penis; urethral abnormalities may sometimes be felt there. The urethra opens into the vertical, slitlike *urethral meatus,* located somewhat ventrally at the tip of the glans.

The *testes* are ovoid, rubbery structures approximately 4.5 cm long, ranging in size from 3.5 cm to 5.5 cm. The left testis usually lies lower than the right. The testes produce spermatozoa and testosterone. Testosterone stimulates the pubertal growth of the male genitalia, prostate, and seminal vesicles. It also stimulates the development of masculine secondary sex characteristics, including facial hair, body hair, musculoskeletal growth, and enlargement of the larynx, with its associated low-pitched voice.

Surrounding or appended to the testes are several structures. The *scrotum* is a loose, wrinkled pouch divided into two compartments, each containing a testis or testicle. Covering the testis, except posteriorly, is the serous membrane of the *tunica vaginalis.* On the posterolateral surface of each testis is the softer, comma-shaped *epididymis,* consisting of tightly coiled spermatic ducts that provide a reservoir for storage, maturation, and transport of sperm from the testis to the *vas deferens.*

During ejaculation, the *vas deferens,* a cordlike structure, transports sperm from the tail of the epididymis along a somewhat circular route to the urethra. The *vas* ascends from the scrotal sac into the pelvic cavity through the external inguinal ring, then loops over the ureter to the prostate behind the bladder. There it merges with the *seminal vesicle* to form the *ejaculatory duct,* which traverses the prostate and empties into the urethra. Secretions from the *vasa deferentia,* the seminal vesicles, and the prostate all contribute to the seminal fluid. Within the scrotum, each vas is closely associated with blood vessels, nerves, and muscle fibers. These structures make up the *spermatic cord.*

Male sexual function depends on normal levels of testosterone, adequate arterial blood flow to the inferior epigastric artery and its cremasteric and pubic branches, and intact neural innervation from α-adrenergic and cholinergic pathways. Erection from venous engorgement of the corpora cavernosa results from two types of stimuli. Visual, auditory, or erotic cues trigger sympathetic outflow from higher brain centers to the T11 through L2 levels of the spinal cord. Tactile stimulation initiates sensory impulses from the genitalia to S_2 to S_4 reflex arcs and parasympathetic pathways through the pudendal nerve. Both sets of stimuli appear to increase levels of nitric oxide and cyclic GMP, resulting in local vasodilation.

Lymphatics. Lymphatics from the penile and scrotal surfaces drain into the inguinal nodes. *When you find an inflammatory or possibly malignant lesion* on these surfaces, *assess the inguinal nodes especially carefully* for enlargement or tenderness. The lymphatics of the testes, however, drain into the abdomen, where enlarged nodes are clinically undetectable. See page 476 for further discussion of the inguinal nodes.

Anatomy of the Groin.   Because hernias are relatively common, it is important to understand the anatomy of the groin. The basic landmarks are the anterior superior iliac spine, the pubic tubercle, and the inguinal ligament that runs between them. Find these on yourself or a colleague.

The *inguinal canal,* which lies above and approximately parallel to the inguinal ligament, forms a tunnel for the vas deferens as it passes through the abdominal muscles. The exterior opening of the tunnel—the *external inguinal ring*—is a triangular, slitlike structure palpable just above and lateral to the pubic tubercle. The internal opening of the canal—or *internal inguinal ring*—is approximately 1 cm above the midpoint of the inguinal ligament. Neither canal nor internal ring is palpable through the abdominal wall. When loops of bowel force their way through weak areas of the inguinal canal, they produce *inguinal hernias,* as illustrated on p. 519.

Another potential route for a herniating mass is the *femoral canal.* This lies below the inguinal ligament. Although you cannot see it, you can estimate its location by placing your right index finger, from below, on the right femoral artery. Your middle finger will then overlie the femoral vein; your ring finger, the femoral canal. Femoral hernias protrude here.

THE HEALTH HISTORY

Common or Concerning Symptoms

- Sexual preference and sexual response
- Penile discharge or lesions
- Scrotal pain, swelling, or lesions

Sexual Preference and Sexual Response. Discussing gender identity and sexual function touches a vital and multifaceted core of your patients' lives. To put your patients at ease, adopt the tips below.

TIPS FOR TAKING THE SEXUAL HISTORY

- Explain why you are taking the sexual history.
- Note that you realize this information is highly personal, and encourage the patient to be open and direct.
- Relate that you gather this history on all your patients.
- Affirm that your conversation is confidential.

For example, you can begin with a general statement such as:

"To provide good care I need to review your sexual health and see if you are at risk for any sexually transmitted diseases. I know this is a sensitive area. Any information you share is confidential and only between us."

Continue with neutral nonjudgmental questions about sexual preference such as "What is your relationship status?" or "Tell me about your sexual preference. Do you prefer partners who are women, men, or both women and men?" Approximately one in ten patients may have same-sex, bisexual, or transgender partner preferences.[1] These patients often experience significant anxiety during clinical encounters, related to fears of clinician acceptance, coexisting mental health conditions, and sparse information about complex issues of hormonal therapy, surgical alterations, and transitions in gender identity.[1]

Continue with questions about sexual function. "How is sexual function for you?" "How is your current relationship?" "Are you satisfied with your relationship and your sexual activity?" "What about your ability to perform sexually?" If the patient expresses relational or sexual concerns, explore both their psychological and physiologic dimensions. Ask about the meaning of the relationship in the patient's life. Also ask about any changes in desire or frequency of sexual activity. What is the patient's view of the cause, what responses has he tried, and what are his hopes?

Direct questions help you to assess each phase of the sexual response. To assess *libido,* or desire, ask "Have you maintained interest in sex?" For the *arousal phase,* ask "Can you achieve and maintain an erection?" Explore the timing, severity, setting, and any other factors that may be contributing to problems. Have any changes in the relationship with his partner or in his life circumstances coincided with onset of a problem? Are there circumstances when erection is normal? On awakening in the early morning or during the night? With other partners? With masturbation?

Lack of libido may arise from psychogenic causes such as depression, endocrine dysfunction, or side effects of medications.

Erectile dysfunction may be from psychogenic causes, especially if early morning erection is preserved; also from decreased testosterone, decreased blood flow in the hypogastric arterial system, or impaired neural innervation.

Other questions relate to the phase of *orgasm* and *ejaculation* of semen. If ejaculation is premature, or early and out of control, ask "About how long does intercourse last?" "Do you climax too soon?" "Do you feel you have control over climaxing?" "Do you think your partner would like intercourse to last longer?" For reduced or absent ejaculation, "Do you find that you cannot have an orgasm even though you can have an erection?" Try to determine whether the problem involves the pleasurable sensation of orgasm, the ejaculation of seminal fluid, or both. Review the frequency and setting of the problem, medications, surgery, and neurologic symptoms.

Premature ejaculation is common, especially in young men. Less common is reduced or absent ejaculation affecting middle-aged or older men. Possible causes are medications, surgery, neurologic deficits, or lack of androgen. Lack of orgasm with ejaculation is usually psychogenic.

Penile Discharge or Lesions.   To assess the possibility of genital infection from sexually transmitted diseases (STDs), ask about any *discharge from the penis,* dripping, or staining of underwear. If penile discharge is present, assess the amount, its color and consistency, and any fever, chills, rash, or associated symptoms.

Penile discharge may accompany gonococcal (usually yellow) and nongonococcal urethritis (may be clear or white).

Scrotal Pain, Swelling, or Lesions.   Inquire about *sores or growths on the penis,* and any *pain or swelling in the scrotum.* Ask about previous genital symptoms or a past history of infections from herpes, gonorrhea, or syphilis. A patient who has multiple partners, is homosexual, uses illicit drugs, or has a prior history of STDs is at increased risk for subsequent STDs.

See Table 13-1, Abnormalities of the Penis and Scrotum (p. 515), Table 13-2, Sexually Transmitted Diseases of Male Genitalia (p. 576), and Table 13-3, Abnormalities of the Testis (p. 517). In addition to STDs, many skin conditions affect the genitalia; likewise, some STDs have minimal symptoms or signs.

Because STDs may involve other parts of the body, additional questions are often indicated. An introductory explanation may be useful. "Sexually transmitted diseases can involve any body opening where you have sex. It's important for you to tell me which openings you use." And further, as needed, "Do you have oral sex? Anal sex?" If the patient's answers are affirmative, ask about symptoms such as sore throat, diarrhea, rectal bleeding, and anal itching or pain.

Infections from oral–penile transmission include gonorrhea, chlamydia, syphilis, and herpes. Symptomatic or asymptomatic proctitis may follow anal intercourse.

For the many patients without symptoms or known risk factors, it is wise to ask "Do you have any concerns about HIV infection?" as an important screening question and to continue with the more general questions suggested on pp. 82–83.

HEALTH PROMOTION AND COUNSELING

Important Topics for Health Promotion and Counseling

- Prevention of STDs and HIV
- Testicular self-examination

Prevention of STDs and HIV Infection. The case for aggressive clinician education, early detection during history taking and physical examination, and treatment for sexually transmitted diseases (STDs) and HIV is compelling. The growing burden of STDs affects the health of all segments of the population, but especially adolescents and young adults. The Institute of Medicine has documented that U.S. rates of STDs are the highest in the industrialized world.[2] In 2005 the Centers for Disease Control and Prevention (CDC) estimated 19 million new STD infections each year, with almost half in the age group 15 to 24 years.[3] Of the 1.3 million new cases reported in 2005, approximately 72% were infections from chlamydia, 25% from gonorrhea, and 3% from syphilis. The CDC notes that these figures represent "only a small proportion of the true national burden of STDs"—many cases are unreported, and viral infections such as human papillomavirus and genital herpes are not subject to requirements for mandatory reporting. Further, more than 1 million Americans are currently infected with HIV, with approximately 40,000 new infections annually. An estimated 25% of infected inhabitants in the United States are unaware of their infected status.[4] Hepatitis B and genital ulcers such as chancroid are also transmitted through sexual contact. The presence of any STD raises the need to investigate co-infection with HIV.

Clinicians must master the skills of eliciting the sexual history and asking frank but tactful questions about sexual practices. Key information includes the patient's sexual orientation, the number of partners in the past month, and any history of past STDs (see also pp. 82–83). Careful screening for alcohol and drug use, especially injection drugs, is also important. Counseling should be interactive and combine messages about general risk reduction relevant to the patient with education about specific actions for reducing the patient's risk (see also Chap. 14, pp. 531–532). Important topics include limiting the number of partners, using condoms, and establishing regular medical care for treatment of STDs and HIV. Men should seek prompt attention for any genital lesions or penile discharge.

In 2006 the CDC issued new recommendations advising universal HIV screening for all people 13 to 64 years, regardless of risk factors. The U.S. Preventive Services Task Force reviewed new evidence about screening in 2007 and continued to affirm screening targeted to those at increased risk and all pregnant women.[5] The Task Force recommends screening and counseling for the following groups: men with male sex partners; men and women having unprotected sex with multiple partners; past or present injection drug users;

sex workers; individuals with past or present sex partners with a history of STDs, HIV infection, injection drug use, or bisexual practice; patients who received blood transfusions between 1978 and 1985; and individuals requesting testing because they may be unwilling to disclose high-risk behaviors.

Testicular Self-examination. In addition, encourage men, especially those between the ages of 15 and 35, to perform monthly *testicular self-examinations* and to seek physician evaluation for the following findings: any painless lump, swelling, or enlargement in either testicle; pain or discomfort in a testicle or the scrotum; a feeling of heaviness or a sudden fluid collection in the scrotum; or a dull ache in the lower abdomen or the groin. (See p. 512 for instructions to patients.)[6]

TECHNIQUES OF EXAMINATION

Many students feel uneasy about examining a man's genitalia. "How will the patient react?" "Will he have an erection?" "Will he let me examine him?" It may be reassuring to explain each step of the examination so that the patient knows what to expect. Request an assistant to accompany you. Occasionally, male patients have erections during the examination. If this happens, explain that this is a normal response, finish your examination, and proceed with an unruffled demeanor. If the man refuses to be examined, you should respect his wishes.

A good genital examination can be done with the patient either standing or supine. To check for hernias or varicoceles, however, the patient should stand, and you should sit comfortably on a chair or stool. A gown conveniently covers the patient's chest and abdomen. *Wear gloves* throughout the examination. Expose the genitalia and inguinal areas. For younger patients, review the sexual maturity ratings on pages 843–844.

 THE PENIS

Inspection

Inspect the penis, including:

See Table 13-1, Abnormalities of the Penis and Scrotum (p. 515).

- The *skin*

- The *prepuce* (foreskin). If present, retract the prepuce or ask the patient to retract it. This step is essential for the detection of many chancres and carcinomas. Smegma, a cheesy, whitish material, may accumulate normally under the foreskin.

Phimosis is a tight prepuce that cannot be retracted over the glans. *Paraphimosis* is a tight prepuce that, once retracted, cannot be returned. Edema ensues.

- The *glans*. Look for any ulcers, scars, nodules, or signs of inflammation.

Balanitis (inflammation of the glans); *balanoposthitis* (inflammation of the glans and prepuce)

Check the skin around the base of the penis for excoriations or inflammation. Look for nits or lice at the bases of the pubic hairs.

Pubic or genital excoriations suggest the possibility of lice (crabs) or sometimes scabies.

Note the location of the urethral meatus.

Compress the glans gently between your index finger above and your thumb below. This maneuver should open the urethral meatus and allow you to inspect it for discharge. Normally there is none.

Hypospadias is a congenital, ventral displacement of the meatus on the penis (p. 515).

Profuse yellow discharge in *gonococcal urethritis*; scanty white or clear discharge in *non-gonococcal urethritis*. Definitive diagnosis requires Gram stain and culture.

If the patient has reported a discharge that you are unable to see, ask him to strip, or milk, the shaft of the penis from its base to the glans. Alternatively, do it yourself. This maneuver may expel some discharge from the urethral meatus for appropriate examination. Have a glass slide and culture materials ready.

Palpation

Palpate any abnormality of the penis, noting any tenderness or induration. Palpate the shaft of the penis between your thumb and first two fingers, noting any induration. Palpation of the shaft may be omitted in a young, asymptomatic male patient.

If you retract the foreskin, replace it before proceeding on to examine the scrotum.

Induration along the ventral surface of the penis suggests a *urethral stricture* or possibly a *carcinoma*. Tenderness of such an indurated area suggests periurethral inflammation secondary to a urethral stricture.

 THE SCROTUM AND ITS CONTENTS

Inspection

Inspect the scrotum, including:

See Table 13-1, Abnormalities of the Penis and Scrotum (p. 515).

● The *skin*. Lift up the scrotum so that you can see its posterior surface.

Rashes, epidermoid cysts, rarely skin cancer

● The *scrotal contours*. Note any swelling, lumps, or veins.

There may be dome-shaped white or yellow papules or nodules formed by occluded follicles filled with keratin debris of desquamated follicular epithelium. Such *epidermoid cysts* are common, frequently multiple, and benign.

A poorly developed scrotum on one or both sides suggests *cryptorchidism* (an undescended testicle). Common scrotal swellings include indirect *inguinal hernias, hydroceles,* and *scrotal edema.*

EPIDERMOID CYSTS

Palpation

Palpate each testis and epididymis between your thumb and first two fingers. Locate the epididymis on the superior posterior surface of each testicle. It feels nodular and cordlike and should not be confused with an abnormal lump.

See Table 13-3, Abnormalities of the Testis (p. 517), and Table 13-4, Abnormalities of the Epididymis and Spermatic Cord (p. 518).

Tender, painful scrotal swelling in *acute epididymitis, acute orchitis, torsion of the spermatic cord,* or a *strangulated inguinal hernia.*

Note size, shape, consistency, and tenderness; feel for any nodules. Pressure on the testis normally produces a deep visceral pain.

Any painless nodule in the testis must raise the possibility of *testicular cancer,* a potentially curable cancer with a peak incidence between the ages of 15 and 35 years.

Palpate each spermatic cord, including the vas deferens, between your thumb and fingers, from the epididymis to the superficial inguinal ring.

Multiple tortuous veins in this area, usually on the left, may be palpable and even visible. They indicate a *varicocele* (p. 518).

Note any nodules or swellings.

The vas deferens, if chronically infected, may feel thickened or beaded. A cystic structure in the spermatic cord suggests a *hydrocele of the cord.*

Swelling in the scrotum other than the testicles can be evaluated by transillumination. After darkening the room, shine the beam of a strong flashlight from behind the scrotum through the mass. Look for transmission of the light as a red glow.

Swellings containing serous fluid, as in hydroceles, light up with a red glow, or transilluminate. Those containing blood or tissue, such as a normal testis, a tumor, or most hernias, do not.

⊚ HERNIAS

Inspection

Sitting comfortably in front of the patient, with the patient standing and an assistant present, *inspect the inguinal regions and genitalia* for bulging areas and asymmetry. As you observe, ask the patient to strain and bear down (the Valsalva maneuver) to increase intra-abdominal pressure, making it easier to detect any hernias.

A bulge that appears on straining suggests a *hernia.*

Palpation

Palpate for an inguinal hernia, using the techniques below. Continue to face the patient; the patient should still be standing.

See Table 13-5, Course, Presentation, and Differentiation of Hernias in the Groin (p. 519).

● To examine for right inguinal hernias, place the tip of your right index finger close to the inferior margin of the scrotal sac, then move your finger upward along the inguinal canal, invaginating the scrotum.

● Follow the spermatic cord upward to the inguinal ligament. Find the triangular slitlike opening of the *external inguinal ring* just above and lateral to the pubic tubercle. Palpate the external inguinal ring and its floor. Ask the patient to bear down. Search for any bulges or masses against the side or pulp of the index finger above the inguinal ligament near the pubic tubercle.

A bulge near the external inguinal ring suggests a *direct inguinal hernia.* A bulge near the internal inguinal ring suggests an *indirect inguinal hernia.* Experts note that distinguishing the type of hernia is difficult, but detecting either type of mass warrants surgical evaluation.[7]

● The external ring may be large enough for you to gently palpate obliquely along the inguinal canal toward the *internal inguinal ring.* Ask the patient to bear down. Check for a bulge that slides down the inguinal canal and taps against the fingertip.

● To examine for left inguinal hernias, use the same techniques with the left index finger.

Inguinal ligament

External inguinal ring

Palpate for a femoral hernia by placing your fingers on the anterior thigh in the region of the femoral canal. Ask the patient to strain down again or cough. Note any swelling or tenderness.

Evaluating a Possible Scrotal Hernia.

If you find a large scrotal mass and suspect that it may be a hernia, ask the patient to lie down. The mass may return to the abdomen by itself. If so, it is a hernia. If not:

● Can you get your fingers above the mass in the scrotum?

If you can, suspect a *hydrocele.*

● Listen to the mass with a stethoscope for bowel sounds.

Bowel sounds may be heard over a hernia, but not over a hydrocele.

If the findings suggest a hernia, gently try to reduce it (return it to the abdominal cavity) by sustained pressure with your fingers. Do not attempt this maneuver if the mass is tender or the patient reports nausea and vomiting.

History may be helpful here. The patient can usually tell you what happens to his swelling on lying down and may be able to demonstrate how he reduces it himself. Remember to ask him.

A hernia is *incarcerated* when its contents cannot be returned to the abdominal cavity. A hernia is *strangulated* when the blood supply to the entrapped contents is compromised. Suspect strangulation in the presence of tenderness, nausea, and vomiting and consider surgical intervention. See Table 13-5, Course, Presentation, and Differentiation of Hernias in the Groin (p. 519)

SPECIAL TECHNIQUES

The Testicular Self-Examination

The incidence of testicular cancer is low, about 4 per 100,000 men, but it is the most common cancer of young men between ages 15 and 35. Although the testicular self-examination (TSE) has not been formally endorsed as a screen for testicular carcinoma, teach your patient the TSE to enhance health awareness and self-care. When detected early, testicular carcinoma has an

---

PATIENT INSTRUCTIONS FOR THE TESTICULAR SELF-EXAMINATION

This examination is best performed after a warm bath or shower. The heat relaxes the scrotum and makes it easier to find anything unusual.

- Standing in front of a mirror, check for any swelling on the skin of the scrotum.
- Examine each testicle with both hands. Cup the index and middle fingers under the testicle and place the thumbs on top.
- Roll the testicle gently between the thumbs and fingers. One testicle may be larger than the other . . . that's normal, but be concerned about any lump or area of pain.

- Find the epididymis. This is a soft, tubelike structure at the back of the testicle that collects and carries sperm, not an abnormal lump.
- If you find any lump, don't wait. See your doctor. The lump may just be an infection, but if it is cancer, it will spread unless stopped by treatment.

(Source: Medline Plus. U.S. National Library of Medicine and National Institutes of Health. Medical Encyclopedia—Testicular self-examination. Available at: www.nlm.nih.gov/medlineplus/ency/article/003909.htm. Accessed June 8, 2007.)

excellent prognosis. Risk factors include cryptorchidism, which confers a high risk for testicular carcinoma in the undescended testicle; a history of carcinoma in the contralateral testicle; mumps orchitis; an inguinal hernia; and a hydrocele in childhood.

RECORDING YOUR FINDINGS

Note that initially you may use sentences to describe your findings; later you will use phrases. The style below contains phrases appropriate for most write-ups.

Recording the Physical Examination— Male Genitalia and Hernias

"Circumcized male. No penile discharge or lesions. No scrotal swelling or discoloration. Testes descended bilaterally, smooth, without masses. Epididymis nontender. No inguinal or femoral hernias."

OR

"Uncircumcized male; prepuce easily retractible. No penile discharge or lesions. No scrotal swelling or discoloration. Testes descended bilaterally; right testicle smooth; 1 × 1 cm firm nodule on left lateral testicle. It is fixed and nontender. Epididymis nontender. No inguinal or femoral hernias."

Suspicious for *testicular carcinoma*, the most common form of cancer in men between the ages of 15 and 35

BIBLIOGRAPHY

CITATIONS

1. Lgbthealthchannel. Available at: http://www.lgbthealthchannel. com/transgender/ht.shtml. Accessed June 6, 2007.
2. Institute of Medicine. Committee on Prevention and Control of Sexually Transmitted Diseases. The Hidden Epidemic: Confronting Sexually Transmitted Diseases. Washington, DC, National Academy Press, 1997:1–432.
3. CDC Trends in Reportable Sexually Transmitted Diseases in the United States 2005. National Surveillance Data for Chlamydia, Gonorrhea, and Syphilis. December 2006. Available at: http:// www.cdc.gov/std/stats/05pdf/trends-2005.pdf   Accessed June 6, 2007.
4. U.S. Preventive Services Task Force. Screening for Genital Herpes Simplex. Available at: http://www.ahrq.gov/clinic/uspstf/ uspsherp.htm. Accessed June 7, 2007.
5. U.S. Preventive Services Task Force. Screening for HIV Recommendation Statement. Release date July 2005; amended April 2007. Available at: http://www.ahrq.gov/clinic/uspstf05/ hiv/hivrs.htm. Accessed June 7, 2007.
6. National Cancer Institute. Cancer Facts. Available at: http:// cis.nih.gov/fact/6_34.htm. Accessed October 31, 2004.
7. Fitzgibbons RJ, Filipi CJ, Quinn TH. Inguinal hernias (Chapter 36). In Brunicardi FC, Andersen DK, Billiar TR, et al (eds). Schwartz's Principles of Surgery, 8th ed. New York, McGraw-Hill, 2005.

ADDITIONAL REFERENCES

Campbell MF, Wein AJ, Kavoussi LR (eds). Campbell-Walsh Urology, 9th ed. Philadelphia: Saunders-Elsevier, 2007.
DeBusk RF. Sexual activity in patients with angina. JAMA 290(23): 3129–3132, 2003.
Delancey JOL, Ashton-Miller JA. Pathophysiology of adult urinary incontinence. Gastroenterology 126(Suppl 1):S23–S32, 2004.
Fitzgibbons RJ, Dilipi CJ, Quinn TH. Inguinal hernias. In: Brunicardi FC, Andersen DK, Billiar TR, et al., eds. Schwartz's Principles of Surgery, 8th ed. New York: McGraw-Hill, 2005.

Gillenwater JY. Adult and Pediatric Urology, 4th ed. Philadelphia, Lippincott Williams & Wilkins, 2002.

Handsfield HH. Color Atlas and Synopsis of Sexually Transmitted Diseases, 2nd ed. New York, McGraw-Hill, 2001.

Institute of Medicine, Committee on Prevention and Control of Sexually Transmitted Diseases. The Hidden Epidemic: Confronting Sexually Transmitted Diseases. Washington, DC: National Academy Press, 1997:1–432.

Malangoni MA, Rosen MJ. Hernias. In: Townsend CM, Beauchamp D, Evers M, et al. Sabiston Textbook of Surgery: The Biological Basis of Modern Surgical Practice, 18th ed. Philadelphia: Elsevier/Saunders, 2008.

National Guideline Clearinghouse. Clinical Prevention Guidance: Sexually Transmitted Diseases Treatment Guidelines 2006. Available at: http://www.guideline.gov/summary/summary.aspx?doc_id=9672&nbr=005181&string=STDs. Accessed June 7, 2007.

Tanagho EA, McAninch JW (eds). Smith's General Urology, 16th ed. New York, Lange Medical Books, McGraw-Hill, 2004.

U.S. Preventive Services Task Force. Screening for genital herpes simplex. March 2005. Available at: http://www.ahrq.gov/clinic/uspstf/uspsherp.htm. Accessed June 7, 2007.

The Bates' suite offers these additional resources to enhance learning and facilitate understanding of this chapter:

- Bates' Pocket Guide to Physical Examination and History Taking, 6th edition
- Bates' Nursing Online
- Bates' Visual Guide to Physical Examination, 4th edition
- thePoint online resources, http://thepoint.lww.com
- Student CD-ROM included with the book

Hypospadias

A congenital displacement of the urethral meatus to the inferior surface of the penis. A groove extends from the actual urethral meatus to its normal location on the tip of the glans.

Scrotal Edema

Pitting edema may make the scrotal skin taut; seen in congestive heart failure or nephrotic syndrome.

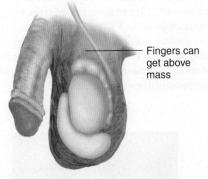

Fingers can get above mass

Peyronie's Disease

Palpable, nontender, hard plaques are found just beneath the skin, usually along the dorsum of the penis. The patient complains of crooked, painful erections.

Hydrocele

A nontender, fluid-filled mass within the tunica vaginalis. It transilluminates, and the examining fingers can get above the mass within the scrotum.

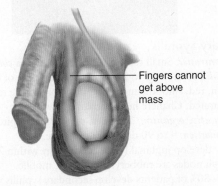

Fingers cannot get above mass

Carcinoma of the Penis

An indurated nodule or ulcer that is usually nontender. Limited almost completely to men who are not circumcised, it may be masked by the prepuce. Any persistent penile sore is suspicious.

Scrotal Hernia

Usually an *indirect inguinal hernia*, that comes through the external inguinal ring, so the examining fingers cannot get above it within the scrotum.

TABLE 13-2

Sexually Transmitted Diseases of Male Genitalia

Genital Warts (condylomata acuminata)

- *Appearance:* Single or multiple papules or plaques of variable shapes; may be round, acuminate (or pointed), or thin and slender. May be raised, flat, or cauliflower-like (verrucous).
- *Causative organism: Human papillomavirus (HPV),* usually from subtypes 6, 11; carcinogenic subtypes rare, approximately 5–10% of all anogenital warts. *Incubation:* weeks to months; infected contact may have no visible warts.
- Can arise on penis, scrotum, groin, thighs, anus; usually asymptomatic, occasionally cause itching and pain.
- May disappear without treatment.

Genital Herpes Simplex

- *Appearance:* Small scattered or grouped vesicles, 1–3 mm in size, on glans or shaft of penis. Appear as erosions if vesicular membrane breaks.
- *Causative organism:* Usually *Herpes simplex virus 2* (90%), a double-stranded DNA virus. *Incubation:* 2 to 7 days after exposure.
- Primary episode may be asymptomatic; recurrence usually less painful, of shorter duration.
- Associated with fever, malaise, headache, arthralgias; local pain and edema, lymphadenopathy.
- Need to distinguish from genital herpes zoster (usually in older patients with dermatomal distribution); candidiasis.

Primary Syphilis

- *Appearance:* Small red papule that becomes a *chancre,* or *painless* erosion up to 2 cm in diameter. Base of chancre is clean, red, smooth, and glistening; borders are raised and indurated. Chancre heals within 3–8 weeks.
- *Causative organism: Treponema pallidum,* a spirochete. *Incubation:* 9 to 90 days after exposure.
- May develop inguinal lymphadenopathy within 7 days; lymph nodes are rubbery, nontender, mobile.
- 20%–30% of patients develop secondary syphilis while chancre still present (suggests co-infection with HIV).
- Distinguish from: genital herpes simplex; chancroid; granuloma inguinale from *Klebsiella granulomatis* (rare in U.S.; 4 variants, so difficult to identify).

Chancroid

- *Appearance:* Red papule or pustule initially, then forms a *painful* deep ulcer with ragged non-indurated margins; contains necrotic exudate, has a friable base.
- *Causative organism: Haemophilus ducreyi,* an anaerobic bacillus. *Incubation:* 3 to 7 days after exposure.
- Painful inguinal adenopathy; suppurative boboes in 25% of patients.
- Need to distinguish from: primary syphilis; genital herpes simplex; lymphomogranuloma venerium, granuloma inguinale from *Klebsiella granulomatis* (both rare in U.S.).

TABLE 13-3
Abnormalities of the Testis

Cryptorchidism

The testis is atrophied and may lie in the inguinal canal or the abdomen, resulting in an unfilled scrotum. As above, there is no palpable left testis or epididymis. Cryptorchidism markedly raises the risk for testicular cancer.

Small Testis

In adults, testicular length is usually ≤3.5 cm. Small, firm testes in *Klinefelter's syndrome,* usually ≤2 cm. Small, soft testes suggesting atrophy are seen in cirrhosis, myotonic dystrophy, use of estrogens, and hypopituitarism; may also follow orchitis.

Acute Orchitis

The testis is acutely inflamed, painful, tender, and swollen. It may be difficult to distinguish from the epididymis. The scrotum may be reddened. Seen in mumps and other viral infections; usually unilateral.

Early

Late

Tumor of the Testis

Usually appears as a painless nodule. Any nodule within the testis warrants investigation for malignancy.

As a testicular neoplasm grows and spreads, it may seem to replace the entire organ. The testicle characteristically feels heavier than normal.

TABLE 13-4

Abnormalities of the Epididymis and Spermatic Cord

Spermatocele and Cyst of the Epididymis

A painless, movable cystic mass just above the testis suggests a spermatocele or an epididymal cyst. Both transilluminate. The former contains sperm, and the latter does not, but they are clinically indistinguishable.

Varicocele of the Spermatic Cord

Varicocele refers to varicose veins of the spermatic cord, usually found on the left. It feels like a soft "bag of worms" separate from the testis, and slowly collapses when the scrotum is elevated in the supine patient. Infertility may be associated.

Acute Epididymitis

An acutely inflamed epididymis is tender and swollen and may be difficult to distinguish from the testis. The scrotum may be reddened and the vas deferens inflamed. It occurs chiefly in adults. Coexisting urinary tract infection or prostatitis supports the diagnosis.

Torsion of the Spermatic Cord

Torsion, or twisting, of the testicle on its spermatic cord produces an acutely painful, tender, and swollen organ that is retracted upward in the scrotum. The scrotum becomes red and edematous. There is no associated urinary infection. Torsion, most common in adolescents, is a surgical emergency because of obstructed circulation.

Tuberculous Epididymitis

The chronic inflammation of tuberculosis produces a firm enlargement of the epididymis, which is sometimes tender, with thickening or beading of the vas deferens.

TABLE
13-5

Course, Presentation, and Differentiation of Hernias in the Groin

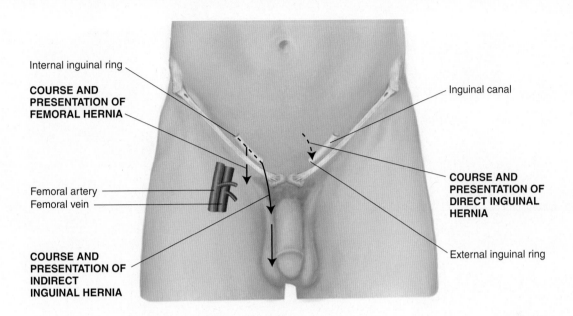

Internal inguinal ring

COURSE AND PRESENTATION OF FEMORAL HERNIA

Femoral artery

Femoral vein

COURSE AND PRESENTATION OF INDIRECT INGUINAL HERNIA

Inguinal canal

COURSE AND PRESENTATION OF DIRECT INGUINAL HERNIA

External inguinal ring

	Inguinal Hernias		Femoral Hernias
	Indirect	*Direct*	
Frequency, Age, and Sex	Most common, all ages, both sexes. Often in children; may be in adults	Less common. Usually in men older than 40; rare in women	Least common. More common in women than in men
Point of Origin	Above inguinal ligament, near its midpoint (the internal inguinal ring)	Above inguinal ligament, close to the pubic tubercle (near the external inguinal ring)	Below the inguinal ligament; appears more lateral than an inguinal hernia. Can be hard to differentiate from lymph nodes
Course	Often into the scrotum	Rarely into the scrotum	Never into the scrotum
(Examining finger in inguinal canal during straining)	The hernia comes down the inguinal canal and touches the fingertip.	The hernia bulges anteriorly and pushes the side of the finger forward.	The inguinal canal is empty.

Female Genitalia

ANATOMY AND PHYSIOLOGY

Review the anatomy of the external female genitalia, or *vulva*, including the *mons pubis*, a hair-covered fat pad overlying the symphysis pubis; the *labia majora*, rounded folds of adipose tissue; the *labia minora*, thinner pinkish-red folds that extend anteriorly to form the *prepuce*; and the *clitoris*. The *vestibule* is the boat-shaped fossa between the labia minora. In its posterior portion lies the vaginal opening, the *introitus*, which in virgins may be hidden by the *hymen*. The term *perineum*, as commonly used clinically, refers to the tissue between the introitus and the anus.

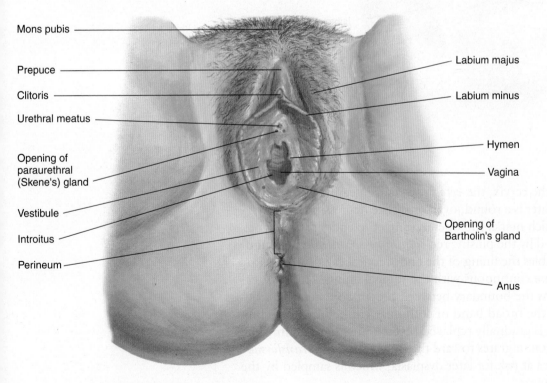

The *urethral meatus* opens into the vestibule between the clitoris and the vagina. Just posterior to it on either side lie the openings of the *paraurethral (Skene's) glands*.

The openings of *Bartholin's glands* are located posteriorly on either side of the vaginal opening but are not usually visible. Bartholin's glands themselves are situated more deeply.

The *vagina* is a musculomembranous tube extending upward and posteriorly between the urethra and the rectum. Its upper third takes a horizontal plane and terminates in the cup-shaped *fornix*. The vaginal mucosa lies in transverse folds, or rugae.

The vagina lies almost at a right angle to the *uterus*, a flattened fibromuscular structure shaped like an inverted pear. The uterus has two parts: the body, or *corpus*, and the cervix, both joined at the *isthmus*. The convex upper surface of the body is termed the uterine *fundus*. The distal cervix protrudes into the vagina, dividing the upper vagina into three recesses, the *anterior*, *posterior*, and *lateral fornices*.

Location of
Bartholin's glands

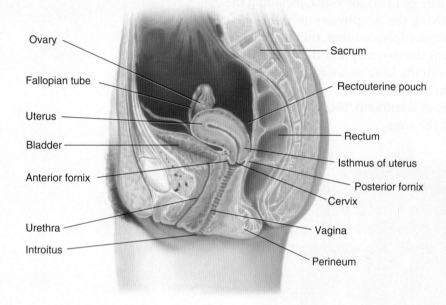

The vaginal surface of the cervix, the *ectocervix*, is seen easily with the help of a speculum. At its center is a round, oval, or slitlike depression, the *external os* of the cervix, which marks the opening into the endocervical canal. The ectocervix is covered by the plushy, red *columnar epithelium* surrounding the os, which resembles the lining of the endocervical canal, and a shiny pink *squamous epithelium* continuous with the vaginal lining. The *squamocolumnar junction* forms the boundary between these two types of epithelium. During puberty, the broad band of columnar epithelium encircling the os, called *ectropion*, is gradually replaced by columnar epithelium. The squamocolumnar junction migrates toward the os, creating the *transformation zone*. This is the area at risk for later dysplasia, which is sampled by the Papanicolaou, or Pap, smear.

A *fallopian tube* with a fanlike tip extends from each side of the uterus toward the ovary. The two ovaries are almond-shaped structures that vary

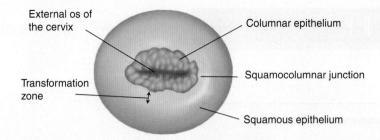

External os of
the cervix

Columnar epithelium

Transformation
zone

Squamocolumnar junction

Squamous epithelium

CERVICAL EPITHELIA AND TRANSFORMATION ZONE

considerably in size but average approximately $3.5 \times 2 \times 1.5$ cm from adult-hood through menopause. The ovaries are palpable on pelvic examination in roughly half of women during the reproductive years. Normally, fallopian tubes cannot be felt. The term *adnexa*, a plural Latin word meaning appendages, refers to the ovaries, tubes, and supporting tissues.

The ovaries have two primary functions: the production of ova and the secretion of hormones, including estrogen, progesterone, and testosterone. Increased hormonal secretions during puberty stimulate the growth of the uterus and its endometrial lining, enlargement of the vagina, and thickening of the vaginal epithelium. They also stimulate the development of secondary sex characteristics, including the breasts and pubic hair.

The parietal peritoneum extends downward behind the uterus into a cul de sac called the *rectouterine pouch* (pouch of Douglas). You can just reach this area on rectovaginal examination.

The pelvic organs are supported by a sling of tissues composed of muscle, ligaments, and fascia, through which the urethra, vagina, and rectum all pass.

Assessment of sexual maturity in girls, as classified by Tanner, depends not on internal examination, but on the growth of pubic hair and the development of breasts. Tanner's stages, or sexual maturity ratings, as they relate to pubic hair and breasts are shown in Chapter 18, Assessing Children: Infancy Through Adolescence, pp. 842–845.

In most women, pubic hair spreads downward in a triangular pattern, pointing toward the vagina. In 10% of women, it may form an inverted triangle, pointing toward the umbilicus. This growth is usually not completed until the middle 20s or later.

Just before menarche, there is a physiologic increase in vaginal secretions—a normal change that sometimes worries a girl or her mother. As menses become established, increased secretions (*leukorrhea*) coincide with ovulation. They also accompany sexual arousal. These normal kinds of discharges must be differentiated from those of infectious processes.

Lymphatics.   Lymph from the vulva and lower vagina drains into the inguinal nodes. Lymph from the internal genitalia, including the upper vagina, flows into the pelvic and abdominal lymph nodes, which are not palpable.

THE HEALTH HISTORY

Common Concerns

- Menarche, menstruation, menopause, postmenopausal bleeding
- Pregnancy
- Vulvovaginal symptoms
- Sexual preference and sexual response

Menarche, Menstruation, Menopause. Learn to recognize patterns of menstrual flow, using the terms below.

THE MENSTRUAL HISTORY—HELPFUL DEFINITIONS

- *Menarche*—age at onset of menses
- *Menopause*—absence of menses for 12 consecutive months, usually occurring between 48 and 55 years
- *Postmenopausal bleeding*—bleeding occurring 6 months or more after cessation of menses
- *Amenorrhea*—absence of menses
- *Dysmenorrhea*—pain with menses, often with bearing down, aching, or cramping sensation in the lower abdomen or pelvis
- *Premenstrual syndrome (PMS)*—a cluster of emotional, behavioral, and physical symptoms occurring 5 days before menses for three consecutive cycles
- *Abnormal uterine bleeding*—bleeding between menses; includes infrequent, excessive, prolonged, or postmenopausal bleeding

Questions about *menarche, menstruation*, and *menopause* often give you an opportunity to explore the patient's concerns and attitude toward her body. When talking with an adolescent girl, for example, opening questions might include: "How did you first learn about monthly periods? How did you feel when they started? Many girls worry when their periods aren't regular or come late. Has anything like that bothered you?" You can explain that girls in the United States usually begin to menstruate between the ages of 9 and 16 years, and often it takes 1 year or more before periods settle into a reasonable, regular pattern. Age at menarche is variable, depending on genetic endowment, socioeconomic status, and nutrition. The interval between periods ranges roughly from 24 to 32 days; flow lasts from 3 to 7 days.

For the menstrual history, ask the patient how old she was when her menstrual periods began, or age at *menarche*. When did her last period start, and, if possible, the one before that? How often does she have periods, as measured by the interval between the first days of successive periods? How regular or irreg-

The dates of previous periods can signal possible pregnancy or menstrual irregularities.

ular are they? How long do they last? How heavy is the flow? What color is it? Flow can be assessed roughly by the number of pads or tampons used daily. Because women vary in their practices for sanitary measures, however, ask the patient whether she usually soaks a pad or tampon, spots it lightly, etc. Further, does she use more than one at a time? Does she have any bleeding between periods? Any bleeding after intercourse?

Ask a middle-aged or older woman if she has stopped menstruating. When? Did any symptoms accompany her changes to menopause? Has she had any bleeding since?

Up to 50% of women report *dysmenorrhea*, or pain with menses. Ask if the patient has any discomfort or pain before or during her periods. If so, what is it like, how long does it last, and does it interfere with usual activities? Are there other associated symptoms? Dysmenorrhea may be *primary*, without an organic cause, or *secondary*, with an organic cause.

Premenstrual syndrome (PMS) includes emotional and behavioral symptoms such as depression, angry outbursts, irritability, anxiety, confusion, crying spells, sleep disturbance, poor concentration, and social withdrawal.[1] Ask about signs such as bloating and weight gain, swelling of the hands and feet, and generalized aches and pains. Criteria for diagnosis are symptoms and signs in the 5 days prior to menses for at least three consecutive cycles; cessation of symptoms and signs within 4 days after onset of menses; and interference with daily activities.

Amenorrhea refers to the absence of periods. Failure of periods to initiate is called *primary amenorrhea*, whereas the cessation of periods after they have been established is termed *secondary amenorrhea*. Pregnancy, lactation, and menopause are physiologic forms of the secondary type.

Ask about any abnormal bleeding. The term *abnormal uterine bleeding* encompasses several patterns:

- *Polymenorrhea*, or fewer than 21-day intervals between menses

- *Oligomenorrhea*, or infrequent bleeding

- *Menorrhagia*, or excessive flow

- *Metorrhagia*, or intermenstrual bleeding

- Postcoital bleeding

Unlike the normal dark red menstrual discharge, excessive flow tends to be bright red and may include "clots" (not true fibrin clots).

Primary dysmenorrhea results from increased prostaglandin production during the luteal phase of the menstrual cycle, when estrogen and progesterone levels decline.

Causes of *secondary dysmenorrhea* include endometriosis, adenomyosis (endometriosis in the muscular layers of the uterus), pelvic inflammatory disease, and endometrial polyps.

Other causes of *secondary amenorrhea* include low body weight from any cause, including malnutrition and anorexia nervosa, stress, chronic illness, and hypothalamic–pituitary–ovarian dysfunction.

Causes vary by age group and include pregnancy, cervical or vaginal infection, or cancer, cervical or endometrial polyps or hyperplasia, fibroids, bleeding disorders, and hormonal contraception or replacement therapy. *Postcoital bleeding* suggests cervical polyps or cancer, or in an older woman, atrophic vaginitis.

Menopause usually occurs between 48 and 55 years, following a period of fluctuation in pituitary secretion of follicle-stimulating hormone (FSH) and luteinizing hormone (LH) and ovarian function.[2] If your patient is *peri-menopausal*, with onset of variable cycle length, ask about such vasomotor symptoms as hot flashes, flushing, and sweating. Sleep disturbances are also common. After menopause, there may be vaginal dryness and *dyspareunia*, or painful intercourse, hair loss, and mild hirsutism as the androgen-to-estrogen ratio increases. Urinary symptoms may also occur in the absence of infection because of atrophy of the urethra and urinary trigone.

Woman may ask about many alternative compounds and botanicals for relief of menopause-related symptoms. Most have not been well-studied or proved to be beneficial. Estrogen replacement relieves symptoms but increases risk of thrombosis. Some evidence shows that some antidepressants and alpha-blockers can be helpful.[3]

Often you will ask, "How do (did) you feel about not having your periods anymore? Has it affected your life in any way?" Ask about any bleeding after menopause.

Postmenopausal bleeding in endometrial cancer, hormone replacement therapy, uterine and cervical polyps

Pregnancy.   Questions relating to pregnancy include "Have you ever been pregnant? How many times? . . . How many living children do you have? . . . Have you ever had a miscarriage or an abortion? How many times?" Ask about any difficulties during pregnancy and the timing and circumstances of any abortion, whether spontaneous or induced. How did the woman experience these losses? Obstetricians commonly record the pregnancy history using the "gravida-para" system.

THE GRAVIDA-PARA NOTATION

- G = gravida, or total number of pregnancies
- P = para, or outcomes of pregnancies. After P, you will often see the notations F (full-term), P (premature), A (abortion), and L (living child).

Inquire about methods of contraception used by the patient and her partner. Is the patient satisfied with the method chosen? Are there any questions about the options available?

If amenorrhea suggests a *current pregnancy*, inquire about the history of intercourse and *common early symptoms:* tenderness, tingling, or increased size of the breasts; urinary frequency; nausea and vomiting; easy fatigability; and feelings that the baby is moving, usually noted at about 20 weeks. Be considerate of the patient's feelings about discussing these topics and explore them when the patient has special concerns. (See also Chapter 19, The Pregnant Woman.)

Amenorrhea followed by heavy bleeding suggests a *threatened abortion* or *dysfunctional uterine bleeding* related to lack of ovulation.

Vulvovaginal Symptoms.   The most common vulvovaginal symptoms are *vaginal discharge* and local *itching.* Follow your usual approach. If the patient reports a discharge, inquire about its amount, color, consistency, and odor. Ask about any local *sores* or *lumps* in the vulvar area. Are they painful or not? Because patients vary in their understanding of anatomical terms, be prepared to try alternative phrasing such as "Any itching (or other symptoms) near your vagina? . . . between your legs? . . . where you urinate?"

See Table 14-1, Lesions of the Vulva, p. 546; and Table 14-6, Vaginal Discharge, p. 550.

Sexual Preference and Sexual Response. Review the Tips for Taking a Sexual History, on p. 504. Using neutral and nonjudgmental questions, ask about your patient's sexual preference and relationship status. Patients with same-sex or transgender preferences may be anxious or fearful during clinical encounters. A reassuring manner will help them express concerns about their sexual health and activity.

Start with general questions such as "How is sex for you?" Or "Are you having any problems with sex?" You can also ask, "Are you satisfied with your sex life as it is now? Has there been any significant change in the last few years? Are you satisfied with you ability to perform sexually? How satisfied do you think your partner is? Do you feel that your partner is satisfied with the frequency of sexual activity?"

If the patient has concerns about sexual activity, ask her to tell you about it. Direct questions help you assess each phase of the sexual response: desire, arousal, and orgasm. "Do you have an interest in (appetite for) sex?" inquires about the desire phase. For the orgasmic phase, "Are you able to reach climax (reach an orgasm or 'come')?" "Is it important for you to reach climax?" For arousal, "Do you get sexually aroused? Do you lubricate easily (get wet or slippery)? Do you stay too dry?"

> Sexual dysfunction is classified by the phase of sexual response. A woman may lack desire, she may fail to become aroused and attain adequate vaginal lubrication, or, despite adequate arousal, she may be unable to reach orgasm. Causes include lack of estrogen, medical illness, and psychiatric conditions.

Ask also about *dyspareunia*. If present, try to localize the symptom. Is it near the outside, occurring at the start of intercourse, or does she feel it farther in, when her partner is pushing deeper? *Vaginismus* refers to an involuntary spasm of the muscles surrounding the vaginal orifice that makes penetration during intercourse painful or impossible.

> Superficial pain suggests local inflammation, atrophic vaginitis, or inadequate lubrication; deeper pain may be from pelvic disorders or pressure on a normal ovary. The cause of *vaginismus* may be physical or psychological.

In addition to ascertaining the nature of a sexual problem, ask about its onset, severity (persistent or sporadic), setting, and factors, if any, that make it better or worse. What does the patient think is the cause of the problem, what has she tried to do about it, and what does she hope for? The setting of sexual dysfunction is an important but complicated topic, involving the patient's general health; medications and drugs, including use of alcohol; her partner's and her own knowledge of sexual practices and techniques; her attitudes, values, and fears; the relationship and communication between partners; and the setting in which sexual activity takes place.

> More commonly, however, a sexual problem is related to situational or psychosocial factors.

Sexually Transmitted Diseases (STDs). Local symptoms or findings on physical examination may raise the possibility of *sexually transmitted diseases*. After establishing the usual attributes of any symptoms, identify sexual preference (male, female, or both). Inquire about sexual contacts and establish the number of sexual partners in the prior month. Ask if the patient has concerns about HIV infection, desires HIV testing, or has current or past partners at risk. Also ask about oral and anal sex and, if indicated, about symptoms involving the mouth, throat, anus, and rectum. Review the past history of venereal disease. "Have you ever had herpes? . . . any other problems such as gonorrhea? . . . syphilis? . . . pelvic infections?" Continue with the more general questions suggested on pp. 82–83.

HEALTH PROMOTION AND COUNSELING

Important Topics for Health Promotion and Counseling

- Cervical cancer screening: Pap smear and HPV infection
- Options for family planning
- Sexually transmitted diseases and HIV
- Changes in menopause

Cervical Cancer Screening: the Pap Smear and Human Papillomavirus (HPV) Infection. Widespread screening by *Papanicolaou (Pap) smear* has contributed to a significant decline in the incidence of and mortality from cervical cancer. The U.S. Preventive Services Task Force notes that "the goal of cytologic screening is to sample the transformation zone, the area where physiologic transformation from columnar endocervical epithelium to squamous (ectocervical) epithelium takes place and where dysplasia and cancer arise."[4] There are two primary types of cervical cancer. Approximately 80% to 90% are squamous cell carcinomas; the remaining 10% to 20% are adenocarcinomas in glandular cells.

Risk factors for cervical cancer are both viral and behavioral. The most important risk factor is infection with the *high-risk strains of HPV*. Genital infection with HPV is the most common STD in the United States.[5] More than 50% of sexually active people contract the infection during their lifetime. Most genital HPV infections are transient and become HPV DNA-negative in 1 to 2 years, possibly from clearance by gradually developing immune antibodies. Persisting HPV is thought to induce precancerous and cancerous lesions, and HPVs cause virtually all cervical cancers.[6] HPV 16 and 18 are responsible for approximately 70% of clinical cancers, and HPV 6 and 11 cause 90% of genital warts.

Other risk factors for cervical cancer include early sexual activity; multiple sexual partners; a history of STDs; failure to undergo screening by Pap smear; age; nutritional status; smoking; immune status; and genetic polymorphisms affecting the entry of HPV DNA into cervical cells.[4]

Pap Smear Screening Guidelines. The American College of Obstetricians and Gynecologists, the American Cancer Society, and the U.S. Preventive Services Task Force have recently issued new recommendations related to screening frequency in different age groups.[4,7,8] These recommendations reflect advances in understanding of the progression from low-grade to high-grade cervical lesions and in the technology of Pap smear testing. Cervical intraepithelial neoplasia progresses slowly and is readily detected on Pap smear. New technologies such as liquid-based cytology, computerized rescreening, and algorithm-based screening may improve detection of abnormal cervical cells, although the U.S. Preventive Services Task Force concluded in 2003 that evidence comparing the accuracy of these new techniques with conventional Pap smears was still insufficient.[4,9]

Recommendations of the American College of Obstetricians and Gynecologists are summarized below.[7] These are in close agreement with the American Cancer Society and the U.S. Preventive Services Task Force (USPSTF). Reviewing the three sets of guidelines is useful and informative.

● Cervical Cancer Screening Guidelines: ACOG[7]

First screen	Screen approximately 3 years after first sexual intercourse or by 21 years of age, whichever comes first.
Women up to age 30	Screen annually with regular test or every 2 years with newer liquid-based cytology test.
Women age 30 or older	• Screen every 2 to 3 years if three consecutive annual cervical cytology results are negative or if combined cytology testing and high-risk HPV testing results are negative. • Screen more frequently in patients with positive Pap or positive high-risk HPV test results; HIV infection; immunosuppression; DES exposure *in utero*; prior history of cervical cancer.
Women with hysterectomy	Discontinue routine screening unless the cervix has been spared or the patient has had cervical dysplasia or neoplasia. Annual screening is recommended for women with such a history until three consecutive tests for vaginal cytology show negative results. (Studies show that 68% of women with hysterectomies for benign cause still report a Pap smear within the prior 3 years.)[10]
Older women	ACOG recommends basing continued screening on clinical assessment of individual health and ability to monitor the patient. The USPSTF found low utility of screening *in women 65 years or older* but recommends continued screening in older women without prior screening or without information about past screening results. The American Cancer Society recommends discontinuing screening in women *older than 70 years* if three consecutive Pap test results are negative and those in the prior 10 years have been negative. The Society states that testing should continue in healthy women with a history of cervical cancer, DES exposure *in utero*, HIV infection, or a weakened immune system.

Take the time to understand how Pap smear results are reported. Current classification and management guidelines are based on the Bethesda System of the National Cancer Institute, revised in 2001.[11,12] The principal categories are provided in the box below. Management depends on the cervical cancer risk and often involves repeat cytology, colposcopy, and DNA testing for human papillomavirus (HPV).

Conventional Pap smears have a sensitivity and specificity for detecting cervical cancer of 30% to 87% and 86% to 100%, respectively. For liquid-based cytology these figures are 61% to 95% and 78% to 82%.[5]

CLASSIFICATION OF PAP SMEAR CYTOLOGY: THE BETHESDA SYSTEM (2001)

- *Negative for intraepithelial lesion or malignancy:* No cellular evidence of neoplasia is present, although other organisms like *Trichomonas, Candida,* or *Actinomyces* may be reported in this category. Shifts in flora consistent with bacterial vaginosis or cellular changes from herpes simplex may also be reported.
- *Epithelial cell abnormalities:* These include precancerous or cancerous lesions:
  - *Squamous cells,* including *atypical squamous cells* (ASC), which may be of undetermined significance (ASC-US); *low-grade squamous intraepithelial lesions* (LSIL), including mild dysplasia; *high-grade squamous intra-epithelial lesions* (HSIL), including moderate and severe dysplasia with features suspicious for invasion; and invasive *squamous cell carcinoma.*
  - *Glandular cells,* including *atypical endocervical cells* or *atypical endometrial cells,* specified or not otherwise specified (NOS); *atypical endocervical cells* or *atypical glandular cells, favor neoplastic; endocervical adeno-carcinoma in situ;* and *adenocarcinoma*
  - *Other malignant neoplasms,* such as sarcomas or lymphomas, both rare

---

The HPV Vaccine. In 2007 the Centers for Disease Control and Prevention recommended administering the *HPV vaccine* to girls and women 11 to 26 years old to reduce the risk of cervical cancer.[13] Studies have shown that the vaccine, which targets HPV types 6, 11, 16, and 18, is almost 100% effective in preventing HPV 16- and 18-related cervical intraepithelial neoplasia grade 2 or 3 and adenocarcinoma in situ in women with no prior exposure to these types.[6] The vaccine also reduces risk of anogenital diseases such as warts, intraepithelial neoplasia, and invasive anogenital cancers.[14] The vaccine is less effective in women already exposed to one of the four HPV types, and it does not treat existing HPV cervical infections, genital warts, precancers, or cancers.[15]

Early vaccination before onset of sexual activity is felt to confer the highest benefit. Approximate initiation of sexual activity in adolescent age groups is 8% before 13 years of age, 33% by ninth grade, and 66% by the end of high school.[16] HPV prevalence is 40% for girls 14 to 19 years.[17] Cervical screening by Pap smear and genital examinations should continue after vaccination to detect changes from new or persisting infection from other oncogenic HPV types. The duration of immunity provided by the HPV vaccine is currently undetermined.

A Note on Ovarian Cancer. Although ovarian cancer is relatively rare, women ask frequently about available screening tests. Currently there are no effective screening tests, although proteomics and CA-125 kinetics may be helpful in the future.[18] The strongest risk factor is a family history of breast or ovarian cancer and BRCA1 and BRCA2 mutations from either parent. CA-125 levels are neither sensitive nor specific. Levels are elevated in more than 80% of women with ovarian cancer and help predict relapse after chemotherapy, but they are also elevated in other conditions and cancers, including pregnancy, endometriosis, uterine fibroids, pelvic inflammatory disease (PID), benign cysts, and pancreatic, breast, lung, gastric, and colon cancers.

STDs and HIV Infection. U.S. rates of STDs are the highest in the industrialized world.[19] *Chlamydia trachomatis* is the most commonly reported STD in the United States and the most common STD in women.[20] Infection rates are highest in women 15 to 19 years and second highest in women 20 to 24 years. African-American women and American Indian/Alaska Native women have the highest infection rates. Most cases are undiagnosed. If untreated, 40% of women will develop PID and 20% will become infertile. Detection, groups most affected, and consequences of underdiagnosis and treatment are similar for *gonorrhea*. Infection with *syphilis* is less common; African-American and Hispanic women are at highest risk. The U.S. Preventive Services Task Force strongly recommends:

- Routine screening for cervical *chlamydia* of all sexually active and pregnant women 24 years or younger and older asymptomatic women at increased risk[21]

- Concurrent chlamydia and Pap smear screening

- Routine screening for cervical *gonorrhea* of all sexually active women at increased risk, including pregnant women[22]

- Routine screening for *syphilis* of women at increased risk and of pregnant women[23]

In the United States, *HIV and AIDS infection* rates are increasing fastest in women, who now account for 30% of cases.[24] Transmission in women is primarily heterosexual. Among infected women, 60% are African-American, 20% are Latina, and 20% are Caucasian. Heterosexual transmission is more likely in the following settings: infected partner with high viral load of HIV-1; cervical ectopy; sex during menstruation; and male partner without circumcision. Recurrent vulvocandidiasis, concurrent STDs, abnormal Pap smears (occurring in 40% of HIV-positive women), and HPV infections are red flags warranting HIV testing. In 2006 the CDC published new guidelines recommending universal HIV testing for all people in the age range of 13 to 64 years, regardless of risk factors. The U.S. Preventive Services Task Force recommendation remains directed at screening those at high risk.[25]

Options for women at high genetic risk include bilateral salpingo-oophorectomy, frequent pelvic examination, CA-125 levels, and transvaginal ultrasound, but none of these are proven screening methods.

As with men, clinicians should assess risk factors for STDs and HIV infection by taking a careful sexual history and counseling patients about spread of disease and how to reduce high-risk practices. Key to effective clinician counseling are respect, compassion, a nonjudgmental attitude, and use of open-ended and understandable questions like "Tell me about any new sex partners" and "Have you ever had anal sex, meaning 'penis in rectum/anus sex'?"[26] The CDC recommends interactive client-centered counseling, tailored to the person's specific risk factors and situation. Training in prevention counseling improves effectiveness. You can begin at the excellent Web sites recommended by the CDC such as http://effectiveinterventions.org or http://depts.washington.edu/nnptc/.

See Chapter 3, Interviewing and the Health History, pp. 82–83, on eliciting the sexual history, and Chapter 13, Male Genitalia and Hernias, pp. 505–507, on risk factors for HIV infection.

Options for Family Planning. It is important to counsel women, particularly adolescents, about the timing of ovulation in the menstrual cycle and how to plan or prevent pregnancy. Survey data indicate that more than half of U.S. pregnancies are unintended, accounting for a high proportion of the 800,000 teen pregnancies each year.[27] Clinicians should be familiar with the numerous options for contraception and their effectiveness. These include natural methods (periodic abstinence, withdrawal, lactation); barrier methods (condom, diaphragm, cervical cap); implantable methods (intrauterine device, subdermal implant); pharmacologic interventions (spermicide, birth control pill, subdermal implant of levonorgestrel, estrogen/progesterone injectables and patch, vaginal ring); and surgery (tubal ligation). Take the time to understand the patient or couple's concerns and preferences and respect these preferences whenever possible. Continued use of a preferred method is superior to a more effective method that is abandoned. For teenagers, a confidential setting eases discussion of topics that may seem private and difficult to explore.

Changes in Menopause. Be familiar with the psychological and physiologic changes of menopause—mood shifts and changes in self-concept, vasomotor changes ("hot flashes"), accelerated bone loss, increases in total and LDL cholesterol, and vulvovaginal atrophy leading to symptoms of vaginal drying, dysuria, and at times dyspareunia.

The clinician must be knowledgeable about the *risks and benefits of estrogen and progesterone replacement therapy,* a common source of questions during office visits. Three major randomized controlled trials since 1998, all with disease-event outcomes, showed that such therapy poses increased risk of stroke and pulmonary embolism and no benefit or increased risk for coronary events.[28–31] Two of the trials showed a 25% increased risk of breast cancer.[28,29,31] A further study showed increased risk of dementia in older postmenopausal women.[32] These risks arise primarily from estrogen effects. Although risks of hip fracture and colon cancer decrease, medical guidelines now caution against using hormone replacement therapy for disease prevention and advise use of minimal doses for menopausal symptoms and for the shortest acceptable duration.[33–35]

TECHNIQUES OF EXAMINATION

Important Areas of Examination

External Examination	Internal Examination
• Mons pubis	• Vagina, vaginal walls
• Labia majora and minora	• Cervix
• Urethral meatus, clitoris	• Uterus, ovaries
• Vaginal introitus	• Pelvic muscles
• Perineum	• Rectovaginal wall

Approach to the Pelvic Examination. Many students feel anxious or uncomfortable when they begin doing pelvic examinations. At the same time, female patients have their own concerns. Some women have had painful, embarrassing, or even demeaning experiences during previous examinations, whereas others may be facing a pelvic examination for the first time. Some are fearful about what the clinician may find and how findings may affect their lives. Asking the patient's permission to perform the examination shows courtesy and respect. If a Pap smear is to be collected using the glass-slide technique, time the examination so that it does not occur during menses, because blood can interfere with interpretation.

In liquid-based cytology, blood cells can be filtered out.[36]

A woman having her first pelvic examination may not know what to expect. Using three-dimensional models, showing her the equipment and letting her handle the speculum, and explaining each step in advance can help her learn about her body and be more comfortable. Careful and gentle technique is especially important in minimizing any pain or discomfort during the first pelvic examination.

The woman's response to the pelvic examination may reveal clues about her feelings about the examination and her sexuality. If she pulls away, adducts her thighs, or reacts negatively to the examination, you can gently comment "I notice you are having some trouble relaxing. Is it just being here, or are you troubled by the examination? . . . Is anything worrying you?" Behaviors that seem to present an obstacle may lead you to a better understanding of your patient's concerns. Adverse reactions may signal prior abuse and should be explored.

Indications for a pelvic examination during adolescence include menstrual abnormalities such as amenorrhea, excessive bleeding, or dysmenorrhea; unexplained abdominal pain; vaginal discharge; the prescription of contraceptives; bacteriologic and cytologic studies in a sexually active girl; and the patient's own desire for assessment.

See Chapter 18, Assessing Children: Infancy Through Adolescence, pp. 826–830.

TIPS FOR THE SUCCESSFUL PELVIC EXAMINATION

The Patient	The Examiner
• Avoids intercourse, douching, or use of vaginal suppositories for 24 to 48 hours before examination	• Obtains permission; selects chaperone
• Empties bladder before examination	• Explains each step of the examination in advance
• Lies supine, with head and shoulders elevated, arms at sides or folded across chest to enhance eye contact and reduce tightening of abdominal muscles	• Drapes patient from midabdomen to knees; depresses drape between knees to provide eye contact with patient
	• Avoids unexpected or sudden movements
	• Chooses a speculum that is the correct size
	• Warms speculum with tap water
	• Monitors comfort of the examination by watching the patient's face
	• Uses excellent but gentle technique, especially when inserting the speculum (see below)

Helping the patient to relax is essential for an adequate examination. Adopting the tips above will help ensure the patient's comfort. Be sure always to wear gloves, both during the examination and when handling equipment and specimens. Plan ahead, so that any needed equipment and culture media are readily at hand.

Note that male examiners should be accompanied by female chaperones. Female examiners should also be assisted if the patient is physically or emotionally disturbed, and to facilitate the examination.

Rape Victims. Regardless of age, *rape* merits special evaluation, usually requiring gynecologic consultation and documentation. Often there is a special rape kit, provided in many emergency departments, that must be used to ensure a chain of custody for evidence. Specimens must be labeled carefully with name, date, and time. Additional information may be needed for further legal investigation.

Choosing Equipment. You should have within reach a good light, a vaginal speculum of appropriate size, water-soluble lubricant, and equipment for taking Papanicolaou smears, bacteriologic cultures and DNA probes, or other diagnostic tests, such as potassium hydroxide or normal saline. Review the supplies and procedures of your own facility before taking cultures and other samples.

Specula are made of metal or plastic and come in two basic shapes, named for Pedersen and Graves. Both are available in small, medium, and large sizes. The medium Pedersen speculum is usually most comfortable for sexually active women. The narrow-bladed Pedersen speculum is best for the patient with a relatively small introitus, such as a virgin or an elderly woman. The Graves specula are best suited for parous women with vaginal prolapse.

Before using a speculum, become thoroughly familiar with how to open and close its blades, lock the blades in an open position, and release them again. Although the instructions in this chapter refer to a metal speculum, you can easily adapt them to a plastic one by handling the speculum before using it.

Plastic specula typically make a loud click or may pinch when locked or released. Forewarning the patient helps to avoid unnecessary surprise.

Positioning the Patient. Drape the patient appropriately and then assist her into the lithotomy position. Help her to place first one heel and then the other into the stirrups. She may be more comfortable with shoes on than with bare feet. Then ask her to slide all the way down the examining table until her buttocks extend slightly beyond the edge. Her thighs should be flexed, abducted, and externally rotated at the hips. A pillow should support her head.

Specula, from left to right: small metal Pedersen, medium metal Pedersen, medium metal Graves, large metal Graves, and large plastic Pedersen

EXTERNAL EXAMINATION

Assess the Sexual Maturity of an Adolescent Patient.   You can assess pubic hair during either the abdominal or the pelvic examination. Note its character and distribution, and rate it according to Tanner's stages, described on p. 845.

Delayed puberty is often familial or related to chronic illness. It may also arise from abnormalities in the hypothalamus, anterior pituitary gland, or ovaries.

Examine the External Genitalia.   Seat yourself comfortably and warn the patient that you will be touching her genital area. Inspect the mons pubis, labia, and perineum. Separate the labia and inspect:

- The labia minora

- The clitoris

Excoriations or itchy, small, red maculopapules suggest *pediculosis pubis* (lice or "crabs"). Look for nits or lice at the bases of the pubic hairs.

Enlarged clitoris in masculinizing conditions

PALPATING BARTHOLIN'S GLAND

● The urethral meatus

● The vaginal opening, or introitus

Note any inflammation, ulceration, discharge, swelling, or nodules. If there are any lesions, palpate them.

If there is a history or an appearance of labial swelling, check Bartholin's glands. Insert your index finger into the vagina near the posterior end of the introitus. Place your thumb outside the posterior part of the labium majus. On each side in turn, palpate between your finger and thumb for swelling or tenderness. Note any discharge exuding from the duct opening of the gland. If any is present, culture it.

Urethral caruncle, prolapse of the urethral mucosa (p. 547)

Herpes simplex, Behcet's disease, syphilitic chancre, epidermoid cyst. See Table 14-1, Lesions of the Vulva (p. 546).

A *Bartholin's gland* may become acutely or chronically infected and then produce a swelling. See Table 14-2, Bulges and Swelling of the Vulva, Vagina, and Urethra (p. 547).

INTERNAL EXAMINATION

Assess the Support of the Vaginal Walls.   With the labia separated by your middle and index fingers, ask the patient to bear down. Note any bulging of the vaginal walls.

Bulging from a *cystocele* or *rectocele*. See Table 14-2, Bulges and Swelling of the Vulva, Vagina, and Urethra (p. 547).

Insert the Speculum.   Select a speculum of appropriate size and shape, and moisten it with warm, but not hot, water. (Lubricants or gels may interfere with cytologic studies and bacterial or viral cultures.) You can enlarge the vaginal introitus by lubricating one finger with water and applying downward pressure at its lower margin. Check the location of the cervix to help angle the speculum more accurately. Enlarging the introitus greatly eases insertion of the speculum and the patient's comfort. With your other hand (usually the left), introduce the closed speculum past your fingers at a somewhat downward slope. Be careful not to pull on the pubic hair or pinch the labia with the speculum. Separating the labia majora with your other hand can help to avoid this.

THE SMALL INTROITUS

Many virginal vaginal orifices admit a single examining finger. Modify your technique so as to use your index finger only. A small Pedersen speculum may make inspection possible. When the vaginal orifice is even smaller, an adequate bimanual examination can be performed by placing one finger in the rectum rather than in the vagina, but warn the patient first!

Similar techniques may be indicated in elderly women if the introitus has become atrophied and tight.

An *imperforate hymen* occasionally delays menarche. Be sure to check for this possibility when menarche seems unduly late in relation to the development of a girl's breasts and pubic hair.

Two methods help you to avoid placing pressure on the sensitive urethra. (1) When inserting the speculum, hold it at an angle (shown below on the left), and then (2) slide the speculum inward along the posterior wall of the vagina, applying downward pressure to keep the vaginal introitus relaxed.

ENTRY ANGLE

ANGLE AT FULL INSERTION

After the speculum has entered the vagina, remove your fingers from the introitus. You may wish to switch the speculum to the right hand to enhance maneuverability of the speculum and subsequent collection of specimens. Rotate the speculum into a horizontal position, maintaining the pressure posteriorly, and insert it to its full length. Be careful not to open the blades of the speculum prematurely.

Inspect the Cervix. Open the speculum carefully. Rotate and adjust the speculum until it cups the cervix and brings it into full view. Position the light until you can visualize the cervix well. When the uterus is retroverted, the cervix points more anteriorly than illustrated. If you have difficulty finding the cervix, withdraw the speculum slightly and reposition it on a different slope. If discharge obscures your view, wipe it away gently with a large cotton swab.

See retroversion of the uterus, p. 537.

Note the color of the cervix, its position, the characteristics of its surface, and any ulcerations, nodules, masses, bleeding, or discharge. Inspect the cervical os for discharge.

See Table 14-3, Variations in the Cervical Surface (p. 548), Table 14-4, Shapes of the Cervical Os (p. 549), and Table 14-5, Abnormalities of the Cervix (p. 549).

Maintain the open position of the speculum by tightening the thumb screw.

A yellowish discharge on the endocervical swab suggests mucopurulent cervicitis, commonly caused by *Chlamydia trachomatis*, *Neisseria gonorrhoeae*, or *herpes simplex* (p. 546). Raised, friable, or lobed wartlike lesions in *condylomata* or *cervical cancer*.

Obtain Specimens for Cervical Cytology (Papanicolaou Smears).

Obtain one specimen from the endocervix and another from the ecto-cervix, or a combination specimen using the cervical brush ("broom"). For best results the patient should not be menstruating. She should avoid intercourse and use of douches, tampons, contraceptive foams or creams, or vaginal suppositories for 48 hours before the examination. In addition to obtaining the Pap smear, for sexually active women age 25 or younger, and for other asymptomatic women at increased risk for infection, plan to culture the cervix routinely for *Chlamydia trachomatis*.[21]

Chlamydial infection is linked to urethritis, cervicitis, pelvic inflammatory disease, ectopic pregnancy, infertility, and chronic pelvic pain. Risk factors include age younger than 25, multiple partners, and prior history of STDs.

OBTAINING THE PAP SMEAR: OPTIONS FOR SPECIMEN COLLECTION

Cervical Scrape and Endocervical Brush

Cervical Scrape. Place the longer end of the scraper in the cervical os. Press, turn, and scrape in a full circle, making sure to include the *transformation zone* and the *squamocolumnar junction.* Smear the specimen on a glass slide. Set the slide in a safe spot that is easy to reach. Note that doing the cervical scrape first reduces obscuring cells with blood, which sometimes appears after use of the endocervical brush.

Endocervical Brush. Take the endocervical brush and place it in the cervical os. Roll it between your thumb and index finger, clockwise and counterclockwise. Remove the brush and pick up the slide you have set aside. Smear the slide with the brush, using a gentle painting motion to avoid destroying any cells. Place the slide into an ether–alcohol solution at once, or spray it promptly with a special fixative.

Note that for pregnant women, a cotton-tip applicator, moistened with saline, is advised in place of the endocervical brush.

Cervical Broom

Many clinicians use a plastic brush tipped with a broomlike fringe for collection of a single specimen containing both squamous and columnar epithelial cells. Rotate the tip of the brush in the cervical os, in a full clockwise direction, then stroke each side of the brush on the glass slide. Promptly place the slide in solution or spray with a fixative as described above.

Alternatively, place the sample directly into preservative so that the laboratory can prepare the slide (liquid-based cytology) (see p. 550).

Inspect the Vagina. Withdraw the speculum slowly while observing the vagina. As the speculum clears the cervix, release the thumb screw and maintain the open position of the speculum with your thumb. Close the speculum as it emerges from the introitus, avoiding both excessive stretching and pinching of the mucosa. During withdrawal, inspect the vaginal mucosa, noting its color and any inflammation, discharge, ulcers, or masses.

See Table 14-6, Vaginal Discharge (p. 550).

Vaginitis with discharge from *Candida, Trichomonas vaginalis,* bacterial vaginosis. Diagnosis depends on laboratory tests because sensitivity and specificity of discharge characteristics are low.[37–39] Vaginal cancer is rare; DES exposure in utero and HPV infection are risk factors.

Perform a Bimanual Examination. Lubricate the index and middle fingers of one of your gloved hands, and *from a standing position,* insert them into the vagina, again exerting pressure primarily posteriorly. Your thumb should be abducted, your ring and little fingers flexed into your palm. Pressing inward on the perineum with your flexed fingers causes little if any discomfort and allows you to position your palpating fingers correctly. Note any nodularity or tenderness in the vaginal wall, including the region of the urethra and the bladder anteriorly.

Stool in the rectum may simulate a rectovaginal mass, but unlike a malignant mass, can usually be dented by digital pressure. Rectovaginal examination confirms the distinction.

Palpate the cervix, noting its position, shape, consistency, regularity, mobility, and tenderness. Normally the cervix can be moved somewhat without pain. Feel the fornices around the cervix.

Pain on movement of the cervix, together with adnexal tenderness, suggest *pelvic inflammatory disease.*

Palpate the uterus. Place your other hand on the abdomen about midway between the umbilicus and the symphysis pubis. While you elevate the cervix and uterus with your pelvic hand, press your abdominal hand in and down, trying to grasp the uterus between your two hands. Note its size, shape, consistency, and mobility, and identify any tenderness or masses.

See Table 14-7, Positions of the Uterus (p. 551), and Table 14-8, Abnormalities of the Uterus (p. 552).

Uterine enlargement suggests pregnancy, uterine myomas (fibroids), or malignancy.

Now slide the fingers of your pelvic hand into the anterior fornix and palpate the body of the uterus between your hands. In this position your pelvic fingers can feel the anterior surface of the uterus, and your abdominal hand can feel part of the posterior surface.

Nodules on the uterine surfaces suggest *myomas* (see p. 552).

If you cannot feel the uterus with either of these maneuvers, it may be tipped posteriorly (retrodisplaced). Slide your pelvic fingers into the posterior fornix and feel for the uterus butting against your fingertips. An obese or poorly relaxed abdominal wall may also prevent you from feeling the uterus even when it is located anteriorly.

See *retroversion* and *retroflexion of the uterus* (p. 551).

Palpate each ovary. Place your abdominal hand on the right lower quadrant, your pelvic hand in the right lateral fornix. Press your abdominal hand in and down, trying to push the adnexal structures toward your pelvic hand. Try to identify the right ovary or any adjacent adnexal masses. By moving your hands slightly, slide the adnexal structures between your fingers, if possible, and note their size, shape, consistency, mobility, and tenderness. Repeat the procedure on the left side.

Three to five years after menopause, ovaries are atrophic and usually nonpalpable. In postmenopausal women, investigate a palpable ovary for possible *ovarian cyst* or *ovarian cancer.* Pelvic pain, bloating, increased abdominal size, and urinary tract symptoms are more common in women with ovarian cancer.[40]

Normal ovaries are somewhat tender. They are usually palpable in slender, relaxed women but are difficult or impossible to feel in others who are obese or poorly relaxed.

Adnexal masses can also arise from a *tubo-ovarian abscess, salpingitis* or inflammation of the fallopian tubes from PID, or ectopic pregnancy. Distinguish such a mass from a uterine myoma. See Table 14-9, Adnexal Masses (p. 553).

Assess the Strength of the Pelvic Muscles. Withdraw your two fingers slightly, just clear of the cervix, and spread them to touch the sides of the vaginal walls. Ask the patient to squeeze her muscles around them as hard and long as she can. A squeeze that compresses your fingers snugly, moves them upward and inward, and lasts 3 seconds or more is full strength.

Impaired strength may be because of age, vaginal deliveries, or neurologic deficits. Weakness may be associated with urinary stress incontinence.

Do a Rectovaginal Examination. The rectovaginal examination has three primary purposes: to palpate a retroverted uterus, the uterosacral ligaments, cul-de-sac, and adnexa; to screen for colorectal cancer in women 50 years or older; and to assess pelvic pathology.[36,41]

After withdrawing your fingers from the bimanual examination, change your gloves and lubricate your fingers as needed (see note below on lubricants). Slowly reintroduce your index finger into the vagina and your middle finger into the rectum. Ask the patient to strain down as you do this to relax her anal sphincter. Mention that this may stimulate an urge to move her bowels, but this will not occur. Apply pressure against the anterior and lateral walls with the examining fingers, and downward pressure with the hand on the abdomen.

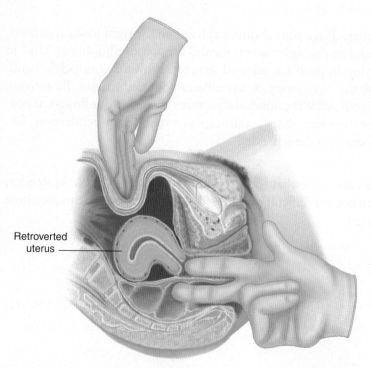

Retroverted uterus

Check the rectal vault for masses (see Chap. 15). If a hemoccult test is planned, you should change gloves to avoid contaminating fecal material with any blood provoked by the Pap smear. After the examination, wipe off the external genitalia and rectum, or offer the patient some tissue so she can do it herself.

See also Chapter 15, The Anus, Rectum, and Prostate, p. 563.

USING LUBRICANTS

If you use a tube of lubricant during a pelvic or rectal examination, you may inadvertently contaminate it by touching the tube with your gloved fingers after touching the patient. To avoid this problem, let the lubricant drop onto your gloved fingers without allowing contact between the tube and the gloves. If you or your assistant should inadvertently contaminate the tube, discard it. Small disposable tubes for use with one patient circumvent this problem.

HERNIAS

Hernias of the groin occur in women as well as in men, but they are much less common. The examination techniques (see pp. 510–512) are basically the same as for men. A woman too should stand up to be examined. To feel an indirect inguinal hernia, however, palpate in the labia majora and upward to just lateral to the pubic tubercles.

An indirect inguinal hernia is the most common hernia that occurs in the female groin. A femoral hernia ranks next in frequency.

SPECIAL TECHNIQUES

If you suspect urethritis or inflammation of the paraurethral glands, insert your index finger into the vagina and milk the urethra gently from inside outward. Note any discharge from or about the urethral meatus. If present, culture it.

Urethritis may arise from infection with *Chlamydia trachomatis* or *Neisseria gonorrhoeae*.

MILKING THE URETHRA

RECORDING YOUR FINDINGS

Note that initially you may use sentences to describe your findings; later you will use phrases. The style below contains phrases appropriate for most write-ups.

Recording the Pelvic Examination—Female Genitalia

"No inguinal adenopathy. External genitalia without erythema, lesions, or masses. Vaginal mucosa pink. Cervix parous, pink, and without discharge. Uterus anterior, midline, smooth, and not enlarged. No adnexal tenderness. Pap smear obtained. Rectovaginal wall intact. Rectal vault without masses. Stool brown and hemoccult negative.

OR

"Bilateral shotty inguinal adenopathy. External genitalia without erythema or lesions. Vaginal mucosa and cervix coated with thin white homogeneous discharge with mild fishy odor. After swabbing cervix, no discharge visible in cervical os. Uterus midline; no adnexal masses. Rectal vault without masses. Stool brown and hemoccult negative."

Suggests bacterial vaginosis

BIBLIOGRAPHY

CITATIONS

1. American College of Obstetricians and Gynecologists. Premenstrual syndrome. Available at: http://www.acog.org/publications/patient_education/bp057.cfm. Accessed November 2, 2007.

2. van Noord PA, Dubas, Dorland M, et al. Age at natural menopause in a population-based screening cohort: the role of menarche, fecundity, and lifestyle factors. Fertil Steril 68(1): 95–102, 1997.

3. NIH State-of-the Science Panel. National Institutes of Health State-of-the-Science Conference Statement: management of menopause-related symptoms. Ann Intern Med 142(12, Part 1): 1003–1013, 2002.

4. U.S. Preventive Services Task Force. Screening for cervical cancer: recommendations and rationale. January 2003. Available at: http://www.ahrq.gov/clinic/3rduspstf/cervcan/cervcanrr.htm. Accessed November 2, 2007.

5. Centers for Disease Control and Prevention. HPV, common infection, common reality. In Human Papillomavirus: HPV Information for Clinicians. November 2006. Available at: http://www.cdc.gov/std/hpv/common-infection/Bro-br.pdf. Accessed November 1, 2007.

6. Future II Study Group. Quadrivalent vaccine against human papillomavirus to prevent high-grade cervical infections. New Engl J Med 356(19):1915–1927, 2007.

7. American College of Obstetricians and Gynecologists (ACOG). Clinical management guidelines for obstetrician-gynecologists: cervical cytology screening. ACOG Practice Bulletin No. 45. Obstet Gynecol 102(2):417–427, 2003. Available at: http://www.ipog.com.br/acog_boletim_31.07.03.pdf. See also: ACOG: Revised cervical cancer screening guidelines require reeducation of women and physicians. News release, May 4, 2004. Available at http://www.acog.org/from_home/publications/press_releases/nr05-04-04-1.cfm; Cervical Cancer Screening Guidelines. Available at: http://www.cdc.gov/std/hpv/ScreeningTables.pdf. Accessed November 2, 2007.

8. American Cancer Society. American Cancer Society Guidelines for Early Detection of Cancer–Cervical Cancer. Available at: http://www.cancer.org/docroot/PED/content/PED_2_3X_ACS_Cancer_Detection_Guidelines_36.asp. See also: Cervical Cancer Screening Guidelines. Available at: http://www.cdc.gov/std/hpv/ScreeningTables.pdf. Accessed November 2, 2007.

9. Marshall AR. The detection of precancerous cervical lesions can be significantly increased. Arch Pathol Lab Med 147(2): 143–145, 2003.

10. Sirovich BE, Welch HG. Cervical cancer screening among women without a cervix. JAMA 291(24):2990–2993, 2004.

11. Solomon D, Davey D, Kurman R, et al. The 2001 Bethesda system: terminology for reporting results of cervical cytology. JAMA 287(16):2114–2119, 2002.

12. Wright TC, Cox JT, Massad JS. 2001 consensus guidelines for the management of women with cervical cytologic abnormalities. JAMA 287(16):2120–2129, 2002.

13. Markowitz LE, Dunne EF, Saraiya M, et al. Quadrivalent human papillomavirus vaccine: recommendations of the Advisory Committee on Immunization Practices (ACIP). MMWR 56(RR-2):1–24, March 12, 2007.

14. Garland SM, Hernandez-Avila M, Wheller CM, et al. Quadrivalent vaccine against human papillomavirus to prevent anogenital diseases. N Engl J Med 356(19):1928–1943, 2007.

15. Hildsheim A, Herrero R, Wacholder S, et al. Effect of human papillomavirus 16/18 L1 viruslike particle vaccine among young women with preexisting infection: a randomized trial. JAMA 298(7):743–752, 2007.

16. Steinbrook R. The potential of human papillomavirus vaccines: perspective. N Engl J Med 354(11):1109–1112, 2007.

17. Dunne EF, Unger ER, Sternberg M, et al. Prevalence of HPV infection among females in the United States. JAMA 297(8): 810–813, 2007.

18. Cannistra SA. Cancer of the ovary. N Engl J Med 351(24): 2519–2529, 2004.

19. Workowski KA, Levine WC, Wasserheit JN. U.S. Centers for Disease Control and Prevention Guidelines for the treatment of sexually transmitted diseases: an opportunity to unify clinical and public health practice. Ann Intern Med 137(4):255–262, 2002.

20. Centers for Disease Control and Prevention. Trends in reportable sexually transmitted diseases in the United States, 2005: national surveillance data for chlamydia, gonorrhea, and syphilis. Available at: http://www.cdc.gov/std/stats/trends2005.htm. Accessed October 31, 2007.

21. U.S. Preventive Services Task Force. Screening for Chlamydial infection. June 2007. Available at: http://www.ahrq.gov/clinic/uspstf/uspschlm.htm. Accessed November 10, 2007.

22. U.S. Preventive Services Task Force. Screening for syphilis infection. July 2004. Available at: http://www.ahrq.gov/clinic/uspstf/uspssyph.htm. Accessed November 10, 2007.

23. U.S. Preventive Services Task Force. Screening for gonorrhea. May 2005. Available at: http://www.ahrq.gov/clinic/uspstf/uspsgono.htm. Accessed November 10, 2007.

24. Levine AM. Evaluation and management of HIV-infected women. Ann Intern Med 136(3):228–242, 2002.

25. U.S. Preventive Services Task Force. Screening for human immunodeficiency virus infection. July 2005, with amendment April 2007. Available at: http://www.ahrq.gov/clinic/uspstf/uspshivi.htm. Accessed November 10, 2007.

26. Workowski KA, Berman SM. Centers for Disease Control and Prevention. Clinical prevention guidance. Sexually transmitted diseases treatment guidelines 2006. MMWR 55(RR-11):2–5, Aug 4 2006.

27. Mosher WD, Martinez GM, Chandra A, et al. Use of contraception and use of family planning services in the United States: 1982–2002. Advance Data from Vital and Health Statistics, No. 350, December 10, 2004, p. 1, Table 9, p. 21. Available at: http://origin.cdc.gov/nchs/data/ad/ad350.pdf. Accessed November 1, 2007.

28. Hulley S, Grady D, Bush T, et al., for the Heart and Estrogen/Progestin Replacement Study Research Group. Randomized trial of estrogen plus progestin for secondary prevention of coronary heart disease in postmenopausal women. JAMA 280(7):605–613, 1998.

29. Writing Group for the Women's Health Initiative Investigators. Risks and benefits of estrogen plus progestin in healthy postmenopausal women. JAMA 288(3):321–333, 2002.

30. Women's Health Initiative Steering Committee. Effects of conjugated equine estrogen in postmenopausal women with hysterectomy. JAMA 291(14):1701–1712, 2004.

31. Hulley SB, Grady D. The WHI estrogen-alone trial—do things look any better? (Editorial). JAMA 291(14):1769–1770, 2004.

32. Shumaker SA, Legault C, Rapp SH, et al. Estrogen plus progestin and the incidence of dementia and mild cognitive impairment in postmenopausal women. JAMA 289(20):2651–2662, 2003.

33. American College of Obstetricians and Gynecologists. ACOG issues state-of-the-art guide to hormone therapy. News release, September 30, 2004. Available at http://www.acog.org/from_home/publications/press_releases/nr09-30-04-2.cfm. Accessed November 11, 2007.

34. American College of Obstetricians and Gynecologists (ACOG) Task Force on Hormone Therapy. Executive summary, supplemental issue: hormone therapy. Obstet Gynecol 104(4):104(suppl)1S–4S, 2004.

35. Mosca L, Collins P, Herrington DM, et al. Hormone replacement therapy and cardiovascular disease. A statement for healthcare professionals from the American Heart Association. Circulation 104(4):499–503, 2001.

36. Edelman A, Anderson J, Lai S, et al. Pelvic examination. N Engl J Med 356(26):e26–28, 2007.

37. Anderson MR, Klink K, Cohrssen A. Evaluation of vaginal complaints. JAMA 291(11):1368–1379, 2004.

38. Eckhert LO. Acute vulvovaginitis. N Engl J Med 355(12):1244–1252, 2006.

39. Bickley LS. Acute vaginitis. In Diagnostic Strategies for the Common Medical Problems. Black ER, Panzer RJ, Bordley DR, et al. (eds). Philadelphia: American College of Physicians, 1999.

40. Goff BA, Mandel LS, Melancon CH, et al. Frequency of symptoms of ovarian cancer in women presenting to primary care clinics. JAMA 291(22):2705–2712, 2004.

41. Padilla LA, Radosevich DM, Milad MP. Accuracy of the pelvic examination in detecting adnexal masses. Obstet Gynecol 96(4):593–598, 2000.

42. Kimberlin DW, Rouse DJ. Genital herpes. N Engl J Med 350(19):1970–1977, 2004.

43. Erhmann DA. Polycystic ovary syndrome. N Engl J Med 352(12):1223–1236, 2005.

ADDITIONAL REFERENCES

Alvarez-Blasco F, Botella-Carretero JI, San Millan JL, et al. Prevalence and characteristics of the polycystic ovary syndrome in overweight and obese women. Arch Intern Med 166:2081–2086, 2006.

Anderson MR, Klink K, Cohrsson A. Evaluation of vaginal complaints. JAMA 291(11):368–379, 2004.

Bent S, Nallamothu BK, Simel DL, et al. Does this woman have an acute uncomplicated urinary tract infection? JAMA 287(20):2701–2710, 2002.

Berek J, Novak E, eds. Berek & Novak's Gynecology, 14th ed. Philadelphia: Lippincott Williams & Wilkins, 2007.

Collaborative Group on Epidemiological Studies of Ovarian Cancer, Beral V, Doll R, et al. Ovarian cancer and oral contraceptives: collaborative reanalysis of data from 45 epidemiological studies

including 23,257 women with ovarian cancer and 87,303 controls. Lancet 371(9609):303–314, 2008.

Datta SD, Sternberg M, Johnson RE, et al. Gonorrhea and chlamydia in the United States among persons 14 to 39 years of age, 1999 to 2002. Ann Intern Med 147(2):89–96, 2007.

Ellis H. Anatomy of the uterus. Anesth Intensive Care Med 6(1):74–75, 2005.

Future II Study Group. Quadrivalent vaccine against human papillomavirus to prevent high-grade cervical lesions. N Engl J Med 356(19):1915–1927, 2007.

Gibbs RS, Danforth DN, eds. Danforth's Obstetrics and Gynecology, 10th ed. Philadelphia: Lippincott Williams & Wilkins, 2008.

Gupta R, Warren T, Wald A. Genital herpes. Lancet 370(9605):2127–2137, 2007.

Hammer SM. Clinical practice: management of newly diagnosed HIV infection. N Engl J Med 353(16):1702–1710, 2005.

Holroyd-Leduc JM, Tannenbaum C, Thorpe KE, et al. What type of urinary incontinence does this woman have? JAMA 299(12):1446–1456, 2008.

Hwang LY, Shafer MA, Pollack LM, et al. Sexual behaviors after universal screening of sexually transmitted infections in healthy young women. Obstet Gynecol 109(1):105–113, 2007.

Katz VL, ed. Comprehensive Gynecology, 5th ed. Philadelphia: Mosby–Elsevier, 2007.

Mayrand MH, Duarte-Franco E, Rodriques I, et al. Human papillomavirus DNA versus Papanicolaou screening tests for cervical cancer. N Engl J Med 357(16):1579–1588, 2007.

Nelson HD. Menopause. Lancet 371(9614):760–770, 2008.

Nyirjesy P, Peyton C, Weitz MV, et al. Causes of chronic vaginitis: analysis of a prospective database of affected women. Obstet Gynecol 108(5):1185–1191, 2006.

Parmigiani G, Chen S, Iversen ES Jr, et al. Validity of models for predicting BRCA1 and BRCA2 mutations. Ann Intern Med 147(7):441–450, 2007.

Peipert JF. Genital chlamydial infections. N Engl J Med 349(25):2424–2430, 2003.

Reif S, Whetten K, Thielman N. Association of race and gender with use of antiretroviral therapy among HIV-infected individuals in the Southeastern United States. South Med J 100(8):775–781, 2007.

Simon V, Ho DD, Abdool Karim Q. HIV/AIDS epidemiology, pathogenesis, prevention, and treatment. Lancet 368(9534):489–504, 2006.

Sirovich BE, Welch HG. Cervical cancer screening among women without a cervix. JAMA 291(24):2990–2993, 2004.

Wooster R, Weber BL. Breast and ovarian cancer. N Engl J Med 348(23):2339–2347, 2003.

Xu F, Sternberg MR, Kottiri BJ, et al. Trends in herpes simplex virus type 1 and type 2 seroprevalence in the United States. JAMA 296(8):964–973, 2006.

The Bates' suite offers these additional resources to enhance learning and facilitate understanding of this chapter:

- Bates' Pocket Guide to Physical Examination and History Taking, 6th edition
- Bates' Nursing Online
- Bates' Visual Guide to Physical Examination, 4th edition
- thePoint online resources, http://thepoint.lww.com
- Student CD-ROM included with the book

Cystic
nodule
in skin

Warts

Epidermoid Cyst

A small, firm, round cystic nodule in the labia suggests an epidermoid cyst. These are yellowish in color. Look for the dark punctum marking the blocked opening of the gland.

Venereal Wart (*Condyloma Acuminatum*)

Warty lesions on the labia and within the vestibule suggest condyloma acuminatum. They result from infection with *human papillomavirus.*

Flat,
gray
papules

Syphilitic Chancre

A firm, painless ulcer suggests the chancre of primary syphilis. Because most chancres in women develop internally, they often go undetected.

Secondary Syphilis (*Condyloma Latum*)

Slightly raised, round or oval, flat-topped papules covered by a gray exudate suggest condylomata lata. These constitute one manifestation of secondary syphilis and are contagious.

Shallow
ulcers on
red bases

Genital Herpes[42]

Shallow, small, painful ulcers on red bases suggest a herpes infection. Initial infection may be extensive, as shown. Recurrent infections usually are confined to a small local patch.

Carcinoma of the Vulva

An ulcerated or raised red vulvar lesion in an elderly woman may indicate vulvar carcinoma.

TABLE 14-2

Bulges and Swelling of the Vulva, Vagina, and Urethra

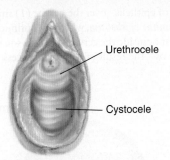

Urethrocele

Cystocele

Cystocele

A cystocele is a bulge of the upper two thirds of the anterior vaginal wall, together with the bladder above it. It results from weakened supporting tissues.

Cystourethrocele

When the entire anterior vaginal wall, together with the bladder and urethra, is involved in the bulge, a cystourethrocele is present. A groove sometimes defines the border between urethrocele and cystocele, but is not always present.

Caruncle

Prolapsed urethral mucosa

Urethral Caruncle

A urethral caruncle is a small, red, benign tumor visible at the posterior part of the urethral meatus. It occurs chiefly in post-menopausal women and usually causes no symptoms. Occasionally, a carcinoma of the urethra is mistaken for a caruncle. To check, palpate the urethra through the vagina for thickening, nodularity, or tenderness, and feel for inguinal lymphadenopathy.

Prolapse of the Urethral Mucosa

Prolapsed urethral mucosa forms a swollen red ring around the urethral meatus. It usually occurs before menarche or after menopause. Identify the urethral meatus at the center of the swelling to make this diagnosis.

Labial swelling

Bulge

Bartholin's Gland Infection

Causes of a Bartholin's gland infection include trauma, gonococci anaerobes like bacteroides and peptostreptococci, and *Chlamydia trachomatis*. Acutely, it appears as a tense, hot, very tender abscess. Look for pus coming out of the duct or erythema around the duct opening. Chronically, a nontender cyst is felt. It may be large or small.

Rectocele

A rectocele is a herniation of the rectum into the posterior wall of the vagina, resulting from a weakness or defect in the endopelvic fascia.

Variations in the Cervical Surface

Two kinds of epithelia cover the cervix: (1) shiny pink *squamous epithelium*, which resembles the vaginal epithelium, and (2) deep red, plushy *columnar epithelium*, which is continuous with the endocervical lining. These meet at the *squamocolumnar junction*. When this junction is at or inside the cervical os, only squamous epithelium is seen. A ring of columnar epithelium is often visible to a varying extent around the os—the result of a normal process that accompanies fetal development, menarche, and the first pregnancy.*

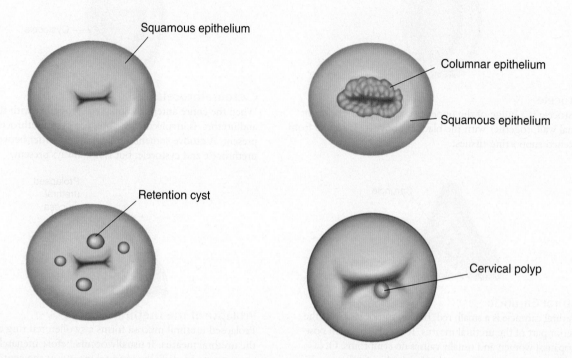

With increasing estrogen stimulation during adolescence, all or part of this columnar epithelium is transformed into squamous epithelium by a process termed *metaplasia*. This change may block the secretions of columnar epithelium and cause *retention cysts*, also called *nabothian cysts*. These appear as translucent nodules on the cervical surface and have no pathologic significance.

A cervical polyp usually arises from the endocervical canal, becoming visible when it protrudes through the cervical os. It is bright red, soft, and rather fragile. When only the tip is seen, it cannot be differentiated clinically from a polyp originating in the endometrium. Polyps are benign but may bleed.

* Terminology is in flux. Other terms for the columnar epithelium that is visible on the ectocervix are *ectropion*, *ectopy*, and *eversion*.

Shapes of the Cervical Os

Normal

Oval   Slit-like

Types of Lacerations from Delivery

Bilateral transverse   Stellate   Unilateral transverse

Abnormalities of the Cervix

Mucopurulent Cervicitis

Mucopurulent cervicitis produces purulent yellow drainage
from the cervical os, usually as a result of infection from
Chlamydia trachomatis, *Neisseria gonorrhoeae*, or herpes.
These infections are sexually transmitted and may occur
without symptoms or signs.

Carcinoma of the Cervix

Carcinoma of the cervix begins in an area of metaplasia. In its earliest
stages, it cannot be distinguished from a normal cervix. In a late stage,
an extensive, irregular, cauliflower-like growth may develop. Early
frequent intercourse, multiple partners, smoking, and infection with
human papillomavirus increase the risk for cervical cancer.

Vaginal adenosis

Columnar epithelium

Collar

Fetal Exposure to Diethylstilbestrol (DES)

Daughters of women who took DES during pregnancy are
at greatly increased risk for several abnormalities, including
(1) columnar epithelium that covers most or all of the cervix,
(2) vaginal adenosis, i.e., extension of this epithelium to the
vaginal wall, and (3) a circular collar or ridge of tissue, of varying
shapes, between the cervix and vagina. Much less common is an
otherwise rare carcinoma of the upper vagina.

TABLE
14-6

Vaginal Discharge

The vaginal discharge from vaginitis must be distinguished from a physiologic discharge. The latter is clear or white and may contain white clumps of epithelial cells; it is not malodorous. It is also important to distinguish vaginal from cervical discharges. Use a large cotton swab to wipe off the cervix. If no cervical discharge is present in the os, suspect a vaginal origin and consider the causes below. Remember that diagnosis of cervicitis or vaginitis hinges on careful collection and analysis of the appropriate laboratory specimens.[37,38]

	Trichomonal Vaginitis	Candidal Vaginitis	Bacterial Vaginosis
Cause	*Trichomonas vaginalis,* a protozoan; often but not always acquired sexually	*Candida albicans,* a yeast (normal overgrowth of vaginal flora); many factors predispose, including antibiotic therapy	Bacterial overgrowth probably from anaerobic bacteria; may be transmitted sexually
Discharge	Yellowish green or gray, possibly frothy; often profuse and pooled in the vaginal fornix; may be malodorous	White and curdy; may be thin but typically thick; not as profuse as in trichomonal infection; not malodorous	Gray or white, thin, homogeneous, malodorous; coats the vaginal walls; usually not profuse, may be minimal
Other Symptoms	Pruritus (though not usually as severe as with *Candida* infection); pain on urination (from skin inflammation or possibly urethritis); dyspareunia	Pruritus; vaginal soreness; pain on urination (from skin inflammation); dyspareunia	Unpleasant fishy or musty genital odor
Vulva and Vaginal Mucosa	Vestibule and labia minora may be reddened. Vaginal mucosa may be diffusively reddened, with small red granular spots or petechiae in the posterior fornix. In mild cases, the mucosa looks normal.	The vulva and even the surrounding skin are often inflamed and sometimes swollen to a variable extent. Vaginal mucosa often reddened, with white, often tenacious patches of discharge. The mucosa may bleed when these patches are scraped off. In mild cases, the mucosa looks normal.	Vulva usually normal. Vaginal mucosa usually normal
Laboratory Evaluation	Scan saline wet mount for trichomonads	Scan potassium hydroxide (KOH) preparation for branching hyphae of *Candida*.	Scan saline wet mount for *clue cells* (epithelial cells with stippled borders); sniff for fishy odor after applying KOH ("whiff test"); vaginal secretions with pH >4.5

Positions of the Uterus

Retroversion and retroflexion are usually normal variants.

Body of the uterus
may not be palpable

Palpable through rectum   Normal angle
maintained

Cervix faces
forward

Retroversion of the Uterus

Retroversion of the uterus refers to a tilting backward of the entire uterus, including both body and cervix. It is a common variant occurring in approximately 20% of women. Early clues on pelvic examination are a cervix that faces forward and a uterine body that cannot be felt by the abdominal hand. In *moderate retroversion*, the body may not be palpable with either hand. In *marked retroversion*, the body can be felt posteriorly, either through the posterior fornix or through the rectum. A retroverted uterus is usually both mobile and asymptomatic. Occasionally, such a uterus is fixed and immobile, held in place by conditions such as endometriosis or pelvic inflammatory disease.

May be palpable
through rectum   Angled back

Retroflexion of the Uterus

Retroflexion of the uterus refers to a backward angulation of the body of the uterus in relation to the cervix. The cervix maintains its usual position. The body of the uterus is often palpable through the posterior fornix or through the rectum.

TABLE	
14-8	**Abnormalities of the Uterus**

Myomas of the Uterus (Fibroids)

Myomas are very common benign uterine tumors. They may be single or multiple and vary greatly in size, occasionally reaching massive proportions. They feel like firm, irregular nodules in continuity with the uterine surface. Occasionally, a myoma projecting laterally can be confused with an ovarian mass; a nodule projecting posteriorly can be mistaken for a retroflexed uterus. Submucous myomas project toward the endometrial cavity and are not themselves palpable, although they may be suspected because of an enlarged uterus.

Myomas

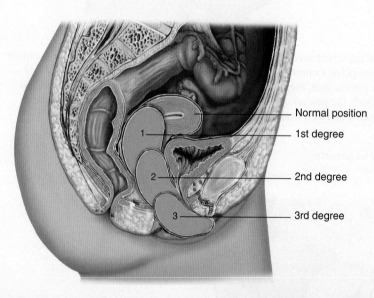

Normal position

1st degree

2nd degree

3rd degree

Prolapse of the Uterus

Prolapse of the uterus results from weakness of the supporting structures of the pelvic floor and is often associated with a cystocele and rectocele. In progressive stages, the uterus becomes retroverted and descends down the vaginal canal to the outside:

- In *first-degree prolapse*, the cervix is still well within the vagina.

- In *second-degree prolapse*, it is at the introitus.

- In *third-degree prolapse* (procidentia), the cervix and vagina are outside the introitus.

TABLE
14-9

Adnexal Masses

Adnexal masses most commonly result from disorders of the fallopian tubes or ovaries. Three examples—often hard to differentiate—are described. In addition, inflammatory disease of the bowel (such as diverticulitis), carcinoma of the colon, and a pedunculated myoma of the uterus may simulate an adnexal mass.

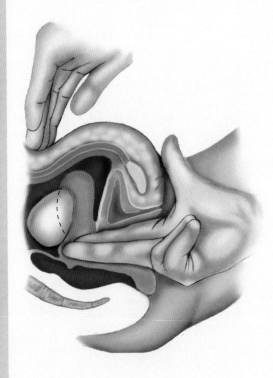

Ovarian Cysts and Ovarian Cancer

Ovarian cysts and tumors may be detected as adnexal masses on one or both sides. Later, they may extend out of the pelvis. Cysts tend to be smooth and compressible, tumors more solid and often nodular. Uncomplicated cysts are not usually tender.

Small (≤6 cm in diameter), mobile, cystic masses in a young woman are usually benign and often disappear after the next menstrual period. Diagnosis of *polycystic ovary syndrome* rests on exclusion of several endocrine disorders and 2 of the 3 features listed: absent or irregular menses; hyperandrogenism (hirsutism, acne, alopecia, elevated serum testosterone); and confirmation of polycystic ovaries on ultrasound. Obesity and absence of lactation outside pregnancy or childbirth are additional predictors.[43]

Ovarian cancer is relatively rare and usually presents at an advanced stage.[18] Symptoms include pelvic pain, bloating, increased abdominal size, and urinary tract symptoms[40]; often there is a palpable ovarian mass. Currently there are no reliable screening tests. A strong family history of breast or ovarian cancer is an important risk factor but occurs in only 5% of cases.

Ruptured Tubal Pregnancy

A ruptured tubal pregnancy spills blood into the peritoneal cavity, causing severe abdominal pain and tenderness. Guarding and rebound tenderness are sometimes associated. A unilateral adnexal mass may be palpable, but tenderness often prevents its detection. Faintness, syncope, nausea, vomiting, tachycardia, and shock may be present, reflecting the hemorrhage. There may be a prior history of amenorrhea or other symptoms of a pregnancy.

Pelvic Inflammatory Disease

Pelvic inflammatory disease (PID) is most often a result of sexually transmitted infection of the fallopian tubes (salpingitis) or of the tubes and ovaries (salpingo-oophoritis). It is caused by *Neisseria gonorrhoeae, Chlamydia trachomatis,* and other organisms. *Acute* disease is associated with very tender, bilateral adnexal masses, although pain and muscle spasm usually make it impossible to delineate them. Movement of the cervix produces pain. If not treated, a *tubo-ovarian abscess* or infertility may ensue.

Infection of the fallopian tubes and ovaries may also follow delivery of a baby or gynecologic surgery.

CHAPTER

15

The Anus, Rectum, and Prostate

ANATOMY AND PHYSIOLOGY

The gastrointestinal tract terminates in a short segment, the *anal canal*. The external margin of the anal canal is poorly demarcated, but the moist, hairless appearance of its skin usually distinguishes it from the surrounding perianal skin. The muscle actions of the voluntary *external anal sphincter* and involuntary *internal anal sphincter* normally hold the anal canal closed. The internal anal sphincter is an extension of the muscular coat of the rectal wall.

Note carefully the angle of the anal canal, on a line roughly between the anus and umbilicus. Unlike the rectum above it, the canal is liberally supplied by

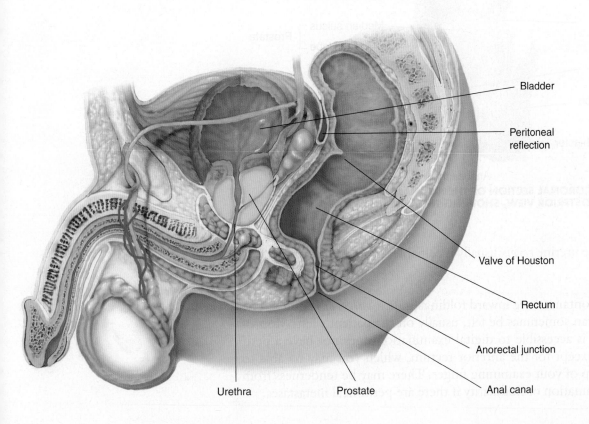

Bladder

Peritoneal reflection

Valve of Houston

Rectum

Anorectal junction

Anal canal

Urethra　　　Prostate

somatic sensory nerves, and a poorly directed finger or instrument will produce pain.

A serrated line marking the change from skin to mucous membrane demarcates the anal canal from the rectum. This anorectal junction, often called the *pectinate* or *dentate line*, is also the boundary between somatic and visceral nerve supplies. It is readily visible on proctoscopic examination, but not palpable.

Above the anorectal junction, the rectum balloons out and turns posteriorly into the hollow of the coccyx and the sacrum. In the male, the three lobes of the *prostate gland* surround the urethra. The prostate gland is small during childhood, but between puberty and approximately 20 years, it increases roughly five-fold in size. Prostate volume further expands as the gland becomes hyperplastic (see p. 567). The two lateral lobes lie against the anterior rectal wall, where they are palpable as a rounded, heart-shaped structure approximately 2.5 cm long. They are separated by a shallow *median sulcus* or groove, also palpable. Note that the third, or median, lobe is anterior to the urethra and cannot be examined. The *seminal vesicles,* shaped like rabbit ears above the prostate, are also not normally palpable.

CORONAL SECTION OF THE ANUS AND RECTUM, POSTERIOR VIEW, SHOWING THE ANTERIOR WALL

In the female, the uterine *cervix* usually is palpable through the anterior wall of the rectum.

The rectal wall contains three inward foldings, called *valves of Houston*. The lowest of these can sometimes be felt, usually on the patient's left. Most of the rectum that is accessible to digital examination does not have a peritoneal surface, except for the anterior rectum, which you may be able to reach with the tip of your examining finger. There may be tenderness from peritoneal inflammation or nodularity if there are peritoneal metastases.

THE HEALTH HISTORY

Common or Concerning Symptoms

- Change in bowel habits
- Blood in the stool
- Pain with defecation; rectal bleeding or tenderness
- Anal warts or fissures
- Weak stream of urine
- Burning with urination

Other chapters have addressed many questions involving symptoms related to the anorectal area and the prostate. For example, you will need to ask if there has been any change in the pattern of bowel function or the size or caliber of the stools. What about diarrhea or constipation? You will need to ask about the color of the stools. Turn to pp. 424–425 and review the health history regarding these symptoms, as well as queries about *blood in the stool,* ranging from black stools, suggesting *melena,* to the red blood of *hematochezia,* to *bright-red blood per rectum.* Also, is any mucus present?

See Table 11-3, Constipation, p. 457, and Table 11-5, Black and Bloody Stools, p. 460.

Change in bowel pattern, especially stools of thin pencil-like caliber, may warn of *colon cancer.* Blood in the stool may be from polyps or cancer, also from gastrointestinal bleeding or local hemorrhoids; mucus may accompany *villous adenoma.*

Be sure to ask about any personal or family history of colonic polyps or colorectal cancer. Is there any history of inflammatory bowel disease?

Positive answers to these questions indicate increased risk for colorectal cancer and need for further testing and surveillance (see screening recommendations, Ch. 11, pp. 431–433).

Is there any pain on defecation? Any itching? Any extreme tenderness in the anus or rectum? Is there any mucopurulent discharge or bleeding? Any ulcerations? Does the patient have anal intercourse?

Proctitis if itching, anorectal pain, tenesmus, or discharge or bleeding from infection or *rectal abscess.* Causes include gonorrhea, chlamydia, lymphogranuloma venereum, receptive anal intercourse, ulcerations of *herpes simplex,* chancre of *primary syphilis* (see Table 13-2 p. 516). Itching in younger patients may be from pinworms.

Is there any history of anal warts or anal fissures?

Genital warts from *human papillomavirus, condylomata lata* in secondary syphilis. Anal fissures in *proctitis, Crohn's disease*

In men, review the pattern of urination (see pp. 427–428). Does the patient have any difficulty starting or holding back the urine stream? Is the flow weak? What about frequent urination, especially at night? Or pain or burning as urine is passed? Any blood in the urine or semen or pain with ejaculation? Is there frequent pain or stiffness in the lower back, hips, or upper thighs?

Also in men, is there any feeling of discomfort or heaviness in the prostate area at the base of the penis? Any associated malaise, fever, or chills?

Suggests possible *prostatitis*

HEALTH PROMOTION AND COUNSELING

Important Topics for Health Promotion and Counseling

- Screening for prostate cancer
- Screening for polyps and colorectal cancer
- Counseling for sexually transmitted diseases

Screening for Prostate Cancer. Prostate cancer is the leading cancer diagnosed in U.S. men, and the third leading cause of death in men following lung and colon cancer.[2] Although lifetime risk of diagnosis is high (approximately 17%), biologic risk and mortality are only approximately 3%. Approximately 60% of cancer cells are "organ-confined" at diagnosis and slow to invade outside the prostate capsule.[3] Age, ethnicity, and family history are the primary risk factors.

- **Age.** Risk of prostate cancer increases sharply with each advancing decade after 50 years. Probability of diagnosis rises by age group, from 2.6% in men 40 to 59 years, to 7% in men 60 to 69 years, to 13% in men 70 years and older.[2]

- **Ethnicity.** For undetermined reasons, incidence rates are significantly higher in African-American men than in Caucasian men: 243 cases per 100,000 compared with 156 cases per 100,000, even after adjustments for access to care.[2] Prostate cancer occurs at an earlier age and more advanced stage in African-American men.

- **Family history.** Approximately 15% of men diagnosed with prostate cancer have an affected first-degree relative.[4] One Scandinavian study of twins ascribed 42% of cases to inheritance.[5] Rare autosomal-dominant alleles appear to contribute to early-onset prostate cancer, and several X-linked alleles are under investigation in families with onset at older ages.[6]

- **Diet.** A series of studies suggests an association between intake of dietary fat, especially saturated fats and fats from animal sources, and risk of prostate cancer. However, the evidence remains inconclusive.[4,6] Other possible influences include selenium, vitamins E and D, lycopene, and isoflavones.[7]

The optimal approach to prostate cancer *screening* remains controversial. The U.S. Preventive Services Task Force in 2002 found insufficient evidence to recommend for or against routine screening using *prostate-specific antigen (PSA) testing* or *digital rectal examination (DRE)*, primarily because of mixed evidence that early detection improves health outcomes.[8] The American Cancer Society and the American Urological Association recommend combining DRE with testing for PSA beginning at 50 years, and at 40 years for African-American men and men with a positive family history, now common clinical practice.[2,9] Overall detection with DRE screening alone is 2.5% to 3.2%, increasing to 4.6% for PSA alone, and 4.5% to 6% for both methods or both methods with additional transurethral ultrasound.[10] DRE detects tumors on the lateral and posterior aspects of the prostate but misses 25% to 35% of cancers in other areas of the prostate gland. Although sensitivity and specificity of the DRE are low, estimated as 59% and 94%, respectively,[11] findings of nodularity, induration, or marked lobe asymmetry should be pursued. The PSA is minimally affected by DRE, so both can be assessed during the same office visit. In large screening populations using a PSA cutoff of 4.0 ng/ml, DRE and PSA are positive in 7% to 11% and 7% to 9%, respectively. As expected, positive rates for both tests increase with age.[12]

Interpreting PSA results is fraught with clinical dilemmas. Since the advent of PSA testing, most men presenting with prostate cancer are now asymptomatic and have nonpalpable tumors. New data have prompted revisions to the initial threshold value of 4.0 ng/ml as the upper limit of "normal." At this threshold for biopsy, approximately one third of tumors have spread to the margins of the prostate gland or beyond (PSA false negatives). In the well-conducted Prostate Cancer Prevention Trial, 15% of men with PSA levels less than 4 ng/ml had biopsy-proven cancer. Cancer was present at all levels of PSA, seen in 10% of men with levels of 0.6 to 1.0 ng/ml, in 24% with levels of 2.1 to 3.0 ng/ml, and in 27% with levels of 3.1 to 4.0 ng/ml.[13] Leading investigators are now advocating baseline PSA screening at 40 years, "a stronger predictor of prostate cancer risk than ethnicity, family history, or digital prostate examination findings"; continued screening after 70 years for those with good life expectancy; a biopsy threshold of 2.5 ng/ml; and attention to *PSA velocity,* namely, the rate of PSA increase in 1 year.[14] Note, however, that benign conditions such as hyperplasia, prostatitis, ejaculation, urinary retention, and prostate biopsy can elevate the PSA (false positives). If the PSA is elevated, repeating the PSA test is prudent.

For men *with symptoms* of prostate disorders, the clinician's role is more straightforward. Review the symptoms of prostate disorders—incomplete emptying of the bladder, urinary frequency or urgency, weak or intermittent stream or straining to initiate flow, hematuria, nocturia, or even bony pains in the pelvis. Men may be reluctant to report such symptoms but should be encouraged to seek evaluation and treatment early.

Screening for Colorectal Cancer.   Screening recommendations to improve detection of colorectal cancer (CRC) have recently been revised, as discussed on pp. 431–433.[15–18] Clinicians have fallen short in rates of CRC screening and should promote screening guidelines more aggressively.[17, 19, 20] In brief:

● Clinicians should first identify whether patients are at average or increased risk for CRC, ideally by approximately age 20 years, but earlier if the patient has a family history of familial adenomatous polyposis (see p. 433).

● Average-risk patients 50 years or older should be offered a range of screening options to increase compliance: annual fecal occult blood testing (FOBT); flexible sigmoidoscopy every 5 years, either alone or combined with annual FOBT; double-contrast barium enema every 5 years; or colonoscopy every 10 years.

● People at increased risk should undergo colonoscopy at intervals ranging from 3 to 5 years.

The 6-sample home FOBT recommended by the U.S. Preventive Services Task Force reduces both mortality and incidence of subsequent new cancer but is underutilized.[21] Too many primary care clinicians are relying on a single office sample for FOBT during DRE, which is well-documented as a poor screening method.[19, 21, 22] Sensitivity and specificity for the 6-sample home test is 24% and 94%, compared with 5% and 98% for the single office FOBT. Moreover, the single office test will detect positive findings in only 5% of patients with advanced neoplasia. Note that DRE, which reaches only 7 to 8 cm of the rectum (usually 12 to 15 cm long), is not a recommended method for CRC screening. Only approximately 10% of CRCs arise in this zone.

Counseling for Sexually Transmitted Diseases (STDs).   Anal intercourse places men and women at risk for perianal and rectal abrasions and transmission of HIV and other STDs. Protective measures include abstinence from high-risk behaviors (see pp. 506–507), use of condoms, and good hygiene.

TECHNIQUES OF EXAMINATION

For many patients, the rectal examination is the least popular segment of the physical examination. It may cause discomfort and even embarrassment for the patient, but if the examination is skillfully done it should not be truly painful. You may choose to omit the rectal examination in adolescents who have no relevant complaints; however, in middle-aged or older adults, omission risks missing an asymptomatic carcinoma. A successful examination requires a calm demeanor, an explanation to the patient of what he or she may feel, gentleness, and slow movement of your finger.

MALE

Choose one of several suitable patient positions for conducting the examination. Often, the clinician asks the patient to stand and lean forward with his upper body resting across the examining table and hips flexed. For most purposes, the side-lying position, depicted below, is satisfactory and allows good visualization of the perianal and sacrococcygeal areas.

No matter how you position the patient, your examining finger cannot reach the full length of the rectum. If a rectosigmoid cancer is suspected or screening is warranted, turn to sigmoidoscopy or colonoscopy.

Ask the patient to lie on his left side with his buttocks close to the edge of the examining table near you. Flexing the patient's hips and knees, especially in the top leg, stabilizes his position and improves visibility. Drape the patient appropriately and adjust the light for the best view. Glove your hands and spread the buttocks apart.

- *Inspect the sacrococcygeal and perianal areas* for lumps, ulcers, inflammation, rashes, or excoriations. Adult perianal skin is normally more pigmented and somewhat coarser than the skin over the buttocks. Palpate any abnormal areas, noting lumps or tenderness.

- *Examine the anus and rectum.* Lubricate your gloved index finger, explain to the patient what you are going to do, and tell him that the examination may make him feel as if he were moving his bowels but that he will not do so. Ask him to strain down. Inspect the anus, noting any lesions.

Anal and perianal lesions include hemorrhoids, venereal warts, herpes, syphilitic chancre, and carcinoma. A linear crack or tear suggests *anal fissure* from large, hard stools, inflammatory bowel disease, or STDs. Consider *pruritus ani* if swollen, thickened, fissured perianal skin with excoriations is noted.

Tender, purulent, reddened mass with fever or chills accompanies an *anal abscess.* Abscesses tunneling to the skin surface from the anus or rectum may form a clogged or draining *anorectal fistula.* Fistulas may ooze blood, pus, or feculent mucus. Consider anoscopy or sigmoidoscopy for better visualization.

As the patient strains, place the pad of your gloved and lubricated index finger over the anus.

As the sphincter relaxes, gently insert your fingertip into the anal canal in the direction pointing toward the umbilicus. If you feel the sphincter tighten, pause and reassure the patient. When in a moment the sphincter relaxes, proceed.

Occasionally, severe tenderness prevents entry and internal examination. Do not try to force it. Instead, place your fingers on both sides of the anus, gently spread the orifice, and ask the patient to strain down. Look for a lesion, such as an anal fissure, that might explain the tenderness.

If you can proceed without undue discomfort, note:

- The sphincter tone of the anus. Normally, the muscles of the anal sphincter close snugly around your finger.

- Tenderness, if any

- Induration

- Irregularities or nodules

Insert your finger into the rectum as far as possible. Rotate your hand clockwise to palpate as much of the rectal surface as possible on the patient's right side, then counterclockwise to palpate the surface posteriorly and on the patient's left side.

Sphincter tightness may occur with anxiety, inflammation, or scarring; laxity appears with some neurologic diseases.

Induration may be caused by inflammation, scarring, or malignancy.

Note any nodules, irregularities, or induration. To bring a possible lesion into reach, take your finger off the rectal surface, ask the patient to strain down, and palpate again.

The irregular border of a rectal cancer is shown below.

Then rotate your hand further counterclockwise so that your finger can examine the *posterior surface of the prostate gland.* By turning your body somewhat away from the patient, you can feel this area more easily. Tell the patient that examining his prostate gland may prompt an urge to urinate.

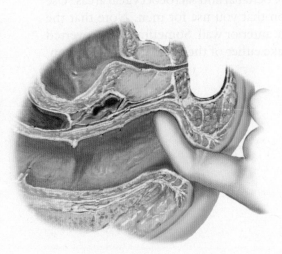

Sweep your finger carefully over the prostate gland, identifying its lateral lobes and the median sulcus between them. Note the size, shape, and consistency of the prostate, and identify any nodules or tenderness. The normal prostate is rubbery and nontender.

See Table 15-3, Abnormalities of the Prostate (p. 570).

If possible, *extend your finger above the prostate* to the region of the seminal vesicles and the peritoneal cavity. Note any nodules or tenderness.

Gently withdraw your finger, and wipe the anus or give the patient tissues. Note the color of any fecal matter on your glove, and test it for occult blood.

A rectal "shelf" of peritoneal metastases (see p. 569) or the tenderness of peritoneal inflammation

A single fecal occult blood test is not an adequate screen for colon cancer, however (see p. 560).[21]

PALPATING THE PROSTATE— VIEW FROM BELOW

FEMALE

The rectum is usually examined after the female genitalia, while the woman is in the lithotomy position. This position allows you to conduct the bimanual examination and delineate a possible adnexal or pelvic mass. It is suitable for testing the integrity of the rectovaginal wall and may also help you to palpate a cancer high in the rectum.

If you need to examine only the rectum, the lateral position is satisfactory and affords a much better view to the perianal and sacrococcygeal areas. Use the same techniques for examination that you use for men. Note that the cervix is readily palpated through the anterior wall. Sometimes a retroverted uterus is also palpable. Do not mistake either of these, or a vaginal tampon, for a tumor.

RECORDING YOUR FINDINGS

Note that initially you may use sentences to describe your findings; later you will use phrases. The style below contains phrases appropriate for most write-ups.

Recording the Physical Examination— The Anus, Rectum, and Prostate

> "No perirectal lesions or fissures. External sphincter tone intact. Rectal vault without masses. Prostate smooth and nontender with palpable median sulcus. (Or in a female, uterine cervix nontender.) Stool brown and hemoccult negative."
>
> **OR**
>
> "Perirectal area inflamed; no ulcerations, warts, or discharge. Unable to examine external sphincter, rectal vault, or prostate because of spasm of external sphincter and marked inflammation and tenderness of anal canal."
>
> **OR**
>
> "No perirectal lesions or fissures. External sphincter tone intact. Rectal vault without masses. Left lateral prostate lobe with 1 × 1 cm firm, hard nodule; right lateral lobe smooth; median sulcus obscured. Stool brown and hemoccult negative."

Raises concern of *proctitis* from infectious cause

Raises concern of *prostate cancer*

BIBLIOGRAPHY

CITATIONS

1. Barry MJ, Fowler FJ, O'Leary M, et al. The American Urological Association symptom index for benign prostatic hyperplasia. J Urol 148(5):1549–1557, 1992.
2. American Cancer Society. Cancer facts and figures 2007. Available at: http://www.cancer.org/downloads/STT/CAFF2007 PWSecured.pdf. Accessed July 5, 2007.
3. National Cancer Institute. Prostate cancer screening. Summary of evidence. Available at: http://www.cancer.gov/cancertopics/pdq/screening/prostate/healthprofessional. Accessed June 6, 2007.
4. National Cancer Institute. Prostate cancer: Prevention. Risk factors for prostate cancer development. Available at: http://www.cancer.gov/cancertopics/pdq/prevention/prostate/HealthProfessional/page3. Accessed June 6, 2007.
5. Lichtenstein P, Holm NV, Verkasalo PK, et al. Environmental and heritable factors in the causation of cancer—analyses of cohorts of twins from Sweden, Denmark, and Finland. N Engl J Med 343(2):78–85, 2000.
6. Nelson WG, DeMarzo AM, Isaacs WB. Prostate cancer. N Engl J Med 349(4):366–381, 2003.
7. National Cancer Institute. Opportunities for Prevention. Available at: http://www.cancer.gov/cancertopics/pdq/prevention/prostate/HealthProfessional/page4. Accessed June 6, 2007.
8. U.S. Preventive Services Task Force. Screening for prostate cancer: recommendation and rationale. Ann Intern Med 137(11):915–916, 2002.
9. AUA Practice Guidelines Committee. AUA guideline on management of benign prostatic hyperplasia. Chapter 1: diagnosis and treatment recommendations. J Urol 170(2 Pt 1):530–547, 2003. Available at: http://www.auanet.org/guidelines/bph.cfm. Accessed July 7, 2007.
10. Murthy GD, Byron DP, Pasquale D. Underutilization of digital rectal examination when screening for prostate cancer. Arch Intern Med 164:313–316, 2004.
11. Hoogendam A, Buntinx F, de Vet HC. The diagnostic value of digital rectal examination in primary care screening for prostate cancer: A meta-analysis. Fam Pract 16:621–626, 1999.
12. Andriole GL, Levin DL, Crawford ED, et al. Prostate cancer screening in the prostate, lung, colorectal and ovarian (PLCO)

cancer screening trial: findings from the initial screening round of a randomized trial. J Natl Cancer Inst 97(6):433–438, 2005.

13. Thompson IM, Pauler DK, Goodman PJ, et al. Prevalence of prostate cancer among men with a prostate-specific antigen level ≤ 4.0 ng per milliliter. N Engl J Med 350(22):2239–2246, 2004.

14. Catalona WJ, Loeb S, Han M. Viewpoint: expanding prostate cancer screening. Ann Intern Med 144(6):441–443, 2006.

15. Winawer S, Fletcher R, Rex D, et al. Gastrointestinal Consortium Panel. Colorectal cancer screening and surveillance: clinical guidelines and rationale. Update based on new evidence. Gastroenterology 124(2):544–560, 2003.

16. Winawer SJ, Zauber AG, Fletcher RH, et al. Guidelines for colonoscopy surveillance after polypectomy: a consensus update. U.S. Multi-Society Task Force on Colorectal Cancer and the American Cancer Society. Gastroenterology 130(6): 1872–1875, 2006.

17. Eisen GM, Weinberg DS. Narrative review: screening for colorectal cancer in patients with a first-degree relative with colonic neoplasia. Ann Intern Med 143(3):190–198, 2005.

18. U.S. Preventive Services Task Force. Routine aspirin or non-steroidal anti-inflammatory drugs for the prevention of colorectal cancer: U.S. Preventive Services Task Force Recommendation Statement. Ann Intern Med 146(5):361–365, 2007.

19. Sox HS. Office-based testing for fecal occult blood: do only in case of emergency [editorial]. Ann Intern Med 142(2): 146–148, 2005.

20. Boolchand V, Olds G, Singh J, et al. Colorectal screening after polypectomy: a national survey study of primary care physicians. Ann Intern Med 145(9):654–659, 2006.

21. Collins JF, Lieberman DA, Durbin TE, et al. Veterans Affairs Cooperative Study #380 Group. Accuracy of screening for fecal occult blood on a single stool sample obtained by digital rectal examination: a comparison with recommended sampling practice. Ann Intern Med 142(2):81–85, 2005.

22. Nadel MR, Shapiro JA, Klabunde CN, et al. A national survey of primary care physicians' methods for screening for fecal occult blood. Ann Intern Med 142(2):86–94, 2005.

ADDITIONAL REFERENCES

Dube C. Rostum A, Lewin G, et al. The use of aspirin for primary prevention of colorectal cancer: a systematic review prepared for the U.S. Preventive Services Task Force. Ann Intern Med 146(5):365–375, 2007.

Hoffman RM. Viewpoint: limiting prostate cancer screening. Ann Intern Med 144(6):438–440, 2006.

Hull TL. Diseases of the anorectum. In: Feldman M, Friedman LS, Brandt LJ, eds. Sleisenger & Fordtran's Gastrointestinal and Liver Disease: Pathophysiology, Diagnosis, Management, 8th ed. Philadelphia: Saunders/Elsevier, 2006.

Philip J, Dutta RS, Ballal M, et al. Is a digital rectal examination necessary in the diagnosis and clinical staging of early prostate cancer? BJU Int 95(7):969–971, 2005.

The Bates' suite offers these additional resources to enhance learning and facilitate understanding of this chapter:

- *Bates' Pocket Guide to Physical Examination and History Taking,* 6th edition
- *Bates' Nursing Online*
- *Bates' Visual Guide to Physical Examination,* 4th edition
- thePoint online resources, http://thepoint.lww.com
- Student CD-ROM included with the book

BPH Symptom Score Index: American Urological Association (AUA)

Score or ask the patient to score each of the questions below. Higher scores (maximum 35) indicate more severe symptoms; scores ≤7 are considered mild and generally do not warrant treatment.

PART A	Not at All	Less Than 1 Time in 5	Less Than Half the Time	About Half the Time	More Than Half the Time	Almost Always	Total Points for Each Row
1. Over the past month, how often have you had a sensation of not emptying your bladder completely after you finished urinating?							
2. Over the past month, how often have you had to urinate again less than two hours after you finished urinating?							
3. Over the past month, how often have you stopped and started again several times when you urinated?							
4. Over the past month, how often have you found it difficult to postpone urination?							
5. Over the past month, how often have you had a weak urinary stream?							
6. Over the past month, how often have you had to push or strain to begin urination?							

PART B	None	1 Time	2 Times	3 Times	4 Times	5 Times	Points for Part B
7. Over the past month, how many times did you most typically get up to urinate from the time you went to bed at night until the time you got up in the morning?							

TOTAL PARTS A and B (maximum 35) _____

(Adapted from: Madsen FA, Bruskewitz RC. Clinical manifestations of benign prostatic hyperplasia. Urol Clin North Am 1995:22:291–298.)

Pilonidal Cyst and Sinus

Location

A pilonidal cyst is a fairly common, probably congenital, abnormality located in the midline superficial to the coccyx or the lower sacrum. Look for the opening of a sinus tract. This opening may exhibit a small tuft of hair and be surrounded by a halo of erythema. Although pilonidal cysts are generally asymptomatic, except perhaps for slight drainage, abscess formation and secondary sinus tracts may complicate the picture.

External Hemorrhoids (*Thrombosed*)

External hemorrhoids are dilated hemorrhoidal veins that originate below the pectinate line and are covered with skin. They seldom produce symptoms unless thrombosis occurs. This causes acute local pain that increases with defecation and sitting. A tender, swollen, bluish, ovoid mass is visible at the anal margin.

Internal Hemorrhoids (*Prolapsed*)

Anterior

Posterior

Internal hemorrhoids are enlargements of the normal vascular cushions located above the pectinate line. Here, they are not usually palpable. Sometimes, especially during defecation, internal hemorrhoids may cause bright-red bleeding. They may also prolapse through the anal canal and appear as reddish, moist, protruding masses, typically located in one or more of the positions illustrated.

Prolapse of the Rectum

On straining for a bowel movement, the rectal mucosa, with or without its muscular wall, may prolapse through the anus, appearing as a doughnut or rosette of red tissue. A prolapse involving only mucosa is relatively small and shows radiating folds, as illustrated. When the entire bowel wall is involved, the prolapse is larger and covered by concentrically circular folds.

(table continues on page 569)

Anal Fissure

Fissure

Sentinel tag

An anal fissure is a very painful oval ulceration of the anal canal, found most commonly in the midline posteriorly, less commonly in the midline anteriorly. Its long axis lies longitudinally. There may be a swollen "sentinel" skin tag just below it. Gentle separation of the anal margins may reveal the lower edge of the fissure. The sphincter is spastic; the examination is painful. Local anesthesia may be required.

Polyps of the Rectum

Polyps of the rectum are fairly common. Variable in size and number, they can develop on a stalk (*pedunculated*) or lie on the mucosal surface (*sessile*). They are soft and may be difficult or impossible to feel even when in reach of the examining finger. Proctoscopy and biopsy are needed for differentiation of benign from malignant lesions.

Rectal Shelf

Anorectal Fistula

Opening

Fistula

An anorectal fistula is an inflammatory tract or tube that opens at one end into the anus or rectum and at the other end onto the skin surface (as shown here) or into another viscus. An abscess usually antedates such a fistula. Look for the fistulous opening or openings anywhere in the skin around the anus.

Cancer of the Rectum

Asymptomatic carcinoma of the rectum makes routine rectal examination important for adults. Illustrated here is the firm, nodular, rolled edge of an ulcerated cancer.

Widespread peritoneal metastases from any source may develop in the area of the peritoneal reflection anterior to the rectum. A firm to hard nodular rectal "shelf" may be just palpable with the tip of the examining finger. In a woman, this shelf of metastatic tissue develops in the rectouterine pouch, behind the cervix and the uterus.

TABLE 15-3

Abnormalities of the Prostate

Normal Prostate Gland

As palpated through the anterior rectal wall, the normal prostate is a rounded, heart-shaped structure approximately 2.5 cm long. The median sulcus can be felt between the two lateral lobes. Only the posterior surface of the prostate is palpable. Anterior lesions, including those that may obstruct the urethra, are not detectable by physical examination.

Prostatitis

Acute bacterial prostatitis, illustrated here, presents with fever and urinary tract symptoms such as frequency, urgency, dysuria, incomplete voiding, and sometimes low back pain. The gland feels tender, swollen, "boggy," and warm. Examine it gently. More than 80% of infections are caused by gram-negative aerobes such as *E. coli, Enterococccus,* and *Proteus.* In men younger than 35, consider sexual transmission of *Neisseria gonorrhea* and *Chlamydia trachomatis.*

Chronic bacterial prostatitis is associated with recurrent urinary tract infections, usually from the same organism. Men may be asymptomatic or have symptoms of dysuria or mild pelvic pain. The prostate gland may feel normal, without tenderness or swelling. Cultures of prostatic fluid usually show infection with *E. coli.*

It may be challenging to distinguish these conditions from the more common *chronic pelvic pain syndrome,* seen in up to 80% of symptomatic men who report obstructive or irritative symptoms on voiding but show no evidence of prostate or urinary tract infection. Physical examination findings are not predictable, but examination is needed to assess any prostate induration or asymmetry suggestive of carcinoma.

Benign Prostatic Hyperplasia

Benign prostatic hyperplasia is a nonmalignant enlargement of the prostate gland that increases with age, present in more than 50% of men by 50 years.[9] Symptoms arise both from smooth-muscle contraction in the prostate and bladder neck and from compression of the urethra. They may be irritative (urgency, frequency, nocturia), obstructive (decreased stream, incomplete emptying, straining), or both, and are seen in more than one-third of men by 65 years. The affected gland may be normal in size, or may feel symmetrically enlarged, smooth, and firm, though slightly elastic; there may be obliteration of the median sulcus and more notable protrusion into the rectal lumen.

Cancer of the Prostate

Cancer of the prostate is suggested by an area of hardness in the gland. A distinct hard nodule that alters the contour of the gland may or may not be palpable. As the cancer enlarges, it feels irregular and may extend beyond the confines of the gland. The median sulcus may be obscured. Hard areas in the prostate are not always malignant. They may also result from prostatic stones, chronic inflammation, and other conditions.

The Musculoskeletal System

ASSESSING THE MUSCULOSKELETAL SYSTEM

OVERVIEW

Musculoskeletal complaints and disorders are leading causes of health care visits in clinical practice. Low back pain alone ranks fifth among reasons for clinical visits and is the second most common symptom of patients seeking care.[1,2]

Prevalence and Age at Onset for Common Musculoskeletal Conditions in the U.S. (1998)

Condition	Prevalence	Age at onset, years
Low back pain	26 million	20–50
Osteoarthritis	17 million	40–80
Fibromyalgia	3.7 million	30–60
RA	2.1 million	30–60
Gout	2.1 million	Men 30–50; Women 55–75
Carpal tunnel	2.0 million	40–60
PMR	450K	50–75
Ankylosing spondylitis	300K	15–35
SLE	239K	15–45
Psoriatic arthritis	160K–275K	5–20
Scleroderma	≤34K	30–55
Myositis	≤25K	DM 5–15; DM/PM 45–65

Source: Cush JJ, Lipsky PE. Approach to articular and musculoskeletal disorders. In: Kasper DL, Braunwald E, Fauci AS, et al., eds. Harrison's Principles of Internal Medicine, 16th ed. New York: McGraw-Hill, 2005. RA, rheumatoid arthritis; PMR, polymyalgia rheumatica; SLE, systemic lupus erythematosus; DM, dermatomyositis; PM, polymyositis.

Because of the specialized nature of joint assessment, the organization of this chapter is a unique departure from other regional examination chapters in this book. Assessment of joints requires both visualization and thorough knowledge of surface landmarks and underlying anatomy. To help students pair their knowledge of joint structure and function with related methods of examination, the Anatomy and Physiology and Techniques of Examination for each joint *are combined*. The format of the chapter is as follows:

CHAPTER ORGANIZATION

- **Joint Structure and Function**
- **The Health History**
- **Health Promotion and Counseling**
- **Examination of Specific Joints: Anatomy and Physiology and Related Techniques of Examination**
  - To promote a systematic approach to examining the joints, the chapter follows a "head-to-toe" sequence, beginning with the jaw and joints of the upper extremities, then proceeding to the spine, hip, and joints of the lower extremities.
  - Sequence: *temporomandibular joint, shoulder, elbow, wrist and hand, spine, hip, knee and lower leg, ankle and foot*
- For each joint there are subsections on *Joint Overview, Bony Structures and Joints, Muscle Groups and Additional Structures,* and *Techniques of Examination.*
  - *Joint Overview* presents the distinguishing anatomical and functional characteristics of each joint.
  - *Techniques of Examination* presents the fundamental steps for examining that joint—*inspection, palpation* of bony landmarks and soft-tissue structures, assessment of *range of motion* (the arc of measurable joint movement in a single plane), and *maneuvers* to test the joint's function and stability.
  - Mastering maneuvers is challenging but increasingly important to diagnosis and office practice and will require both supervision and practice.

JOINT STRUCTURE AND FUNCTION

It is helpful to begin by reviewing some anatomical terminology.

- *Articular structures* include the joint capsule and articular cartilage, the synovium and synovial fluid, intra-articular ligaments, and juxta-articular bone.

  Articular disease typically involves swelling and tenderness of the entire joint and limits both active and passive range of motion.

- *Extra-articular structures* include periarticular ligaments, tendons, bursae, muscle, fascia, bone, nerve, and overlying skin.

  Extra-articular disease typically involves selected regions of the joint and types of movement.

  - *Ligaments* are ropelike bundles of collagen fibrils that connect bone to bone.

- *Tendons* are collagen fibers connecting muscle to bone. Another type of collagen matrix forms the *cartilage* that overlies bony surfaces.

- *Bursae* are pouches of synovial fluid that cushion the movement of tendons and muscles over bone or other joint structures.

To understand joint function, study the various types of joints and how they articulate, or interconnect, and the role of bursae in easing joint movement.

TYPES OF JOINT ARTICULATION

There are three primary types of joint articulation—synovial, cartilaginous, and fibrous—allowing varying degrees of joint movement.

SYNOVIAL

● Joints

Type of Joint	Extent of Movement	Example
Synovial	Freely movable	Knee, shoulder
Cartilaginous	Slightly movable	Vertebral bodies of the spine
Fibrous	Immovable	Skull sutures

Synovial Joints.   The bones do not touch each other, and the joint articulations are *freely moveable*. The bones are covered by *articular cartilage* and separated by a *synovial cavity* that cushions joint movement, as shown. A *synovial membrane* lines the synovial cavity and secretes a small amount of viscous lubricating fluid—the *synovial fluid*. The membrane is attached at the margins of the articular cartilage and pouched or folded to accommodate joint movement. Surrounding the synovial membrane is a fibrous *joint capsule*, which is strengthened by ligaments extending from bone to bone.

CARTILAGINOUS

Cartilaginous Joints.   These joints, such as those between vertebrae and the symphysis pubis, are *slightly moveable*. Fibrocartilaginous discs separate the bony surfaces. At the center of each disc is the *nucleus pulposus,* fibrocartilaginous material that serves as a cushion or shock absorber between bony surfaces.

Fibrous Joints.   In these joints, such as the sutures of the skull, intervening layers of fibrous tissue or cartilage hold the bones together. The bones are almost in direct contact, which allows *no appreciable movement.*

FIBROUS

STRUCTURE OF SYNOVIAL JOINTS

As you learn about the examination of the musculoskeletal system, think about how the anatomy of the joint relates to its movement.

● Synovial Joints

Type of Joint	Articular Shape	Movement	Example
Spheroidal (ball and socket)	Convex surface in concave cavity	Wide-ranging flexion, extension, abduction, adduction, rotation, circumduction	Shoulder, hip
Hinge	Flat, planar	Motion in one plane; flexion, extension	Interphalangeal joints of hand and foot; elbow
Condylar	Convex or concave	Movement of two articulating surfaces not dissociable	Knee; temporo-mandibular joint

SPHEROIDAL JOINT (BALL AND SOCKET)

Many of the joints we examine are *synovial,* or movable, *joints.* The shape of the articulating surfaces of synovial joints determines the direction and extent of joint motion.

- *Spheroidal joints* have a ball-and-socket configuration—a rounded, convex surface articulating with a cuplike cavity, allowing a wide range of rotatory movement, as in the shoulder and hip.

- *Hinge joints* are flat, planar, or slightly curved, allowing only a gliding motion in a single plane, as in flexion and extension of the digits.

HINGE JOINT

- In *condylar joints,* such as the knee, the articulating surfaces are convex or concave, termed condyles.

Bursae. Easing joint action are *bursae,* roughly disc-shaped synovial sacs that allow adjacent muscles or muscles and tendons to glide over each other during movement. They lie between the skin and the convex surface of a bone or joint (as in the prepatellar bursa of the knee, p. 627) or in areas where tendons or muscles rub against bone, ligaments, or other tendons or muscles (as in the subacromial bursa of the shoulder, pp. 590–591).

Knowledge of the underlying joint anatomy and movement will help you assess joints subjected to trauma. Your knowledge of the soft-tissue structures, ligaments, tendons, and bursae will help you evaluate the changes of aging, as well as arthritis.

CONDYLAR JOINT

THE HEALTH HISTORY

Common or Concerning Symptoms

- Low back pain
- Neck pain
- Monoarticular or polyarticular joint pain
- Inflammatory or infectious joint pain
- Joint pain with systemic features such as fever, chills, rash, anorexia, weight loss, weakness
- Joint pain with symptoms from other organ systems

Joint pain is one of the leading complaints of patients seeking health care. In addition to obtaining the seven features of any joint pain, three tips help guide your subsequent examination and diagnosis:

TIPS FOR ASSESSING JOINT PAIN

- Ask the patient to *"point to the pain."* This may save considerable time because the patient's verbal description may be imprecise.
- Clarify and record the *mechanism of injury,* particularly if there is a history of trauma.
- Determine whether the pain is *localized or diffuse, acute or chronic, inflammatory or noninflammatory.*

Low Back Pain.   You may wish to begin with "Any pains in your back?" because two-thirds of adults have low back pain at least once during their lifetime.[3] Low back pain is the second most common reason for office visits. Using open-ended questions, get a clear picture of the problem, especially location of the pain.

See Table 16-1, Low Back Pain, p. 642.

Approximately 85% of patients have *idiopathic low back pain* without a precise underlying cause (this term is preferred to "sprain" or "strain").[4]

Determine if the pain is *on the midline,* over the vertebrae, or *off the midline.*

For *midline back pain,* assess for musculoligamentous injury, disc herniation, vertebral collapse, spinal cord metastases, or rarely *epidural abscess.* For *pain off the midline,* assess for sacroiliitis, trochanteric bursitis, sciatica, or hip arthritis.

Is there radiation into the leg? If yes, is there any associated numbness or paresthesia?

Radicular gluteal and posterior leg pain in the S1 distribution in *sciatica* that increases with cough or Valsalva (see pp. 703–704 for related neurologic findings). Leg pain that resolves with rest and/or lumbar forward flexion in *spinal stenosis.*

What about associated bladder or bowel dysfunction?

Elicit any *"red flags" for serious underlying systemic disease:* age older than 50 years, history of cancer, unexplained weight loss, pain lasting more than 1 month or not responding to treatment, pain at night or increased by rest, history of intravenous drug use, or presence of infection.[3,5]

Consider *cauda equina syndrome* from S2–4 midline disc or tumor if bowel or bladder dysfunction (usually urinary retention and overflow incontinence).[3]

In cases of low back pain plus a red flag, there is a 10% probability of serious systemic disease.[3,5]

Neck Pain.

Neck pain is also common. Although usually self-limited, it is important to ask about radiation into the arm, arm or leg weakness or paresthesias, or change in bladder or bowel function. Be sure to elicit symptoms related to the "red flags" listed above. Persisting pain after blunt trauma or a motor vehicle accident warrants further evaluation.[6]

See Table 16-2, Pains in the Neck, p. 643.

Radicular pain from spinal nerve compression, most commonly C7 followed by C6. Unlike low back pain, usually from foraminal impingement from degenerative joint changes (70% to 75%) rather than disc herniation (20% to 25%).[7,8]

Joint Pain.

To pursue other musculoskeletal disorders, ask "Do you have any pains in your joints?" Joint pain may be *localized, diffuse, or systemic.* Ask the patient to *point to the pain.*

- If the joint pain is localized and involves only one joint, it is *monoarticular.* Pain originating in the small joints of the hands and feet is more sharply localized than pain from larger joints. Pain from the hip joint is especially deceptive. Although typically in the groin or buttock, it is sometimes felt in the anterior thigh or partly or solely in the knee.

Pain in one joint suggests trauma, monoarticular arthritis, possible tendinitis, or bursitis. Lateral hip pain near the greater trochanter suggests *trochanteric bursitis.*

- Patients may report joint pain that is *polyarticular,* involving several joints. If polyarticular, what is the *pattern of involvement* . . . migrating from joint to joint or steadily spreading from one joint to multiple joints? Is the involvement symmetric, affecting similar joints on both sides of the body?

Migratory pattern of spread in *rheumatic fever* or *gonococcal arthritis*; progressive additive pattern with symmetric involvement in *rheumatoid arthritis*

● Joint pain may also be *extra-articular*, involving bones, muscles, and tissues around the joint such as the tendons, bursae, or even overlying skin. Generalized "aches and pains" are called *myalgias* if in muscles and *arthralgias* if there is pain but no evidence of arthritis.

Extra-articular pain in inflammation of bursae (*bursitis*), tendons (*tendinitis*), or tendon sheaths (*tenosynovitis*); also *sprains* from stretching or tearing of ligaments

Timing. Assess the chronicity, quality, and severity of the joint symptoms. *Timing* is especially important. Did the pain or discomfort develop rapidly over the course of a few hours or insidiously over weeks or even months? Has the pain progressed slowly or fluctuated, with periods of improvement and worsening? How long has the pain lasted? What is it like over the course of a day? . . . In the morning? . . . As the day wears on?

Severe pain of rapid onset in a red, swollen joint in *acute septic arthritis* or *gout*.[9,10] In children consider *osteomyelitis* in bone contiguous to a joint.

If more rapid in onset, how did the pain arise? Was there an acute injury or overuse from repetitive motion of the same part of the body? If the pain comes from trauma, what was the *mechanism of injury* or the series of events that caused the joint pain? Further, what aggravates or relieves the pain? What are the effects of exercise, rest, and treatment?

See Table 16-3, Patterns of Pain In and Around the Joints, pp. 644–645.

Inflammation. Try to determine whether the problem is *inflammatory* or *noninflammatory*. Is there *tenderness, warmth,* or *redness*? These features are best assessed on examination, but patients can sometimes guide you to points of tenderness. Ask about systemic symptoms such as fever or chills.

Fever, chills, warmth, redness in *septic arthritis;* also consider *gout* or possible *rheumatic fever*

Swelling and Stiffness. Additional symptoms can help you decide if the pain is *articular* in origin, such as *swelling, stiffness,* or *decreased range of motion*. Localize any *swelling* as accurately as possible. If *stiffness* is present, it may be difficult to assess because people use the term differently. Musculoskeletal stiffness refers to a perceived tightness or resistance to movement, the opposite of feeling limber. It is often associated with discomfort or pain. If the patient does not report stiffness spontaneously, ask about it and try to calculate its duration. Find out when the patient gets up in the morning and when the joints feel the most limber. Healthy people experience stiffness and muscular soreness after unusually strenuous muscular exertion, usually peaking within 2 days.

Pain, swelling, loss of active and passive motion, "locking," deformity in *articular joint pain;* loss of active but not passive motion, tenderness outside the joint, absence of deformity often in *nonarticular pain*

To assess *limitations of motion,* ask about changes in level of activity because of problems with the involved joint. When relevant, inquire specifically about the patient's ability to walk, stand, lean over, sit, sit up, rise from a sitting position, climb, pinch, grasp, turn a page, open a door handle or jar, and daily activities such as combing hair, brushing teeth, eating, dressing, and bathing.

Stiffness and limited motion after inactivity, sometimes called *gelling,* in degenerative joint disease but usually lasts only a few minutes; stiffness lasting 30 minutes or more in *rheumatoid arthritis* and other inflammatory arthritides. Stiffness also with *fibromyalgia* and *polymyalgia rheumatica (PMR)*

Systemic Features. Finally, some joint problems have *systemic* features such as fever, chills, rash, anorexia, weight loss, and weakness.

Generalized symptoms are common in *rheumatoid arthritis, systemic lupus erythematosus (SLE), PMR,* and other inflammatory arthritides. High fever and chills suggest an infectious cause.

Other joint disorders may be linked to *organ systems outside the musculo-skeletal system.* Symptoms elsewhere in the body can give important clues to these conditions. Be alert to the symptoms and disorders below.

● Joint Pain and Systemic Disorders

- *Skin conditions*

  A butterfly rash on the cheeks

  The scaly rash and pitted nails of psoriasis

  A few papules, pustules, or vesicles on reddened bases, located on the distal extremities

  An expanding erythematous patch early in an illness

  Hives

  Erosions or scale on the penis and crusted, scaling papules on the soles and palms

  The maculopapular rash of rubella

  Clubbing of the fingernails (see p. 193)

- Red, burning, and itchy eyes (*conjunctivitis*)
- Preceding *sore throat*

- *Diarrhea, abdominal pain, cramping*

- Symptoms of *urethritis*

- Mental status change, facial or other weakness, stiff neck

Systemic lupus erythematosus
Psoriatic arthritis
Gonococcal arthritis

Lyme disease
Serum sickness, drug reaction
Reiter's syndrome, which also includes arthritis, urethritis, and uveitis
Arthritis of *rubella*
Hypertrophic osteoarthropathy
Reiter's syndrome, Behçet's syndrome[11]
Acute rheumatic fever or *gonococcal arthritis*
Arthritis with *ulcerative colitis, regional enteritis, scleroderma*
Reiter's syndrome or possibly *gonococcal arthritis*
Lyme disease with central nervous system involvement

HEALTH PROMOTION AND COUNSELING

Important Topics for Health Promotion and Counseling

- Nutrition, exercise, and weight
- Low back: lifting and biomechanics
- Preventing falls
- Osteoporosis: screening and prevention

Maintaining the integrity of the musculoskeletal system brings many features of daily life into play—balanced nutrition, regular exercise, appropriate weight. As described later in this chapter, each joint has its own specific vulnerabilities to trauma and wear. Care with lifting, avoidance of falls, household safety measures, and exercise help to protect and preserve well-functioning muscles and joints.

Nutrition, Exercise, and Weight. The habits of a healthy lifestyle convey direct benefit to the skeleton. Good nutrition supplies calcium needed for bone mineralization and bone density. Exercise appears to maintain and possibly increase bone mass, in addition to improving outlook and management of stress. Weight appropriate to height and body frame reduces excess mechanical wear on weight-bearing joints such as hips and knees. Regular physical activity has been shown to help prevent osteoporosis, obesity, cardiovascular disease, hypertension, and type 2 diabetes, and may reduce all-cause morbidity and lengthen life span.[12] Even modest activity, such as walking or bicycling 30 minutes each day, benefits health. Twenty to 30% of adult Americans report sedentary lifestyles and may benefit from routine counseling, although evidence linking counseling to behavior change is still preliminary.

Low Back: Lifting and Biomechanics. One of the most vulnerable parts of the skeleton is the low back, especially L5–S1, where the sacral vertebrae take a sharp posterior angle. From 60% to 80% of the population experiences *low back pain* at least once in a lifetime.[13] Usually symptoms are short lived, but 30% to 60% of people experience recurrences when onset is work related. Exercises to strengthen the low back, especially in flexion and extension, and risk factor modification are often recommended (although studies have not demonstrated a consistent benefit for these interventions).[3,14,15] Alternatively, fitness exercises appear equally effective. Education on lifting strategies, posture, and the biomechanics of injury is prudent for patients doing repetitive lifting such as nurses, heavy-machinery operators, and construction workers. For occupational back pain, increasing graded physical activity and behavioral counseling show promise in improving functional status and return to work.[16] Such programs focus on improvements in function and do not make pain relief a condition for resuming work.

Preventing Falls. Among elderly people in the United States, *falls* exact a heavy toll in morbidity and mortality. They are the leading cause of nonfatal injuries and account for a dramatic rise in death rates after 65 years, increasing from approximately 5/100,000 in the general population to 10/100,000 between the ages of 65 and 74 years, to approximately 147/100,000 after age 85 years.[17] Approximately 5% of falls result in fractures, usually of the wrist, hip, pelvis, or femur. Only one third of fracture patients regain their prior level of function, and one third require nursing home placement.[18] Risk factors are both cognitive and physiologic, including unstable gait, imbalanced posture, reduced strength, cognitive loss as in dementia, deficits in vision and proprioception, and osteoporosis. Poor lighting, stairs, chairs at awkward heights, slippery or irregular surfaces, and ill-fitting shoes are environmental dangers that can often be corrected. Clinicians should work with patients and families to help modify such risks whenever possible. Home health assessments have proven useful in reducing environmental hazards, as have exercise programs to improve patient balance and strength. (See Chapter 20, The Older Adult, pp. 910–911.)

Osteoporosis: Screening and Prevention. Osteoporosis is a major threat to U.S. public health.[18–21]

- 10 million Americans have osteoporosis, and 34 million are at increased risk because of low bone mass.

- Osteoporosis can occur at any age, and 42% of those at risk are men. Prevalence in U.S. white women increases from 15% at ages 50 to 59 years to 70% in women older than 80 years. Prevalence in African-American women older than 50 years is 12%, and in Mexican-American women, 18%.

- One of every two women and one in four men older than 50 years will have a fracture related to osteoporosis. Approximately one third of fractures occur in younger women.

- 20% of patients with osteoporotic hip fractures die within 1 year.

The National Institutes of Health define osteoporosis as a "skeletal disorder characterized by compromised bone strength predisposing a person to an increased risk of fracture."[19] *Bone strength* reflects both *bone density* and *bone quality*. *Bone density* is determined by the interaction of bone mass (highest in the second decade), new bone formation, and bone resorption or loss. *Bone quality* refers to "architecture, turnover, damage accumulation from microfractures, and mineralization." Osteoporosis typically arises from bone loss during aging, but reduced bone mass from suboptimal bone growth in childhood and adolescence can also cause osteoporosis.

There is no direct measurement of bone strength. Bone mineral density, which accounts for approximately 70% of bone strength, is used as a proxy measure.[19] The World Health Organization uses bone density to define osteopenia and osteoporosis:

- *Osteopenia* is bone density 1.0–2.5 standard deviations below the mean for young adult white women (T score between –2.5 and –1.0).

- *Osteoporosis* is bone density 2.5 or more standard deviations below the mean for young adult white women (T score less than –2.5).

Z scores for age-matched controls are more useful for young people, because they allow comparison with those of similar age, height, and weight. Bone density is measured at the hip, femoral neck, Ward's triangle at the femoral neck, the greater trochanter, and the total hip, which includes all the measurements. A 10% drop in bone density, equivalent to 1.0 standard deviation, is associated with a 20% increase in risk for fracture.

The U.S. Preventive Services Task Force recommends routine bone density screening for women 65 years or older and for younger women with risk factors.[22] The relative fracture risk is higher in those with osteoporosis; however, almost half of all fragility fractures occur in the osteopenic group, which is larger.[23]

RISK FACTORS FOR OSTEOPOROSIS[19,23]

- Postmenopausal status in white women
- Age older than 50 years
- Weight less than 70 kg
- Family history of fracture in a first-degree relative
- History of fracture
- Higher intakes of alcohol
- Women with delayed menarche or early menopause
- Current smokers
- Low levels of 25-hydroxyvitamin D
- Use of corticosteroids for more than 2 months
- Inflammatory disorders of the musculoskeletal, pulmonary, or gastro-intestinal systems, including celiac sprue, chronic renal disease, organ transplantation, hypogonadism, anorexia nervosa

Basic screening questions for older women include the following: Have you ever had a fracture? Did either parent ever have a fracture? Do you smoke? What is your weight? Have you ever taken estrogen replacement therapy?[21] Screening should be expanded to younger women and men with risk factors. Low body weight is the single best predictor of low bone density, and bone density at the femoral neck is the best predictor of subsequent hip fracture.[22,24] Falls increase risk of fracture, so assess the risk factors for falls: impaired cognition, vision, or gait; neuromuscular deficits; and medications affecting balance.

Learn the therapeutic uses of available agents and options for treating osteoporosis, briefly summarized here:[25]

- Increased *calcium* intake reduces age-related hyperparathyroidism and increases mineralization of newly formed bone.

- Up to two thirds of patients with hip fractures are deficient in *vitamin D*, essential for calcium absorption and muscle strength.[25]

- *Antiresorptive agents* inhibit osteoclast activity and slow bone remodeling, allowing better mineralization of bone matrix and stabilization of the trabecular microarchitecture. These agents include bisphosphonates, selective estrogen-receptor modulators (SERMs), calcitonin, and postmenopausal estrogen, now in question because of associated risks of breast cancer and vascular problems.

- *Anabolic agents* such as parathyroid hormone stimulate bone formation by acting primarily on osteoblasts but require subcutaneous administration and monitoring for hypercalcemia. They are reserved for moderate to severe cases of osteoporosis.

● *Regular exercise* that includes weight-bearing and resistance training can increase bone density and muscle strength but has not yet been shown to reduce fracture risk.[19] Multidisciplinary programs to improve strength, balance, and home and medication safety can help prevent falls.

Despite the benefits of estrogen on bone density, three recent trials have shown increased risk of stroke for women taking hormone replacement therapy and failure to reduce risk of coronary heart disease; two of the trials found an increased risk of breast cancer.[26–28] The U.S. Preventive Services Task Force now recommends against routine use of estrogen and progestin for the prevention of chronic conditions in postmenopausal women.[29] Despite public interest, natural estrogens, including plant-derived phyto-estrogens, have not been shown to reduce fracture risk.[19]

EXAMINATION OF SPECIFIC JOINTS: ANATOMY AND PHYSIOLOGY AND TECHNIQUES OF EXAMINATION

Important Areas of Examination for Each of the Major Joints

- Inspection for joint symmetry, alignment, bony deformities
- Inspection and palpation of surrounding tissues for skin changes, nodules, muscle atrophy, crepitus
- Range of motion and maneuvers to test joint function and stability, and integrity of ligaments, tendons, bursae, especially if pain or trauma
- Assessment of inflammation or arthritis, especially swelling, warmth, tenderness, redness

During the interview you have evaluated the patient's ability to carry out normal activities of daily living. Keep these abilities in mind during your physical examination.

In your general survey of the patient you have assessed general appearance, body proportions, and ease of movement. Now visualize the underlying anatomy of the musculoskeletal system and recall the key elements of the history—for example, the mechanism of injury if there is trauma, or the time course of symptoms and limitations in function in arthritis.

Your examination should be systematic. It should include inspection, palpation of bony landmarks as well as related joint and soft-tissue structures, assessment of range of motion, and *special maneuvers* to test specific movements. Recall that the anatomical shape of each joint determines its range of motion. There are two phases to *range of motion*: *active* (by the patient) and *passive* (by the examiner).

TIPS FOR SUCCESSFUL EXAMINATION OF THE MUSCULOSKELETAL SYSTEM

- During inspection, look for *symmetry* of involvement. Is there a symmetric change in joints on both sides of the body, or is the change only in one or two joints?

  Note any *joint deformities* or *malalignment of bones*.

  (continued)

Acute involvement of only one joint suggests trauma, septic arthritis, gout. *Rheumatoid arthritis* typically involves several joints, symmetrically distributed.[30–32]

Dupuytren's contracture (p. 650), bowlegs or knock-knees

> ## Tips for Successful Examination of the Musculoskeletal System (continued)
>
> - Use inspection and palpation to assess the *surrounding tissues,* noting skin changes, subcutaneous nodules, and muscle atrophy. Note any *crepitus,* an audible or palpable crunching during movement of tendons or ligaments over bone. This may occur in normal joints but is more significant when associated with symptoms or signs.
>
> - Test range of motion and maneuvers (described for each joint) to demonstrate *limitations in range of motion* or joint instability from excess mobility of joint ligaments, called *ligamentous laxity.*
>
> - Finally, test *muscle strength* to aid in the assessment of joint function (for these techniques, see Chap. 17).
>
> Be especially alert to *signs of inflammation and arthritis.*
>
> - *Swelling.* Palpable swelling may involve: (1) the synovial membrane, which can feel boggy or doughy; (2) effusion from excess synovial fluid within the joint space; or (3) soft-tissue structures such as bursae, tendons, and tendon sheaths.
>
> - *Warmth.* Use the backs of your fingers to compare the involved joint with its unaffected contralateral joint, or with nearby tissues if both joints are involved.
>
> - *Tenderness.* Try to identify the specific anatomical structure that is tender. Trauma may also cause tenderness.
>
> - *Redness.* Redness of the overlying skin is the *least* common sign of inflammation near the joints.

Subcutaneous nodules in *rheumatoid arthritis* or *rheumatic fever;* effusions in trauma; crepitus over inflamed joints, in *osteoarthritis,* or inflamed tendon sheaths

Decreased range of motion in arthritis, inflammation of tissues around a joint, fibrosis in or around a joint, or bony fixation (*ankylosis*). Ligamentous laxity of the ACL in knee trauma

Muscle atrophy or weakness in *rheumatoid arthritis*

Palpable bogginess or doughiness of the synovial membrane indicates *synovitis,* which is often accompanied by effusion. Palpable joint fluid in effusion, tenderness over the tendon sheaths in *tendinitis*

Arthritis, tendinitis, bursitis, *osteomyelitis*

Tenderness and warmth over a thickened synovium suggest arthritis or infection.

Redness over a tender joint suggests septic or gouty arthritis, or possibly *rheumatoid arthritis.*

If the person has painful joints, move the person gently. Patients may move more comfortably by themselves. Let them show you how they manage. If joint trauma is present, consider an x-ray before attempting movement.

The detail needed for examination of the musculoskeletal system varies widely. This section presents examination techniques for both comprehensive and targeted assessment of joint function. Patients with extensive or severe musculoskeletal problems will require more time. A briefer survey for those without musculoskeletal symptoms is outlined in Chapter 4 (see p. 111).

To help organize your approach to the musculoskeletal examination, study the following flowchart on musculoskeletal complaints.

APPROACH TO MUSCULOSKELETAL COMPLAINTS

Musculoskeletal complaint

Initial rheumatic history and physical
exam to determine
1. Is it articular?
2. Is it acute or chronic?
3. Is inflammation present?
4. How many/which joints are involved?

Is it articular? — No →

Nonarticular condition
Consider
- *Trauma/fracture*
- *Fibromyalgia*
- *Polymyalgia rheumatica*
- *Bursitis*
- *Tendinitis*

Yes ↓

Is complaint > 6 wk?

No → **Acute**   Yes → **Chronic**

Consider
- Acute arthritis
  - *Infectious arthritis*
  - *Gout*
  - *Pseudogout*
  - *Reiter's syndrome*
- Initial presentation
  of chronic arthritis

Chronic

Is inflammation present?
1. Is there prolonged morning stiffness?
2. Is there soft tissue swelling?
3. Are there systemic symptoms?
4. Is the ESR or CRP elevated?

No → **Chronic noninflammatory arthritis**   Yes → **Chronic inflammatory arthritis**

Chronic inflammatory arthritis → **How many joints involved?**

1-3 → **Chronic inflammatory mono/oligoarthritis**
Consider
- *Indolent infection*
- *Psoriatic arthritis*
- *Reiter's syndrome*
- *Pauciarticular JA*

>3 → **Chronic inflammatory polyarthritis**

Chronic noninflammatory arthritis → **Are DIP, CMC1, hip or knee joints involved?**

No → Unlikely to be osteoarthritis
Consider
- *Osteonecrosis*
- *Charcot arthritis*

Yes → **Osteoarthritis**

Chronic inflammatory polyarthritis → **Is involvement symmetric?**

No → Consider
- *Psoriatic arthritis*
- *Reiter's syndrome*

Yes → **Are PIP, MCP, or MTP joints involved?**

No → Unlikely to be rheumatoid arthritis
Consider
- *SLE*
- *Scleroderma*
- *Polymyositis*

Yes → **Rheumatoid arthritis**

From Kasper DL, Braunwald E, Fauci AS, et al., eds. Harrison's Principles of Internal Medicine, 16th ed. New York: McGraw-Hill, 2005. ESR, erythrocyte sedimentation rate; CRP, C-reactive protein; DIP, distal interphalangeal; CMC, carpometacarpal; PIP, proximal interphalangeal; MCP, metacarpophalangeal; MTP, metatarsophalangeal; PMR, polymyalgia rheumatica; SLE, systemic lupus erythematosus; JA, juvenile arthritis.

TEMPOROMANDIBULAR JOINT (TMJ)

Overview, Bony Structures, and Joints

The temporomandibular joint is the most active joint in the body, opening and closing up to 2000 times a day. It is formed by the fossa and articular tubercle of the temporal bone and the condyle of the mandible. It lies midway between the external acoustic meatus and the zygomatic arch.

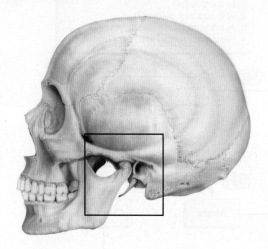

A fibrocartilaginous disc cushions the action of the condyle of the mandible against the synovial membrane and capsule of the articulating surfaces of the temporal bone. Hence, it is a condylar synovial joint.

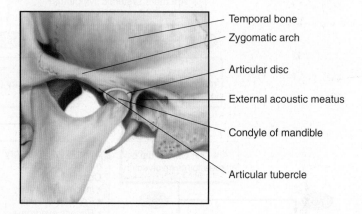

Temporal bone

Zygomatic arch

Articular disc

External acoustic meatus

Condyle of mandible

Articular tubercle

Muscle Groups and Additional Structures

The principal muscles opening the mouth are the *external pterygoids*. Closing the mouth are the muscles innervated by Cranial Nerve V, the trigeminal nerve (see p. 659)—the *masseter*, the *temporalis*, and the *internal pterygoids*.

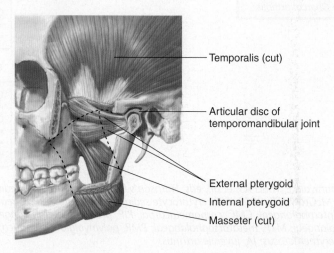

Temporalis (cut)

Articular disc of temporomandibular joint

External pterygoid

Internal pterygoid

Masseter (cut)

Techniques of Examination

Inspection and Palpation. Inspect the face for symmetry. Inspect the TMJ for swelling or redness. Swelling may appear as a rounded bulge approximately ½ cm anterior to the external auditory meatus.

Facial asymmetry associated with *TMJ syndrome*. Typical features are unilateral chronic pain with chewing, jaw clenching, or teeth grinding, often associated with stress (may also present as headache). Pain with chewing also in *trigeminal neuralgia, temporal arteritis*.

Swelling, tenderness, and decreased range of motion in inflammation or arthritis

To locate and palpate the joint, place the tips of your index fingers just in front of the tragus of each ear and ask the patient to open his or her mouth. The fingertips should drop into the joint spaces as the mouth opens. Check for smooth range of motion; note any swelling or tenderness. Snapping or clicking may be felt or heard in normal people.

Dislocation of the TMJ may be seen in trauma.

Palpable crepitus or clicking in poor occlusion, meniscus injury, or synovial swelling from trauma

Palpate the muscles of mastication:

- The *masseters*, externally at the angle of the mandible

- The *temporal muscles*, externally during clenching and relaxation of the jaw

- The *pterygoid muscles*, internally between the tonsillar pillars at the mandible

Pain and tenderness on palpation in *TMJ syndrome*

Range of Motion and Maneuvers. The temporomandibular joint has glide and hinge motions in its upper and lower portions, respectively. Grinding or chewing consists primarily of gliding movements in the upper compartments.

Range of motion is three-fold: ask the patient to demonstrate opening and closing, protrusion and retraction (by jutting the jaw forward), and lateral, or side-to-side, motion. Normally as the mouth is opened wide, three fingers can be inserted between incisors. During normal protrusion of the jaw, the bottom teeth can be placed in front of the upper teeth.

THE SHOULDER

Overview

The glenohumeral joint of the shoulder is distinguished by wide-ranging movement in all directions. This joint is largely uninhibited by bony structures. The humeral head contacts less than one third of the surface area of the glenoid fossa and virtually dangles from the scapula, attached by the joint capsule, the intra-articular capsular ligaments, the glenoid labrum, and a meshwork of muscles and tendons.

The shoulder derives its mobility from a complex interconnected structure of four joints, three large bones, and three principal muscle groups, often referred to as the *shoulder girdle*. These structures are viewed as *dynamic stabilizers*, or those capable of movement, or *static stabilizers*, those incapable of movement.

- *Dynamic stabilizers:* the SITS muscles of the rotator cuff (supraspinatus, infraspinatus, teres minor, and subscapularis), which move the humerus and depress and stabilize the humeral head within the glenoid fossa

- *Static stabilizers:* the bony structures of the shoulder girdle, the labrum, the articular capsule, and the glenohumeral ligaments. The *labrum* is a fibrocartilaginous ring that surrounds the glenoid and deepens its socket, providing greater stability to the humeral head. The *articular capsule*, formed by tendons of the rotator cuff and other capsular muscles and strengthened by the glenohumeral ligaments, also adds to joint stability.

Bony Structures

The bony structures of the shoulder include the humerus, the clavicle, and the scapula. The scapula is anchored to the axial skeleton only by the sternoclavicular joint and inserting muscles, often called the *scapulothoracic articulation* because it is not a true joint.

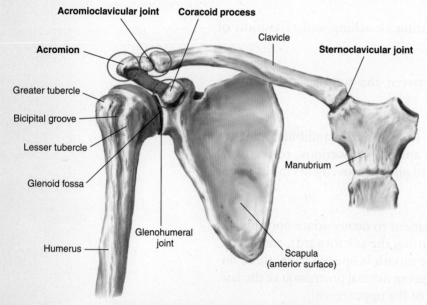

IMPORTANT BONES OF THE SHOULDER

Identify the *manubrium*, the *sternoclavicular joint*, and the *clavicle*. Also identify the *tip of the acromion*, the *greater tubercle of the humerus*, and the *coracoid process*, which are important landmarks for shoulder anatomy.

Joints

Three different joints articulate at the shoulder:

- The *glenohumeral joint*. In this joint, the head of the humerus articulates with the shallow glenoid fossa of the scapula. This joint is deeply situated and not normally palpable. It is a ball-and-socket joint, allowing the arm its wide arc of movement—flexion, extension, abduction (movement away from the trunk), adduction (movement toward the trunk), rotation, and circumduction.

- The *sternoclavicular joint*. The convex medial end of the clavicle articulates with the concave hollow in the upper sternum.

- The *acromioclavicular joint*. The lateral end of the clavicle articulates with the acromion process of the scapula.

Muscle Groups

Three groups of muscles attach at the shoulder:

The Scapulohumeral Group. This group extends from the scapula to the humerus and includes the muscles inserting directly on the humerus, known as *"SITS muscles"* of the *rotator cuff*:

- *Supraspinatus*—runs above the glenohumeral joint; inserts on the greater tubercle

- *Infraspinatus* and *teres minor*—cross the glenohumeral joint posteriorly; insert on the greater tubercle

- *Subscapularis* (not illustrated)—originates on the anterior surface of the scapula and crosses the joint anteriorly; inserts on the lesser tubercle.

Posterior view
Axioscapular group (pulls shoulder backward)
Scapulohumeral group (rotates shoulder laterally; includes rotator cuff)

Axioscapular group
Scapulohumeral group
Levator scapulae
Rhomboids
Trapezius
Supraspinatus
Infraspinatus
Deltoid
Teres minor
Latissimus dorsi

The scapulohumeral group rotates the shoulder laterally (the *rotator cuff*) and depresses and rotates the head of the humerus. (See pp. 593–596 for discussion of rotator cuff injuries.)

The Axioscapular Group. This group attaches the trunk to the scapula and includes the trapezius, rhomboids, serratus anterior, and levator scapulae. These muscles rotate the scapula.

The Axiohumeral Group. This group attaches the trunk to the humerus and includes the pectoralis major and minor and the latissimus dorsi. These muscles produce internal rotation of the shoulder.

Anterior view
Axiohumeral group (rotates shoulder internally)

The biceps and triceps, which connect the scapula to the bones of the forearm, are also involved in shoulder movement, particularly abduction.

Additional Structures

Also important to shoulder movement are the *articular capsule and bursae*. Surrounding the glenohumeral joint is a fibrous articular capsule formed by the tendon insertions of the rotator cuff and other capsular muscles. The loose fit of the capsule allows the shoulder bones to separate, and contributes to the shoulder's wide range of movement. The capsule is lined by a synovial membrane with two outpouchings—the *subscapular bursa* and the *synovial sheath of the tendon of the long head of the biceps*.

To locate the biceps tendon, rotate your arm externally and find the tendinous cord that runs just medial to the greater tubercle. Roll it under your fingers. This is the tendon of the long head of the biceps. It runs in the bicipital groove between the greater and lesser tubercles.

The principal bursa of the shoulder is the *subacromial bursa,* positioned between the acromion and the head of the humerus and overlying the supraspinatus tendon. Abduction of the shoulder compresses this bursa. Normally, the supraspinatus tendon and the subacromial bursa are not palpable. However, if the bursal surfaces are inflamed (subacromial bursitis), there may be tenderness just below the tip of the acromion, pain with abduction and rotation, and loss of smooth movement.

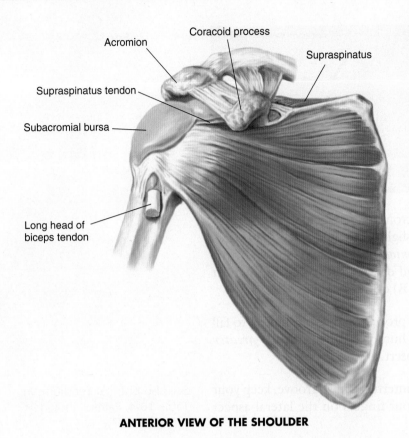

Acromion

Coracoid process

Supraspinatus

Supraspinatus tendon

Subacromial bursa

Long head of
biceps tendon

shoulder

ANTERIOR VIEW OF THE SHOULDER

Techniques of Examination

Inspection.   Observe the shoulder and shoulder girdle anteriorly, and inspect the scapulae and related muscles posteriorly.

Scoliosis may cause elevation of one shoulder. With *anterior dislocation of the shoulder*, the rounded lateral aspect of the shoulder appears flattened.[33,34]

Note any swelling, deformity, muscle atrophy or fasciculations (fine tremors of the muscles), or abnormal positioning.

Atrophy of supraspinatus and infraspinatus over posterior scapula with increased prominence of scapular spine within 2 to 3 weeks of *rotator cuff tear*.

Look for swelling of the joint capsule anteriorly or a bulge in the subacromial bursa under the deltoid muscle. Survey the entire upper extremity for color change, skin alteration, or unusual bony contours.

A significant amount of synovial fluid is needed before the joint capsule appears distended.

Palpation.   Begin by palpating the bony landmarks of the shoulder; then palpate any area of pain.

See Table 16-4, Painful Shoulders, (pp. 646–647).

● Beginning medially, at the *sternoclavicular joint,* trace the clavicle laterally with your fingers.

- Now, from behind, follow the bony spine of the scapula laterally and upward until it becomes the acromion (**A**), the summit of the shoulder. Its upper surface is rough and slightly convex. Identify the anterior tip of the acromion.

- With your index finger on top of the acromion, just behind its tip, press medially with your thumb to find the slightly elevated ridge that marks the distal end of the clavicle at the *acromioclavicular joint* (shown by the arrow). Move your thumb medially and down a short step to the next bony prominence, the *coracoid process* (**B**) of the scapula.

- Now, with your thumb on the coracoid process, allow your fingers to fall on and grasp the lateral aspect of the humerus to palpate the *greater tubercle* (**C**), where the SITS muscles insert.

- Next, to palpate the *biceps tendon* in the intertubercular groove, keep your thumb on the coracoid process and your fingers on the lateral aspect of the humerus. Remove your index finger and place it halfway in between the coracoid process and the greater tubercle on the anterior surface of the arm. As you check for tendon tenderness, rolling the tendon under the fingertips may be helpful. You can also rotate the forearm externally, locate the muscle distally near the elbow, and track the muscle and its tendon proximally into the intertubercular groove.

See also Bicipital Tendinitis in Table 16-4, Painful Shoulders (pp. 646–647).

PALPATION OF THE BICIPITAL GROOVE AND TENDON

- To examine the subacromial and subdeltoid bursae and the SITS muscles, first passively extend the humerus by lifting the elbow posteriorly. This rotates these structures so that they are anterior to the acromion. Palpate carefully over the subacromial and subdeltoid bursae. The underlying palpable SITS muscles are:

Localized tenderness arises from *subacromial* or *subdeltoid bursitis,* degenerative changes, or calcific deposits in the rotator cuff.

Swelling suggests a *bursal tear* that communicates with the articular cavity.

  - Supraspinatus—directly under the acromion

  - Infraspinatus—posterior to supraspinatus

  - Teres minor—posterior and inferior to the supraspinatus rupture of the rotator

  - (The fourth muscle, the subscapularis, inserts anteriorly and is not palpable.)

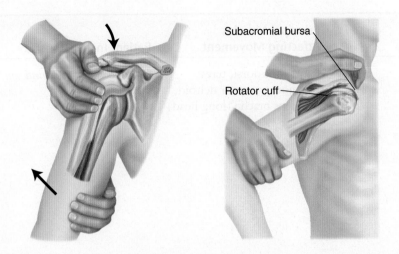

Subacromial bursa

Rotator cuff

Tenderness over the "SITS" muscle insertions and inability to lift the arm above shoulder level are seen in sprains, tears, and tendon rupture of the rotator cuff, most commonly the *supraspinatus*. See Table 16-4, Painful Shoulders (pp. 646–647).

● The fibrous articular capsule and the broad, flat tendons of the rotator cuff are so closely associated that they must be examined simultaneously. Swelling in the capsule and synovial membrane is often best detected by looking down on the shoulder from above. Palpate the capsule and synovial membrane beneath the anterior and posterior acromion.

Tenderness and effusion suggest synovitis of the glenohumeral joint. If the margins of the capsule and synovial membrane are palpable, a moderate to large effusion is present. Minimal degrees of synovitis at the glenohumeral joint cannot be detected on palpation.

Range of Motion and Maneuvers

Range of Motion.   The six motions of the shoulder girdle are flexion, extension, abduction, adduction, and internal and external rotation.

Standing in front of the patient, watch for smooth fluid movement as the patient performs the motions listed in the table below. Note the specific muscles responsible for each motion and clear simple instructions that prompt the requested patient response.

Restricted range of motion in *bursitis, capsulitis, rotator cuff tears* or *sprains*, or *tendinitis*.

Shoulder Movement		Principal Muscles Affecting Movement	Patient Instructions
Flexion	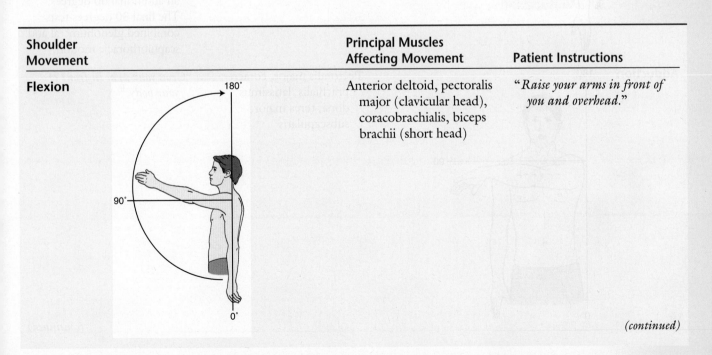	Anterior deltoid, pectoralis major (clavicular head), coracobrachialis, biceps brachii (short head)	*"Raise your arms in front of you and overhead."*

(continued)

Shoulder Movement	Principal Muscles Affecting Movement	Patient Instructions
Extension	Latissimus dorsi, teres major, posterior deltoid, triceps brachii (long head)	*"Raise your arms behind you."*
Abduction	Supraspinatus, middle deltoid, serratus anterior (via upward rotation of the scapula)	*"Raise your arms out to the side and overhead."* Note that to test *pure gleno-humeral motion*, the patient should raise the arms to shoulder level at 90 degrees, with palms facing down. To test *scapulothoracic motion*, the patient should turn the palms up and raise the arms an additional 60 degrees. The final 30 degrees tests combined glenohumeral and scapulothoracic motion.
Adduction	Pectoralis major, coraco-brachialis, latissimus dorsi, teres major, subscapularis	*"Cross your arm in front of your body."*

(continued)

Shoulder Movement		Principal Muscles Affecting Movement	Patient Instructions
Internal Rotation		Subscapularis, anterior deltoid, pectoralis major, teres major, latissimus dorsi	*"Place one hand behind your back and touch your shoulder blade."*
			Identify the highest midline spinous process the patient is able to reach.
External Rotation		Infraspinatus, teres minor, posterior deltoid	*"Raise your arm to shoulder level; bend your elbow and rotate your forearm toward the ceiling."*
			or
			"Place one hand behind your neck or head as if you are brushing your hair."

90°

Maneuvers. The examination of the shoulder often requires selective evaluation of specific motions and structures. There are more than 20 different maneuvers for testing shoulder function, not all well-studied.[35] Common recommended maneuvers, with evidence when available, are described on pp. 596–599. Using these maneuvers will take practice with supervision, but you will find them helpful in identifying shoulder pathology.

Note that the most common cause of shoulder pain involves the rotator cuff, usually involving the supraspinatus tendon with later possible progression posteriorly and anteriorly. Compression of the rotator cuff muscles and tendons between head of the humerus and the acromion cause "impingement signs" during frequently performed maneuvers such as Neer's, Hawkins, and the dropped-arm tests. However, the best predictors of rotator cuff tear are supraspinatus weakness on abduction, infraspinatus weakness during external rotation, and a positive impingement sign.[35,36]

Age 60 years or older and a positive dropped-arm test are the individual findings most likely to identify a rotator cuff tear, with likelihood ratios (LRs) of 3.2 and 5.0, respectively. The combined findings of supraspinatus weakness, infraspinatus weakness, and a positive impingement sign increase the likelihood of a tear to 48.0; when all three are absent, the LR falls to 0.02, virtually ruling out the diagnosis.[35,36]

● Maneuvers for Examining the Shoulder

Structure	Technique
Acromioclavicular Joint	Palpate and compare both joints for swelling or tenderness. Adduct the patient's arm across the chest, sometimes called the *"crossover test."*

See Table 16-4, Painful Shoulders (pp. 646–647). Localized tenderness or pain with *adduction* suggests inflammation or arthritis of the acromioclavicular joint. But sensitivity and specificity of tenderness is ~95% and 10%; of adduction, ~80% and 50%.

(continued)

● Maneuvers for Examining the Shoulder (continued)

Structure	Technique	
Overall Shoulder Rotation	Ask the patient to touch the opposite scapula using the two motions shown below (the Apley scratch test).	Difficulty with these motions suggests rotator cuff disorder.

Tests abduction and external rotation.

Tests adduction and internal rotation.

Rotator Cuff — Test *Neer's impingement sign*. Press on the scapula to prevent scapular motion with one hand, and raise the patient's arm with the other. This compresses the greater tuberosity of the humerus against the acromion.

Pain during this maneuver is a *positive test* indicating possible *rotator cuff tear*.

Test *Hawkin's impingement sign*. Flex the patient's shoulder and elbow to 90° with the palm facing down. Then, with one hand on the forearm and one on the arm, rotate the arm internally. This compresses the greater tuberosity against the coracoacromial ligament.

Pain during this maneuver is a *positive test* indicating possible *rotator cuff tear*.

(continued)

● Maneuvers for Examining the Shoulder (continued)

Structure	Technique	
	Test *supraspinatus strength* (sometimes called the "empty can test"). Elevate the arms to 90° and internally rotate the arms with the thumbs pointing down, as if emptying a can. Ask the patient to resist as you place downward pressure on the arms.	Weakness during this maneuver is a *positive test* indicating possible *rotator cuff tear.*
	Test *infraspinatus strength.* Ask the patient to place arms at the side and flex the elbows to 90° with the thumbs turned up. Provide resistance as the patient presses the forearms outward.	Weakness during this maneuver is a *positive test* indicating possible *rotator cuff tear* or *bicipital tendinitis.*
	Test *forearm supination.* Flex the patient's forearm to 90° at the elbow and pronate the patient's wrist. Provide resistance when the patient supinates the forearm.	Pain during this maneuver is a *positive test* indicating inflammation of the long head of the biceps tendon and possible *rotator cuff tear.*

(continued)

● Maneuvers for Examining the Shoulder (continued)

Structure	Technique	
	Test the *"drop-arm" sign*. Ask the patient to fully abduct the arm to shoulder level (or up to 90°) and lower it slowly. (Note that abduction above shoulder level, from 90° to 120°, reflects action of the deltoid muscle.)	If the patient cannot hold the arm fully abducted at shoulder level, the test is *positive*, indicating a *rotator cuff tear* (LR, 5.0).[35]

THE ELBOW

Overview, Bony Structures, and Joints

The elbow helps position the hand in space and stabilizes the lever action of the forearm. The elbow joint is formed by the humerus and the two bones of the forearm, the radius, and the ulna. Identify the medial and lateral epicondyles of the humerus and the olecranon process of the ulna.

These bones have three articulations: the *humeroulnar joint*, the *radiohumeral joint*, and the *radioulnar joint*. All three share a large common articular cavity and an extensive synovial lining.

Muscle Groups and Additional Structures

Muscles traversing the elbow include the *biceps* and *brachioradialis* (flexion), the *triceps* (extension), the *pronator teres* (pronation), and the *supinator* (supination).

Humerus — Lateral epicondyle
Medial epicondyle — **Radiohumeral joint**
Humeroulnar joint
Radioulnar joint
Supinator
Pronator teres
Brachioradialis
Ulna — Radius

LEFT ANTERIOR ELBOW

Note the location of the *olecranon bursa* between the olecranon process and the skin. The bursa is not normally palpable but swells and becomes tender when inflamed. The *ulnar nerve* runs posteriorly in the ulnar groove between the medial epicondyle and the olecranon process. On the ventral forearm, the *median nerve* is just medial to the brachial artery.

Ulnar nerve

Olecranon process

Synovial membrane (distended)

Medial epicondyle

Radial nerve

Olecranon bursa

LEFT POSTERIOR ELBOW

Techniques of Examination

Inspection. Support the patient's forearm with your opposite hand so the elbow is flexed to about 70°. Identify the medial and lateral epicondyles and the olecranon process of the ulna. Inspect the contours of the elbow, including the extensor surface of the ulna and the olecranon process. Note any nodules or swelling.

See Table 16-5, Swollen or Tender Elbows (p. 648).

Swelling over the olecranon process in olecranon bursitis (see p. 648); inflammation or synovial fluid in arthritis.

Palpation. Palpate the olecranon process and press over the epicondyles for tenderness. Note any displacement of the olecranon.

Tenderness distal to the epicondyle in *lateral epicondylitis* (tennis elbow) and less commonly in *medial epicondylitis* (pitcher's or golfer's elbow)

The olecranon is displaced posteriorly in *posterior dislocation of the elbow* and *supracondylar fracture*.

Palpate the grooves between the epicondyles and the olecranon, noting any tenderness, swelling, or thickening. The synovium is most accessible to examination between the olecranon and the epicondyles. (Normally neither synovium nor bursa is palpable.) The sensitive ulnar nerve can be felt posteriorly between the olecranon process and the medial epicondyle.

POSTERIOR DISLOCATION OF THE ELBOW

SUPRACONDYLAR FRACTURE OF THE ELBOW

Range of Motion and Maneuvers. Range of motion includes *flexion* and *extension* at the elbow and *pronation* and *supination* of the forearm. In the table following, note the specific muscles responsible for each motion and clear, simple instructions that prompt the requested patient response.

Full elbow extension makes intra-articular effusion or hemarthrosis unlikely.

Elbow Movement	Primary Muscles Affecting Movement	Patient Instructions
Flexion	Biceps brachii, brachialis, brachioradialis	*"Bend your elbow."*
Extension	Triceps brachii, anconeus	*"Straighten your elbow."*
Supination	Biceps brachii, supinator	*"Turn your palms up, as if carrying a bowl of soup."*
Pronation	Pronator teres, pronator quadratus	*"Turn your palms down."*

THE WRIST AND HANDS

Overview

The wrist and hands form a complex unit of small, highly active joints used almost continuously during waking hours. There is little protection from overlying soft tissue, increasing vulnerability to trauma and disability.

Bony Structures

The wrist includes the distal radius and ulna and eight small carpal bones. At the wrist, identify the bony tips of the radius and the ulna.

The carpal bones lie distal to the wrist joint within each hand. Identify the carpal bones, each of the five metacarpals, and the proximal, middle, and distal phalanges. Note that the thumb lacks a middle phalanx.

Joints

The numerous joints of the wrist and hand lend unusual dexterity to the hands.

- *Wrist joints.* The wrist joints include the *radiocarpal* or *wrist joint*, the *distal radioulnar joint*, and the *intercarpal joints*. The joint capsule, articular disc, and synovial membrane of the wrist join the radius to the ulna and to the proximal carpal bones. On the dorsum of the wrist, locate the groove of the *radiocarpal joint*, which provides most of the flexion and extension at the wrist because the ulna does not articulate directly with the carpal bones.

- *Hand joints.* The joints of the hand include the *metacarpophalangeal joints* (MCPs), the *proximal interphalangeal joints* (PIPs), and the *distal interphalangeal joints* (DIPs). Flex the hand and find the groove marking the MCP joint of each finger. It is distal to the knuckle and is best felt on either side of the extensor tendon.

Distal interphalangeal joint (DIP)
Proximal interphalangeal joint (PIP)
Metacarpophalangeal joint (MCP)
Phalanges
Metacarpal
Hamate
Trapezoid
Trapezium
Capitate
Scaphoid
Carpal
Triquetrum
Lunate
Radius
Ulna

Radiocarpal joint
Intercarpal joints
Distal radioulnar joint

Metacarpophalangeal joint

Muscle Groups

Wrist flexion arises from the two carpal muscles, located on the radial and ulnar surfaces. Two radial and one ulnar muscle provide wrist extension. Supination and pronation result from muscle contraction in the forearm.

The thumb is powered by three muscles that form the thenar eminence and provide flexion, abduction, and opposition. The muscles of extension are at the base of the thumb along the radial margin. Movement in the digits depends on action of the flexor and extensor tendons of muscles in the forearm and wrist.

The intrinsic muscles of the hand attaching to the metacarpal bones are involved in flexion (*lumbricals*), abduction (*dorsal interossei*), and adduction (*palmar interossei*) of the fingers.

Additional Structures

Soft-tissue structures, especially tendons and tendon sheaths, are especially important to movement of the wrist and hand. Six extensor tendons and two flexor tendons pass across the wrist and hand to insert on the fingers. Through much of their course these tendons travel in tunnel-like sheaths, generally palpable only when swollen or inflamed.

Be familiar with the structures in the *carpal tunnel*, a channel beneath the palmar surface of the wrist and prox-imal hand. The channel contains the sheath and flexor tendons of the fore-arm muscles and the *median nerve*.

Holding the tendons and tendon sheath in place is a transverse liga-ment, the *flexor retinaculum*. The median nerve lies between the flexor retinaculum and the tendon sheath. It provides sensation to the palm and the palmar surface of most of the thumb, the second and third digits, and half of the fourth digit. It also innervates the thumb muscles of flex-ion, abduction, and opposition.

- Flexor retinaculum
- Carpal tunnel
- Median nerve

Techniques of Examination

Inspection. Observe the position of the hands in motion to see if move-ments are smooth and natural. At rest, the fingers should be slightly flexed and aligned almost in parallel.

Guarded movement suggests injury. Poor finger alignment is seen in flexor tendon damage.

Inspect the palmar and dorsal surfaces of the wrist and hand carefully for swelling over the joints.

Diffuse swelling in arthritis or infection; local swelling from cystic ganglion. See Table 16-6, Arthritis in the Hands (p. 649), and Table 16-7, Swellings and Deformities of the Hands (p. 650).

Note any deformities of the wrist, hand, or finger bones, as well as any angulation from radial or ulnar deviation.

In *osteoarthritis,* Heberden's nodes at the DIP joints, Bouchard's nodes at the PIP joints. In *rheumatoid arthritis,* symmetric deformity in the PIP, MCP, and wrist joints, with ulnar deviation

Observe the contours of the palm, namely the thenar and hypothenar eminences.

Thenar atrophy in median nerve compression from *carpal tunnel syndrome;* hypothenar atrophy in *ulnar nerve compression.*

Note any thickening of the flexor tendons or flexion contractures in the fingers.

Flexion contractures in the ring, 5th, and 3rd fingers, or *Dupuytren's contractures,* arise from thickening of the palmar fascia (see p. 649).

Palpation. At the wrist, palpate the distal radius and ulna on the lateral and medial surfaces. Palpate the groove of each wrist joint with your thumbs on the dorsum of the wrist, your fingers beneath it. Note any swelling, bogginess, or tenderness.

Tenderness over the distal radius in *Colles' fracture.* Any tenderness or bony step-offs are suspicious for fracture.

Swelling and/or tenderness suggests *rheumatoid arthritis* if bilateral and of several weeks' duration.

Palpate the radial styloid bone and the *anatomical snuffbox,* a hollowed depression just distal to the radial styloid process formed by the abductor and extensor muscles of the thumb. The "snuffbox" becomes more visible with lateral extension of the thumb away from the hand.

Tenderness over the extensor and abductor tendons of the thumb at the radial styloid in *de Quervain's tenosynovitis* and *gonococcal tenosynovitis.* See Table 16-8, Tendon Sheath, Palmar Space, and Finger Infections (p. 651).

Tenderness over the "snuffbox" in *scaphoid fracture,* the most common injury of the carpal bones. Poor blood supply puts the scaphoid bone at risk for *avascular necrosis.*

Palpate the eight carpal bones lying distal to the wrist joint, and then each of the five metacarpals and the proximal, middle, and distal phalanges.

Synovitis in the MCPs is painful with this pressure—a point to remember when shaking hands.

Palpate any other area where you suspect an abnormality.

Compress the MCP joints by squeezing the hand from each side between the thumb and fingers. Alternatively, use your thumb to palpate each MCP joint just distal to and on each side of the knuckle as your index finger feels the head of the metacarpal in the palm. Note any swelling, bogginess, or tenderness.

The MCPs are often boggy or tender in *rheumatoid arthritis* (but rarely involved in osteoarthritis). Pain with compression also in *posttraumatic arthritis.*

Now examine the fingers and thumb. Palpate the medial and lateral aspects of each PIP joint between your thumb and index finger, again checking for swelling, bogginess, bony enlargement, or tenderness.

PIP changes seen in *rheumatoid arthritis*, Bouchard's nodes in *osteoarthritis*. Pain at the base of the thumb in first *carpometacarpal arthritis.*

Hard dorsolateral nodules on the DIP joints, or *Heberden's nodes,* common in osteoarthritis; DIP joint involvement in *psoriatic arthritis*

Using the same techniques, examine the DIP joints.

HEBERDEN'S NODES

In any area of swelling or inflammation, palpate along the tendons inserting on the thumb and fingers.

Tenderness and swelling in *tenosynovitis,* or inflammation of the tendon sheaths. *De Quervain's tenosynovitis* over the extensor and abductor tendons of the thumb as they cross the radial styloid. See Table 16-8, Tendon Sheath, Palmar Space, and Finger Infections (p. 651).

Wrists: Range of Motion and Maneuvers

Range of Motion.   Refer to the table below for specific muscles responsible for each movement and clear, simple instructions that prompt the patient to properly follow your directions. For techniques of testing wrist muscle strength, turn to Chapter 17, The Nervous System, pp. 680–683.

Conditions that impair range of motion include *arthritis, tenosynovitis, Dupuytren's contracture.* See Table 16-7, Swellings and Deformities of the Hands (p. 650).

Wrist Movement	Primary Muscles Affecting Movement	Patient Instructions
Flexion	Flexor carpi radialis, flexor carpi ulnaris	*"With palms down, point your fingers toward the floor."*
Extension	Extensor carpi ulnaris, extensor carpi radialis longus, extensor carpi radialis brevis	*"With palms down, point your fingers toward the ceiling."*
Adduction (radial deviation)	Flexor carpi ulnaris	*"With palms down, bring your fingers toward the midline."*
Abduction (ulnar deviation)	Flexor carpi radialis	*"With palms down, bring your fingers away from the midline."*

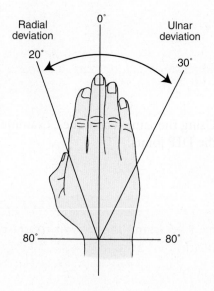

Maneuvers.   Several maneuvers useful for assessing common office complaints relating to the wrist are listed on the next page. For complaints of dropping objects, inability to twist lids off jars, aching at the wrist or even the forearm, and numbness of the first three digits, learn the tests on the next page for assessing *carpal tunnel syndrome.* Note the distribution of the median, radial, and ulnar nerve innervations of the wrist and hand on the next page.

Onset of *carpal tunnel syndrome* often related to repetitive motion with wrists flexed (as in keyboard use, mail-sorting), pregnancy, rheumatoid arthritis, diabetes, hypothyroidism

Thenar atrophy may also be present.

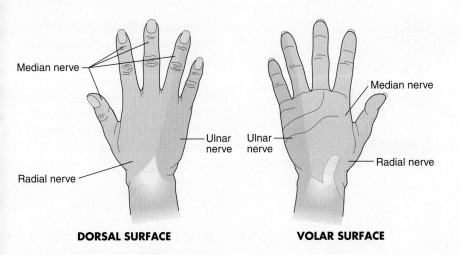

DORSAL SURFACE   **VOLAR SURFACE**

Decreased sensation in the median nerve distribution in *carpal tunnel syndrome*

You can test sensation as follows:

● Pulp of the index finger—median nerve

● Pulp of the 5th finger—ulnar nerve

● Dorsal web space of the thumb and index finger—radial nerve

HAND GRIP. Test *hand grip strength* by asking the patient to grasp your second and third fingers. This tests function of wrist joints, the finger flexors, and the intrinsic muscles and joints of the hand.

Decreased grip strength is a *positive test* for weakness of the finger flexors and/or intrinsic muscles of the hand.

Wrist pain and grip weakness in *de Quervain's tenosynovitis*. Decreased grip strength in *arthritis*, *carpal tunnel syndrome*, epicondylitis, and *cervical radiculopathy*.

THUMB MOVEMENT. Test the thumb function if there is wrist pain by asking the patient to grasp the thumb against the palm and then move the wrist toward the midline in ulnar deviation (commonly called *Finkelstein's test*).

Tendon

Pain during this maneuver identifies *de Quervain's tenosynovitis* from inflammation of the abductor pollicis longus and extensor pollicis brevis tendons and tendon sheaths.

CARPAL TUNNEL—THUMB ABDUCTION, TINEL'S TEST, AND PHALEN'S TEST.[37–39] Test *thumb abduction* by asking the patient to raise the thumb straight up as you apply downward resistance.

Weakness on thumb abduction is a *positive test*—the abductor pollicis longus is innervated only by the median nerve. Weak thumb abduction, hand symptom diagrams, and decreased sensation roughly double the likelihood of carpal tunnel disease.[37]

Test *Tinel's sign* for median nerve compression by tapping lightly over the course of the median nerve in the carpal tunnel as shown.

Aching and numbness in the median nerve distribution is a *positive test*.

Test *Phalen's sign* for median nerve compression by asking the patient to hold the wrists in flexion for 60 seconds. Alternatively, ask the patient to press the backs of both hands together to form right angles. These maneuvers compress the median nerve.

Numbness and tingling in the median nerve distribution within 60 seconds is a *positive test*.

Tinel's and Phalen's signs do not reliably predict positive electro-diagnosis of carpal tunnel disease.[37]

Fingers and Thumbs: Range of Motion and Maneuvers

Range of Motion.   Assess *flexion*, *extension*, *abduction*, and *adduction* of the fingers.

● *Flexion and extension.* For *flexion*, to test the lumbricals and finger flexor muscles, ask the patient to *"Make a tight fist with each hand, thumb across the knuckles."* For *extension*, to test the finger extensor muscles, ask the patient to *"Extend and spread the fingers."*

At the MCPs, the fingers may extend beyond the neutral position. Also test the flexion and extension of the PIP and DIP joints (lumbrical muscles). The fingers should open and close easily.

● *Abduction and adduction.* Ask the patient to spread the fingers apart (abduction from dorsal interossei) and back together (adduction from palmar interossei). Check for smooth, coordinated movement.

Impaired hand movement in arthritis, trigger finger, Dupuytren's contracture

Thumbs.   At the *thumb,* assess *flexion, extension, abduction, adduction,* and *opposition.* Each of these movements is powered by a related muscle of the thumb.

Ask the patient to move the thumb across the palm and touch the base of the 5th finger to test *flexion,* and then to move the thumb back across the palm and away from the fingers to test *extension.*

FLEXION   **EXTENSION**

Next, ask the patient to place the fingers and thumb in the neutral position with the palm up, then have the patient move the thumb anteriorly away from the palm to assess abduction and back down for adduction. To test opposition, or movements of the thumb across the palm, ask the patient to touch the thumb to each of the other fingertips.

ABDUCTION AND   **OPPOSITION**
ADDUCTION

A full examination of the wrist and hand involves detailed testing of muscle strength and sensation, found in Chapter 17, The Nervous System, pp. 680–683.

 THE SPINE

Overview

The vertebral column, or spine, is the central supporting structure of the trunk and back. Note the *concave curves* of the cervical and lumbar spine and the *convex curves* of the thoracic and sacrococcygeal spine. These curves help distribute upper body weight to the pelvis and lower extremities and cushion the concussive impact of walking or running.

The complex mechanics of the back reflect the coordinated action of:

- The vertebrae and intervertebral discs

- An interconnecting system of ligaments between anterior vertebrae and posterior vertebrae, ligaments between the spinous processes, and ligaments between the lamina of two adjacent vertebrae

- Large superficial muscles, deeper intrinsic muscles, and muscles of the abdominal wall

Bony Structures

The vertebral column contains 24 vertebrae stacked on the sacrum and coccyx. A typical vertebra contains sites for joint articulations, weight bearing, and muscle attachments, as well as foramina for the spinal nerve roots and peripheral nerves. Anteriorly, the *vertebral body* supports weight bearing. The posterior *vertebral arch* encloses the spinal cord. Review the location of the vertebral processes and foramina, with particular attention to:

- The *spinous process* projecting posteriorly in the midline and the two transverse processes at the junction of the *pedicle* and the *lamina*. Muscles attach at these processes.

- The *articular processes*—two on each side of the vertebra, one facing up and one facing down, at the junction of the pedicles and laminae, often called *articular facets.*

- The *vertebral foramen,* which encloses the spinal cord, the *intervertebral foramen,* formed by the inferior and superior articulating process of adjacent vertebrae, creating a channel for the spinal nerve roots; and in the cervical vertebrae, the *transverse foramen* for the vertebral artery.

REPRESENTATIVE CERVICAL AND LUMBAR VERTEBRAE

C4–5 Coronal and Lateral Views

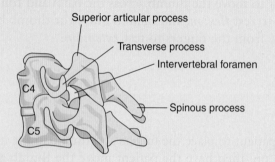

T12–L1 Coronal and Lateral Views

The proximity of the spinal cord and spinal nerve roots to their bony vertebral casing and the intervertebral discs makes them especially vulnerable to disc herniation, impingement from degenerative changes in the vertebrae, and trauma.

Joints

The spine has slightly movable cartilaginous joints between the vertebral bodies and between the articular facets. Between the vertebral bodies are the *intervertebral discs,* each consisting of a soft mucoid central core, the *nucleus pulposus,* rimmed by the tough fibrous tissue of the *annulus fibrosis.* The intervertebral discs cushion movement between vertebrae and allow the vertebral column to curve, flex, and bend. The flexibility of the spine is largely determined by the angle of the articular facet joints relative to the plane of the vertebral body, and varies at different levels of the spine. Note that the vertebral column angles sharply posterior at the *lumbosacral junction* and becomes immovable. The mechanical stress at this angulation contributes to the risk for disc herniation and subluxation, or slippage, of L5 on S1.

Muscle Groups

The *trapezius* and *latissimus dorsi* form the large outer layer of muscles attaching to each side of the spine. They overlie two deeper muscle layers—a layer attaching to the head, neck, and spinous processes (*splenius capitis, splenius cervicis,* and *sacrospinalis*) and a layer of smaller intrinsic muscles between vertebrae. Muscles attaching to the anterior surface of the vertebrae, including the *psoas* muscle and muscles of the abdominal wall, assist with flexion.

Muscles moving the neck and lower vertebral column are summarized in the table on p. 613.

Techniques of Examination

Inspection. Begin by observing the patient's posture, including the position of both the neck and trunk, when entering the room.

Trapezius (neck extension; overlies small intrinsic neck muscles of neck extension and rotation)

Sternocleidomastoid (neck flexion, rotation)

Splenius capitis (neck extension)

Deltoid

Teres minor

Teres major

Spinous process T12

Latissimus dorsi

External abdominal oblique

Iliac crest

Gluteus maximus

Assess the patient for erect position of the head, smooth, coordinated neck movement, and ease of gait.

Neck stiffness signals arthritis, muscle strain, or other underlying pathology that should be pursued.

Drape or gown the patient to expose the entire back for complete inspection. If possible, the patient should be upright in the natural standing position—with feet together and arms hanging at the sides. The head should be midline in the same plane as the sacrum, and the shoulders and pelvis should be level.

Viewing the patient from behind, identify the following landmarks:

● Spinous processes, usually more prominent at C7 and T1 and more evident on forward flexion

● Paravertebral muscles on either side of the midline

● Iliac crests

● Posterior superior iliac spines, usually marked by skin dimples.

A line drawn above the posterior iliac crests crosses the spinous process of L4.

Inspect the patient from the side and from behind. Evaluate the spinal curvatures and the features described in the table on the next page.

Lateral deviation and rotation of the head suggest *torticollis*, from contraction of the sternocleidomastoid muscle.

Spinous process of L4

Posterior superior iliac spine

Sacroiliac joint

Ischial tuberosity and site of ischial bursa

Paravertebral muscles

Iliac crest

Sciatic nerve

Palpation. From a sitting or standing position, palpate the *spinous processes* of each vertebra with your thumb.

In the neck, also palpate the *facet joints* that lie between the cervical vertebrae about 1 inch lateral to the spinous processes of C2–C7. These joints lie deep to the trapezius muscle and may not be palpable unless the neck muscles are relaxed.

In the lower lumbar area, check carefully for any vertebral "step-offs" to determine whether one spinous process seems unusually prominent (or recessed) in relation to the one above it. Identify any tenderness.

Palpate over the *sacroiliac joint,* often identified by the dimple overlying the posterior superior iliac spine.

You may wish to percuss the spine for tenderness by thumping, but not too roughly, with the ulnar surface of your fist.

Tenderness suggests fracture or dislocation if preceded by trauma, underlying infection, or arthritis.

Tenderness in arthritis, especially at the facet joints between C5 and C6

Step-offs in *spondylolisthesis,* or forward slippage of one vertebra, which may compress the spinal cord. Vertebral tenderness is suspicious for fracture or infection.

Tenderness over the sacroiliac joint in sacroiliitis. *Ankylosing spondylitis* may produce sacroiliac tenderness.[40]

Pain on percussion may arise from *osteoporosis, infection,* or *malignancy.*

● Inspection of the Spine

View of Patient	Focus of Inspection

From the side — Cervical, thoracic, and lumbar curves.

Cervical concavity

Thoracic convexity

Lumbar concavity

Increased *thoracic kyphosis* occurs with aging. In children a correctable structural deformity should be pursued.

From behind — Upright spinal column (an imaginary line should fall from C7 through the gluteal cleft)

Alignment of the shoulders, the iliac crests, and the skin creases below the buttocks (gluteal folds)

In *scoliosis,* there is lateral and rotatory curvature of the spine to bring the head back to midline. Scoliosis often becomes evident during adolescence, before symptoms appear.

Unequal shoulder heights seen in: scoliosis; Sprengel's deformity of the scapula (from the attachment of an extra bone or band between the upper scapula and C7); in "winging" of the scapula (from loss of innervation of the serratus anterior muscle by the long thoracic nerve); and in contralateral weakness of the trapezius.

Unequal heights of the iliac crests, or *pelvic tilt,* suggest unequal lengths of the legs and disappear when a block is placed under the short leg and foot. Scoliosis and hip abduction or adduction may also cause a pelvic tilt. "Listing" of the trunk to one side is seen with a herniated lumbar disc.

Skin markings, tags, or masses

Birthmarks, port-wine stains, hairy patches, and lipomas often overlie bony defects such as *spina bifida.*

Café-au-lait spots (discolored patches of skin), skin tags, and fibrous tumors in *neurofibromatosis*

Inspect and palpate the *paravertebral muscles* for tenderness and spasm. Muscles in spasm feel firm and knotted and may be visible.

Spasm occurs in degenerative and inflammatory processes of muscles, prolonged contraction from abnormal posture, or anxiety.

With the hip flexed and the patient lying on the opposite side, palpate the *sciatic nerve*, the largest nerve in the body, consisting of nerve roots from L4, L5, S1, S2, and S3. The nerve lies midway between the greater trochanter and the ischial tuberosity as it leaves the pelvis through the sciatic notch.

Sciatic nerve tenderness suggests a herniated disc or mass lesion impinging on the contributing nerve roots.

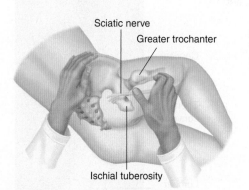

Sciatic nerve
Greater trochanter
Ischial tuberosity

Palpate for tenderness in any other areas that are suggested by the patient's symptoms. Recall that low back pain warrants careful assessment for cord compression, the most serious cause of pain, because of risk for paralysis of the affected limb.

Herniated intervertebral discs, most common at L5–S1 or L4–L5, may produce tenderness of the spinous processes, the intervertebral joints, the paravertebral muscles, the sacrosciatic notch, and the sciatic nerve.

Rheumatoid arthritis may also cause tenderness of the intervertebral joints.

Remember that tenderness in the costovertebral angles may signify kidney infection rather than a musculoskeletal problem.

See Table 16-1, Low Back Pain (p. 642).

Spinous process of L5 vertebra

Intervertebral joint between L5 and sacrum

Posterior superior iliac spine

Sacroiliac joint

Ischial tuberosity and site of ischial bursa

Paravertebral muscles

Sacroiliac notch

Sciatic nerve

Range of Motion and Maneuvers

Range of Motion: Neck.   The neck is the most mobile portion of the spine, remarkable for its seven fragile vertebrae supporting the 10- to 15-pound head. *Flexion* and *extension* occur primarily between the skull and C1, the atlas; *rotation* at C1–C2; the axis, and *lateral bending* at C2–C7.

Limitations in range of motion can arise from stiffness from arthritis, pain from trauma, or muscle spasm such as *torticollis*.

In the table below, note the specific muscles responsible for each motion and clear, simple instructions that prompt the requested patient response.

Neck Movement	Primary Muscles Affecting Movement	Patient Instructions
Flexion	Sternocleidomastoid, scalene, prevertebral muscles	*"Bring your chin to your chest."*
Extension	Splenius capitus and cervicis, small intrinsic neck muscles	*"Look up at the ceiling."*
Rotation	Sternocleidomastoid, small intrinsic neck muscles	*"Look over one shoulder, and then the other."*
Lateral Bending	Scalenes and small intrinsic neck muscles	*"Bring your ear to your shoulder."*

It is important to assess any complaints or findings of neck, shoulder, or arm pain or numbness for possible cervical cord or nerve root compression. See Table 16-2, Pains in the Neck (p. 643).

Tenderness, loss of sensation, or impaired movement warrants careful neurologic testing of the neck and upper extremities.

Tenderness at C1–C2 in *rheumatoid arthritis* suggests possible risk for subluxation and high cervical cord compression.

Range of Motion: Spinal Column.   Now assess range of motion in the spinal column. In the table below, note the specific muscles responsible for each motion and clear, simple instructions that prompt the requested patient response.

Back Movement	Primary Muscles Affecting Movement	Patient Instructions
Flexion	Psoas major, psoas minor, quadratus lumborum; abdominal muscles attaching to the anterior vertebrae, such as the internal and external obliques and rectus abdominis	*"Bend forward and try to touch your toes."* Note the smoothness and symmetry of movement, the range of motion, and the curve in the lumbar area. As flexion proceeds, the lumbar concavity should flatten out.

Deformity of the thorax on forward bending in *scoliosis*.

To measure flexion of the spine, mark the spine at the lumbosacral junction, then 10 cm above and 5 cm below this point. A 4-cm increase between the two upper marks is normal; the distance between the lower two marks should be unchanged.

10+ cm

5 cm

Normally increased by up to 4 cm

Persistence of lumbar lordosis suggests muscle spasm or *ankylosing spondylitis*.

(continued)

Back Movement	Primary Muscles Affecting Movement	Patient Instructions	
Extension	Deep intrinsic muscles of the back, such as the erector spinae and transversospinalis groups	*"Bend back as far as possible."* Support the patient by placing your hand on the posterior superior iliac spine, with your fingers pointing toward the midline.	Decreased *spinal mobility* in *osteoarthritis,* and *ankylosing spondylitis,*[40,41] among other conditions
Rotation	Abdominal muscles, intrinsic muscles of the back	*"Rotate from side to side."* Stabilize the patient's pelvis by placing one hand on the patient's hip and the other on the opposite shoulder. Then rotate the trunk by pulling the shoulder and then the hip posteriorly. Repeat these maneuvers for the opposite side.	
Lateral Bending	Abdominal muscles, intrinsic muscles of the back	*"Bend to the side from the waist."* Stabilize the patient's pelvis by placing your hand on the patient's hip. Repeat for the opposite side.	

As with the neck, pain or tenderness with these maneuvers, particularly with radiation into the leg, warrants careful neurologic testing of the lower extremities. See Chapter 17, the Nervous System, for the Straight Leg Raise Test, pp. 703–704.

Underlying cord or nerve root compression should be considered. Note that arthritis or infection in the hip, rectum, or pelvis may cause symptoms in the lumbar spine. See Table 16-1, Low Back Pain (p. 642).

THE HIP

Overview

The hip joint is deeply embedded in the pelvis and is notable for its strength, stability, and wide range of motion. The stability of the hip joint, so essential for weight bearing, arises from the deep fit of the head of the femur into the *acetabulum*, its strong fibrous articular capsule, and the powerful muscles crossing the joint and inserting below the femoral head, providing leverage for movement of the femur.

Bony Structures and Joints

The hip joint lies below the middle third of the inguinal ligament but in a deeper plane. It is a ball-and-socket joint—note how the rounded head of the femur articulates with the cuplike cavity of the acetabulum. Because of its overlying muscles and depth, it is not readily palpable. Review the bones of the pelvis—the *acetabulum*, the *ilium*, and the *ischium*—and the connection inferiorly at the *symphysis pubis* and posteriorly with the sacroiliac bone.

On the *anterior surface of the hip*, locate the following bony landmarks:

- The iliac crest at the level of L4

- The iliac tubercle

- The anterior superior iliac spine

- The greater trochanter

- The pubic symphysis

ANTERIOR VIEW

On the *posterior surface of the hip,* locate the following:

● The posterior superior iliac spine

● The greater trochanter

● The ischial tuberosity

● The sacroiliac joint

Note that an imaginary line between the posterior superior iliac spines crosses the joint at S2.

Muscle Groups

Four powerful muscle groups move the hip. Picture these groups as you examine patients, and remember that to move the femur or any bone in a given direction, the proximal and distal muscle insertions must **extend across the joint line.**

The *flexor group* lies anteriorly and flexes the thigh. The primary hip flexor is the *iliopsoas,* extending from above the iliac crest to the lesser trochanter. The *extensor group* lies posteriorly and extends the thigh. The *gluteus maximus* is the primary extensor of the hip. It forms a band crossing from its origin along the medial pelvis to its insertion below the trochanter.

The *adductor group* is medial and swings the thigh toward the body. The muscles in this group arise from the rami of the pubis and ischium and insert on the posteromedial aspect of the femur. The *abductor group* is lateral, extending from the iliac crest to the head of the femur, and moves the thigh away from the body. This group includes the *gluteus medius* and *minimus.* These muscles help stabilize the pelvis during the stance phase of gait.

POSTERIOR VIEW

Flexor Group

Extensor Group

Adductor Group

Abductor Group

Additional Structures

A strong, dense articular capsule, extending from the acetabulum to the femoral neck, encases and strengthens the hip joint, reinforced by three overlying ligaments and lined with synovial membrane. There are three principal bursae at the hip. Anterior to the joint is the *psoas* (also termed *iliopectineal* or *iliopsoas*) *bursa*, overlying the articular capsule and the psoas muscle. Find the bony prominence lateral to the hip joint—the *greater trochanter* of the femur. The large multilocular *trochanteric bursa* lies on its posterior surface. The *ischial* (or *ischiogluteal*) *bursa*—not always present—lies under the *ischeal tuberosity*, on which a person sits. Note its proximity to the sciatic nerve, as shown on p. 621.

Techniques of Examination

Inspection.   Inspection of the hip begins with careful observation of the patient's gait on entering the room. Observe the two phases of gait:

- *Stance*—when the foot is on the ground and bears weight (60% of the walking cycle)

    Most problems appear during the weight-bearing stance phase.

| Heelstrike | Foot flat | Midstance | Push-off |

THE STANCE PHASE OF GAIT

- *Swing*—when the foot moves forward and does not bear weight (40% of the cycle)

Observe the gait for the width of the base, the shift of the pelvis, and flexion of the knee. The width of the base should be 2 to 4 inches from heel to heel. Normal gait has a smooth, continuous rhythm, achieved in part by contraction of the abductors of the weight-bearing limb. Abductor contraction stabilizes the pelvis and helps maintain balance, raising the opposite hip. The knee should be flexed throughout the stance phase, except when the heel strikes the ground to counteract motion at the ankle.

A wide base suggests cerebellar disease or foot problems.

Hip dislocation, arthritis, or abductor weakness can cause the pelvis to drop on the opposite side, producing a waddling gait.

Lack of knee flexion interrupts the smooth pattern of gait.

2"–4"

Observe the lumbar portion of the spine for slight lordosis and, with the patient supine, assess the length of the legs for symmetry. (To measure leg length, see Special Techniques, pp. 637–638).

Inspect the anterior and posterior surfaces of the hip for any areas of muscle atrophy or bruising.

Palpation

Bony Landmarks.   Palpate the surface landmarks of the hip, identified on pp. 617–618. On the *anterior aspect* of the hips, palpate the key structures listed below.

- Identify the *iliac crest* at the upper margin of the pelvis at the level of L4.

- Follow the downward anterior curve and locate the *iliac tubercle,* marking the widest point of the crest, and continue tracking downward to the *anterior–superior iliac spine.*

- Place your thumbs on the anterior superior spines and move your fingers downward from the iliac tubercles to the *greater trochanter* of the femur.

- Then move your thumbs medially and obliquely to the *pubic symphysis,* which lies at the same level as the greater trochanter.

On the *posterior aspect* of the hips, palpate the bony landmarks below.

- Palpate the *posterior–superior iliac spine* directly underneath the visible dimples just above the buttocks.

- Placing your left thumb and index finger over the posterior superior iliac spine, next locate the *greater trochanter* laterally with your fingers at the level of the gluteal fold, and place your thumb medially on the *ischial tuberosity.* The *sacroiliac joint* is not always palpable. Note that an imaginary line along the posterior–superior iliac spines crosses the joint at S2.

Loss of lordosis may reflect *paravertebral spasm;* excess lordosis suggests a *flexion deformity* of the hip.

Changes in leg length are seen in abduction or adduction deformities and scoliosis. Leg shortening and external rotation suggest *hip fracture.*

Inguinal Structures. With the patient supine, ask the patient to place the heel of the leg being examined on the opposite knee. Then palpate along the *inguinal ligament*, which extends from the anterior–superior iliac spine to the pubic tubercle. The femoral nerve, artery, and vein bisect the overlying inguinal ligament; lymph nodes lie medially. The mnemonic **NAVEL** may help you remember the lateral-to-medial sequence of **N**erve—**A**rtery—**V**ein—**E**mpty space—**L**ymph node.

Bursae. If the hip is painful, palpate the *(psoas) bursa*, below the inguinal ligament but on a deeper plane.

Inguinal
ligament

Femoral **nerve**
Femoral **artery**
Femoral **vein**

Bulges along the ligament may suggest an *inguinal hernia* or, on occasion, an *aneurysm*.

Enlarged lymph nodes suggest infection in the lower extremity or pelvis.

Tenderness in the groin area may be from *synovitis* of the hip joint, *bursitis*, or possibly *psoas abscess*.

Trochanteric bursa

Ischiogluteal bursa

TROCHANTERIC BURSA

Focal tenderness over the trochanter in *trochanteric bursitis*. Tenderness over the posterolateral surface of the greater trochanter in localized tendinitis or muscle spasm from referred hip pain

With the patient resting on one side and the hip flexed and internally rotated, palpate the *trochanteric bursa* lying over the greater trochanter. Normally, the *ischiogluteal bursa*, over the ischial tuberosity, is not palpable unless inflamed.

ISCHIOGLUTEAL BURSA

Tenderness in *ischiogluteal bursitis* or "weaver's bottom"—because of the adjacent sciatic nerve, this may mimic sciatica.

Range of Motion and Maneuvers

Range of Motion. Now assess hip range of motion, referring to the table below for specific muscles responsible for each movement and clear, simple instructions that prompt the patient to properly follow your directions.

Hip Movement	Primary Muscles Affecting Movement	Patient Instructions
Flexion	Iliopsoas	*"Bend your knee to your chest and pull it against your abdomen."*
Extension (actually hyperextension)	Gluteus maximus	*"Lie face down, then bend your knee and lift it up."*
		Or *"Lying flat, move your lower leg away from the midline and down over the side of the table."*
Abduction	Gluteus medius and minimus	*"Lying flat, move your lower leg away from the midline."*
Adduction	Adductor brevis, adductor longus, adductor magnus, pectineus, gracilis	*"Lying flat, bend your knee and move your lower leg toward the midline."*
External Rotation	Internal and external obturators, quadratus femoris, superior and inferior gemelli	*"Lying flat, bend your knee and turn your lower leg and foot across the midline."*
Internal Rotation	Gluteus medius and minimus	*"Lying flat, bend your knee and turn your lower leg and foot away from the midline."*

Maneuvers. Often the examiner must assist the patient with movements of the hip, so further detail is provided below for knee flexion, abduction, adduction, and external and internal rotation.

- *Flexion*. With the patient supine, place your hand under the patient's lumbar spine. Ask the patient to bend each knee in turn up to the chest and pull it firmly against the abdomen. Note that the hip can flex further when the knee is flexed. When the back touches your hand, indicating normal flattening of the lumbar lordosis—further flexion must arise from the hip joint itself.

In *flexion deformity of the hip,* as the opposite hip is flexed (with the thigh against the chest), the affected hip does not allow full leg extension, and the affected thigh appears flexed.

HIP FLEXION AND FLATTENING OF LUMBAR LORDOSIS

As the thigh is held against the abdomen, observe the degree of flexion at the hip and knee. Normally the anterior portion of the thigh can almost touch the chest wall. Note whether the opposite thigh remains fully extended, resting on the table.

Flexion deformity may be masked by an increase, rather than flattening, in lumbar lordosis and an anterior pelvic tilt.

- *Extension.* With the patient lying face down, extend the thigh toward you in a posterior direction. Alternatively, carefully position the supine patient near the edge of the table and extend the leg posteriorly.

- *Abduction.* Stabilize the pelvis by pressing down on the opposite anterior superior iliac spine with one hand. With the other hand, grasp the ankle and abduct the extended leg until you feel the iliac spine move. This movement marks the limit of hip abduction.

Restricted abduction is common in hip osteoarthritis.

Alternatively, stand at the foot of the table, grasp both ankles, and spread them maximally, abducting both extended legs at the hips. This method provides easy comparison of two sides when movements are restricted, but it is impractical when range of motion is full.

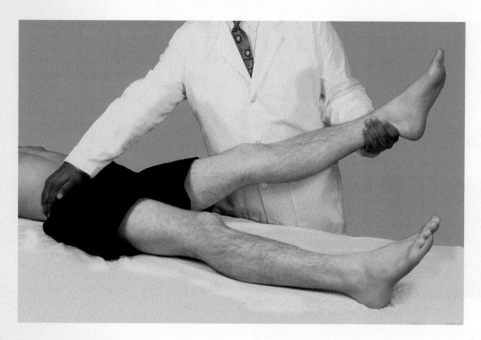

- *Adduction.* With the patient supine, stabilize the pelvis, hold one ankle, and move the leg medially across the body and over the opposite extremity.

- *External and internal rotation.* Flex the leg to 90° at hip and knee, stabilize the thigh with one hand, grasp the ankle with the other, and swing the lower leg—medially for external rotation at the hip and laterally for internal rotation. Although confusing at first, it is the motion of the head of the femur in the acetabulum that identifies these movements.

Restrictions of internal and external rotation are sensitive indicators of hip disease such as arthritis.[42]

THE KNEE

Overview

The knee joint is the largest joint in the body. It is a hinge joint involving three bones: the femur, the tibia, and the patella (or knee cap), with three articular surfaces, two between the femur and the tibia and one between the femur and the patella. Note how the two rounded condyles of the femur rest on the relatively flat tibial plateau. There is no inherent stability in the knee joint itself, making it dependent on ligaments to hold its articulating bones in place. This feature, in addition to the lever action of the femur on the tibia and lack of padding from fat or muscle, makes the knee highly vulnerable to injury.

Bony Structures

Learn the bony landmarks in and around the knee. These will guide your examination of this complicated joint.

- On the *medial surface*, identify the *adductor tubercle*, the *medial epicondyle* of the femur, and the *medial condyle* of the tibia.

- On the *anterior surface,* identify the patella, which rests on the anterior articulating surface of the femur midway between the epicondyles, embedded in the tendon of the quadriceps muscle. This tendon continues below the knee joint as the *patellar tendon,* which inserts distally on the *tibial tuberosity.*

- On the *lateral surface,* find the *lateral epicondyle* of the femur and the *lateral condyle* of the tibia.

ANTERIOR ASPECT OF THE KNEE

Joints

Two condylar *tibiofemoral joints* are formed by the convex curves of the medial and lateral condyles of the femur as they articulate with the concave condyles of the tibia. The third articular surface is the *patellofemoral joint.* The patella slides on the groove of the anterior aspect of the distal femur, called the *trochlear groove,* during flexion and extension of the knee.

Muscle Groups

Powerful muscles move and support the knee. The *quadriceps femoris* extends the leg, covering the anterior, medial, and lateral aspects of the thigh. The *hamstring muscles* lie on the posterior aspect of the thigh and flex the knee.

Quadriceps femoris

Rectus femoris

Vastus lateralis

Vastus medialis

Hamstring muscles

Semimembranosus

Gracilis

Sartorius

Semitendinosus

ANTERIOR VIEW   **MEDIAL VIEW**

Additional Structures

The menisci and two important pairs of ligaments, the collaterals and the cruciates, are crucial to stability of the knee. Identify these structures on the illustrations on p. 625 and below.

- The *medial and lateral menisci* cushion the action of the femur on the tibia. These crescent-shaped fibrocartilaginous discs add a cup-like surface to the otherwise flat tibial plateau.

- The *medial collateral ligament (MCL)*, not easily palpable, is a broad, flat ligament connecting the medial femoral epicondyle to the medial condyle of the tibia. The medial portion of the MCL also attaches to the medial meniscus.

Femur

Semimembranosus bursa (synovial cavity distended)

Medial collateral ligament

Medial meniscus

Fibula

Vastus medialis

Suprapatellar pouch

Prepatella bursa

Patella

Patellar tendon

Tibial tuberosity

Anserine bursa

Tibia

LEFT KNEE—MEDIAL VIEW

● The *lateral collateral ligament (LCL)* connects the lateral femoral epicondyle and the head of the fibula. The MCL and LCL provide medial and lateral stability to the knee joint.

● The *anterior cruciate ligament (ACL)* crosses obliquely from the anterior medial tibia to the lateral femoral condyle, preventing the tibia from sliding forward on the femur.

● The *posterior cruciate ligament (PCL)* crosses from the *posterior* tibia and lateral meniscus to the medial femoral condyle, preventing the tibia from slipping backward on the femur. Because these ligaments lie within the knee joint, they are not palpable. They are nonetheless crucial to the anteroposterior stability of the knee.

Observe the concavities that are usually evident at each side of the patella and also above it. Occupying these areas is the synovial cavity of the knee, the largest joint cavity in the body. This cavity includes an extension 6 centimeters above the upper border of the patella, lying upward and deep to the quadriceps muscle—the *suprapatellar pouch.* The joint cavity covers the anterior, medial, and lateral surfaces of the knee, as well as the condyles of the femur and tibia posteriorly. Although the synovium is not normally detectable, these areas may become swollen and tender when the joint is inflamed.

Several bursae lie near the knee. The *prepatellar bursa* lies between the patella and the overlying skin. The *anserine bursa* lies 1 to 2 inches below the knee joint on the medial surface, proximal and medial to the attachments of the medial hamstring muscles on the proximal tibia. It cannot be palpated due to these overlying tendons. Now identify the large *semimembranosus bursa* that communicates with the joint cavity, also on the posterior and medial surfaces of the knee.

Techniques of Examination

Inspection. Observe the gait for a smooth, rhythmic flow as the patient enters the room. The knee should be extended at heel strike and flexed at all other phases of swing and stance.

Stumbling or pushing the knee into extension with the hand during heel strike suggests *quadriceps weakness.*

Check the alignment and contours of the knees. Observe any atrophy of the quadriceps muscles.

Bowlegs (*genu varum*) and knock-knees (*genu valgum*) are common; flexion contracture (inability to extend fully) in limb paralysis

Look for loss of the normal hollows around the patella, a sign of swelling in the knee joint and suprapatellar pouch; note any other swelling in or around the knee.

Swelling over the patella suggests *prepatellar bursitis.* Swelling over the tibial tubercle suggests *infrapatellar* or, if more medial, *anserine bursitis.*

Palpation. Ask the patient to sit on the edge of the examining table with the knees in flexion. In this position, bony landmarks are more visible, and the muscles, tendons, and ligaments are more relaxed, making them easier to palpate.

Pay special attention to any areas of tenderness. Pain is a common complaint in knee problems, and localizing the structure causing pain is important for accurate evaluation.

The Tibiofemoral Joint.
Palpate the *tibiofemoral joint*. Facing the knee, place your thumbs in the soft tissue depressions on either side of the *patellar tendon*. Identify the groove of the tibiofemoral joint. Note that the patella lies just above this joint line. As you press your thumbs downward, you can feel the edge of the tibial plateau. Follow it medially, then laterally, until you are stopped by the converging femur and tibia. By moving your thumbs upward toward the midline to the top of the patella, you can follow the articulating surface of the femur and identify the margins of the joint.

Note any irregular bony ridges along the joint margins.

Osteoarthritis if tender bony ridges along the joint margins, genu varum deformity, and stiffness 30 minutes or less (likelihood ratios: 11.8, 3.4, and 3.0).[43–46] Crepitus may also be present.

Palpate the *medial meniscus* by pressing on the medial soft-tissue depression along the upper edge of the tibial plateau. It is easier to palpate the medial meniscus if the tibia is slightly internally rotated. Place the knee in slight flexion and palpate the *lateral meniscus* along the lateral joint line.

Meniscus tear with tenderness after trauma more common in medial meniscus.

Assess *the medial and lateral joint compartments* of the tibiofemoral joint with the knee flexed on the examining table to approximately 90°. Pay special attention to any areas of pain or tenderness.

- *Medial compartment.* Medially, move your thumbs upward to palpate the *medial femoral condyle*. The *adductor tubercle* is posterior to the medial femoral condyle. Move your thumbs downward to palpate the *medial tibial plateau*.

Medial femoral condyle

Adductor tubercle

Medial femoral epicondyle

Medial collateral ligament

Anserine bursa

Patellar tendon

Medial tibial plateau

Tibial tuberosity

Also medially, palpate along the joint line and identify the *medial collateral ligament*, which connects the medial epicondyle of the femur to the medial condyle and superior medial surface of the tibia. Palpate along this broad, flat ligament from its origin to insertion.

MCL tenderness after injury suspicious for an MCL tear; LCL injuries less frequent

- *Lateral compartment.* Lateral to the patellar tendon, move your thumbs upward to palpate the *lateral femoral condyle* and downward to palpate the *lateral tibial plateau.* When the knee is flexed, the femoral epicondyles are lateral to the femoral condyles.

  Also on the lateral surface, ask the patient to cross one leg so the ankle rests on the opposite knee and find the *lateral collateral ligament,* a firm cord that runs from the lateral femoral epicondyle to the head of the fibula.

Assess the *patellofemoral compartment.* Now locate the *patella* and trace the *patellar tendon* distally until you palpate the *tibial tuberosity.* Ask the patient to extend the leg to make sure the patellar tendon is intact.

Tenderness over the tendon or inability to extend the leg suggests a partial or complete tear of the patellar tendon.

With the patient supine and the knee extended, compress the patella against the underlying femur. Ask the patient to tighten the quadriceps as the patella moves distally in the trochlear groove. Check for a smooth sliding motion (the *patellofemoral grinding test*).

Pain and crepitus suggest roughening of the patellar undersurface that articulates with the femur. Similar pain may occur with climbing stairs or getting up from a chair.

Pain with compression and with patellar movement during quadriceps contraction suggests *chondromalacia,* or degenerative patella (the *patellofemoral syndrome*).

The Suprapatellar Pouch, Prepatellar Bursa, and Anserine Bursa. Try to palpate any thickening or swelling in the *suprapatellar pouch* and along the margins of the patella. Start 10 centimeters above the superior border of the patella, well above the pouch, and feel the soft tissues between your thumb and fingers. Move your hand distally in progressive steps, trying to identify the pouch. Continue your palpation along the sides of the patella. Note any tenderness or warmth greater than in the surrounding tissues.

Swelling above and adjacent to the patella suggests synovial thickening or effusion in the knee joint.

Thickening, bogginess, or warmth in these areas indicate synovitis or nontender effusions from osteoarthritis.

Check three other bursae for bogginess or swelling. Palpate the *prepatellar bursa,* and over the *anserine bursa* on the posteromedial side of the knee between the medial collateral ligament and the tendons inserting on the medial tibial and plateau. On the posterior surface, with the leg extended, check the medial aspect of the popliteal fossa.

Prepatellar bursitis ("housemaid's knee") from excessive kneeling. *Anserine bursitis* from running, valgus knee deformity, fibromyalgias, osteoarthritis. A *popliteal or "baker's" cyst* from distention of the gastrocnemius semimembranosus bursa

Palpation Tests for Effusion in the Knee Joint. Learn to apply three tests for detecting fluid in the knee joint: the bulge sign, the balloon sign, and balloting the patella.

- The *Bulge Sign (for minor effusions).* With the knee extended, place the left hand above the knee and apply pressure on the suprapatellar pouch, displacing or "milking" fluid downward. Stroke downward on the medial aspect of the knee and apply pressure to force fluid into the lateral area. Tap the knee just behind the lateral margin of the patella with the right hand.

A fluid wave or bulge on the medial side between the patella and the femur is considered a positive bulge sign consistent with an effusion.

Milk downward   Apply medial pressure   Tap and watch for fluid wave

- The *Balloon Sign (for major effusions).* Place the thumb and index finger of your right hand on each side of the patella; with the left hand, compress the suprapatellar pouch against the femur. Feel for fluid entering (or ballooning into) the spaces next to the patella under your right thumb and index finger.

When the knee joint contains a large effusion, suprapatellar compression ejects fluid into the spaces adjacent to the patella. A palpable fluid wave signifies a positive "balloon sign." A returning fluid wave into the suprapatellar pouch confirms an effusion.

● *Ballotting the patella.* To assess large effusions, you can also compress the suprapatellar pouch and "ballotte" or push the patella sharply against the femur. Watch for fluid returning to the suprapatellar pouch.

Palpable fluid returning into the pouch further confirms the presence of a large effusion.

A palpable patellar click with compression may also occur, but yields more false positives.

Gastrocnemius and Soleus Muscles, Achilles Tendon. Palpate the *gastrocnemius* and *soleus muscles* on the posterior surface of the lower leg. Their common tendon, the Achilles, is palpable from about the lower third of the calf to its insertion on the calcaneus.

A defect in the muscles with tenderness and swelling in a *ruptured Achilles tendon;* tenderness and thickening of the tendon above the calcaneus, sometimes with a protuberant posterolateral bony process of the calcaneus in *Achilles tendinitis*

To test the integrity of the *Achilles tendon,* place the patient prone with the knee and ankle flexed at 90°, or alternatively, ask the patient to kneel on a chair. Squeeze the calf and watch for plantar flexion at the ankle.

Absence of plantar flexion is a positive test indicating rupture of the Achilles tendon. Sudden severe pain "like a gunshot wound," an ecchymosis from the calf into the heel, and a flat-footed gait with absence of "toe-off" may also be present.

Range of Motion and Maneuvers

Range of Motion.   Now assess knee range of motion, referring to the table below for specific muscles responsible for each movement and clear, simple instructions that prompt the patient to properly follow your directions.

Knee Movement	Primary Muscles Affecting Movement	Patient Instructions
Flexion	Hamstring group: biceps femoris, semitendinosus, and semimembranosus	*"Bend or flex your knee." Or "Squat down to the floor."*
Extension	Quadriceps: rectus femoris, vastus medialis, lateralis, and intermedius	*"Straighten your leg." Or "After you squat down to the floor, stand up."*
Internal Rotation	Sartorius, gracilis, semitendinosus, semimembranosus	*"While sitting, swing your lower leg toward the midline."*
External Rotation	Biceps femoris	*"While sitting, swing your lower leg away from the midline."*

Crepitus with flexion and extension in osteoarthritis.[44,45]

Maneuvers.   You will often need to test ligamentous stability and integrity of the menisci, particularly when there is a history of trauma or palpable tenderness.[47,48] Always examine both knees and compare findings.

● Maneuvers for Examining the Knee

Structure	Maneuver
Medial meniscus and lateral meniscus	*McMurray Test.* If a click is felt or heard at the joint line during flexion and extension of the knee, or if tenderness is noted along the joint line, further assess the meniscus for a posterior tear. With the patient supine, grasp the heel and flex the knee. Cup your other hand over the knee joint with fingers and thumb along the medial and lateral joint line. From the heel, rotate the lower leg internally and externally. Then push on the lateral side to apply a valgus stress on the medial side of the joint. At the same time, rotate the leg externally and slowly extend it.

(continued)

A click or pop along the medial joint with valgus stress, external rotation, and leg extension suggests a probable *tear of the posterior portion of the medial meniscus.* The tear may displace meniscal tissue, causing "locking" on full knee extension.

A McMurray sign and locking make a medial meniscus tear 8.2 and 3.2 times more likely.[43]

● **Maneuvers for Examining the Knee** (continued)

Structure	Maneuver	
Medial collateral ligament (MCL)	*Abduction (or Valgus) Stress Test.* With the patient supine and the knee slightly flexed, move the thigh about 30° laterally to the side of the table. Place one hand against the lateral knee to stabilize the femur and the other hand around the medial ankle. Push medially against the knee and pull laterally at the ankle to open the knee joint on the medial side (*valgus stress*).	Pain or a gap in the medial joint line points to ligamentous laxity and a partial tear of the *medial collateral ligament*. Most injuries are on the medial side.
Lateral collateral ligament (LCL)	*Adduction (or Varus) Stress Test.* Now, with the thigh and knee in the same position, change your position so you can place one hand against the medial surface of the knee and the other around the lateral ankle. Push medially against the knee and pull laterally at the ankle to open the knee joint on the lateral side (*varus stress*).	Pain or a gap in the lateral joint line points to ligamentous laxity and a partial tear of the *lateral collateral ligament*.
Anterior cruciate ligament (ACL)	*Anterior Drawer Sign.* With the patient supine, hips flexed and knees flexed to 90° and feet flat on the table, cup your hands around the knee with the thumbs on the medial and lateral joint line and the fingers on the medial and lateral insertions of the hamstrings. Draw the tibia forward and observe if it slides forward (like a drawer) from under the femur. Compare the degree of forward movement with that of the opposite knee.	A few degrees of forward movement are normal if equally present on the opposite side. A forward jerk showing the contours of the upper tibia is a *positive anterior drawer sign,* making an ACL tear 11.5 times more likely.[43]
	Lachman Test. Place the knee in 15° of flexion and external rotation. Grasp the distal femur with one hand and the upper tibia with the other. With the thumb of the tibial hand on the joint line, simultaneously move the tibia forward and the femur back. Estimate the degree of forward excursion.	Significant forward excursion indicates an *ACL tear* (likelihood increases by 17.0 if *positive test*).[43]

(continued)

● Maneuvers for Examining the Knee (continued)

Structure	Maneuver
Posterior cruciate ligament (PCL)	*Posterior Drawer Sign.* Position the patient and place your hands in the positions described for the anterior drawer test. Push the tibia posteriorly and observe the degree of backward movement in the femur.

Isolated *PCL tears* are rare.

THE ANKLE AND FOOT

Overview

The total weight of the body is transmitted through the ankle to the foot. The ankle and foot must balance the body and absorb the impact of the heel strike and gait. Despite thick padding along the toes, sole, and heel and stabilizing ligaments at the ankles, the ankle and foot are frequent sites of sprain and bony injury.

Bony Structures and Joints

The ankle is a hinge joint formed by the *tibia,* the *fibula,* and the *talus.* The tibia and fibula act as a mortise, stabilizing the joint while bracing the talus like an inverted cup.

The principal joints of the ankle are the *tibiotalar joint,* between the tibia and the talus, and the *subtalar (talocalcaneal) joint.*

Note the principal landmarks of the ankle: the *medial malleolus,* the bony prominence at the distal end of the tibia, and the *lateral malleolus,* at the distal end of the fibula. Lodged under the talus and jutting posteriorly is the *calcaneus,* or heel.

MEDIAL VIEW

An imaginary line, the *longitudinal arch,* spans the foot, extending from the calcaneus of the hind foot along the tarsal bones of the midfoot (see cuneiforms, navicular, and cuboid bones on the next page) to the forefoot metatarsals and toes. The *heads of the metatarsals* are palpable in the ball of the foot. In the forefoot, identify the *metatarsophalangeal joints,* proximal to the webs of the toes, and the *proximal and distal interphalangeal joints* of the toes.

Muscle Groups and Additional Structures

Movement at the ankle joint is limited to dorsiflexion and plantar flexion. *Plantar flexion* is powered by the gastrocnemius, the posterior tibial muscle, and the toe flexors. Their tendons run behind the malleoli. The *dorsiflexors* include the anterior tibial muscle and the toe extensors. They lie prominently on the anterior surface, or dorsum, of the ankle, anterior to the malleoli.

Ligaments extend from each malleolus onto the foot.

LATERAL VIEW

- Medially, the triangle-shaped *deltoid ligament* fans out from the inferior surface of the medial malleolus to the talus and proximal tarsal bones, protecting against stress from eversion (ankle bows inward).

- Laterally, the three ligaments are less substantial, with higher risk for injury: the *anterior talofibular ligament*—most at risk in injury from inversion (ankle bows outward) injuries; the *calcaneofibular ligament*; and the *posterior talofibular ligament*. The strong Achilles tendon attaches the gastrocnemius and soleus muscles to the posterior calcaneus. The plantar fascia inserts on the medial tubercle of the calcaneus.

Techniques of Examination

Inspection.   Observe all surfaces of the ankles and feet, noting any deformities, nodules, swelling, calluses, or corns.

See Table 16-9, Abnormalities of the Feet (p. 652) and Table 16-10, Abnormalities of the Toes and Soles (p. 653).

Palpation.   With your thumbs, palpate the anterior aspect of each *ankle joint*, noting any bogginess, swelling, or tenderness.

Localized tenderness in arthritis, ligamentous injury, or infection of the ankle

Feel along the *Achilles tendon* for nodules and tenderness.

Rheumatoid nodules; tenderness in Achilles tendinitis, bursitis, or partial tear from trauma

Palpate the heel, especially the posterior and inferior calcaneus, and the plantar fascia for tenderness.

Bone spurs may be present on the calcaneus. Focal heel pain on palpation of the plantar fascia suggests *plantar fasciitis;* seen in prolonged standing or heel-strike exercise, also in *rheumatoid arthritis, gout.*[49,50]

Palpate for tenderness over the medial and lateral malleolus, especially in cases of trauma.

After trauma, inability to bear weight after 4 steps and tenderness over the posterior aspects of either malleolus, especially the medial malleolus, is suspicious for ankle fracture (known as the Ottowa ankle rule).[51]

Palpate the *metatarsophalangeal joints* for tenderness. Compress the forefoot between the thumb and fingers. Exert pressure just proximal to the heads of the 1st and 5th metatarsals.

Tenderness on compression is an early sign of *rheumatoid arthritis.* Acute inflammation of the first metatarsophalangeal joint in *gout.*

Palpate the heads of the five metatarsals and the grooves between them with your thumb and index finger. Place your thumb on the dorsum of the foot and your index finger on the plantar surface.

Pain and tenderness, called *metatarsalgia,* in trauma, arthritis, vascular compromise

Tenderness over the 3rd and 4th metatarsal heads on the plantar surface in *Morton's neuroma* (see p. 652).

Range of Motion and Maneuvers

Range of Motion.   Assess flexion and extension at the tibiotalar (ankle) joint. In the foot, assess inversion and eversion at the subtalar and transverse tarsal joints.

Ankle and Foot Movement	Primary Muscles Affecting Movement	Patient Instructions
Ankle Flexion (plantar flexion)	Gastrocnemius, soleus, plantaris, tibialis posterior	*"Point your foot toward the floor."*
Ankle Extension (dorsiflexion)	Tibialis anterior, extensor digitorum longus, and extensor hallucis longus	*"Point your foot toward the ceiling."*
Inversion	Tibialis posterior and anterior	*"Bend your heel inward."*
Eversion	Peroneus longus and brevis	*"Bend your heel outward."*

Maneuvers

- *The Ankle (Tibiotalar) Joint.* Dorsiflex and plantar flex the foot at the ankle.

- *The Subtalar (Talocalcaneal) Joint.* Stabilize the ankle with one hand, grasp the heel with the other, and invert and evert the foot.

Pain during movements of the ankle and the foot helps to localize possible arthritis.

An arthritic joint is frequently painful when moved in any direction, whereas a ligamentous sprain produces maximal pain when the ligament is stretched. For example, in a common form of sprained ankle, inversion and plantar flexion of the foot cause pain, whereas eversion and plantar flexion are relatively pain free.

INVERSION

EVERSION

- *The Transverse Tarsal Joint.* Stabilize the heel and invert and evert the forefoot.

- *The Metatarsophalangeal Joints.* Flex the toes in relation to the feet.

INVERSION

EVERSION

SPECIAL TECHNIQUES

Measuring the Length of Legs. If you suspect that the patient's legs are unequal in length, measure them. Get the patient relaxed in the supine position and symmetrically aligned with legs extended. With a tape, measure the distance between the anterior superior iliac spine and the medial malleolus. The tape should cross the knee on its medial side.

Unequal leg length may explain a scoliosis.

Describing Limited Motion of a Joint. Although measurement of motion is seldom necessary, limitations can be described in degrees. Pocket goniometers are available for this purpose. In the two examples shown below, the red lines indicate the range of the patient's movement, and the black lines suggest the normal range.

Observations may be described in several ways. The numbers in parentheses are suitably abbreviated recordings.

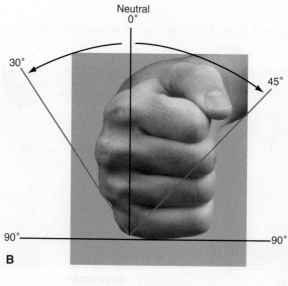

A. The elbow flexes from 45° to 90° (45° → 90°),

    -or-

The elbow has a flexion deformity of 45° and can be flexed farther to 90° (45° → 90°).

B. Supination at elbow = 30° (0° → 30°)

Pronation at elbow = 45° (0° → 45°)

RECORDING YOUR FINDINGS

The examples below contain phrases appropriate for most write-ups. Note that use of the anatomical terms specific to the structure and function of individual joint problems makes your write-up of musculoskeletal findings more meaningful and informative.

Recording the Examination—The Musculoskeletal System

"Full range of motion in all joints. No evidence of swelling or deformity."

OR

"Full range of motion in all joints. Hand with degenerative changes of Heberden's nodes at the distal interphalangeal joints, Bouchard's nodes at proximal interphalangeal joints. Mild pain with flexion, extension, and rotation of both hips. Full range of motion in the knees, with moderate crepitus; no effusion but boggy synovium and osteophytes along the tibiofemoral joint line bilaterally. Both feet with hallux valgus at the first metatarsophalangeal joints."

Suggests osteoarthritis

OR

"Right knee with moderate effusion and tenderness over medial meniscus along the joint line. Moderate laxity of anterior cruciate ligament (ACL) on anterior drawer test; posterior cruciate ligament (PCL) and medial and lateral collateral ligaments (MCL, LCL) intact—no posterior drawer sign or tenderness with varus or valgus stress. Patellar tendon intact—patient able to extend lower extremity. All other joints with good range of motion, no other deformity or swelling."

Suggests partial tear of medial meniscus and ACL, possibly from sports injury or trauma

BIBLIOGRAPHY

CITATIONS

1. Atlas SJ, Deyo RA. Evaluating and managing acute low back pain in the primary care setting. J Gen Intern Med 16(2): 129–131, 2001.
2. Cush JJ, Lipsky PE. Approach to articular and musculoskeletal disorders. In: Kasper DL, Braunwald E, Fauci AS, et al., eds. Harrison's Principles of Internal Medicine, 16th ed. New York: McGraw-Hill, 2005:2029–2036.
3. Deyo RA, Weinstein JN. Low back pain. N Engl J Med 344(5):363–370, 2001.
4. Deyo RA. Diagnostic evaluation of LBP: reaching a specific diagnosis is often impossible. Arch Intern Med 162(13): 1444–1447, 2002.
5. Lurie JD, Gerber PD, Sox HC. A pain in the back. N Engl J Med 343(10):723–726, 2000.
6. Hoffman JR, Mower WR, Wolfson AB, et al. Validity of a set of clinical criteria to rule out injury to the cervical spine in patients with blunt trauma. N Engl J Med 343(2):94–99, 2000.
7. Devereaux MW. Neck and low back pain. Med Clin North Am 87(3):643–662, 2003.
8. Carette S, Fehlings MG. Cervical radiculopathy. N Engl J Med 353(4):392–399, 2005.
9. Margaretten ME, Kohlwes J, Moore D, et al. Does this adult patient have septic arthritis? JAMA 297(13):1478–1488, 2007.
10. Terkeltaub RA. Gout. N Engl J Med 249(17):1647–1655, 2003.
11. Sakane T, Takleno M, Suzuke N, et al. Bechet's disease. N Engl J Med 341(17):1284–1291, 1999.
12. U.S. Preventive Services Task Force. Behavioral counseling in primary care to promote physical activity: recommendations and rationale. Rockville, MD: Agency for Healthcare Research

and Quality, July 2002. Available at: http://www.ahrq.gov/clinic/3rduspstf/physactivity/physactrr.htm. Accessed December 10, 2007.

13. U.S. Preventive Services Task Force. Counseling to prevent low back pain. In: Guide to Clinical Preventive Services, 2nd ed. Baltimore: Williams & Wilkins, 1996:600–709.

14. U.S. Preventive Services Task Force. Primary care interventions to prevent low back pain in adults: recommendation statement. Rockville MD: Agency for Healthcare Research and Quality, February 2004. Available at: http://www.ahrq.gov/clinic/uspstf/uspsback.htm. Accessed December 10, 2007.

15. Caragee EJ. Persistent low back pain. N Engl J Med 352(18):1891–1898, 2005.

16. Staal JB, Hlobil H, Twoisk JWR, et al. Graded activity for low back pain in occupational health care. Ann Intern Med 140(2):77–84, 2004.

17. U.S. Preventive Services Task Force. Counseling to prevent household and recreational injuries. In: Guide to Clinical Preventive Services, 2nd ed. Baltimore: Williams & Wilkins, 1996:659–686.

18. National Institutes of Health Osteoporosis and Related Bone Disease National Resource Center. Osteoporosis overview: facts and figures. Available at: http://www.niams.nih.gov/Health_Info/Bone/Osteoporosis/default.asp. Accessed December 9, 2007.

19. NIH Consensus Development Panel on Osteoporosis Prevention, Diagnosis, and Therapy. Osteoporosis prevention, diagnosis, and therapy. JAMA 285(6):785–795, 2001.

20. Green CJ. Postmenopausal osteoporosis. N Engl J Med 353(6):595–603, 2005.

21. Kuehn BM. Evidence-based guidelines needed for osteoporosis screening and treatment. JAMA 294(1):34, 2005.

22. U.S. Preventive Services Task Force. Screening for osteoporosis in postmenopausal women: recommendations and rationale. Rockville, MD: Agency for Healthcare Research and Quality, September 2002. Available at: http://www.ahrq.gov/clinic/3rduspstf/osteoporosis/osteorr.htm. Accessed December 10, 2007.

23. Raisz LG. Screening for osteoporosis. N Engl J Med 353(2):164–171, 2005.

24. Margolis KL, Ensrud KE, Schreiner PJ, et al. Body size and risk for clinical fractures in older women. Ann Intern Med 133(2):123–127, 2000.

25. Rosen CJ. Postmenopausal osteoporosis. N Engl J Med 353(6):595–603, 2005.

26. Hulley S, Grady D, Bush T, et al. Randomized trial of estrogen plus progestin for secondary prevention of coronary heart disease in postmenopausal women. Heart and Estrogen/Progestin Replacement Study (HERS) Research Group. JAMA 280(7): 605–613, 1998.

27. Writing Group for the Women's Health Initiative Investigators. Risks and benefits of estrogen plus progestin in healthy postmenopausal women: principal results from the Women's Health Initiative randomized controlled trial. JAMA 288: 321–333, 2002.

28. Women's Health Initiative Steering Committee. Effects of conjugated equine estrogen in postmenopausal women with hysterectomy: the Women's Health Initiative randomized controlled trial. JAMA 291:1701–1712, 2004.

29. U.S. Preventive Services Task Force. Hormone replacement therapy for primary prevention of chronic conditions: recommendations and rationale. Rockville MD: Agency for Healthcare Research and Quality, May 2005. Available at: http://www.ahrq.gov/clinic/uspstf05/ht/htpostmenrs.htm. Accessed December 10, 2007.

30. Arnett FC, Edworthy SM, Bloch DA, et al. The American Rheumatism Association 1987 revised criteria for the classification of rheumatoid arthritis. Arthritis Rheum 31:315–324, 1988.

31. Goldring SR. A 55-year-old woman with rheumatoid arthritis. JAMA 283(4):524–529, 2000.

32. Lee DM, Weinblatt ME. Rheumatoid arthritis. Lancet 358:903–911, 2001.

33. Woodward TW, Best TM. The painful shoulder. Part II. Acute and chronic disorders. Am Fam Phys 61(11):3291–3300, 2000.

34. Liume JJ, Verhagen AP, Meidema HS, et al. Does this patient have an instability of the shoulder or a labrum lesion? The rational clinical examination. JAMA 292:1989–1999, 2004.

35. McGee S. Examination of the musculoskeletal system: the shoulder. In: Evidence-based Physical Diagnosis, 2nd ed. St. Louis: Saunders, 2007:628–638.

36. Murrell GA. Diagnosis of rotator cuff tears. Lancet 357: 769–770, 2001.

37. D'Arcy CA, McGee S. Does this patient have carpal tunnel syndrome? The rational clinical examination. JAMA 283(23): 3110–3117, 2000.

38. Griffin LY, ed. Hand and wrist. In: Essentials of Musculoskeletal Care 3. Rosemont, IL: American Academy of Orthopedic Surgeons, 2005:297–299, 321–327.

39. Katz JN, Simmons BP. Carpal tunnel syndrome. N Engl J Med 346(23):1807–1811, 2002.

40. Haywood KL, Garratt AM, Jordan K, et al. Spinal mobility in ankylosing spondylitis: reliability, validity and responsiveness. Rheumatology 43(6):750–757, 2004.

41. Laine C, Goldmann D, eds. In the clinic: osteoarthritis. Ann Intern Med 147(3):ITC8-1–ITC8-16, 2007.

42. Steultjens MPM, Dekker J, van Baar ME, et al. Range of joint motion and disability in patients with osteoarthritis of the knee or hip. Rheumatology 39(9):955–961, 2000.

43. McGee S. Examination of the musculoskeletal system: the knee. In: Evidence-based Physical Diagnosis, 2nd ed. St. Louis: Saunders, 2007:638–652.

44. Altman R, Asch E, Bloch D, et al. Development of criteria for the classification and reporting of osteoarthritis: classification of osteoarthritis of the knee. Arthritis Rheum 29(8): 1039–1049, 1986.

45. Cibere J, Bellamy N, Thorne A, et al. Reliability of the knee examination in osteoarthritis. Arthritis Rheum 50(2): 458–468, 2004.

46. Felson DT. Osteoarthritis of the knee. N Engl J Med 354(8):841–848, 2006.

47. Solomon DH, Simel DL, Bates DW, et al. Does this patient have a torn meniscus or ligament of the knee? Value of the physical examination. The rational physical examination. JAMA 286(13):1610–1620, 2001.

48. Jackson JL, O'Malley PG, Kroenke K. Evaluation of acute knee pain in primary care. Ann Intern Med 139(7):575–588, 2003.

49. Young CC, Rutherford DS, Niedfeldt MW. Treatment of plantar fasciitis. Am Fam Phys 63:467–474, 477–478, 2001.

50. Buchbinder R. Plantar fasciitis. N Engl J Med 350(21): 2159–2166, 2004.

51. Stiell IG, Greenberg GH, McKnight RD, et al. Decision rules for the use of radiography in acute ankle injuries: refinement and prospective validation. JAMA 269(9):1127–1132, 1993.

52. Chou R, Qaseem A, Sonow V, et al. Diagnosis and treatment of low back pain: a joint clinical practice guideline from the American College of Physicians and the American Pain Society. Ann Intern Med 147(7):478–491, 2007.

53. McGee S. Disorders of the nerve roots, plexi, and peripheral nerves. In: Evidence-based Physical Diagnosis, 2nd ed. St. Louis: Saunders, 2007:777–788.

54. Kyle RA, Rajkumar SV. Multiple myeloma. N Engl J Med 351(18):1860–1873, 2004.

55. Davis BT, Pasternak MS. Case 19-2007: a 19-year-old college student with fever and joint pain. N Engl J Med 356(25): 2631–2637, 2007.

56. Goldenberg DL, Burckhardt C, Crofford L. Management of fibromyalgia syndrome. JAMA 292(19):2388–2395, 2004.

57. Levanthal LJ. Management of bromyalgia. Ann Intern Med 131(11):850–858, 1999.

58. Wolfe F, Smythe HA, Yunus MB, et al. The American College of Rheumatology 1990 criteria for the classification of fibromyalgia. Report of the Multicenter Criteria Committee. Arthritis Rheum 33(2):160–172, 1990.

59. Griffin LY, ed. Shoulder. In: Essentials of Musculoskeletal Care 3. Rosemont, IL: American Academy of Orthopedic Surgeons, 2005:155, 214–221.

ADDITIONAL REFERENCES

Chou R, Huffman AH. Nonpharmacologic therapies for acute and chronic low back pain: a review of the evidence for an American Pain Society/American College of Physicians Clinical Practice Guideline. Ann Intern Med 147(7):492–504, 2007.

Clegg DO, Reda DJ, Harria CL. Glucosamine, chondroitin sulfate, and the two in combination for painful knee osteoarthritis. N Engl J Med 354(8):795–808, 2006.

Darouiche RO. Spinal epidural abscess. N Engl J Med 355(19): 2012–2020, 2006.

Firestein GS, Kelley WN. Kelley's Textbook of Rheumatology, 8th ed. Philadelphia: Saunders–Elsevier, 2008.

Fransen M, Nairn L, Winstanley J, et al. Physical activity for osteoarthritis management: a randomized controlled clinical trial evaluating hydrotherapy or Tai Chi classes. Arthritis Rheum 57(3):407–414, 2007.

Griffin LY, ed. Essentials of Musculoskeletal Care, 3rd ed. Rosemont, IL: American Academy of Orthopedic Surgeons, 2005.

Hoppenfeld S, Hutton R. Physical Examination of the Spine and Extremities. New York: Appleton–Century–Crofts, 1976.

Koopman WJ, Moreland LW. Arthritis and Allied Conditions: A Textbook of Rheumatology, 15th ed. Philadelphia: Lippincott Williams & Wilkins, 2005.

Lane NE. Osteoarthritis of the hip. N Engl J Med 357(14): 1413–1421, 2007.

Lew DP, Waldvogel FA. Osteomyelitis. Lancet 364(9431): 369–379, 2004.

Matsen FA. Rotator-cuff failure. N Engl J Med 358(20): 2138–2147, 2008.

Murrell GAC, Walton JR. Diagnosis of rotator cuff tears. Lancet 357(9258):769–770, 2001.

O'Dell JR. Therapeutic strategies for rheumatoid arthritis. N Engl J Med 350(25):2591–2602, 2004.

Peul WC, van Houwelingen HC, van den Hout WB, et al. Surgery versus prolonged conservative treatment for sciatica. N Engl J Med 356(22):2245–2256, 2007.

Porcheret M, Jordan K, Croft P. Treatment of knee pain in older adults in primary care: development of an evidence-based model of care. Rheumatology 46(4):638–648, 2007.

Scholten RJ, Deville W, Opstelten W, et al. The accuracy of physical diagnostic tests for assessing meniscal lesions of the knee: a meta-analysis. J Fam Pract 50(11):938–944, 2001.

Walton J, Mahajan S, Paxinos A, et al. Diagnostic values of tests for acromioclavicular joint pain. J Bone Joint Surg 86(4):807–812, 2004.

> **The Bates' suite offers these additional resources to enhance learning and facilitate understanding of this chapter:**

- Bates' Pocket Guide to Physical Examination and History Taking, 6th edition
- Bates' Nursing Online
- Bates' Visual Guide to Physical Examination, 4th edition
- thePoint online resources, http://thepoint.lww.com
- Student CD-ROM included with the book

TABLE
16-1

Low Back Pain[52]

Patterns	Possible Causes	Physical Signs
Mechanical Low Back Pain Aching pain in the lumbosacral area; may radiate into lower leg, especially along L5 (lateral leg) or S1 (posterior leg) dermatomes. Refers to anatomic or functional abnormality in absence of neoplastic, infectious, or inflammatory disease.[3] Usually acute (<3 months), idiopathic, benign, and self-limiting; represents 97% of symptomatic low back pain. Commonly work-related and occurring in patients 30 to 50 years. Risk factors include heavy lifting, poor conditioning, obesity.	Often arises from muscle and ligament injuries (~70%) or age-related intervertebral disc or facet disease (~4%).[3] Causes also include herniated disc (~4%), spinal stenosis (~3%), compression fractures (~4%), and spondylolisthesis (2%).	Paraspinal muscle or facet tenderness, pain with back movement, loss of normal lumbar lordosis, but no motor or sensory loss or reflex abnormalities. In osteoporosis, check for thoracic kyphosis, percussion tenderness over a spinous process, or fractures in the thoracic spine or hip.
Sciatica (Radicular Low Back Pain) Shooting pain below the knee, commonly into the lateral leg (L5) or posterior calf (S1); typically accompanies low back pain. Patients report associated paresthesias and weakness. Bending, sneezing, coughing, straining during bowel movements often worsen pain.[1]	Sciatic pain very sensitive, ~95%, and specific, ~88%, for disc herniation. Usually from herniated intervertebral disc with compression or traction of nerve root(s) in people 50 years or older. Involves L5 and S1 roots in ~95% of disc herniations.[3] Root or spinal cord compression from neoplastic conditions in fewer than 1% of cases. Tumor or midline disc herniation in bowel or bladder dysfunction, leg weakness from cauda equina syndrome (S2–4).	Disc herniation most likely if calf wasting, weak ankle dorsiflexion, absent ankle jerk, positive crossed straight-leg raise (pain in affected leg when healthy leg tested); negative straight-leg raise makes diagnosis highly unlikely. Ipsilateral straight-leg raise sensitive, ~65–98%, but not specific, ~10–60%.[53]
Lumbar Spinal Stenosis "Pseudoclaudication" pain in the back or legs with walking that improves with rest, lumbar flexion (which decompresses spinal cord), or both. Pain vague but usually bilateral, with paresthesias in one or both legs.	Arises from hypertrophic degenerative disease of one or more vertebral, facets and thickening of the ligamentum flavum causing, narrowing of the spinal canal centrally or in lateral recesses. More common after age 60 years.	Posture may be flexed forward, with lower extremity weakness and hyporeflexia. Straight-leg raise usually negative.
Chronic Back Stiffness	*Ankylosing spondylitis*, an inflammatory polyarthritis, most common in men younger than 40 years.[40] *Diffuse idiopathic hyperostosis (DISH);* affects men > women, usually 50 years or older	Loss of the normal lumbar lordosis, muscle spasm, limited anterior and lateral flexion. Improves with exercise. Lateral immobility of the spine, especially in thoracic area.
Nocturnal Back Pain, Unrelieved by Rest	Consider *metastatic malignancy* to the spine from cancer of the prostate, breast, lung, thyroid, and kidney, and multiple myeloma.[54]	Variable with the source. Local vertebral tenderness may be present.
Pain Referred from the Abdomen or Pelvis Usually a deep, aching pain; the level varies with the source. Accounts for approximately 1% of low back pain.	Peptic ulcer, pancreatitis, pancreatic cancer, chronic prostatitis, endometriosis, dissecting aortic aneurysm, retroperitoneal tumor, and other causes.	Spinal movements are not painful and range of motion is not affected. Look for signs of the primary disorder.

TABLE

16-2

Pains in the Neck

Patterns	Possible Causes	Physical Signs
Mechanical Neck Pain Aching pain in the cervical paraspinal muscles and ligaments with associated muscle spasm, with associated stiffness and tightness in the upper back and shoulder, lasting up to 6 weeks. No associated radiation, paresthesias, or weakness. Headache may be present.	Mechanism poorly understood, possibly sustained muscle contraction. Associated with poor posture, stress, poor sleep, poor head position during activities such as computer use, watching television, driving.	Local muscle tenderness, pain on movement. No neurologic deficits. Possible trigger points in *fibromyalgia*. *Torticollis* if prolonged abnormal neck posture and muscle spasm.
Mechanical Neck Pain—Whiplash[7] Also mechanical neck pain with aching paracervical pain and stiffness, often beginning the day after injury. Occipital headache, dizziness, malaise, and fatigue may be present. Chronic whiplash syndrome if symptoms last more than 6 months, present in 20% to 40% of injuries.	Musculoligamental sprain or strain from forced hyperflection–hyperextension injury to the neck, as in rear-end collisions.	Localized paracervical tenderness, decreased neck range of motion, perceived weakness of the upper extremities. Causes of cervical cord compression such as fracture, herniation, head injury, or altered consciousness are excluded.
Cervical Radiculopathy—from nerve root compression[7,8] Sharp burning or tingling pain in the neck and one arm, with associated parathesias and weakness. Sensory symptoms often in myotomal pattern, deep in muscle, rather than dermatomal pattern.	Dysfunction of cervical spinal nerve, nerve roots, or both from foraminal encroachment of the spinal nerve (~75%), herniated cervical disc (~25%). Rarely from tumor, syrinx, multiple sclerosis. Mechanisms may involve hypoxia of the nerve root and dorsal ganglion, release of inflammatory mediators.	C7 nerve root affected most often (45%–60%), with weakness in triceps and finger flexors and extensors. C6 nerve root involvement also common, with weakness in biceps, brachioradialis, wrist extensors.
Cervical Myelopathy—from cervical cord compression[7] Neck pain with bilateral weakness and parathesias in both upper and lower extremities, often with urinary frequency. Hand clumsiness, palmar paresthesias, and gait changes may be subtle. Neck flexion often exacerbates symptoms.	Usually from cervical *spondylosis*, defined as cervical degenerative disc disease from spurs, protrusion of ligamentum flavum, and/or disc herniation (~80%); also from cervical stenosis from osteophytes, ossification of ligamentum flavum. Large central or paracentral disc herniation may also compress cord.	Hyperreflexia; clonus at the wrist, knee, or ankle; extensor plantar reflexes (positive Babinski signs); and gait disturbances. May also see *Lhermitte's sign:* neck flexion with resulting sensation of electrical shock radiating down the spine. Confirmation of cervical myelopathy warrants neck immobilization and neurosurgical evaluation.

Patterns of Pain In and Around the Joints

Problem	Process	Common Locations	Pattern of Spread	Onset	Progression and Duration
Rheumatoid Arthritis[30–32,55]	Chronic inflammation of *synovial membranes* with secondary erosion of adjacent cartilage and bone, and damage to ligaments and tendons	Hands (proximal interphalangeal and metacarpopha-langeal joints), feet (metatarsopha-langeal joints), wrists, knees, elbows, ankles	Symmetrically additive: progresses to other joints while persisting in the initial ones	Usually insidious	Often chronic, with remissions and exacerbations
Osteoarthritis (*degenerative joint disease*)[41]	Degeneration and progressive loss of *cartilage* within the joints, damage to underlying bone, and formation of new bone at the margins of the cartilage	Knees, hips, hands (distal, sometimes proximal inter-phalangeal joints), cervical and lumbar spine, and wrists (first carpometa-carpal joint); also joints previously injured or diseased	Additive; however, only one joint may be involved.	Usually insidious	Slowly progressive, with temporary exacerbations after periods of overuse
Gouty Arthritis[10] *Acute Gout*	An inflammatory reaction to microcrystals of sodium urate	Base of the big toe (the first metatarso-phalangeal joint), the instep or dorsa of feet, the ankles, knees, and elbows	Early attacks usually confined to one joint	Sudden, often at night, often after injury, surgery, fasting, or excessive food or alcohol intake	Occasional isolated attacks lasting days up to 2 weeks; they may get more frequent and severe, with persisting symptoms.
Chronic Tophaceous Gout	Multiple local accumulations of sodium urate in the joints and other tissues (*tophi*), with or without inflammation	Feet, ankles, wrists, fingers, and elbows	Additive, not so symmetric as rheumatoid arthritis	Gradual develop-ment of chronicity with repeated attacks	Chronic symptoms with acute exacerbations
Polymyalgia Rheumatica	A disease of unclear etiology in people >age 50, especially women; may be associated with giant cell arteritis	Muscles of the hip girdle and shoulder girdle; symmetric		Insidious or abrupt, even appearing overnight	Chronic but ultimately self-limiting
Fibromyalgia Syndrome[56–58]	Widespread musculoskeletal pain and tender points. May accompany other diseases. Mechanisms unclear	"All over," but especially in the neck, shoulders, hands, low back, and knees	Shifts unpredict-ably or worsens in response to immobility, excessive use, or chilling	Variable	Chronic, with "ups and downs"

The vagueness of these characteristics is in itself a clue to the fibromyalgia syndrome.

Associated Symptoms

Swelling	Redness, Warmth, and Tenderness	Stiffness	Limitation of Motion	Generalized Symptoms
Frequent swelling of synovial tissue in joints or tendon sheaths; also subcutaneous nodules	Tender, often warm, but seldom red	Prominent, often for an hour or more in the mornings, also after inactivity	Often develops	Weakness, fatigue, weight loss, and low fever are common.
Small effusions in the joints may be present, especially in the knees; also bony enlargement	Possibly tender, seldom warm, and rarely red	Frequent but brief (usually 5–10 min), in the morning and after inactivity	Often develops	Usually absent
Present, within and around the involved joint	Exquisitely tender, hot, and red	Not evident	Motion is limited primarily by pain.	Fever may be present.
Present as tophi in joints, bursae, and subcutaneous tissues	Tenderness, warmth, and redness may be present during exacerbations.	Present	Present	Possibly fever; patient may also develop symptoms of renal failure and renal stones.
None	Muscles often tender, but not warm or red	Prominent, especially in the morning	Usually none	Malaise, a sense of depression, possibly anorexia, weight loss, and fever, but no true weakness
None	Multiple specific and symmetric tender "trigger points," often not recognized until the examination	Present, especially in the morning	Absent, though stiffness is greater at the extremes of movement	A disturbance of sleep, usually associated with morning fatigue

TABLE
16-4

Painful Shoulders[33,45,59]

Rotator Cuff Tendinitis

Repeated shoulder motion, as in throwing or swimming, can cause edema and hemorrhage followed by inflammation, most commonly involving the supraspinatus tendon. Acute, recurrent, or chronic pain may result, often aggravated by activity. Patients report sharp catches of pain, grating, and weakness when lifting the arm overhead. When the supraspinatus tendon is involved, tenderness is maximal just below the tip of the acromion. Patients are typically athletically active.

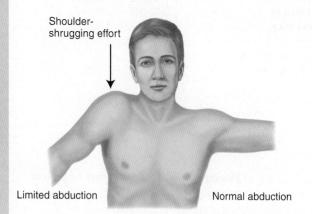

Shoulder-shrugging effort

Limited abduction   Normal abduction

Rotator Cuff Tears

When the arm is raised in forward flexion, the rotator cuff may impinge against the undersurface of the acromion and the coracoacromial ligament. Injury from a fall or repeated impingement may weaken the rotator cuff, causing a partial or complete tear, usually after age 40. Weakness, atrophy of the supraspinatus and infraspinatus muscles, pain, and tenderness may ensue. In a complete tear of the supraspinatus tendon (illustrated), active abduction and forward flexion at the glenohumeral joint are severely impaired, producing a characteristic shrugging of the shoulder and a positive "drop arm" test (see p. 599).

Calcific Tendinitis

Calcific tendinitis is a degenerative process in the tendon associated with the deposition of calcium salts. Usually involves the supraspinatus tendon. Acute, disabling attacks of shoulder pain may occur, usually in patients > age 30, more often in women. The arm is held close to the side, and all motions are severely limited by pain. Tenderness is maximal below the tip of the acromion. The subacromial bursa, which overlies the supraspinatus tendon, may be inflamed. Chronic, less severe pain may also occur.

Bicipital Tendinitis

Inflammation of the long head of the biceps tendon and tendon sheath causes anterior shoulder pain resembling and often coexisting with rotator cuff tendinitis. Both conditions may involve impingement injury. Tenderness is maximal in the bicipital groove. Externally rotate and abduct the arm to separate this area from the subacromial tenderness of supraspinatus tendinitis. With the patient's arm at the side, elbow flexed to 90°, ask the patient to supinate the forearm against your resistance. Increased pain in the bicipital groove confirms this condition.

Adhesive Capsulitis (Frozen Shoulder)

Adhesive capsulitis refers to fibrosis of the glenohumeral joint capsule, manifested by diffuse, dull, aching pain in the shoulder and progressive restriction of active and passive range of motion, but usually no localized tenderness. The condition is usually unilateral and occurs in people aged 50 to 70. There is often an antecedent painful disorder of the shoulder or another condition (such as myocardial infarction) that has decreased shoulder movements. The course is chronic, lasting months to years. The disorder may resolve spontaneously, at least partially.

Acromioclavicular Arthritis

Acromioclavicular arthritis is uncommon, usually arising from direct injury to the shoulder girdle with resulting degenerative changes. Tenderness is localized over the acromioclavicular joint. Glenohumeral joint motion is not painful, but movement of the scapula, as in shoulder shrugging, is painful.

Coracoid process

Acromion

Glenoid fossa

Humerus

Anterior Dislocation of the Humerus[33,34,59]

Shoulder instability from anterior dislocation of the humerus usually results from a fall or forceful throwing motion, then becomes recurrent. The shoulder seems to "slip out of the joint" when the arm is abducted and externally rotated, causing a *positive apprehension sign* for anterior instability when the examiner places the arm in this position. Any shoulder movement may cause pain, and patients hold the arm in a neutral position. The rounded lateral aspect of the shoulder appears flattened. Dislocations may also be inferior, posterior (relatively rare), and multidirectional.

| TABLE 16-5 | **Swollen or Tender Elbows** |

Olecranon bursitis

Olecranon Bursitis

Swelling and inflammation of the olecranon bursa may result from trauma or may be associated with rheumatoid or gouty arthritis. The swelling is superficial to the olecranon process.

Arthritis

Arthritis of the Elbow

Synovial inflammation or fluid is felt best in the grooves between the olecranon process and the epicondyles on either side. Palpate for a boggy, soft, or fluctuant swelling and for tenderness.

Rheumatoid nodules

Rheumatoid Nodules

Subcutaneous nodules may develop at pressure points along the extensor surface of the ulna in patients with rheumatoid arthritis or acute rheumatic fever. They are firm and nontender, and are not attached to the overlying skin. They may or may not be attached to the underlying periosteum. They may develop in the area of the olecranon bursa, but often occur more distally.

Epicondylitis

Epicondylitis

Lateral epicondylitis (tennis elbow) follows repetitive extension of the wrist or pronation–supination of the forearm. Pain and tenderness develop 1 cm distal to the lateral epicondyle and possibly in the extensor muscles close to it. When the patient tries to extend the wrist against resistance, pain increases.

Medial epicondylitis (pitcher's, golfer's, or Little League elbow) follows repetitive wrist flexion, as in throwing. Tenderness is maximal just lateral and distal to the medial epicondyle. Wrist flexion against resistance increases the pain.

TABLE
16-6

Arthritis in the Hands

Acute Rheumatoid Arthritis

Tender, swollen

Tender, painful, stiff joints in *rheumatoid arthritis*, usually with *symmetric* involvement on both sides of the body. The proximal interphalangeal, metacarpophalangeal, and wrist joints are the most frequently affected. Note the fusiform or spindle-shaped swelling of the proximal interphalangeal joints in acute disease.

Chronic Rheumatoid Arthritis

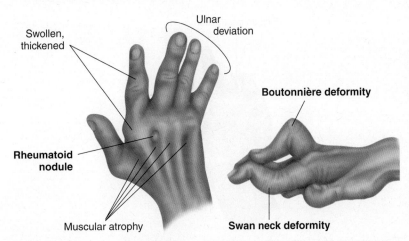

Swollen, thickened

Ulnar deviation

Boutonnière deformity

Rheumatoid nodule

Muscular atrophy

Swan neck deformity

In chronic disease, note the swelling and thickening of the metacarpophalangeal and proximal interphalangeal joints. Range of motion becomes limited, and fingers may deviate toward the ulnar side. The interosseous muscles atrophy. The fingers may show *"swan neck" deformities* (hyperextension of the proximal interphalangeal joints with fixed flexion of the distal interphalangeal joints). Less common is a *boutonnière deformity* (persistent flexion of the proximal interphalangeal joint with hyperextension of the distal interphalangeal joint). Rheumatoid nodules are seen in the acute or the chronic stage.

Osteoarthritis (*Degenerative Joint Disease*)

Radial deviation of distal phalanx

Heberden's node

Bouchard's node

Metacarpophalangeal joints uninvolved

Heberden's nodes on the dorsolateral aspects of the distal interphalangeal joints from bony overgrowth of osteoarthritis. Usually hard and painless, they affect the middle-aged or elderly; often associated with arthritic changes in other joints. Flexion and deviation deformities may develop. *Bouchard's nodes* on the proximal interphalangeal joints are less common. The metacarpophalangeal joints are spared.

Chronic Tophaceous Gout

Swollen

Draining tophus

Knobby swelling

The deformities of long-standing chronic tophaceous gout can mimic rheumatoid arthritis and osteoarthritis. Joint involvement is usually not as symmetric as in rheumatoid arthritis. Acute inflammation may be present. Knobby swellings around the joints ulcerate and discharge white chalklike urates.

TABLE
16-7

Swellings and Deformities of the Hands

Dupuytren's Contracture

Flexion contraction

Cord

The first sign of a *Dupuytren's contracture* is a thickened plaque overlying the flexor tendon of the ring finger and possibly the little finger at the level of the distal palmar crease. Subsequently, the skin in this area puckers, and a thickened fibrotic cord develops between palm and finger. Flexion contracture of the fingers may gradually ensue.

Trigger Finger

Caused by a painless nodule in a flexor tendon in the palm, near the metacarpal head. The nodule is too big to enter easily into the tendon sheath during extension of the fingers from a flexed position. With extra effort or assistance, the finger extends and flexes with a palpable and audible snap as the nodule pops into the tendon sheath. Watch, listen, and palpate the nodule as the patient flexes and extends the fingers.

Thenar Atrophy

Normal hypothenar eminence

Flattened thenar eminence

Thenar atrophy suggests a *median nerve disorder* such as *carpal tunnel syndrome* (see p. 608). Hypothenar atrophy suggests an *ulnar nerve disorder*.

Ganglion

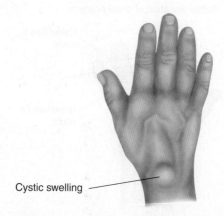

Cystic swelling

Ganglia are cystic, round, usually nontender swellings along tendon sheaths or joint capsules, frequently at the dorsum of the wrist. Flexion of the wrist makes ganglia more prominent; extension tends to obscure them. Ganglia may also develop elsewhere on the hands, wrists, ankles, and feet.

TABLE **16-8**	## Tendon Sheath, Palmar Space, and Finger Infections

Acute Tenosynovitis

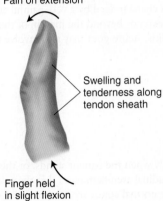

Pain on extension

Swelling and tenderness along tendon sheath

Finger held in slight flexion

Infection of the flexor tendon sheaths, *acute tenosynovitis*, may follow local injury, even when trivial in nature. Unlike arthritis, tenderness and swelling develop not in the joint but along the course of the tendon sheath, from the distal phalanx to the level of the metacarpophalangeal joint. The finger is held in slight flexion; finger extension is very painful.

Acute Tenosynovitis and Thenar Space Involvement

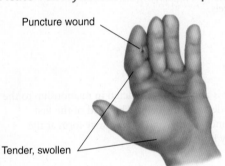

Puncture wound

Tender, swollen

If the infection progresses, it may extend from the tendon sheath into the adjacent fascial spaces within the palm. Infections of the index finger and thenar space are illustrated. Early diagnosis and treatment are important.

Felon

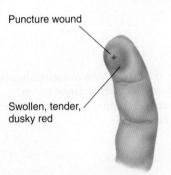

Puncture wound

Swollen, tender, dusky red

Injury to the fingertip may result in infection in the enclosed fascial spaces of the finger pad. Severe pain, localized tenderness, swelling, and dusky redness are characteristic. Early diagnosis and treatment are important.

| TABLE
16-9

Abnormalities of the Feet

Hot, red, tender, swollen

Acute Gouty Arthritis

The metatarsophalangeal joint of the great toe may be the first joint involved in *acute gouty arthritis.* It is characterized by a very painful and tender, hot, dusky red swelling that extends beyond the margin of the joint. It is easily mistaken for a cellulitis. Acute gout may also involve the dorsum of the foot.

Medial border becomes convex

Sole touches floor

Flat Feet

Signs of *flat feet* may be apparent only when the patient stands, or they may become permanent. The longitudinal arch flattens so that the sole approaches or touches the floor. The normal concavity on the medial side of the foot becomes convex. Tenderness may be present from the medial malleolus down along the medial-plantar surface of the foot. Swelling may develop anterior to the malleoli. Inspect the shoes for excess wear on the inner sides of the soles and heels.

Hallux Valgus

In *hallux valgus,* the great toe is abnormally abducted in relationship to the first metatarsal, which itself is deviated medially. The head of the first metatarsal may enlarge on its medial side, and a bursa may form at the pressure point. This bursa may become inflamed.

Morton's
neuroma

Morton's Neuroma

Tenderness over the plantar surface, third and fourth metatarsal heads, from probable entrapment of the medial and lateral plantar nerves. Symptoms include hyperesthesia, numbness, aching, and burning from the metatarsal heads into the third and fourth toes.

TABLE
16-10

Abnormalities of the Toes and Soles

Red, tender

Granulation
tissue

Hyperextended

Flexed

Red, thickened

Ingrown Toenail

The sharp edge of a toenail may dig into and injure the lateral nail fold, resulting in inflammation and infection. A tender, reddened, overhanging nail fold, sometimes with granulation tissue and purulent discharge, results. The great toe is most often affected.

Hammer Toe

Most commonly involving the second toe, a hammer toe is characterized by hyperextension at the metatarso-phalangeal joint with flexion at the proximal interphalangeal joint. A corn frequently develops at the pressure point over the proximal interphalangeal joint.

Corn

A corn is a painful conical thickening of skin that results from recurrent pressure on normally thin skin. The apex of the cone points inward and causes pain. Corns characteristically occur over bony prominences such as the 5th toe. When located in moist areas such as pressure points between the 4th and 5th toes, they are called soft corns.

Callus

Like a corn, a callus is an area of greatly thickened skin that develops in a region of recurrent pressure. Unlike a corn, a callus involves skin that is normally thick, such as the sole, and is usually painless. If a callus is painful, suspect an underlying plantar wart.

Plantar Wart

A plantar wart is a common wart, *verruca vulgaris,* located in the thickened skin of the sole. It may look like a callus or even be covered by one. Look for the characteristic small dark spots that give a stippled appearance to a wart. Normal skin lines stop at the wart's edge.

Neuropathic Ulcer

When pain sensation is diminished or absent, as in diabetic neuropathy, neuropathic ulcers may develop at pressure points on the feet. Although often deep, infected, and indolent, they are painless. Callus formation about the ulcer is diagnostically helpful. Like the ulcer itself, it results from chronic pressure.

The Nervous System

Assessment of the nervous system calls for many complex skills of examination and clinical reasoning. You have already learned the principles and techniques for assessing mental status, a critical component of the nervous system examination. As you saw in Chapter 5, Behavior and Mental Status, often the patient's mental status gives clues about delirium, memory disorders, and other neurologic conditions. As you study this chapter, let three important questions guide your approach to this challenging clinical area:

● Is the mental status intact?

● Are right-sided and left-sided examination findings symmetric?

● If the findings are asymmetric or otherwise abnormal, does the lesion lie in the *central nervous system*, consisting of the brain and spinal cord, or in the *peripheral nervous system*, consisting of the 12 pairs of cranial nerves and the spinal and peripheral nerves?

In this chapter, the section on *Anatomy and Physiology* briefly describes the principal structures and functions of the brain (shown below), spinal cord, cranial and peripheral nerves, and reflexes, with summaries of the important motor and sensory pathways. Following the *Health History* and *Health*

Frontal lobe
Parietal lobe
Occipital lobe
Diencephalon
Pituitary gland
Midbrain
Pons
Medulla
Brainstem
Cerebellum

RIGHT HALF OF THE BRAIN, MEDIAL VIEW

Promotion and Counseling sections, *Techniques of Examination* details how to examine the cranial nerves, the motor and sensory systems, and reflexes. As you will see in *Recording Your Findings,* the mental status examination begins the written record for examination findings.

ANATOMY AND PHYSIOLOGY

CENTRAL NERVOUS SYSTEM

The Brain

The brain has four regions: the cerebrum, the diencephalon, the brainstem, and the cerebellum. The cerebral hemispheres contain the greatest mass of brain tissue. Each hemisphere is subdivided into frontal, parietal, temporal, and occipital lobes, as shown below.

LEFT LATERAL VIEW OF THE BRAIN

The brain is a vast network of interconnecting *neurons* (nerve cells). These consist of cell bodies and their *axons*—single long fibers that conduct impulses to other parts of the nervous system.

Brain tissue may be gray or white. *Gray matter* consists of aggregations of neuronal cell bodies. It rims the surfaces of the cerebral hemispheres, forming the cerebral cortex. *White matter* consists of neuronal axons that are coated with myelin. The myelin sheaths, which create the white color, allow nerve impulses to travel more rapidly.

Deep in the brain lie additional clusters of gray matter. These include the *basal ganglia,* which affect movement, and the thalamus and the hypothalamus, structures in the diencephalon. The *thalamus* processes sensory impulses and relays them to the cerebral cortex. The *hypothalamus* maintains homeostasis and regulates temperature, heart rate, and blood pressure. The hypothalamus affects the endocrine system and governs emotional behaviors such as anger and sexual drive. Hormones secreted in the hypothalamus act directly on the pituitary gland.

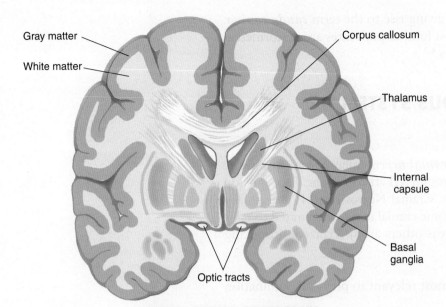

Gray matter

White matter

Corpus callosum

Thalamus

Internal capsule

Basal ganglia

Optic tracts

CORONAL SECTION OF THE BRAIN

In contrast, note the *internal capsule,* a white-matter structure where myelinated fibers converge from all parts of the cerebral cortex and descend into the brainstem. The *brainstem,* which connects the upper part of the brain with the spinal cord, has three sections: the midbrain, the pons, and the medulla.

Consciousness depends on the interaction between intact cerebral hemispheres and an important structure in the diencephalon and upper brainstem, the *reticular activating (arousal) system.*

The *cerebellum,* which lies at the base of the brain, coordinates all movement and helps maintain the body upright in space.

The Spinal Cord

Below the medulla, the central nervous system extends itself as the elongated *spinal cord,* encased within the bony vertebral column and terminating at the first or second lumbar vertebra. The cord provides a series of segmental relays with the periphery, serving as a conduit for information flow to and from the brain. The motor and sensory nerve pathways relay neural signals that enter and exit the cord through posterior and anterior nerve roots through the spinal and peripheral nerves.

The spinal cord is divided into five segments: cervical, from C1 to C8; thoracic, from T1 to T12; lumbar, from L1 to L5; sacral, from S1 to S5; and coccygeal.

Note that the spinal cord is not as long as the vertebral canal. The lumbar and sacral roots travel the longest intraspinal distance and

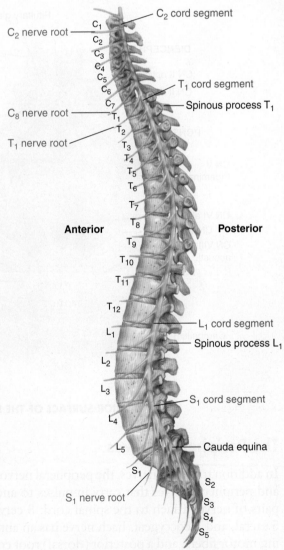

C_2 cord segment

C_1
C_2 nerve root — C_2
C_3
C_4
C_5
C_6
C_7
C_8 nerve root — T_1

T_1 cord segment

Spinous process T_1

T_1 nerve root — T_2
T_3
T_4
T_5
T_6
T_7

Anterior T_8 **Posterior**
T_9
T_{10}
T_{11}
T_{12}
L_1

L_1 cord segment
Spinous process L_1

L_2
L_3

S_1 cord segment

L_4
L_5

Cauda equina

S_1
S_1 nerve root
S_2
S_3
S_4
S_5

THE SPINAL CORD, LATERAL VIEW

fan out like a horse's tail at L1 to L2, giving rise to the term *cauda equina*. To avoid injury to the spinal cord, most lumbar punctures are performed at the L3–4 or L4–5 vertebral interspaces.[1,2]

PERIPHERAL NERVOUS SYSTEM

The Cranial Nerves

Twelve pairs of special nerves called *cranial nerves* emerge from within the skull or *cranium*. Cranial Nerves III through XII arise from the diencephalon and the brainstem, as illustrated below. Cranial Nerves I and II are actually fiber tracts emerging from the brain. Some cranial nerves are limited to general motor or sensory functions, whereas others are specialized, producing smell, vision, or hearing (I, II, VIII).

Functions of the cranial nerves (CN) most relevant to physical examination are summarized on the next page.

Pituitary gland

DIENCEPHALON

CN II optic nerve
CN II optic tract

CN I olfactory

MIDBRAIN

CN III oculomotor

CN IV trochlear

PONS

CN V trigeminal

CN VI abducens
CN VII facial
CN VIII acoustic

MEDULLA

CN IX glossopharyngeal

CN X vagus

CN XI spinal accessory

CN XII hypoglossal

Cerebellum

S. Shapley Bowman

INFERIOR SURFACE OF THE BRAIN

The Peripheral Nerves

In addition to cranial nerves, the peripheral nervous system also includes spinal and peripheral nerves that carry impulses to and from the cord. Thirty-one pairs of nerves attach to the spinal cord: 8 cervical, 12 thoracic, 5 lumbar, 5 sacral, and 1 coccygeal. Each nerve has an anterior (ventral) root containing motor fibers, and a posterior (dorsal) root containing sensory fibers. The anterior and posterior roots merge to form a short *spinal nerve*, less than 5 mm

● Cranial Nerves

No.	Name	Function
I	**Olfactory**	Sense of smell
II	**Optic**	Vision
III	**Oculomotor**	Pupillary constriction, opening the eye (lid elevation), and most extraocular movements
IV	**Trochlear**	Downward, internal rotation of the eye
V	**Trigeminal**	*Motor*—temporal and masseter muscles (jaw clenching), lateral pterygoids (lateral jaw movement) *Sensory*—facial. The nerve has three divisions: (1) ophthalmic, (2) maxillary, and (3) mandibular.
VI	**Abducens**	Lateral deviation of the eye

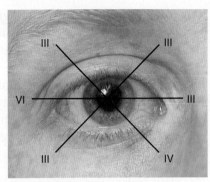

RIGHT EYE (CN III, IV, VI)

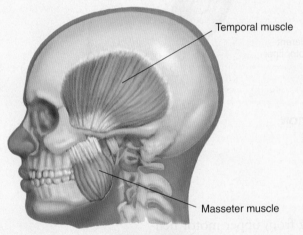

Temporal muscle

Masseter muscle

CN V—MOTOR

(1)

(2)

(3)

C2

CN V—SENSORY

VII	**Facial**	*Motor*—facial movements, including those of facial expression, closing the eye, and closing the mouth *Sensory*—taste for salty, sweet, sour, and bitter substances on the anterior two thirds of the tongue
VIII	**Acoustic**	Hearing (cochlear division) and balance (vestibular division)
IX	**Glossopharyngeal**	*Motor*—pharynx *Sensory*—posterior portions of the eardrum and ear canal, the pharynx, and the posterior tongue, including taste (salty, sweet, sour, bitter)
X	**Vagus**	*Motor*—palate, pharynx, and larynx *Sensory*—pharynx and larynx
XI	**Spinal accessory**	*Motor*—the sternomastoid and upper portion of the trapezius
XII	**Hypoglossal**	*Motor*—tongue

Sternomastoid muscle

Trapezius muscle

CN XI—MOTOR

long. Spinal nerve fibers commingle with similar fibers from other levels in plexuses outside the cord, from which *peripheral nerves emerge*. Most peripheral nerves contain both *sensory* (afferent) and *motor* (efferent) fibers.

Like the brain, the spinal cord contains both gray matter and white matter. Nuclei of gray matter, which are aggregations of nerve cell bodies, are surrounded by white tracts of nerve fibers connecting the brain to the peripheral nervous system. Note the butterfly appearance of the gray-matter nuclei, with anterior and posterior horns.

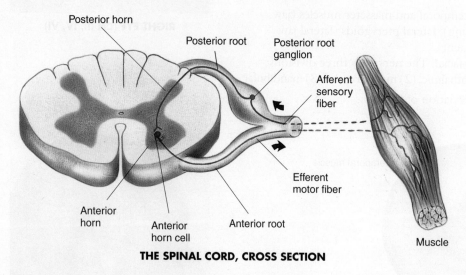

THE SPINAL CORD, CROSS SECTION

 MOTOR PATHWAYS

Motor pathways are complex avenues, extending from upper motor neurons through long white matter tracts, to synapses with lower motor neurons, and into the periphery through peripheral nerve structures. Nerve cell bodies or *upper motor neurons* lie in the motor strip of the cerebral cortex and in several brainstem nuclei; their axons synapse with motor nuclei in the brainstem (for cranial nerves) and in the spinal cord (for peripheral nerves). *Lower motor neurons* have cell bodies in the spinal cord, termed anterior horn cells; their axons transmit impulses through the anterior roots and spinal nerves into peripheral nerves, terminating at the neuromuscular junction.

THE PRINCIPAL MOTOR PATHWAYS

- The **corticospinal (pyramidal) tract**. The corticospinal tracts mediate voluntary movement and integrate skilled, complicated, or delicate movements by stimulating selected muscular actions and inhibiting others. They also carry impulses that inhibit *muscle tone,* the slight tension maintained by normal muscle even when it is relaxed. The corticospinal tracts originate in the motor cortex of the brain. Motor fibers travel down into

(continued)

THE PRINCIPAL MOTOR PATHWAYS (CONTINUED)

the lower medulla, where they form an anatomical structure resembling a pyramid. There, most of these fibers cross to the opposite or *contralateral* side of the medulla, continue downward, and synapse with anterior horn cells or with intermediate neurons. Tracts synapsing in the brainstem with motor nuclei of the cranial nerves are termed *corticobulbar*.

- The **basal ganglia system**. This exceedingly complex system includes motor pathways between the cerebral cortex, basal ganglia, brainstem, and spinal cord. It helps to maintain muscle tone and to control body movements, especially gross automatic movements such as walking.
- The **cerebellar system**. The cerebellum receives both sensory and motor input and coordinates motor activity, maintains equilibrium, and helps to control posture.

Three kinds of motor pathways impinge on the anterior horn cells: the corticospinal tract, the basal ganglia system, and the cerebellar system. Additional pathways originating in the brainstem mediate flexor and extensor tone in limb movement and posture, most notably in coma (see Table 17-13, p. 733).

All of these higher motor pathways affect movement only through the lower motor neuron systems—sometimes called the "final common pathway." Any movement, whether initiated voluntarily in the cortex, "automatically" in the basal ganglia, or reflexly in the sensory receptors, must ultimately be translated into action via the anterior horn cells. A lesion in any of these areas will affect movement or reflex activity.

When the corticospinal tract is damaged or destroyed, its functions are reduced or lost below the level of injury. *When upper motor neuron systems are damaged above the crossover of its tracts in the medulla, motor impairment develops on the opposite or contralateral side. In damage below the crossover, motor impairment occurs on the same or ipsilateral side of the body.* The affected limb becomes weak or paralyzed, and skilled, complicated, or delicate movements are performed especially poorly when compared with gross movements.

In upper motor neuron lesions, muscle tone is increased and deep tendon reflexes are

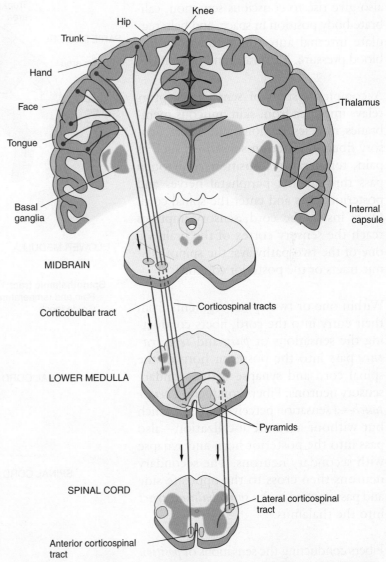

MOTOR PATHWAYS: CORTICOSPINAL AND CORTICOBULBAR TRACTS

exaggerated. Damage to the lower motor neuron systems causes ipsilateral weakness and paralysis, but in this case, muscle tone and reflexes are decreased or absent.

Disease of the basal ganglia system or cerebellar system does not cause paralysis but can be disabling. Damage to the basal ganglia system produces changes in muscle tone (most often an increase), disturbances in posture and gait, a slowness or lack of spontaneous and automatic movements termed *bradykinesia*, and various involuntary movements. Cerebellar damage impairs coordination, gait, and equilibrium and decreases muscle tone.

SENSORY PATHWAYS

Sensory impulses not only participate in reflex activity, as previously described, but also give rise to conscious sensation, calibrate body position in space, and help regulate internal autonomic functions like blood pressure, heart rate, and respiration.

A complex system of sensory receptors relays impulses from skin, mucous membranes, muscles, tendons, and viscera. Sensory fibers registering sensations such as pain, temperature, position, and touch pass through the peripheral nerves and posterior roots and enter the spinal cord. Once inside the cord, sensory impulses reach the sensory cortex of the brain via one of the two pathways: the spinothalamic tracts or the posterior columns.

Within one or two spinal segments from their entry into the cord, fibers conducting the sensations of *pain* and *temperature* pass into the posterior horn of the spinal cord and synapse with secondary sensory neurons. Fibers conducting *crude touch*—a sensation perceived as light touch but without accurate localization—also pass into the posterior horn and synapse with secondary neurons. The secondary neurons then cross to the opposite side and pass upward in the *spinothalamic tract* into the thalamus.

Fibers conducting the sensations of *position* and *vibration* pass directly into the *posterior*

SENSORY PATHWAYS: SPINOTHALAMIC TRACT AND POSTERIOR COLUMNS

columns of the cord and travel upward to the medulla, together with fibers transmitting *fine touch*—touch that is accurately localized and finely discriminating. These fibers synapse in the medulla with secondary sensory neurons. Fibers projecting from secondary neurons cross to the opposite side at the medullary level and continue on to the thalamus.

At the *thalamic level,* the general quality of sensation is perceived (e.g., pain, cold, pleasant, unpleasant), but fine distinctions are not made. For full perception, a third group of sensory neurons sends impulses from the thalamus to the *sensory cortex* of the brain. Here stimuli are localized and higher-order discriminations are made.

Lesions at different points in the sensory pathways produce different kinds of sensory loss. Patterns of sensory loss, together with their associated motor findings, help you to identify where the causative lesions might be. A lesion in the sensory cortex may not impair the perception of pain, touch, and position, for example, but does impair finer discrimination. A person so affected cannot appreciate the size, shape, or texture of an object by feeling it and therefore cannot identify it. Loss of position and vibration sense with preservation of other sensations points to disease of the posterior columns, whereas loss of all sensations from the waist down, together with paralysis and hyperactive reflexes in the legs, indicates transection of the spinal cord (see Table 17-11, p. 731). Crude and light touch are often preserved despite partial damage to the cord, because impulses originating on one side of the body travel up both sides of the cord.

Dermatomes.   A *dermatome* is the band of skin innervated by the sensory root of a single spinal nerve. Knowledge and testing of dermatomes help localize a lesion to a specific spinal cord segment. The dermatome "maps" are on pp. 694–695.

SPINAL REFLEXES: THE DEEP TENDON RESPONSE

The deep tendon or muscle stretch reflexes are relayed over structures of both the central and peripheral nervous systems. Recall that a *reflex* is an involuntary stereotypical response that may involve as few as two neurons, one afferent (sensory) and one efferent (motor), across a single synapse. The deep tendon reflexes in the arms and legs are such monosynaptic reflexes. They illustrate the simplest unit of sensory and motor function. (Other reflexes are polysynaptic, involving interneurons interposed between sensory and motor neurons.)

To elicit a deep tendon reflex, briskly tap the tendon of a partially stretched muscle. For the reflex to fire, all components of the reflex arc must be intact: sensory nerve fibers, spinal cord synapse, motor nerve fibers, neuromuscular junction, and muscle fibers. Tapping the tendon activates special sensory fibers in the partially stretched muscle, triggering a sensory impulse that travels to the spinal cord via a peripheral nerve. The stimulated sensory fiber synapses directly with the anterior horn cell innervating the same muscle.

When the impulse crosses the neuromuscular junction, the muscle suddenly contracts, completing the reflex arc.

Because each deep tendon reflex involves specific spinal segments, together with their sensory and motor fibers, an abnormal reflex can help you to locate a pathologic lesion. Learn the segmental levels of the deep tendon reflexes. You can remember them easily by their numerical sequence in ascending order from ankle to triceps: S1–L2, 3, 4–C5, 6, 7.

● Deep Tendon Reflexes

Ankle reflex	Sacral 1 primarily
Knee reflex	Lumbar 2, 3, 4
Supinator (brachioradialis) reflex	Cervical 5, 6
Biceps reflex	Cervical 5, 6
Triceps reflex	Cervical 6, 7

Reflexes may be initiated by stimulating skin as well as muscle. Stroking the skin of the abdomen, for example, produces a localized muscular twitch. These superficial (cutaneous) reflexes and their corresponding spinal segments include the following:

● Cutaneous Stimulation Reflexes

Abdominal reflexes—upper	Thoracic 8, 9, 10
—lower	Thoracic 10, 11, 12
Plantar responses	Lumbar 5, Sacral 1
Anal reflex	Sacral 2, 3, 4

THE HEALTH HISTORY

Common or Concerning Symptoms

- Headache
- Dizziness or vertigo
- Generalized, proximal, or distal weakness
- Numbness, abnormal or loss of sensations
- Loss of consciousness, syncope, or near-syncope
- Seizures
- Tremors or involuntary movements

Two of the most common symptoms in neurologic disorders are *headache* and *dizziness*. Turn to the next page to review the health history pertinent to these symptoms.

See Table 7-1, Primary Headaches, p. 249, and Table 7-2, Secondary Headaches, pp. 250–251.

Headache.   For headache, be sure to ask about severity, location, duration, and any associated symptoms such as visual changes, weakness, or loss of sensation. Ask if the headache is affected by coughing, sneezing, or sudden movement of the head, which can increase intracranial pressure.

Be alert to the many atypical presentations of migraine headaches and screen accordingly.[6–9]

Subarachnoid hemorrhage may present as "the worst headache of my life."[3,4] Severe headache in *meningitis*.[5] Dull headache affected by the actions listed, especially in the same location, in mass lesions such as *brain* or *abscess*.

Dizziness or Vertigo.   The complaint of *dizziness* can have many meanings. You will need to elicit exactly what the patient has experienced. Is the patient light-headed or feeling faint? Or is there *vertigo*, a perception that the room is spinning or rotating?

Light-headedness in palpitations, near syncope from vasovagal stimulation, low blood pressure, febrile illness, and others. Vertigo in inner-ear conditions, brainstem tumor. See Table 7-3, Dizziness and Vertigo, p. 252.

Especially in older patients, are any medications contributing to the dizziness? Are there any associated symptoms such as double vision, or *diplopia*, difficulty forming words, or *dysarthria*, or difficulty with gait or balance, or *ataxia*?

Diplopia, dysarthria, ataxia in vertebrobasilar *transient ischemic attack* (TIA) or *stroke*.[10] See Table 17-1, Types of Stroke, pp. 714–715.

Weakness.   What about any associated *weakness,* either generalized or in the face or a part of the body? Weakness is another common symptom and requires careful attention to detail. Probe for exactly what it means to the patient. Explore whether there is *paralysis,* or inability to move a part or side of the body. Did the weakness start slowly or suddenly? Has it progressed? How? What areas of the body are involved? Does the weakness affect one or both sides? What movements are affected?

Weakness or paralysis in *transient ischemic attack* or *stroke*[11]

Focal weakness may arise from ischemic, vascular, or mass lesions in the central nervous system; also from peripheral nervous system disorders, neuromuscular disorders, or diseases in the muscles themselves.

For weakness without light-headedness, try to distinguish between *proximal* and *distal weakness.* For proximal weakness, ask about combing hair, trying to reach something on a high shelf, or difficulty getting up out of a chair or taking a high step up. Does the weakness increase with repeated effort and improve after rest? Are there associated sensory or other symptoms? For distal weakness in the arms, inquire about hand movements such as opening a jar or can, or using hand tools such as scissors, pliers, or a screwdriver. For distal weakness in the legs, ask about frequent tripping.

Bilateral proximal weakness in myopathy. Bilateral, predominantly distal weakness in polyneuropathy. Weakness made worse with repeated effort and improved with rest suggests *myasthenia gravis*.[12]

Loss of Sensation.   Find out if the patient has had any *loss of sensation.* Ask if there has been any *numbness,* but clarify its meaning and location. Has there been loss of sensation, difficulty moving a limb, or altered sensations such as tingling or pins and needles? There may be peculiar sensations without an obvious stimulus, called *paresthesias.* These occur commonly when an arm or leg "goes to sleep" following compression of a nerve, and may be described as tingling, prickling, or feelings of warmth, coldness, or pressure. *Dysesthesias* are distorted sensations in response to a stimulus and may last longer than the stimulus itself. For example, a person may perceive a light touch or pinprick as a burning or tingling sensation that is irritating

Loss of sensation, paresthesias, and dysesthesias in central lesions in the brain and spinal cord, as well as disorders of peripheral sensory roots and nerves; paresthesias in the hands and around the mouth in hyperventilation. Burning pain in painful sensory neuropathy.[13]

or unpleasant. *Pain* may arise from neurologic causes but is usually reported with symptoms of other body systems, such as the head and neck or the musculoskeletal system.

See Table 16-1, Low Back Pain, p. 642, and Table 16-2, Pains in the Neck, p. 643.

Loss of Consciousness (Fainting). "Have you ever fainted or passed out?" leads the discussion to any *loss of consciousness*. Begin by exploring what the patient means by loss of consciousness. Did the patient black out completely, or could he or she hear voices throughout the episode, indicating some consciousness? Be sure to use descriptive terms carefully and precisely. *Syncope* is the sudden but temporary loss of consciousness and postural tone that occur with decreased blood flow to the brain, commonly described as *fainting*. Symptoms of feeling faint, light-headed, or weak, but without actual loss of consciousness, are called *near syncope* or *presyncope*.

See Table 17-2, Syncope and Similar Disorders, pp. 716–717.

Get as complete and unbiased a description of the event as you can. What brought on the episode? Were there any warning symptoms? Was the patient standing, sitting, or lying down when the episode began? How long did it last? Could voices be heard while passing out and coming to? How rapidly did the patient recover? In retrospect, were onset and offset slow or fast?

Young people with emotional stress and warning symptoms of flushing, warmth, or nausea may have *vasodepressor (or vasovagal) syncope* of slow onset, slow offset. *Cardiac syncope* from arrhythmias, more common in older patients, often with sudden onset, sudden offset.[14]

Also ask if anyone observed the episode. If so, what did the patient look like before losing consciousness, during the episode, and afterward? Was there any seizure-like movement of the arms or legs? Any incontinence of the bladder or bowel? Any drowsiness or impaired memory after the episode ended?

Tonic–clonic motor activity, bladder or bowel incontinence, and *postictal state* suggest a generalized *seizure*. Unlike syncope, injury such as tongue biting or bruising of limbs may occur.[15]

Seizures. A *seizure* is a paroxysmal disorder caused by sudden excessive electrical discharge in the cerebral cortex or its underlying structures. Seizures can be of several types.[15] Depending on the type, there may or may not be loss of consciousness. With some types of seizures, there may be abnormal feelings, thought processes, and sensations, including smells, as well as abnormal movements. Asking "Have you ever had any seizures or 'spells'?" . . . "Any fits or convulsions?" can open the discussion. As with syncope, aim for a full and complete description, including precipitating circumstances, warnings, and behavior and feelings both during the attack and afterward. Ask about age at onset, frequency, any change in frequency or symptom pattern, and use of medications. Is there any history of prior head injury or other conditions that may be causally related?

See Table 17-3, Seizure Disorders, pp. 718–719.

Tremors. *Tremors* and other *involuntary movements* occur with or without additional neurologic manifestations. Ask about any trembling, shakiness, or body movements that the patient seems unable to control.

See Table 17-4, Tremors and Involuntary Movements, pp. 720–721. Tremor, rigidity, and bradykinesia in Parkinson disease [16,17]

Distinct from these symptoms is an almost indescribable *restlessness of the legs* that typically develops at rest and is accompanied by an urge to move about. Walking gives relief.

The common but often overlooked *restless legs syndrome*, usually benign[18]

HEALTH PROMOTION AND COUNSELING

Important Topics for Health Promotion and Counseling

- Preventing stroke or transient ischemic attack (TIA)
- Reducing risk of peripheral neuropathy
- Detecting the "three D's": delirium, dementia, and depression

Preventing Stroke and Transient Ischemic Attack (TIA). Stroke from cerebrovascular disease is the third leading cause of death in the United States and the leading cause of long-term disability in the workforce and general population. Learn the causes and time course of stroke and TIAs.

- *Stroke* is a sudden neurologic deficit caused by cerebrovascular ischemia (80% to 85%) or hemorrhage (15% to 20%). *Hemorrhagic strokes* may be *intracerebral* (10% to 15% of all strokes) or *subarachnoid* (5% of all strokes).[19,20]

- *TIA* is a sudden focal neurologic deficit defined in the past as lasting less than 24 hours, but more recently defined as lasting less than 1 hour and without underlying structural defects.[21–23] A TIA is an important harbinger of stroke—in the first 3 months after a TIA, 15% of patients will progress to stroke, especially those with diabetes, age older than 60 years, or changes in speech or motor function.[23] Risk of stroke is highest in the first 30 days after a TIA.

STROKE AT A GLANCE

Key Facts for Prevention and Patient Education[19]

- Stroke is the third leading cause of U.S. deaths after heart disease and cancer and affects more than 5,700,000 people.
- Stroke incidence and mortality are disproportionately higher in African-Americans compared to whites:
  - *Incidence, black vs. white, ages 45 to 84 years:* 6.6 vs. 3.6 per 1000 (men); 4.9 vs. 2.3 per 1000 (women)
  - *Mortality, black vs. white, ages 45 to 84 years:* 73.9 vs. 48.1 (men); 64.9 vs. 47.4 (women)
- Crude cumulative incidence of stroke is disproportionately higher in Mexican Americans compared to non-Hispanic whites: 16.8 vs. 13.6 per 1000.
- One-year mortality after TIA is approximately 25%.
- Public awareness of stroke warning signs is high, but only 17% would call 911 if they thought someone was having a stroke.
- Stroke outcomes markedly improve if therapy is given within 3 hours of onset of symptoms; however, the median emergency-room arrival time from onset of symptoms is 3 to 6 hours.
- Physician awareness of warning signs, risk factors, and prevention remains insufficient.

Symptoms and signs of stroke depend on the vascular territory affected in the brain. The most common cause of ischemic symptoms and signs is occlusion of the *middle cerebral artery*, which causes visual field cuts and contralateral hemiparesis and sensory deficits. In the left hemisphere, occlusion of the middle cerebral artery often produces *aphasia*, and in the right hemisphere, *neglect* or *inattention* to the opposite side of the body.

See Table 17-1, Types of Stroke, pp. 714–715.

See pp. 147–148 and Table 17-5, Disorders of Speech, p. 722, for discussion of *aphasia*.

Stroke Warning Signs. The American Heart Association and the American Stroke Association urge patients to seek immediate care for any of the following critical warning signs:

● Sudden numbness or weakness of the face, arm, or leg

● Sudden confusion, trouble speaking or understanding

● Sudden trouble walking, dizziness, or loss of balance or coordination

● Sudden trouble seeing in one or both eyes

● Sudden severe headache

Teach these warning signs of "stroke attack" to your patients, especially those with risk factors.

Stroke Risk Factors—Primary Prevention. Primary prevention targets *modifiable risk factors for ischemic stroke*, namely hypertension, smoking, hyperlipidemia, diabetes, excess weight, lack of exercise, and heavy alcohol use. Careful management of atrial fibrillation and asymptomatic carotid artery disease reduces disease-specific risk of stroke. To prevent hemorrhagic stroke from intracerebral hemorrhage, control of hypertension is key. Rupture of saccular aneurysms in the circle of Willis is the most common cause of hemorrhagic stroke from subarachnoid hemorrhage—risk factors are smoking, hypertension, alcohol abuse, and family history in a first-degree relative.

In Chapter 4, see Blood Pressure Classification in Adults, p. 118.

Stroke Risk Factors—Secondary Prevention. Once a patient has experienced an ischemic stroke or TIA, focus on addressing any secondary risk factors, depending on the etiology. Causes of ischemic stroke are atherosclerotic large vessel disease, cardiac emboli, small vessel lacunar disease, other/unusual causes, and idiopathic (no mechanism identified). As you gain clinical experience, you will turn to the extensive literature that establishes treatment guidelines, risks, and benefits for this group of patients.[27,35] Note that younger patients are most likely to have strokes that are cryptogenic or from other or unusual causes such as collagen vascular disease, Takayasu's arteritis, arterial dissection, fibromuscular dysplasia, and cocaine and illicit drug use. Learn the indications for preventive therapy with aspirin or coumadin.[27]

See Table 17-1, Types of Stroke, pp. 714–715, for further discussion of lacunar and other types of stroke.

● Stroke Risk Factors—Primary Prevention for Ischemic Stoke

Behavioral Risk Factors

- Hypertension

  Hypertension is the leading determinant of risk for both ischemic and hemorrhagic stroke. Patients with blood pressure less than 120/80 have half the lifetime risk of stroke compared to those with hypertension.[19] Optimal blood pressure control is especially important for African-Americans because of their higher risk of stroke.[24]

- Smoking

  Heavy *smoking*, or smoking more than 40 cigarettes a day, doubles the risk of stroke compared to light smoking, or smoking fewer than 10 cigarettes a day. It takes 5 years for ex-smokers to drop to the same risk level as nonsmokers.

- Hyperlipidemia

  Growing evidence from cardiovascular studies using statin agents shows that reducing *hyperlipidemia* lowers stroke risk by 25%.[25,26]

- Diabetes

  Diabetes increases risk of ischemic stroke, hypertension, and hyperlipidemia. Guidelines recommend tight control to prevent the microvascular complications of diabetes, but studies do not yet consistently show that improved glucose control reduces risk of stroke. Noteworthy is the United Kingdom Prospective Diabetes Study, in which patients with hypertension and type 2 diabetes and aggressive blood pressure control had a 44% reduction in the risk of fatal and nonfatal stroke.[27,28]

- Weight

  Obesity doubles risk of stroke.

- Exercise

  As with other conditions like coronary heart disease, hypertension, and diabetes, moderate *exercise*, namely 30 minutes of brisk walking or its equivalent on most days, reduces risk of stroke.[19] Evidence of a consistent "dose-response" benefit between amount of physical activity and stroke risk is still inconclusive.[28]

- Alcohol use

  Heavy alcohol use has a "direct dose-dependent effect on the risk of hemorrhagic stroke" and appears to increase risk of ischemic stroke through the interaction of its effects on hypertension, hypercoagulable states, cardiac arrhythmias, and reductions in cerebral blood flow.[27]

Disease-Specific Risk Factors

- Atrial fibrillation

  Valvular (rheumatic) and nonvalvular *atrial fibrillation* increases risk of stroke 5- and 17-fold, respectively, compared to controls.[27] Risk reductions for ischemic stroke with warfarin therapy at INR values of 2 to 3 and with aspirin therapy are 68% and 20%, respectively, but individual risk levels vary. When considering anti-thrombotic therapy, experts recommend individual risk stratification into high, moderate, and low risk groups to balance risk of stroke against risk of bleeding. Improved risk assessment tools using community-based scoring systems are now emerging.[29–31] Patients with atrial

(continued)

● Stroke Risk Factors—Primary Prevention for Ischemic Stoke (continued)

Disease-Specific Risk Factors

fibrillation at highest risk for stroke are those with additional risk factors: prior TIA or stroke, hypertension, diabetes, poor left ventricular function, rheumatic mitral valve disease, and female gender if older than 75 years.

- Carotid artery disease

The prevalence of *carotid artery disease* from atherosclerotic disease of the extracranial carotid arteries in the U.S. population older than 65 years is 1%.[32] Carotid endarterectomy in asymptomatic patients with more than 60% carotid stenosis reduces stroke risk over 5 years from 11% to 5%, even with a perioperative stroke or death rate of 3%.[32,33] No single risk factor or risk assessment tool currently identifies people with clinically significant high-risk carotid disease. In 2007 the U.S. Preventive Services Task Force recommended against screening in the general population because of risks of false positives using carotid ultrasound for screening, risk of stroke using angiography, and the need for surgical risk of endarterectomy to be less than 3%.[34]

Reducing Risk of Peripheral Neuropathies. Diabetes is the most common cause of peripheral neuropathy, present in 10% of patients at diagnosis and rising to 50% within 5 years.[36] Diabetes causes several types of neuropathy, including a slowly progressive *distal symmetric sensorimotor polyneuropathy*, the "stocking" of the "stocking-glove" changes and the most common of the diabetic neuropathies; *autonomic dysfunction* leading to erectile dysfunction, orthostatic hypotension, and gastroparesis; *mononeuritis multiplex*, causing patchy sensory and motor deficits in at least two separate nerve areas; and *diabetic amyotrophy*, causing thigh pain and proximal lower extremity weakness, initially unilateral. Counsel patients to achieve optimal glycemic control. When HgA1C is less than or equal to 7.4%, onset of diabetic neuropathy drops by 50% to 60%.[37]

Detecting the "Three D's": Delirium, Dementia, and Depression. Delirium and dementia are increasingly common in clinical practice, with subtle presentations that call for early detection. Because delirium and dementia occur primarily in older adults, turn to Chapter 20, The Older Adult, for discussion of relevant measures for Health Promotion and Counseling. Screening and risk-factor intervention for depression, which is easily confused with delirium and depression, are found in Chapter 5, Behavior and Mental Status.

See Chapter 20, The Older Adult, pp. 911–912, and Table 20-2, Delirium and Dementia, p. 931.

See also Chapter 5, Behavior and Mental Status, pp. 135–162.

TECHNIQUES OF EXAMINATION

Important Areas of Examination

- Mental status—see Chapter 5, Behavior and Mental Status
- Cranial Nerves I through XII
- Motor system: muscle bulk, tone, and strength; coordination, gait, and stance
- Sensory system: pain and temperature, position and vibration, light touch, discrimination
- Deep tendon, abdominal, and plantar reflexes

Now return to the three important questions that govern the neurologic examination:

- Is the mental status intact?

- Are right-sided and left-sided findings symmetric?

- If the findings are asymmetric or otherwise abnormal, does the causative lesion lie in the *central nervous system* or the *peripheral nervous system*?

In this section, you will learn the techniques for a practical and reasonably comprehensive examination of the nervous system. It is important to master the techniques for a thorough examination. At first these techniques may seem difficult, but with practice, dedication, and supervision, you will come to feel comfortable evaluating neurologic symptoms and disease. You should be active in your learning and ask your instructors or even neurologists to review your skills.

The detail of an appropriate neurologic examination varies widely. As you gain experience, you will find that in healthy people, your examination will come to be relatively brief. When you detect abnormal findings, your examination will become more comprehensive. Be aware that neurologists may use many other techniques in specific situations.

For efficiency, you should integrate the neurologic assessment with other parts of your examination. Survey the patient's mental status and speech during the interview, for example, even though you may wish to do further testing during your neurologic evaluation. Assess some of the cranial nerves as you examine the head and neck, and inspect the arms and legs for neurologic abnormalities while you also observe the peripheral vascular and musculoskeletal systems. Chapter 1 provides an outline for this kind of integrated approach. Think about and describe your findings, however, in terms of the nervous system as a unit.

GUIDELINES FOR A SCREENING NEUROLOGIC EXAMINATION FROM THE AMERICAN ACADEMY OF NEUROLOGY

Students should be able to perform a brief screening neurologic examination that is sufficient to detect significant neurologic disease even in patients with no neurologic complaints. Although the exact sequence of such screening may vary, it should contain at least some assessment of mental status, cranial nerves, strength, gait and coordination, sensation and reflexes. One example of a screening examination is given here.

Mental Status—level of alertness, appropriateness of responses, orientation to date and place

Cranial Nerves

- Visual acuity
- Pupillary light reflex
- Eye movements
- Hearing
- Facial strength—smile, eye closure

Motor System

- Strength—shoulder abduction, elbow extension, wrist extension, finger abduction, hip flexion, knee flexion, ankle dorsiflexion
- Gait—casual, tandem
- Coordination—fine finger movements, finger-to-nose

Sensory System—one modality at toes—can be light touch, pain/ temperature, or proprioception

Reflexes

- Deep tendon reflexes—biceps, patellar, Achilles
- Plantar responses

Note: If there is reason to suspect neurologic disease based on the patient's history or the results of any components of the screening examination, a more complete neurologic examination may be necessary.

(Source: Adapted from the American Academy of Neurology. Available at: http://www.aan.com/globals/axon/assets/2770.pdf. Accessed January 2, 2008.)

Whether you conduct a comprehensive or screening examination, organize your thinking into five categories: (1) mental status, speech, and language; (2) cranial nerves; (3) the motor system; (4) the sensory system; and (5) reflexes. If your findings are abnormal, begin to group them into patterns of central or peripheral disorders.

THE CRANIAL NERVES

Overview. The examination of the cranial nerves (abbreviated as CN) can be summarized as follows.

SUMMARY: CRANIAL NERVES I–XII

I	Smell
II	Visual acuity, visual fields, and ocular fundi
II, III	Pupillary reactions
III, IV, VI	Extraocular movements
V	Corneal reflexes, facial sensation, and jaw movements
VII	Facial movements
VIII	Hearing
IX, X	Swallowing and rise of the palate, gag reflex
V, VII, X, XII	Voice and speech
XI	Shoulder and neck movements
XII	Tongue symmetry and position

Cranial Nerve I—Olfactory.   Test the *sense of smell* by presenting the patient with familiar and nonirritating odors. First be sure that each nasal passage is open by compressing one side of the nose and asking the patient to sniff through the other. The patient should then close both eyes. Occlude one nostril and test smell in the other with such substances as cloves, coffee, soap, or vanilla. (Avoid noxious triggers like ammonia that might stimulate CNV.) Ask if the patient smells anything and, if so, what. Test the other side. A person normally perceives odor on each side and can often identify it.

Loss of smell in sinus conditions, head trauma, smoking, aging, and the use of cocaine. Also in *Parkinson disease.*

Cranial Nerve II—Optic.   Test *visual acuity* (see pp. 211–212).

Inspect the *optic fundi* with your ophthalmoscope, paying special attention to the optic discs (see pp. 218–222).

Disc pallor in optic atrophy; disc bulging in papilledema (see p. 220)

Test the visual fields by confrontation (see pp. 212–213). Occasionally—in stroke patients for example—patients will complain of partial loss of vision, and testing of both eyes reveals a *visual field defect*, or abnormality in peripheral vision, such as *homonymous hemianopsia.* Testing one eye would not confirm the finding.

See Table 7-5, Visual Field Defects, p. 254. Prechiasmal, or anterior defects, in *glaucoma, retinal emboli, optic neuritis* (visual acuity poor). Bitemporal hemianopsias from defects at the optic chiasm, usually from *pituitary tumor.* Homonymous hemianopsias or quadrantanopsia in postchiasmal lesions, usually in the *parietal lobe,* with associated findings of stroke (visual acuity normal)[38]

Cranial Nerves II and III—Optic and Oculomotor.   Inspect the size and shape of the pupils, and compare one side with the other. *Anisocoria,* or a difference of >0.4 mm in the diameter of one pupil compared to the other, is seen in up to 38% of healthy individuals. Test the *pupillary reactions to light.*

See Table 7-10, Pupillary Abnormalities, p. 259. Minimal constriction in the larger pupil if abnormality of the pupillary *constrictor* muscle from iris disorder or *CN III palsy* with parasympathetic denervation, ptosis, and ophthalmoplegia (eyes not aligned). Pupils constrict

Also check the *near response* (p. 216), which tests pupillary constriction (pupillary constrictor muscle), convergence (medial rectus muscles), and accommodation of the lens (ciliary muscle).

to light in *Horner's syndrome*, but due to sympathetic degeneration, the affected pupil remains small (miosis) due to abnormal pupillary *dilator* muscle.[38]

Cranial Nerves III, IV, and VI—Oculomotor, Trochlear, and Abducens.

Test the *extraocular movements* in the six cardinal directions of gaze, and look for loss of conjugate movements in any of the six directions, which causes *diplopia*. Ask the patient which direction makes the diplopia worse and inspect the eye closely for asymmetric deviation of movement. Determine if the diplopia is *monocular* or *binocular* by asking the patient to cover one eye, or perform the cover-uncover test (see Table 7-11, p. 260).

See Table 7-11, Dysconjugate Gaze, p. 260. Monocular diplopia in local problems with glasses or contact lenses; cataracts; astigmatism; ptosis. Binocular diplopia in *CN III, IV, VI neuropathy* (40% of patients), eye muscle disease from *myasthenia gravis*, *trauma*, *thyroid ophthalmopathy*, *internuclear ophthalmoplegia*[38]

Check convergence of the eyes. Identify any *nystagmus*, an involuntary jerking movement of the eyes with quick and slow components. Note the direction of gaze in which it appears, the plane of the nystagmus (horizontal, vertical, rotary, or mixed), and the direction of the quick and slow components (see p. 218). *Nystagmus is named for the direction of the quick component.*

See Table 17-6, Nystagmus, p. 723. Nystagmus in *cerebellar disease*, especially with gait ataxia and dysarthria (increases with retinal fixation) and *vestibular disorders* (decreases with retinal fixation). Also in *internuclear ophthalmoplegia*

Ask the patient to fix his or her vision on a distant object and observe if the nystagmus increases or decreases.

Look for *ptosis* (drooping of the upper eyelids). A slight difference in the width of the palpebral fissures may be a normal variation in approximately one third of all people.

Ptosis in *3rd nerve palsy* (CN III), *Horner's syndrome* (ptosis, meiosis, anhidrosis), *myasthenia gravis*

Cranial Nerve V—Trigeminal

Motor. While palpating the temporal and masseter muscles in turn, ask the patient to clench his or her teeth. Note the strength of muscle contraction. Ask the patient to move the jaw side to side.

Difficulty clenching the jaw or moving it to the opposite side in masseter and lateral pterygoid weakness, respectively

Unilateral weakness in CNV pontine lesions; bilateral weakness in cerebral hemispheric disease because of bilateral cortical innervation

Central nervous system patterns from stroke include facial and body sensory loss on same side but from contralateral cortical or thalamic lesion; ipsilateral face but contralateral body sensory loss in brainstem lesions

PALPATING TEMPORAL MUSCLES

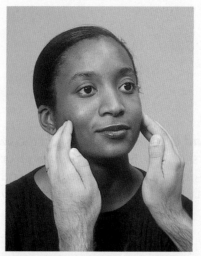

PALPATING MASSETER MUSCLES

Sensory. After explaining what you plan to do, test the forehead, cheeks, and jaw on each side for *pain sensation*. Suggested areas are indicated by the circles. The patient's eyes should be closed. Use a safety pin or other suitable sharp object,* occasionally substituting the blunt end for the point as a stimulus. Ask the patient to report whether it is "sharp" or "dull" and to compare sides.

Isolated facial sensory loss in peripheral nerve disorders like *trigeminal neuralgia*

If you find an abnormality, confirm it by testing *temperature sensation*. Two test tubes, filled with hot and ice-cold water, are the traditional stimuli. A tuning fork may also be used. It usually feels cool. If you are near running water, the fork is easily made colder or warm. Dry it before use. Touch the skin and ask the patient to identify "hot" or "cold."

Then test for *light touch,* using a fine wisp of cotton. Ask the patient to respond whenever you touch the skin.

Corneal Reflex. Test the *corneal reflex.* Ask the patient to look up and away from you. Approaching from the other side, out of the patient's line of vision, and avoiding the eyelashes, touch the cornea (not just the conjunc-

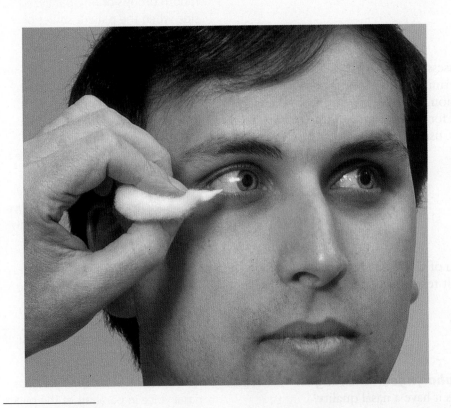

---

*To avoid transmitting infection, use a new object with each patient. You can create a sharp wood splinter by breaking or twisting a cotton swab. The cotton end of the swab can also be used as a dull stimulus.

tiva) lightly with a fine wisp of cotton. If the patient is apprehensive, however, first touching the conjunctiva may allay fear.

Look for blinking of the eyes, the normal reaction to this stimulus. The sensory limb of this reflex is carried in CN V, and the motor response, in CN VII. Use of contact lenses frequently diminishes or abolishes this reflex.

Absent blinking from CN V or VII lesion. Absent blinking and sensorineural hearing loss in *acoustic neuroma.*

Cranial Nerve VII—Facial.

Inspect the face, both at rest and during conversation with the patient. Note any asymmetry (e.g., of the nasolabial folds), and observe any tics or other abnormal movements.

Flattening of the nasolabial fold and drooping of the lower eyelid suggest facial weakness.

A peripheral injury to CN VII, as in *Bell's palsy,* affects both the upper and lower face; a central lesion affects mainly the lower face. Loss of taste, hyperacusis, increased or decreased tearing also in *Bell's palsy.* See Table 17-7, Types of Facial Paralysis, p. 725.

Ask the patient to:

1. Raise both eyebrows.

2. Frown.

3. Close both eyes tightly so that you cannot open them. Test muscular strength by trying to open them, as illustrated.

4. Show both upper and lower teeth.

5. Smile.

6. Puff out both cheeks.

In unilateral facial paralysis, the mouth droops on the paralyzed side when the patient smiles or grimaces.

Cranial Nerve VIII—Acoustic.

Assess hearing with the whispered voice test. If hearing loss is present, determine if the loss is *conductive,* from impaired "air through ear" transmission, or *sensorineural,* from damage to the cochlear branch of CN VIII. Test for (1) *air and bone conduction,* using the Rinne test, and (2) *lateralization,* using the Weber test.

See techniques for Weber and Rinne test on pp. 226–227 and Table 7-21, Patterns of Hearing Loss, p. 271. The whispered voice test is both sensitive (>90%) and specific (>80%) when assessing presence or absence of hearing loss.[38] Excess cerumen, otosclerosis, *otitis media* in conductive hearing loss; *presbyacusis* from aging, most commonly in sensorineural hearing loss

Specific tests of the vestibular function of CN VIII are rarely included in the usual neurologic examination. Consult textbooks of neurology or otolaryngology as the need arises.

Vertigo with hearing loss and nystagmus in *Meniere's disease*—see Table 7-3, Dizziness and Vertigo, p. 252, Table 17-6, Nystagmus, pp. 723–724 for caloric stimulation in comatose patients.

Cranial Nerves IX and X—Glossopharyngeal and Vagus.

Listen to the patient's *voice.* Is it hoarse, or does it have a nasal quality?

Hoarseness in vocal cord paralysis; nasal voice in paralysis of the palate

Is there difficulty in swallowing?

Pharyngeal or palatal weakness

Ask the patient to say "ah" or to yawn as you watch the *movements of the soft palate and the pharynx.* The soft palate normally rises symmetrically, the uvula remains in the midline, and each side of the posterior pharynx moves medially, like a curtain. The slightly curved uvula seen occasionally as a normal variation should not be mistaken for a uvula deviated by a lesion of CN X.

The palate fails to rise with a bilateral lesion of the vagus nerve. In unilateral paralysis, one side of the palate fails to rise and, together with the uvula, is pulled toward the normal side (see p. 236).

Warn the patient that you are going to test the *gag reflex,* which consists of elevation of the tongue and soft palate and constriction of the pharyngeal muscles. Stimulate the back of the throat lightly on each side in turn and note the gag reflex. It may be symmetrically diminished or absent in some normal people.

Unilateral absence of this reflex suggests a lesion of CN IX, perhaps CN X.

Cranial Nerve XI—Spinal Accessory. From behind, look for atrophy or *fasciculations* in the trapezius muscles, and compare one side with the other. Fasciculations are fine flickering irregular movements in small groups of muscle fibers. Ask the patient to shrug both shoulders upward against your hands. Note the strength and contraction of the trapezii.

Trapezius weakness with atrophy and fasciculations indicates a peripheral nerve disorder. In trapezius muscle paralysis, the shoulder droops, and the scapula is displaced downward and laterally.

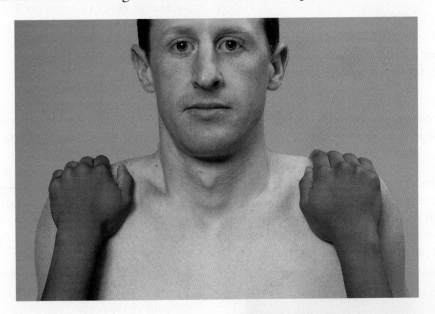

Ask the patient to turn his or her head to each side against your hand. Observe the contraction of the opposite sternomastoid and note the force of the movement against your hand.

A supine patient with bilateral weakness of the sternomastoids has difficulty raising the head off the pillow.

Cranial Nerve XII—Hypoglossal. Listen to the articulation of the patient's words. This depends on Cranial Nerves V, VII, and X as well as XII. Inspect the patient's tongue as it lies on the floor of the mouth. Look for any atrophy or *fasciculations.* Some coarser restless movements are often seen in a normal tongue. Then,

For poor articulation, or *dysarthria,* see Table 17-5, Disorders of Speech (p. 722). Tongue atrophy and fasciculations in *amyotrophic lateral sclerosis, polio*

with the patient's tongue protruded, look for asymmetry, atrophy, or deviation from the midline. Ask the patient to move the tongue from side to side, and note the symmetry of the movement. In ambiguous cases, ask the patient to push the tongue against the inside of each cheek in turn as you palpate externally for strength.

 THE MOTOR SYSTEM

As you assess the motor system, focus on body position, involuntary movements, characteristics of the muscles (bulk, tone, and strength), and coordination. These components are described below in sequence. You may either use this sequence or check each component in the arms, legs, and trunk in turn. If you see an abnormality, identify the muscle(s) involved. Determine whether the abnormality is central or peripheral in origin, and begin to learn which nerves innervate the affected muscles.

Body Position. Observe the patient's body position during movement and at rest.

Involuntary Movements. Watch for involuntary movements such as tremors, tics, or fasciculations. Note their location, quality, rate, rhythm, and amplitude, and their relation to posture, activity, fatigue, emotion, and other factors.

Muscle Bulk. Inspect the size and contours of muscles. Do the muscles look flat or concave, suggesting atrophy? If so, is the process unilateral or bilateral? Is it proximal or distal?

When looking for atrophy, pay particular attention to the hands, shoulders, and thighs. The thenar and hypothenar eminences should be full and convex, and the spaces between the metacarpals, where the dorsal interosseous muscles lie, should be full or only slightly depressed. Atrophy of hand muscles may occur with normal aging, however, as shown on the right below.

In a unilateral cortical lesion, the protruded tongue deviates transiently in a direction away from the side of the cortical lesion, toward the side of weakness.

Abnormal positions alert you to neurologic deficits such as paralysis.

See Table 17-4, Tremors and Involuntary Movements (pp. 720–721).

Muscular *atrophy* refers to a loss of muscle bulk, or wasting. It results from diseases of the peripheral nervous system such as diabetic neuropathy, as well as diseases of the muscles themselves. *Hypertrophy* is an increase in bulk with proportionate strength, whereas increased bulk with diminished strength is called *pseudohypertrophy* (seen in the *Duchenne form of muscular dystrophy*).

Atrophy

Hand of a 44-year-old woman

Hand of an 84-year-old woman

Flattening of the thenar and hypothenar eminences and furrowing between the metacarpals suggest atrophy. Localized atrophy of the thenar and hypothenar eminences in median and ulnar nerve damage, respectively

— Hypothenar eminence

— Flattening of the thenar
eminence due to mild atrophy

Hand of a 44-year-old woman

Hand of an 84-year-old woman

Be alert for fasciculations in atrophic muscles. If absent, tap on the muscle with a reflex hammer to try to stimulate them.

Muscle Tone. When a normal muscle with an intact nerve supply is relaxed voluntarily, it maintains a slight residual tension known as muscle tone. This can be assessed best by feeling the muscle's resistance to passive stretch. Persuade the patient to relax. Take one hand with yours and, while supporting the elbow, flex and extend the patient's fingers, wrist, and elbow, and put the shoulder through a moderate range of motion. With practice, these actions can be combined into a single smooth movement. On each side, note muscle tone—the resistance offered to your movements. Tense patients may show increased resistance. You will learn the feel of normal resistance only with repeated practice.

If you suspect decreased resistance, hold the forearm and shake the hand loosely back and forth. Normally the hand moves back and forth freely but is not completely floppy.

If resistance is increased, determine whether it varies as you move the limb or whether it persists throughout the range of movement and in both directions, for example, during both flexion and extension. Feel for any jerkiness in the resistance.

To assess muscle tone in the legs, support the patient's thigh with one hand, grasp the foot with the other, and flex and extend the patient's knee and ankle on each side. Note the resistance to your movements.

Other causes of muscular atrophy include motor neuron diseases, any disease that affects the peripheral motor system projecting from the spinal cord, rheumatoid arthritis, and protein-calorie malnutrition.

Fasciculations with atrophy and muscle weakness suggest disease of the peripheral motor unit.

Decreased resistance suggests disease of the peripheral nervous system, cerebellar disease, or the acute stages of spinal cord injury. See Table 17-8, Disorders of Muscle Tone (p. 726)

Marked floppiness indicates muscle *hypotonia* or *flaccidity*, usually from a disorder of the peripheral motor system.

Spasticity is increased resistance that worsens at the extremes of range. Spasticity, seen in central corticospinal tract diseases, is rate-dependent, increasing with rapid movement. *Rigidity* is increased resistance throughout the range of movement and in both directions (not rate-dependent).

Muscle Strength. Normal people vary widely in their strength, and your standard of normal, while admittedly rough, should allow for such variables as age, sex, and muscular training. A person's dominant side is usually slightly stronger than the other side. Keep this difference in mind when you compare sides.

Test muscle strength by asking the patient to move actively against your resistance or to resist your movement. Remember that a muscle is strongest when shortest, and weakest when longest.

If the muscles are too weak to overcome resistance, test them against gravity alone or with gravity eliminated. When the forearm rests in a pronated position, for example, dorsiflexion at the wrist can be tested against gravity alone. When the forearm is midway between pronation and supination, extension at the wrist can be tested with gravity eliminated. Finally, if the patient fails to move the body part, watch or feel for weak muscular contraction.

Impaired strength is called weakness, or *paresis*. Absence of strength is called paralysis, or *plegia*. *Hemiparesis* refers to weakness of one half of the body; *hemiplegia* to paralysis of one half of the body. *Paraplegia* means paralysis of the legs; *quadriplegia*, paralysis of all four limbs.

See Table 17-9, Disorders of the Central and Peripheral Nervous Systems (pp. 727–729).

SCALE FOR GRADING MUSCLE STRENGTH

Muscle strength is graded on a 0 to 5 scale:

0—No muscular contraction detected
1—A barely detectable flicker or trace of contraction
2—Active movement of the body part with gravity eliminated
3—Active movement against gravity
4—Active movement against gravity and some resistance
5—Active movement against full resistance without evident fatigue. This is normal muscle strength.

More experienced clinicians make further distinctions by using plus or minus signs toward the stronger end of this scale. Thus 4+ indicates good but not full strength, while 5− means a trace of weakness.

Methods for testing the major muscle groups are described below. The spinal root innervations and the muscles affected are shown in parentheses. To localize lesions in the spinal cord or the peripheral nervous system more precisely, additional testing may be necessary. For these specialized methods, refer to texts of neurology.

Test flexion (C5, C6—biceps) *and extension* (C6, C7, C8—triceps) *at the elbow* by having the patient pull and push against your hand.

FLEXION AT ELBOW

EXTENSION AT ELBOW

Test extension at the wrist (C6, C7, C8, radial nerve—extensor carpi radialis longus and brevis) by asking the patient to make a fist and resist your pulling it down.

Weakness of extension is seen in peripheral nerve disease such as radial nerve damage and in central nervous system disease producing hemiplegia, as in *stroke* or *multiple sclerosis*.

EXTENSION AT WRIST

Test the grip (C7, C8, T1). Ask the patient to squeeze two of your fingers as hard as possible and not let them go. (To avoid getting hurt by hard squeezes, place your own middle finger on top of your index finger.) You should normally have difficulty removing your fingers from the patient's grip. Testing both grips simultaneously with arms extended or in the lap facilitates comparison.

A weak grip in cervical radiculopathy, *de Quervain's tenosynovitis, carpal tunnel syndrome,* arthritis, epicondylitis

TEST OF GRIP

Test finger abduction (C8, T1, ulnar nerve). Position the patient's hand with palm down and fingers spread. Instructing the patient not to let you move the fingers, try to force them together.

Weak finger abduction in ulnar nerve disorders

FINGER ABDUCTION

Test opposition of the thumb (C8, T1, median nerve). The patient should try to touch the tip of the little finger with the thumb, against your resistance.

Weak opposition of the thumb in median nerve disorders such as *carpal tunnel syndrome* (see p. 608)

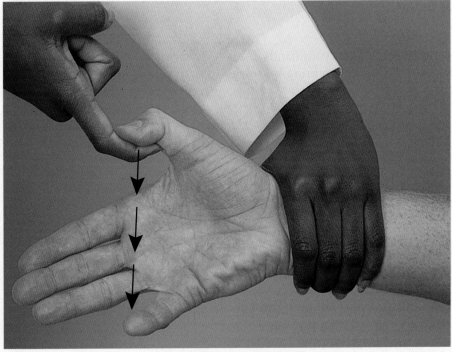

OPPOSITION OF THE THUMB

You may already have assessed *muscle strength of the trunk* during other segments of the examination, namely:

● Flexion, extension, and lateral bending of the spine, and

● Thoracic expansion and diaphragmatic excursion during respiration

Test flexion at the hip (L2, L3, L4—iliopsoas) by placing your hand on the patient's thigh and asking the patient to raise the leg against your hand.

FLEXION OF THE HIP

Test adduction at the hips (L2, L3, L4—adductors). Place your hands firmly on the bed between the patient's knees. Ask the patient to bring both legs together.

Symmetric weakness of the proximal muscles suggests a *myopathy* or muscle disorder; symmetric weakness of distal muscles suggests a *polyneuropathy*, or disorder of peripheral nerves.

Test abduction at the hips (L4, L5, S1—gluteus medius and minimus). Place your hands firmly on the bed outside the patient's knees. Ask the patient to spread both legs against your hands.

Test extension at the hips (S1—gluteus maximus). Have the patient push the posterior thigh down against your hand.

Test extension at the knee (L2, L3, L4—quadriceps). Support the knee in flexion and ask the patient to straighten the leg against your hand. The quadriceps is the strongest muscle in the body, so expect a forceful response.

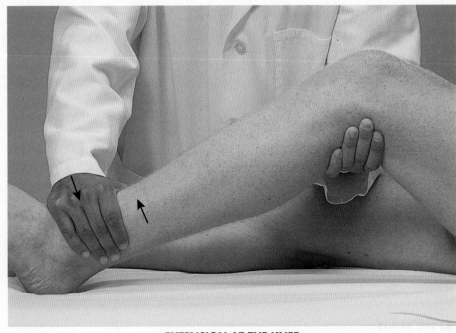

EXTENSION AT THE KNEE

Test flexion at the knee (L4, L5, S1, S2—hamstrings) as shown below. Place the patient's leg so that the knee is flexed with the foot resting on the bed. Tell the patient to keep the foot down as you try to straighten the leg.

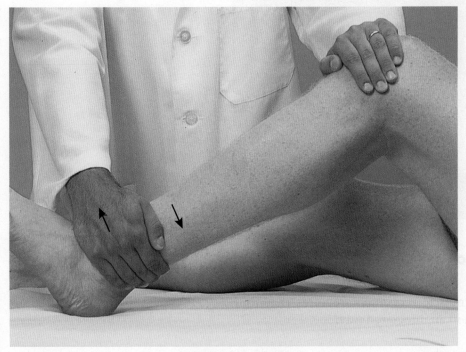

FLEXION AT THE KNEE

Test dorsiflexion (mainly L4, L5—tibialis anterior) and *plantar flexion* (mainly S1—gastrocnemius, soleus) at the ankle by asking the patient to pull up and push down against your hand.

DORSIFLEXION AT THE ANKLE

PLANTAR FLEXION AT THE ANKLE

Coordination. Coordination of muscle movement requires that four areas of the nervous system function in an integrated way:

- The motor system, for muscle strength

- The cerebellar system (also part of the motor system), for rhythmic movement and steady posture

In cerebellar disease look for nystagmus, dysarthria, hypotonia, and ataxia.

- The vestibular system, for balance and for coordinating eye, head, and body movements

- The sensory system, for position sense

To assess coordination, observe the patient's performance in:

- Rapid alternating movements

- Point-to-point movements

- Gait and other related body movements

- Standing in specified ways

Rapid Alternating Movements

ARMS.   Show the patient how to strike one hand on the thigh, raise the hand, turn it over, and then strike the back of the hand down on the same place. Urge the patient to repeat these alternating movements as rapidly as possible.

Observe the speed, rhythm, and smoothness of the movements. Repeat with the other hand. The non-dominant hand often performs somewhat less well.

In cerebellar disease, one movement cannot be followed quickly by its opposite and movements are slow, irregular, and clumsy. This abnormality is called *dysdiadochokinesis.* Upper motor neuron weakness and basal ganglia disease may also impair rapid alternating movements, but not in the same manner.

Show the patient how to tap the distal joint of the thumb with the tip of the index finger, again as rapidly as possible. Again, observe the speed, rhythm, and smoothness of the movements. The nondominant side often performs less well.

LEGS.   Ask the patient to tap your hand as quickly as possible with the ball of each foot in turn. Note any slowness or awkwardness. The feet normally perform less well than the hands.

Dysdiadochokinesis in cerebellar disease

Point-to-Point Movements

ARMS—FINGER-TO-NOSE TEST.   Ask the patient to touch your index finger and then his or her nose alternately several times. Move your finger about so that the patient has to alter directions and extend the arm fully to reach it. Observe the accuracy and smoothness of movements and watch for any tremor. Normally the patient's movements are smooth and accurate.

In cerebellar disease, movements are clumsy, unsteady, and inappropriately varying in their speed, force, and direction. The finger may initially overshoot its mark, but finally reaches it fairly well, termed *dysmetria.* An *intention tremor* may appear toward the end of the movement (see p. 720).

Now hold your finger in one place so that the patient can touch it with one arm and finger outstretched. Ask the patient to raise the arm overhead and lower it again to touch your finger. After several repeats, ask the patient to close both eyes and try several more times. Repeat on the other side. Normally a person can touch the examiner's finger successfully with eyes open or closed. These maneuvers test position sense and the functions of both the labyrinth and the cerebellum.

Cerebellar disease causes incoordination that worsens with eyes closed. If present, this suggests loss of position sense. Repetitive and consistent deviation to one side, referred to as *past pointing,* worse with the eyes closed, suggests cerebellar or vestibular disease.

LEGS—HEEL-TO-SHIN TEST.   Ask the patient to place one heel on the opposite knee, and then run it down the shin to the big toe. Note the smoothness and accuracy of the movements. Repetition with the patient's eyes closed tests for position sense. Repeat on the other side.

In cerebellar disease, the heel may overshoot the knee and then oscillate from side to side down the shin. When position sense is lost, the heel is lifted too high and the patient tries to look. With eyes closed, performance is poor.

Gait.   Ask the patient to:

Abnormalities of gait increase risk of falls.

- *Walk across the room* or down the hall, then turn, and come back. Observe posture, balance, swinging of the arms, and movements of the legs. Normally balance is easy, the arms swing at the sides, and turns are accomplished smoothly.

A gait that lacks coordination, with reeling and instability, is called *ataxic.* Ataxia may be due to cerebellar disease, loss of position sense, or intoxication. See Table 17-10, Abnormalities of Gait and Posture (p. 730).

- *Walk heel-to-toe* in a straight line— a pattern called *tandem walking.*

Tandem walking may reveal an ataxia not previously obvious.

- *Walk on the toes,* then *on the heels*— sensitive tests, respectively, for plantar flexion and dorsiflexion of the ankles, as well as for balance.

Walking on toes and heels may reveal distal muscular weakness in the legs. Inability to heel-walk is a sensitive test for corticospinal tract damage.

- *Hop in place* on each foot in turn (if the patient is not too ill). Hopping involves the proximal muscles of the legs as well as the distal ones and requires both good position sense and normal cerebellar function.

Difficulty with hopping may be due to weakness, lack of position sense, or cerebellar dysfunction.

- *Do a shallow knee bend,* first on one leg, then on the other. Support the patient's elbow if you think the patient is in danger of falling.

Difficulty here suggests proximal weakness (extensors of the hip), weakness of the quadriceps (the extensor of the knee), or both.

- *Rising from a sitting position* without arm support and *stepping up* on a sturdy stool are more suitable tests than hopping or knee bends when patients are old or less robust.

Proximal muscle weakness involving the pelvic girdle and legs causes difficulty with both of these activities.

Stance.   The following two tests can often be performed concurrently. They differ only in the patient's arm position and in what you are looking for. In each case, stand close enough to the patient to prevent a fall.

THE ROMBERG TEST.   This is mainly a test of position sense. The patient should first stand with feet together and eyes open and then close both eyes for 30 to 60 seconds without support. Note the patient's ability to maintain an upright posture. Normally only minimal swaying occurs.

In ataxia from dorsal column disease and loss of position sense, vision compensates for the sensory loss. The patient stands fairly well with eyes open but loses balance when they are closed, a *positive Romberg sign.* In *cerebellar ataxia,* the patient has difficulty standing with feet together whether the eyes are open or closed.

TEST FOR PRONATOR DRIFT.   The patient should stand for 20 to 30 seconds with both arms straight forward, palms up, and with eyes closed. A person who cannot stand may be tested for a pronator drift in the sitting position. In either case, a normal person can hold this arm position well.

Now, instructing the patient to keep the arms up and eyes shut, as shown on the next page, *tap the arms briskly downward.* The arms normally return smoothly to the horizontal position. This response requires muscular strength, coordination, and a good sense of position.

Pronator drift is the pronation of one forearm. It is both sensitive and specific for a corticospinal tract lesion originating in the contralateral hemisphere. Downward drift of the arm with flexion of fingers and elbow may also occur.[39]

A sideward or upward drift, sometimes with searching, writhing movements of the hands, suggests loss of position sense—the patient may not recognize the displacement and, if told to correct it, does so poorly. In cerebellar incoordination, the arm returns to its original position but overshoots and bounces.

THE SENSORY SYSTEM

To evaluate the sensory system, you will test several kinds of sensation:

● Pain and temperature (spinothalamic tracts)

● Position and vibration (posterior columns)

● Light touch (both of these pathways)

● Discriminative sensations, which depend on some of the above sensations but also involve the cortex

Familiarize yourself with each kind of test so that you can use it as indicated. When you detect abnormal findings, correlate them with motor and reflex activity. Assess the patient carefully as you consider the following questions: Is the underlying lesion central or peripheral? Is the sensory loss bilateral or unilateral? Does it have a pattern suggesting a dermatomal distribution, a polyneuropathy, or a spinal cord syndrome with a loss of pain and temperature sensation but intact touch and vibration? To advance in physical diagnosis of nervous system disorders, you will need to work with specialists to further refine your examination and learn the complex presentation of many of the sensory syndromes.

See Table 17-9, Disorders of the Central and Peripheral Nervous Systems (pp. 727–729).

See textbooks in Additional References, pp. 712–713, for discussion of *spinal cord syndromes* with crossed sensory findings, both ipsilateral and contralateral to the cord injury.

Patterns of Testing. Because sensory testing quickly fatigues many patients, producing unreliable results, conduct the examination as efficiently as possible. Pay special attention to those areas (1) where there are symptoms such as numbness or pain, (2) where there are motor or reflex abnormalities that suggest a lesion of the spinal cord or peripheral nervous system, and (3) where there are trophic changes, such as absent or excessive sweating, atrophic skin, or cutaneous ulceration. Repeat testing at another time is often required to confirm abnormalities.

The following patterns of testing help you to identify sensory deficits accurately and efficiently.

- *Compare symmetric areas* on the two sides of the body, including the arms, legs, and trunk.

- When testing pain, temperature, and touch sensation, also *compare the distal with the proximal areas* of the extremities. Further, scatter the stimuli so as to sample most of the dermatomes and major peripheral nerves (see pp. 694–695). One suggested pattern includes both shoulders (C4), the inner and outer aspects of the forearms (C6 and T1), the thumbs and little fingers (C6 and C8), the fronts of both thighs (L2), the medial and lateral aspects of both calves (L4 and L5), the little toes (S1), and the medial aspect of each buttock (S3).

- When testing vibration and position sensation, first test the fingers and toes. If these are normal, you may safely assume that more proximal areas will also be normal.

- *Vary the pace of your testing.* This is important so that the patient does not merely respond to your repetitive rhythm.

- When you detect an area of sensory loss or hypersensitivity, *map out its boundaries* in detail. Stimulate first at a point of reduced sensation, and move by progressive steps until the patient detects the change. An example is shown at right.

By identifying the distribution of sensory abnormalities and the kinds of sensations affected, you can infer where the causative lesion might be. Any motor deficit or reflex abnormality also helps in this localizing process.

Meticulous sensory mapping helps to establish the level of a spinal cord lesion and to determine whether a more peripheral lesion is in a nerve root, a major peripheral nerve, or one of its branches.

Hemisensory loss from a lesion in the spinal cord or higher pathways

Symmetric distal sensory loss suggests a *polyneuropathy*, as described in the example on the next page. You may miss this finding unless you compare distal and proximal areas.

Here all sensation in the hand is lost. Repetitive testing in a proximal direction reveals a gradual change to normal sensation at the wrist. This pattern fits neither a peripheral nerve nor a dermatome (see pp. 694–695). If bilateral, it suggests the "glove and stocking" sensory loss of a *polyneuropathy*, often seen in *alcoholism* and *diabetes*.

Before each of the following tests, show the patient what you plan to do and what responses you want. Unless otherwise specified, the patient's eyes should be closed during actual testing.

Pain.   Use a sharp safety pin, a broken cotton swab, or other suitable tool. Occasionally, substitute the blunt end for the point. Ask the patient, "Is this sharp or dull?" or, when making comparisons, "Does this feel the same as this?" Apply the lightest pressure needed for the stimulus to feel sharp, and try not to draw blood.

To prevent transmitting a blood-borne infection, *discard the pin or other device safely. Do not reuse it on another person.*

Temperature.   Testing is often omitted if pain sensation is normal, but include it if there is any question. Use two test tubes, filled with hot and cold water, or a tuning fork heated or cooled by water. Touch the skin and ask the patient to identify "hot" or "cold."

Light Touch.   With a fine wisp of cotton, touch the skin lightly, avoiding pressure. Ask the patient to respond whenever a touch is felt, and to compare one area with another. Calloused skin is normally relatively insensitive and should be avoided.

Vibration.   Use a relatively low-pitched tuning fork of 128 Hz. Tap it on the heel of your hand and place it firmly over a distal interphalangeal joint of the patient's finger, then over the interphalangeal joint of the big toe. Ask what the patient feels. If you are uncertain whether it is pressure or vibration, ask the patient to tell you when the vibration stops, and then touch the fork to stop it. If vibration sense is impaired, proceed to more proximal bony prominences (e.g., wrist, elbow, medial malleolus, patella, anterior superior iliac spine, spinous processes, and clavicles).

TUNING FORK ON PAD OF LARGE TOE, NOT BONE

Proprioception (Position).   Grasp the patient's big toe, *holding it by its sides* between your thumb and index finger, and then pull it away from the other toes. (These precautions prevent extraneous tactile stimuli from revealing position changes that might not otherwise be detected.) Demonstrate "up" and "down" as you move the patient's toe clearly upward and downward. Then, with the patient's eyes closed, ask for a response of "up" or "down" when moving the large toe in a small arc.

Repeat several times on each side, avoiding simple alternation of the stimuli. If position sense is impaired, move proximally to test it at the ankle joint. In a similar fashion, test

Analgesia refers to absence of pain sensation, *hypalgesia* to decreased sensitivity to pain, and *hyperalgesia* to increased sensitivity.

Anesthesia is absence of touch sensation, *hypesthesia* is decreased sensitivity, and *hyperesthesia* is increased sensitivity.

Vibration sense is often the first sensation to be lost in a peripheral neuropathy. Common causes include *diabetes* and *alcoholism.* Vibration sense is also lost in posterior column disease, as in *tertiary syphilis* or *vitamin B$_{12}$ deficiency.*

Testing vibration sense in the trunk may be useful in estimating the level of a cord lesion.

Loss of position sense, like loss of vibration sense, in *tabes dorsalis, multiple sclerosis,* or *B$_{12}$ deficiency* from posterior column disease; and in peripheral neuropathy from diabetes.

position in the fingers, moving proximally if indicated to the metacarpopha-langeal joints, wrist, and elbow.

Discriminative Sensations.   Several additional techniques test the ability of the sensory cortex to correlate, analyze, and interpret sensations. Because discriminative sensations depend on touch and position sense, they are useful only when these sensations are either intact or only slightly impaired.

Screen a patient with *stereognosis,* and proceed to other methods if indicated. The patient's eyes should be closed during all these tests.

- *Stereognosis.* Stereognosis refers to the ability to identify an object by feeling it. Place in the patient's hand a familiar object such as a coin, paper clip, key, pencil, or cotton ball, and ask the patient to tell you what it is. Normally a patient will manipulate it skillfully and identify it correctly within 5 seconds. Asking the patient to distinguish "heads" from "tails" on a coin is a sensitive test of stereognosis.

- *Number identification (graphesthesia).* When motor impairment, arthritis, or other conditions prevent the patient from manipulating an object well enough to identify it, test the ability to identify numbers. With the blunt end of a pen or pencil, draw a large number in the patient's palm. A normal person can identify most such numbers.

- *Two-point discrimination.* Using the two ends of an opened paper clip, or the sides of two pins, touch a finger pad in two places simultaneously. Alternate the double stimulus irregularly with a one-point touch. Be careful not to cause pain.

Find the minimal distance at which the patient can discriminate one from two points (normally less than 5 mm on the finger pads). This test may be used on other parts of the body, but normal distances vary widely from one body region to another.

- *Point localization.* Briefly touch a point on the patient's skin. Then ask the patient to open both eyes and point to the place touched. Normally a person can do so accurately. This test, together with the test for extinction, is especially useful on the trunk and the legs.

When touch and position sense are normal or only slightly impaired, a disproportionate decrease in or loss of discriminative sensations suggests disease of the sensory cortex. Stereognosis, number identification, and two-point discrimination are also impaired in posterior column disease.

Astereognosis refers to the inability to recognize objects placed in the hand.

The inability to recognize numbers, like astereognosis, suggests a lesion in the sensory cortex.

Lesions of the sensory cortex increase the distance between two recognizable points.

Lesions of the sensory cortex impair the ability to localize points accurately.

- *Extinction.* Simultaneously stimulate corresponding areas on both sides of the body. Ask where the patient feels your touch. Normally both stimuli are felt.

With lesions of the sensory cortex, only one stimulus may be recognized. The stimulus on the side opposite the damaged cortex is extinguished.

Dermatomes. Knowledge of dermatomes helps you localize neurologic lesions to a specific level of the spinal cord, particularly in spinal cord injury. *A dermatome is the band of skin innervated by the sensory root of a single spinal nerve.* Dermatome patterns are mapped in the next two figures, using the

In spinal cord injury, the sensory level may be several segments *lower* than the spinal lesion, for reasons that are not well understood. Tapping for the level of vertebral pain may be helpful.[38]

AREAS INNERVATED BY PERIPHERAL NERVES

DERMATOMES INNERVATED BY POSTERIOR ROOTS

international standard recommended by the American Spinal Injury Association.[40] Dermatome levels are more variable than these diagrams suggest. They overlap at their upper and lower margins and also slightly across the midline.

Do not try to memorize all the dermatomes. Instead, focus on learning selected dermatomes such as those shaded in green on the right side of the diagrams. The distribution of a few key peripheral nerves is shown in the inserts on the left.

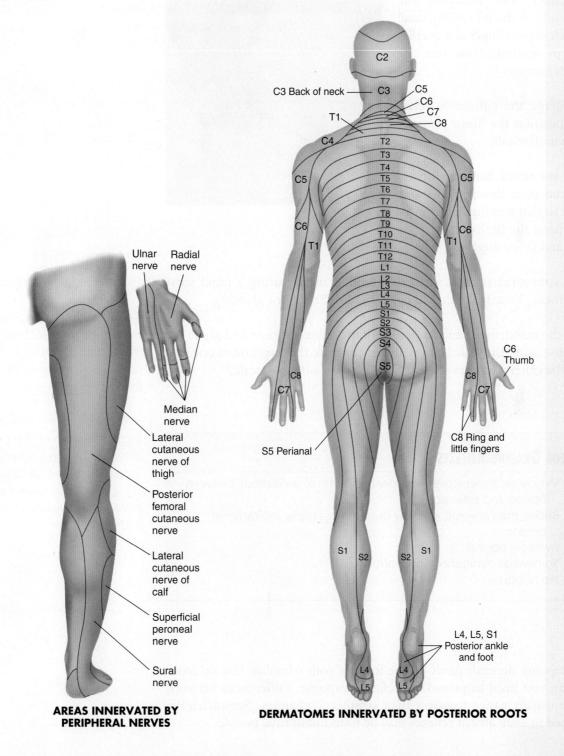

AREAS INNERVATED BY PERIPHERAL NERVES

DERMATOMES INNERVATED BY POSTERIOR ROOTS

DEEP TENDON REFLEXES

Eliciting the *deep tendon reflexes* involves a series of examiner skills. Be sure to select a properly weighted reflex hammer. Learn when to use either the pointed or the flat end of the hammer. For example, the pointed end is useful for striking small areas, such as your finger as it overlies the biceps tendon. Now test the reflexes as follows:

● Encourage the patient to relax, then position the limbs properly and symmetrically.

● Hold the reflex hammer loosely between your thumb and index finger so that it swings freely in an arc within the limits set by your palm and other fingers.

● With your wrist relaxed, strike the tendon briskly using a rapid wrist movement. Your strike should be quick and direct, not glancing.

● Note the speed, force, and amplitude of the reflex response and grade the response using the scale below. Always compare the response of one side with the other. Reflexes are usually graded on a 0 to 4+ scale.[41]

Hyperactive reflexes (hyperreflexia) in central nervous system lesions along the descending corticospinal tract. Look for associated upper motor neuron findings of weakness, spasticity, or a positive Babinski sign.

Hypoactive or *absent reflexes (hyporeflexia)* in diseases of spinal nerve roots, spinal nerves, plexuses, or peripheral nerves. Look for associated findings of lower motor unit disease, namely weakness, atrophy, and fasciculations.[38]

SCALE FOR GRADING REFLEXES

4+	Very brisk, hyperactive, with *clonus* (rhythmic oscillations between flexion and extension)
3+	Brisker than average; possibly but not necessarily indicative of disease
2+	Average; normal
1+	Somewhat diminished; low normal
0	No response

Reflex response depends partly on the force of your stimulus. Use no more force than you need to provoke a definite response. Differences between sides are usually easier to assess than symmetric changes. Symmetrically diminished or even absent reflexes may be found in normal people.

Reinforcement.   If the patient's reflexes are symmetrically diminished or absent, use *reinforcement,* a technique involving isometric contraction of other muscles for up to 10 seconds that may increase reflex activity. In testing arm reflexes, for example, ask the patient to clench his or her teeth or to squeeze one thigh with the opposite hand. If leg reflexes are diminished or absent, reinforce them by asking the patient to lock fingers and pull one hand against the other. Tell the patient to pull just before you strike the tendon.

REINFORCEMENT OF KNEE REFLEX

The Biceps Reflex (C5, C6).   The patient's arm should be partially flexed at the elbow with palm down. Place your thumb or finger firmly on the biceps tendon. Strike with the reflex hammer so that the blow is aimed directly through your digit toward the biceps tendon.

PATIENT SITTING

PATIENT LYING DOWN

Observe flexion at the elbow, and watch for and feel the contraction of the biceps muscle.

The Triceps Reflex (C6, C7). The patient may be sitting or supine. Flex the patient's arm at the elbow, with palm toward the body, and pull it slightly across the chest. Strike the triceps tendon above the elbow. Use a direct blow from directly behind it. Watch for contraction of the triceps muscle and extension at the elbow.

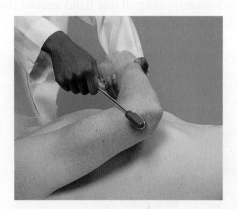

If you have difficulty getting the patient to relax, try supporting the upper arm as illustrated on the right. Ask the patient to let the arm go limp, as if it were "hung up to dry." Then strike the triceps tendon.

The Supinator or Brachioradialis Reflex (C5, C6). The patient's hand should rest on the abdomen or the lap, with the forearm partly pronated. Strike the radius with the point or flat edge of the reflex hammer, about 1 to 2 inches above the wrist. Watch for flexion and supination of the forearm.

The Knee Reflex (L2, L3, L4).   The patient may be either sitting or lying down as long as the knee is flexed. Briskly tap the patellar tendon just below the patella. Note contraction of the quadriceps with extension at the knee. A hand on the patient's anterior thigh lets you feel this reflex.

PATIENT SITTING

Two methods are useful when examining the supine patient. Supporting both knees at once, as shown below on the left, allows you to assess small differences between knee reflexes by repeatedly testing one reflex and then the other. Sometimes, however, supporting both legs is uncomfortable for both the examiner and the patient. You may wish to rest your supporting arm under the patient's leg, as shown below on the right. Some patients find it easier to relax with this method.

The Ankle Reflex (primarily S1).   If the patient is sitting, dorsiflex the foot at the ankle. Persuade the patient to relax. Strike the Achilles tendon. Watch and feel for plantar flexion at the ankle. Note also the speed of relaxation after muscular contraction.

The slowed relaxation phase of reflexes in *hypothyroidism* is often easily seen and felt in the ankle reflex.

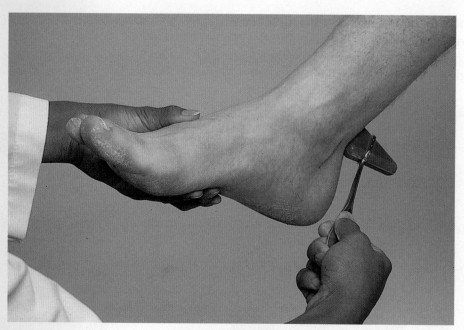

PATIENT SITTING

When the patient is lying down, flex one leg at both hip and knee and rotate it externally so that the lower leg rests across the opposite shin. Then dorsiflex the foot at the ankle and strike the Achilles tendon.

PATIENT LYING DOWN

Clonus. If the reflexes seem hyperactive, test for *ankle clonus.* Support the knee in a partly flexed position. With your other hand, dorsiflex and plantar flex the foot a few times while encouraging the patient to relax, and then sharply dorsiflex the foot and maintain it in dorsiflexion. Look and feel for rhythmic oscillations between dorsiflexion and plantar flexion. In most nor-

Sustained clonus indicates central nervous system disease. The ankle plantar flexes and dorsiflexes repetitively and rhythmically.

mal people, the ankle does not react to this stimulus. A few clonic beats may be seen and felt, especially when the patient is tense or has exercised.

Clonus may also be elicited at other joints. A sharp downward displacement of the patella, for example, may elicit patellar clonus in the extended knee.

CUTANEOUS STIMULATION REFLEXES

The Abdominal Reflexes.

Test the abdominal reflexes by lightly but briskly stroking each side of the abdomen, above (T8, T9, T10) and below (T10, T11, T12) the umbilicus, in the directions illustrated. Use a key, the wooden end of a cotton-tipped applicator, or a tongue blade twisted and split longitudinally. Note the contraction of the abdominal muscles and deviation of the umbilicus toward the stimulus. Obesity may mask an abdominal reflex. In this situation, use your finger to retract the patient's umbilicus away from the side to be stimulated. Feel with your retracting finger for the muscular contraction.

Abdominal reflexes may be absent in both central and peripheral nerve disorders.

The Plantar Response (L5, S1).

With an object such as a key or the wooden end of an applicator stick, stroke the lateral aspect of the sole from the heel to the ball of the foot, curving medially across the ball. Use the lightest stimulus that will provoke a response, but be increasingly firm if necessary. Note movement of the big toe, normally plantar flexion.

Dorsiflexion of the big toe is a *positive Babinski response* from a central nervous system lesion in the corticospinal tract; also seen in unconscious states from drug or alcohol intoxication or the postictal period following a seizure.

Some patients withdraw from this stimulus by flexing the hip and the knee. Hold the ankle, if necessary, to complete your observation. It is sometimes difficult to distinguish withdrawal from a Babinski response.

The Anal Reflex.   Using a dull object, such as a cotton swab, stroke outward in the four quadrants from the anus. Watch for reflex contraction of the anal musculature.

A marked Babinski response is occasionally accompanied by reflex flexion at hip and knee.

Loss of the anal reflex suggests a lesion in the S2–3–4 reflex arc, as in a cauda equina lesion.

 ## SPECIAL TECHNIQUES

Meningeal Signs.   Testing for these signs is important if you suspect meningeal inflammation from central nervous system infection or subarachnoid hemorrhage.

Neck Mobility.   First make sure there is no injury to the cervical vertebrae or cervical cord. (In settings of trauma, this may require evaluation by x-ray.) Then, with the patient supine, place your hands behind the patient's head and flex the neck forward, until the chin touches the chest if possible. Normally the neck is supple, and the patient can easily bend the head and neck forward.

Neck stiffness and resistance to flexion in 90% of patients with acute bacterial meningitis and in 20% to 85% with subarachnoid hemorrhage.[38] Also in arthritis and neck injury

Brudzinski's Sign. As you flex the neck, watch the hips and knees in reaction to your maneuver. Normally they should remain relaxed and motionless.

Kernig's Sign. Flex the patient's leg at both the hip and the knee, and then straighten the knee. Discomfort behind the knee during full extension occurs in many normal people, but this maneuver should not produce pain.

Flexion of the hips and knees is a *positive Brudzinski's sign* and suggests meningeal inflammation.

Pain and increased resistance to extending the knee are a *positive Kernig's sign.* When bilateral, it suggests meningeal irritation.

Compression of a lumbosacral nerve root may also cause resistance, together with pain in the low back and the posterior thigh. Only one leg is usually involved.

Lumbosacral Radiculopathy: Straight-Leg Raise. If the patient has low back pain with nerve pain that radiates down the leg, commonly called

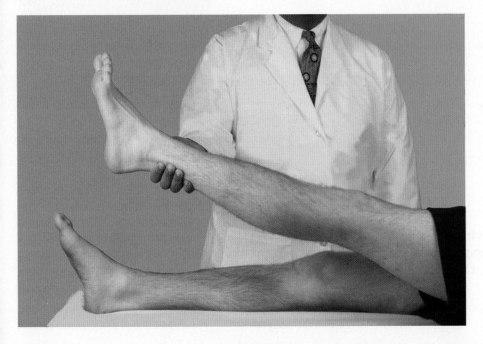

See Table 16-1, Low Back Pain, p. 642. Compression of the spinal nerve root as it exits through the vertebral foramen causes a painful *radiculopathy* with associated muscle weakness and dermatomal sensory loss, usually from a herniated disc. More than 95% of disc herniations occur at L5–S1, where the spine angles sharply posterior. Look for confirming ipsilateral calf wasting and weak ankle dorsiflexion, which make the diagnosis five times more likely.[38]

sciatica if in the S₁ distribution. Test straight-leg raising on each side in turn. Place the patient in the supine position. Raise the patient's relaxed and straightened leg, flexing the leg at the hip, then dorsiflex the foot. Some examiners first raise the patient's leg with the knee flexed, then extend the leg.

Assess the degree of elevation at which pain occurs, the quality and distribution of the pain, and the effects of dorsiflexion. Tightness or discomfort in the buttocks or hamstrings is common during these maneuvers—do not interpret this as "radicular pain" or a positive test.

Pain radiating into the ipsilateral leg is a *positive straight-leg test* for *lumbosacral radiculopathy*. Foot dorsiflexion can further increase leg pain in *lumbosacral radiculopathy, sciatic neuropathy*, or both. Increased pain when the contralateral healthy leg is raised is a *positive crossed straight-leg-raising sign*. These maneuvers stretch the affected nerve roots and sciatic nerve.

In addition, be sure to examine motor and sensory function and reflexes at the lumbosacral levels.

Sensitivity and specificity of positive ipsilateral straight-leg raise for disc herniation is roughly 95% and 25%; of crossed straight-leg raise, 40% and 90%.[42]

Asterixis. Asterixis helps identify metabolic encephalopathy in patients whose mental functions are impaired. Ask the patient to "stop traffic" by extending both arms, with hands cocked up and fingers spread. Watch for 1 to 2 minutes, coaxing the patient as necessary to maintain this position.

Sudden, brief, nonrhythmic flexion of the hands and fingers indicates asterixis, seen in liver disease, uremia, and hypercapnia.

Winging of the Scapula. When the shoulder muscles seem weak or atrophic, look for winging. Ask the patient to extend both arms and push against your hand or against a wall. Observe the scapulae. Normally they lie close to the thorax.

In winging, shown next, the medial border of the scapula juts backward. It suggests weakness of the serratus anterior muscle, seen in *muscular dystrophy* or injury to the long thoracic nerve.

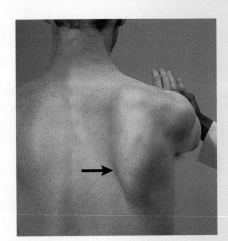

In very thin but normal people, the scapulae may appear "winged" even when the musculature is intact.

The Stuporous or Comatose Patient. Coma signals a potentially life-threatening event affecting the two hemispheres, the brainstem, or both. The usual sequence of history, physical examination, and laboratory evaluation does not apply. Instead, you must:

See Table 17-11, Metabolic and Structural Coma (p. 731).

- First assess the ABCs (airway, breathing, and circulation)

- Establish the patient's level of consciousness

- Examine the patient neurologically. Look for focal or asymmetric findings, and determine whether impaired consciousness arises from a metabolic or a structural cause.

Five clinical signs strongly predict death or poor outcome, with likelihood ratios of 5 to 12: at 24 hours—absent corneal response, absent pupillary response, absent withdrawal response to pain, no motor response; at 72 hours—no motor response.[45]

Interview relatives, friends, or witnesses to establish the speed of onset and duration of unconsciousness, any warning symptoms, precipitating factors, or previous episodes, and the prior appearance and behavior of the patient. Any history of past medical and psychiatric illnesses is also useful.

As you proceed to the examination, remember two cardinal DON'Ts:

"DON'T'S" WHEN ASSESSING THE COMATOSE PATIENT

- *Don't* dilate the pupils, the single most important clue to the underlying cause of coma (structural vs. metabolic), and
- *Don't* flex the neck if there is any question of trauma to the head or neck. Immobilize the cervical spine and get an x-ray first to rule out fractures of the cervical vertebrae that could compress and damage the spinal cord.

Airway, Breathing, and Circulation. Quickly check the patient's color and pattern of breathing. Inspect the posterior pharynx and listen over the trachea for stridor to make sure the airway is clear. If respirations are slowed or shallow, or if the airway is obstructed by secretions, consider intubating the patient as soon as possible while stabilizing the cervical spine.

Assess the remaining vital signs: pulse, blood pressure, and *rectal* temperature. If hypotension or hemorrhage is present, establish intravenous access and begin intravenous fluids. (Further emergency management and laboratory studies are beyond the scope of this text.)

Level of Consciousness. Level of consciousness primarily reflects the patient's capacity for arousal, or wakefulness. It is determined by the level of activity that the patient can be aroused to perform in response to escalating stimuli from the examiner.

Five clinical levels of consciousness are described in the table below, together with related techniques for examination. Increase your stimuli in a stepwise manner, depending on the patient's response.

When you examine patients with an altered level of consciousness, describe and record exactly what you see and hear. Imprecise use of terms such as lethargy, obtundation, stupor, or coma may mislead other examiners.

● Level of Consciousness (Arousal): Techniques and Patient Response

Level	Technique	Abnormal Response
Alertness	Speak to the patient in a normal tone of voice. An alert patient opens the eyes, looks at you, and responds fully and appropriately to stimuli (arousal intact).	
Lethargy	Speak to the patient in a loud voice. For example, call the patient's name or ask "How are you?"	A lethargic patient appears drowsy but opens the eyes and looks at you, responds to questions, and then falls asleep.
Obtundation	Shake the patient gently as if awakening a sleeper.	An obtunded patient opens the eyes and looks at you, but responds slowly and is somewhat confused. Alertness and interest in the environment are decreased.
Stupor	Apply a painful stimulus. For example, pinch a tendon, rub the sternum, or roll a pencil across a nail bed. (No stronger stimuli needed!)	A stuporous patient arouses from sleep only after painful stimuli. Verbal responses are slow or even absent. The patient lapses into an unresponsive state when the stimulus ceases. There is minimal awareness of self or the environment.
Coma	Apply repeated painful stimuli.	A comatose patient remains unarousable with eyes closed. There is no evident response to inner need or external stimuli.

Neurologic Evaluation

RESPIRATIONS.   Observe the rate, rhythm, and pattern of respirations. Because neural structures that govern breathing in the cortex and brainstem overlap those that govern consciousness, abnormalities of respiration often occur in coma.

See Table 17-11, Metabolic and Structural Coma (p. 731), and Table 4-8, Abnormalities in Rate and Rhythm of Breathing (p. 134).

PUPILS.   Observe the size and equality of the pupils and test their reaction to light. The presence or absence of the light reaction is one of the most important signs distinguishing structural from metabolic causes of coma. The light reaction often remains intact in metabolic coma.

See Table 17-12, Pupils in Comatose Patients (p. 732).

Structural lesions from stroke, abscess, or tumor mass may lead to asymmetrical pupils and loss of light reaction.

OCULAR MOVEMENT.   Observe the position of the eyes and eyelids at rest. Check for horizontal deviation of the eyes to one side (*gaze preference*). When the oculomotor pathways are intact, the eyes look straight ahead.

In structural hemispheric lesions, the eyes "look at the lesion" in the affected hemisphere.

In irritative lesions from epilepsy or early cerebral hemorrhage, the eyes "look away" from the affected hemisphere.

OCULOCEPHALIC REFLEX (DOLL'S EYE MOVEMENTS).   This reflex helps to assess brainstem function in a comatose patient. Holding open the upper eyelids so that you can see the eyes, turn the head quickly, first to one side and then to the other. (Make sure the patient has no neck injury before performing this test.)

In a comatose patient with absence of doll's eye movements, shown below, the ability to move both eyes to one side is lost, suggesting a lesion of the midbrain or pons.

In a comatose patient with an intact brainstem, as the head is turned, the eyes move toward the opposite side (the doll's eye movements). In the adjacent photo, for example, the patient's head has been turned to the right; her eyes have moved to the left. Her eyes still seem to gaze at the camera. The doll's eye movements are intact.

OCULOVESTIBULAR REFLEX (WITH CALORIC STIMULATION).   If the oculocephalic reflex is absent and you seek further assessment of brainstem function, test the oculovestibular reflex. Note that this test is almost never performed in an awake patient.

Make sure the eardrums are intact and the canals clear. You must elevate the patient's head to 30° to perform the test accurately. Place a kidney basin under the ear to catch any overflowing water. With a large syringe, inject ice water through a small catheter that is lying in (but not plugging) the ear canal. Watch for deviation of the eyes in the horizontal plane. You may need to use up to 120 ml of ice water to elicit a response. In the comatose patient with an *intact brainstem*, the eyes drift *toward* the irrigated ear. Repeat on the opposite side, waiting 3 to 5 minutes if necessary for the first response to disappear.

No response to stimulation suggests brainstem injury.

POSTURE AND MUSCLE TONE.   Observe the patient's posture. If there is no spontaneous movement, you may need to apply a painful stimulus (see p. 706). Classify the resulting pattern of movement as:

See Table 17-13, Abnormal Postures in Comatose Patients (p. 733).

● *Normal–avoidant*—the patient pushes the stimulus away or withdraws.

● *Stereotypic*—the stimulus evokes abnormal postural responses of the trunk and extremities.

Two stereotypic responses predominate: *decorticate rigidity* and *decerebrate rigidity* (see Table 17-13, Abnormal Postures in Comatose Patients, p. 733).

● *Flaccid paralysis or no response*

No response on one side suggests a corticospinal tract lesion.

Test muscle tone by grasping each forearm near the wrist and raising it to a vertical position. Note the position of the hand, which is usually only slightly flexed at the wrist.

The hemiplegia of sudden cerebral accidents is usually flaccid at first. The limp hand drops to form a right angle with the wrist.

Then lower the arm to about 12 or 18 inches off the bed and drop it. Watch how it falls. A normal arm drops somewhat slowly.

A flaccid arm drops rapidly, like a flail.

Support the patient's flexed knees. Then extend one leg at a time at the knee and let it fall (see below). Compare the speed with which each leg falls.

In *acute hemiplegia*, the flaccid leg falls more rapidly.

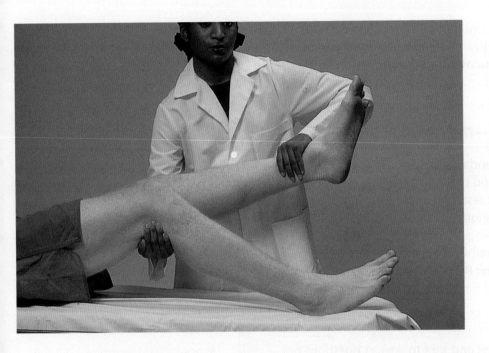

Flex both legs so that the heels rest on the bed and then release them. The normal leg returns slowly to its original extended position.

In acute hemiplegia, the flaccid leg falls rapidly into extension, with external rotation at the hip.

Further Examination. As you complete the neurologic examination, check for facial asymmetry and asymmetries in motor, sensory, and reflex function. Test for meningeal signs if indicated.

Meningitis, subarachnoid hemorrhage[3]

As you proceed to the general physical examination, check for unusual odors.

Alcohol, liver failure, uremia

Look for abnormalities of the skin, including color, moisture, evidence of bleeding disorders, needle marks, and other lesions.

Jaundice, cyanosis, cherry red color of carbon monoxide poisoning

Examine the scalp and skull for signs of trauma.

Bruises, lacerations, swelling

Examine the fundi carefully.

Papilledema, hypertensive retinopathy

Check to make sure the corneal reflexes are intact. (Remember that use of contact lenses may abolish these reflexes.)

Reflex loss in coma and lesions affecting CN V or CN VII

Inspect the ears and nose, and examine the mouth and throat.

Blood or cerebrospinal fluid in the nose or the ears suggests a skull fracture; otitis media suggests a possible brain abscess.

Be sure to evaluate the heart, lungs, and abdomen.

Tongue injury suggests a seizure.

RECORDING YOUR FINDINGS

Note that initially you may use sentences to describe your findings; later you will use phrases. The style below contains phrases appropriate for most write-ups. Note the **five components** of the examination and write-up of the nervous system.

Recording the Examination—The Nervous System

"**Mental Status:** Alert, relaxed, and cooperative. Thought process coherent. Oriented to person, place, and time. Detailed cognitive testing deferred. **Cranial Nerves:** I—not tested; II through XII intact. **Motor:** Good muscle bulk and tone. Strength 5/5 throughout. Cerebellar—Rapid alternating movements (RAMs), finger-to-nose (F→N), heel-to-shin (H→S) intact. Gait with normal base. Romberg—maintains balance with eyes closed. No pronator drift. **Sensory:** Pinprick, light touch, position, and vibration intact. **Reflexes:** 2+ and symmetric with plantar reflexes downgoing."

OR

"*Mental Status:* The patient is alert and tries to answer questions but has difficulty finding words. *Cranial Nerves:* I—not tested; II—visual acuity intact; visual fields full; III, IV, VI—extraocular movements intact; V motor—temporal and masseter strength intact, sensory corneal reflexes present; VII motor—prominent right facial droop and flattening of right nasolabial fold, left facial movements intact, sensory—taste not tested; VIII—hearing intact bilaterally to whispered voice; IX, X—gag intact; XI—strength of sternomastoid and trapezius muscles 5/5; XII—tongue midline. *Motor:* strength in right biceps, triceps, iliopsoas, gluteals, quadriceps, hamstring, and ankle flexor and extensor muscles 3/5 with good bulk but increased tone and spasticity; strength in comparable muscle groups on the left 5/5 with good bulk and tone. Gait—unable to test. Cerebellar—unable to test on right due to right arm and leg weakness; RAMs, F→N, H→S intact on left. Romberg—unable to test due to right leg weakness. Right pronator drift present. *Sensory:* decreased sensation to pinprick over right face, arm, and leg; intact on the left. Stereognosis and two-point discrimination not tested. *Reflexes* (can record in two ways):

	Biceps	Triceps	Brach	Knee	Ankle	Plantar
RT	4+	4+	4+	4+	4+	↑
LT	2+	2+	2+	2+	1+	↓

Suggests left hemispheric CVA in distribution of the left middle cerebral artery, with right-sided hemiparesis

BIBLIOGRAPHY

CITATIONS

1. Straus SE, Thorpe KE, Holroyd-Leduc J. How do I perform a lumbar puncture and analyze the results to diagnose bacterial meningitis? JAMA 296(16):2012–2022, 2006.

2. Ellenby MS, Tegtmeyer K, Lai S, et al. Lumbar puncture. N Engl J Med 355(13):e12, 2006.

3. Suarez JI, Tarr RW, Selman WR. Aneurysmal subarachnoid hemorrhage. N Engl J Med 354(4):387–396, 2006.

4. Brisman JL, Song JK, Newell DW. Cerebral aneurysms. N Engl J Med 355(9):928–939, 2006.

5. Van de Beek D, de Gans J, Spanjaard L, et al. Clinical features and prognostic factors in adults with bacterial meningitis. N Engl Med 351(18):1849–1859, 2004.

6. Goadsby PJ, Lifton RB, Ferrari MD. Migraine: current understanding and treatment. N Engl J Med 346(4):257–269, 2002.

7. Kaniecki R. Headache assessment and management. JAMA 289(11):1430–1433, 2003.

8. Maizels M, Burchette R. A rapid and sensitive paradigm for screening headache patients in primary care. Headache 43(5):441–450, 2003.

9. American Academy of Neurology. AAN encounter kit for headache. Available at: http://www.aan.com/go/practice/quality/headache. Accessed January 13, 2008.

10. Savitz SI, Caplan LR. Vertebrobasilar disease. N Engl J Med 352(25):2618–2626, 2005.

11. Johnston SC. Transient ischemic attack. N Engl J Med 347(21):1687–1692, 2002.

12. Scherer K, Bedlack RS, Simel DL. Does this patient have myasthenia gravis? JAMA 293(15):1906–1914, 2005.

13. Mendell JR, Sahenk Z. Painful sensory neuropathy. N Engl J Med 348(13):1243–1255, 2003.

14. Kapoor WN. Syncope. N Engl J Med 343(25):1856–1862, 2000.

15. Browne TR, Holmes GL. Epilepsy. N Engl J Med 344(15):1145–1151, 2001.

16. Rao G, Fisch L, Srinivasan S, et al. Does this patient have Parkinson disease? JAMA 289(3):347–353, 2003.

17. Louis ED. Essential tremor. N Engl J Med 345(12):887–891, 2001.

18. Earley CJ. Restless legs syndrome. N Engl J Med 348(21):2103–2109, 2003.

19. American Heart Association. Heart Disease and Stroke Statistics—2007 Update. Available at: http://www.americanheart.org/downloadable/heart/1166712318459HS_Stats InsideText.pdf. Accessed December 7, 2007.

20. Van der Worp HB, van Gijn J. Acute ischemic stroke. N Engl J Med 357(6):572–570, 2007.

21. Kidwell CS, Warach S. Acute ischemic cerebrovascular syndrome: diagnostic criteria. Stroke 34(12):2995–2998, 2003.

22. Albers GW, Caplan LR, Easton JD, et al. Transient ischemic attack: proposal for a new definition. N Engl J Med 347(21):1713–1716, 2002.

23. Johnston SC, Gress DR, Browner WS, et al. Short-term prognosis after emergency department diagnosis of TIA. JAMA 284(22):2901–2906, 2000.

24. Douglas JG, Bakris GL, Epstein M, et al. Management of high blood pressure in African Americans: consensus statement of the Hypertension in African Americans Working Group of the International Society on Hypertension in Blacks. Arch Intern Med 163(5):525–541, 2003.

25. Corvol JC, Bouzamondo A, Sirol M, et al. Differential effects of lipid-lowering therapies on stroke prevention: a meta-analysis of randomized trials. Arch Intern Med 163(6):669–676, 2003.

26. Collins R, Armitage J, Parish S, et al. Effects of cholesterol lowering with simvastatin on stroke and other major vascular events in 20,536 people with cerebrovascular disease or other high-risk conditions. Lancet 363(9411):757–767, 2004.

27. Straus SE, Majumdar SR, McAlister FA. New evidence for stroke prevention: scientific review. JAMA 288(11):1388–1395, 2002.

28. Gorelick PB, Sacco RL, Smith DB, et al. Prevention of a first stroke: a review of the guidelines and a multidisciplinary consensus statement from the National Stroke Association. JAMA 281(12):1112–1120, 1999.

29. Waldo AL. Stroke prevention after atrial fibrillation. JAMA 290(8):1093–1094, 2003.

30. Wang TJ, Massaro JM, Levy D, et al. A risk score for predicting stroke or death in individuals with new-onset atrial fibrillation in the community. The Framingham Heart Study. JAMA 290(8):1049–1056, 2003.

31. Hart RG. Atrial fibrillation and stroke prevention. JAMA 349(11):1015–1016, 2003.

32. Wolff T, Guirgulis-Blake J, Miller T, et al. Screening for carotid artery stenosis: an update of the evidence for the U.S. Preventive Services Task Force. Ann Intern Med 147(12):860–870, 2007.

33. Halliday I, Mansfield A, Marro J, et al. Prevention of disabling and fatal strokes by successful carotid endarterectomy in patients without recent neurological symptoms: randomized controlled trial. Lancet 363(9420):1491–1502, 2004.

34. U.S. Preventive Services Task Force. Screening for Carotid Artery Stenosis. Rockville, MD: Agency for Healthcare Research and Quality, December 2007. Available at: http://www.ahrq.gov/clinic/uspstf/uspsacas.htm. Accessed December 30, 2007.

35. American College of Physicians. Stroke in Neurology: Medical Knowledge Self-Assessment Program (MKSAP) 14. Philadelphia: American College of Physicians, 2006:52–68.

36. Boulton AJ, Vinik AT, Arezzo JC, et al. Diabetic neuropathies: A statement by the American Diabetes Association. Diabetes Care 28(4):956–962, 2005.

37. Martin CL, Albers J, Herman WH, et al. Neuropathy among the Diabetes Control and Complications Trial Cohort 8 years after trial completion. Diabetes Care 29(2):340–344, 2006.

38. McGee S. Evidence-Based Physical Diagnosis, 2nd ed. St. Louis: Saunders, 2005. See especially Visual field defects, pp. 663–670; The pupils, pp. 203–233; Nerves of the eye muscles (III, IV, and VI): approach to diplopia, pp. 671–689; Coordination and cerebellar testing, pp. 793–800; Miscellaneous cranial nerves, pp. 690–706; Hearing, pp. 242–249; Stance and gait, pp. 57–74; Examination of the sensory system, pp. 736–753; Examination of the reflexes, pp. 754–771; Disorders of the nerve roots, plexi, and peripheral nerves, pp. 772–792; and Meninges, pp. 277–282.

39. Teitelbaum JS, Eliasziw M, Garner M. Tests of motor function in patients suspected of having mild unilateral cerebral lesions. Can J Neurol Sci 29(4):337–344, 2002.

40. Maynard FM, Bracken MB, Creasey G, et al. International standards for neurological and functional classification of spinal cord injury. Spinal Cord 35(5):266–274, 1997. See diagram, American Spinal Cord Injury Association, Available at http://www.asia-spinalinjury.org/publications/2006_Classif_worksheet.pdf. Accessed January 7, 2008.

41. Hallett M. NINDS myotatic reflex scale. Neurology 43(12): 2723, 1993.

42. Sabatine MS. Pocket Medicine, 2nd ed. Philadelphia: Lippincott Williams & Wilkins, 2004.

43. Bateman DE. Neurological assessment of coma. J Neurol Neurosurg Psychiatry 71(Suppl 1):i13–i37, 2001.

44. Laureys S, Owen AM, Schiff ND. Brain function in coma, vegetative state, and related disorders. Lancet Neurol 3(9):537–546, 2004.

45. Booth CM, Boone RH, Tomlinson G, et al. Is this patient dead, vegetative, or severely neurologically impaired? Assessing outcome for comatose survivors of cardiac arrest. JAMA 291(7):870–879, 2004.

46. Goldstein LB, Matchar DB. Clinical assessment of stroke. JAMA 271(14):1114–1120, 1994.

47. Goldstein LB, Simel DL. Is this patient having a stroke? JAMA 293(19):2391–2402, 2005.

48. Grubb BP. Neurocardiogenic syncope. N Engl J Med 352(10): 1004–1010, 2004.

49. Soteriades ES, Evans JC, Larson MG, et al. Incidence and prognosis of syncope. N Engl J Med 347(12):878–885, 2002.

ADDITIONAL REFERENCES

Aids to the Examination of the Peripheral Nervous System: Medical Research Council Memorandum No. 45. London: Her Majesty's Stationery Office, 1976.

Booth CN, Boone RH, Tomlinson G, et al. Is this patient dead, vegetative, or severely neurologically impaired? JAMA 291(7): 870–879, 2004.

Boyer EW, Shannon M. The serotonin syndrome. N Engl J Med 352(11):1112–1120, 2005.

Budson AE, Price BH. Memory dysfunction. N Engl J Med 352(7):692–699, 2005.

Campbell WW, DeJong RN, Haerer AF. DeJong's The Neurologic Examination, 6th ed. Philadelphia: Lippincott Williams & Wilkins, 2005.

Chang BS, Lowenstein DH. Epilepsy. N Engl J Med 349(13): 1257–1266, 2003.

Chimowitz MI. The accuracy of bedside neurological diagnoses. Ann Neurol 28(1):78–85, 1990.

Darouiche RO. Spinal epidural abscess. N Engl J Med 355(19): 2012–2020, 2006.

Detsky ME, McDonald DR, Baerlocher MO, et al. Does this patient with headache have a migraine or need neuroimaging? JAMA 296(10):1272–1283, 2006.

Freeman R. Clinical practice: neurogenic orthostatic hypotension. N Engl J Med 358(6):615–624, 2008.

Gardner P. Prevention of meningococcal disease. N Engl J Med 355(14):1466–1473, 2006.

Gilden DH. Bell's palsy. N Engl J Med 351(13):1323–1331, 2004.

Gilman S, Manter JT, Gatz AJ, et al. Manter and Gatz's Essentials of Clinical Neuroanatomy and Neurophysiology, 10th ed. Philadelphia: FA Davis, 2003.

Gilron I, Watson PN, Cahill C, et al. Neuropathic pain: a practical guide for the clinician. CMAJ 175(3):265–275, 2006.

Griggs RC, Joynt RJ, eds. Baker and Joynt's Clinical Neurology on CD-ROM. Philadelphia: Lippincott Williams & Wilkins, 2003.

Jeha LE, Sila CA, Lederman RJ, et al. West Nile virus infection: a new acute paralytic illness. Neurology 61(1):55–59, 2003.

Katz JN. Carpal tunnel syndrome. N Engl J Med 346(23):1807–1812, 2002.

Lavan ZP. Stroke prevention through community action. J Community Nurs 19(3):4, 6, 8–10, 2005.

Louis ED. Essential tremor. N Engl J Med 345(12):887–891, 2001.

Magnetic Resonance Angiography in Relatives of Patients with Subarachnoid Hemorrhage Study Group. Risks and benefits of screening for intracranial aneurysms in first-degree relatives of patients with sporadic subarachnoid hemorrhage. N Engl J Med 341(18):1344–1350, 1999.

McGill M, Molyneaux L, Spencer R, et al. Possible sources of discrepancies in the use of the Semmes-Weinstein monofilament. Diabetes Care 22(4):598–602, 1999.

Mendell JR, Sahenk Z. Painful sensory neuropathy. N Engl. J Med 348(13):1243–1294, 2003.

Nutt JG, Wooten GF. Clinical practice: diagnosis and initial management of Parkinson's disease. N Engl J Med 353(10): 1021–1027, 2005.

Partanen J, Kiskanen L, Leghtinen J, et al. Natural history of peripheral neuropathic pain patients with non-insulin-dependent diabetes mellitus. N Engl J Med 333(2):89–94, 1995.

Plum F, Posner JB. Plum and Posner's Diagnosis of Stupor and Coma, 4th ed. Oxford, New York: Oxford University Press, 2007.

Ropper AH, Adams RD, Victor MV, et al. Adams and Victor's Principles of Neurology, 8th ed. New York: McGraw-Hill, 2005.

Rosenberg RN. Atlas of Clinical Neurology, 3rd ed. Philadelphia: Current Medicine Group, 2008.

Rowland LP, Merritt HH. Merritt's Neurology, 11th ed. Philadelphia: Lippincott Williams & Wilkins, 2005.

Saltzman CL, Rashid R, Hayes A, et al. 4.5 Gram monofilament sensation beneath both first metatarsal heads indicates protective foot sensation in diabetic patients. J Bone Joint Surg 86(4):717–723, 2004.

Tan MP, Parry SW. Vasovagal syncope in the older patient. J Am Coll Cardiol 51(6):599–606, 2008.

Tarsy D, Simon DK. Dystonia. N Engl J Med 355(8):818–829, 2006.

Van de Beek D, de Gans J, Tunkel AR, et al. Community-acquired bacterial meningitis in adults. N Engl J Med 354(1):44–53, 2006.

The Bates' suite offers these additional resources to enhance learning and facilitate understanding of this chapter:

- *Bates' Pocket Guide to Physical Examination and History Taking,* 6th edition
- *Bates' Nursing Online*
- *Bates' Visual Guide to Physical Examination,* 4th edition
- thePoint online resources, http://thepoint.lww.com
- Student CD-ROM included with the book

TABLE
17-1

Types of Stroke

Assessing patients with stroke involves three fundamental questions based on a careful history and detailed physical examination: *What brain area and related vascular territory explain the patient's findings? Is the stroke ischemic or hemorrhagic? If ischemic, is the mechanism thrombus or embolus?* Stroke is a medical emergency, and timing is of the essence. Answers to these questions are critical to patient outcomes and use of antithrombotic therapies in acute ischemic stroke.

In *acute ischemic stroke,* ischemic brain injury begins with a central core of very low perfusion and often irreversible cell death. This core is surrounded by an *ischemic penumbra* of metabolically disturbed cells that are still potentially viable, depending on restoration of blood flow and duration of ischemia. Because most irreversible damage occurs in the first 3 to 6 hours after onset of symptoms, therapies targeted to the 3-hour window achieve the best outcomes, with recovery in up to 50% of patients in some studies.[20]

Clinician performance in diagnosing stroke improves with training.[46] Understanding the pathophysiology of stroke takes dedication, expert supervision to improve techniques of neurologic examination, and perseverance. *This brief overview is intended to prompt further study and practice.* Accuracy in clinical examination is achievable, and more important than ever in determining patient therapy.[47] (See also pp. 667–668 for discussion of *stroke risk factors–primary and secondary prevention.*)

Clinical Features and Vascular Territories of Stroke

Clinical Finding	Vascular Territory	Additional Comments
Contralateral leg weakness	*Anterior circulation*—anterior cerebral artery (ACA)	Includes stem of circle of Willis connecting internal carotid artery to ACA, and the segment distal to ACA and its anterior choroidal branch
Contralateral face, arm > leg weakness, sensory loss, field cut, aphasia (left MCA) or neglect, apraxia (right MCA)	*Anterior circulation*—middle cerebral artery (MCA)	Largest vascular bed for stroke
Contralateral motor or sensory deficit without cortical signs	*Subcortical circulation*—lenticulostriate deep penetrating branches of MCA	Small vessel subcortical *lacunar infarcts* in internal capsule, thalamus, or brainstem. Four common syndromes: pure motor hemiparesis; pure sensory hemianesthesia; ataxic hemiparesis; clumsy hand–dysarthria syndrome
Contralateral field cut	*Posterior circulation*—posterior cerebral artery (PCA)	Includes paired vertebral and basilar artery, paired posterior cerebral arteries. Bilateral PCA infarction causes cortical blindness but preserved pupillary light reaction.
Dysphagia, dysarthria, tongue/palate deviation and/or ataxia with crossed sensory/motor deficits (= ipsilateral face with contralateral body)	*Posterior circulation*—brainstem, vertebral, or basilar artery branches	
Oculomotor deficits and/or ataxia with crossed sensory/motor deficits	*Posterior circulation*—basilar artery	Complete basilar artery occlusion—"locked-in syndrome" with intact consciousness but with inability to speak and quadriplegia

*Learn to differentiate cortical from subcortical involvement. *Subcortical or lacunar syndromes* do not affect higher cognitive function, language, or visual fields.

(Source: Adapted from American College of Physicians. Stroke, in Neurology. Medical Knowledge Self-Assessment Program (MKSAP) 14. Philadelphia: American College of Physicians, 2006. pp. 52–68.)

(table continues on page 715)

Lateral
ventrical

Body of
caudate

Internal
capsule

Anterior cerebral
artery

Anterior choroidal
artery

Middle cerebral
artery

Posterior cerebral
artery

Putamen

Thalamus

Globus
pallidus

Uncus

Prefrontal area

Motor speech
(Broca's) area

Taste area

Sensory speech
(Wernike's) area

Premotor area

Primary somatic
sensory cortex

Primary
auditory cortex

Reading compre-
hension area

Primary motor
cortex

Somatic sensory
association area

Auditory
association area

Visual association
area

Visual cortex

Syncope and Similar Disorders[48,49]

Problem	Mechanism	Precipitating Factors
Vasodepressor or Vasovagal Syncope *(the common faint)*	Sudden peripheral vasodilatation, especially in the skeletal muscles, without a compensatory rise in cardiac output. Blood pressure falls. Often slow onset, slow offset.	A strong emotion such as fear or pain
Postural *(orthostatic)* **Hypotension**	• *Inadequate vasoconstrictor reflexes* in both arterioles and veins, with resultant venous pooling, decreased cardiac output, and low blood pressure • *Hypovolemia,* a diminished blood volume insufficient to maintain cardiac output and blood pressure, especially in the upright position	• Standing up • Standing up after hemorrhage or dehydration
Cough Syncope	Several possible mechanisms associated with increased intrathoracic pressure	Severe paroxysm of coughing
Micturition Syncope	Unclear	Emptying the bladder after getting out of bed to void
Cardiovascular Disorders		
Arrhythmias	Decreased cardiac output secondary to rhythms that are too fast (usually more than 180) or too slow (less than 35–40). Often sudden onset; sudden offset.	A sudden change in rhythm
Aortic Stenosis and Hypertrophic Cardiomyopathy	Vascular resistance falls with exercise, but cardiac output cannot rise.	Exercise
Myocardial Infarction	Sudden arrhythmia or decreased cardiac output	Variable
Massive Pulmonary Embolism	Sudden hypoxia or decreased cardiac output	Variable, including prolonged bed rest and clotting disorders
Disorders Resembling Syncope		
Hypocapnia due to Hyperventilation	Constriction of cerebral blood vessels secondary to hypocapnia that is induced by hyperventilation	Possibly a stressful situation
Hypoglycemia	Insufficient glucose to maintain cerebral metabolism; secretion of epinephrine contributes to symptoms. True syncope is uncommon.	Variable, including fasting
Hysterical Fainting from Conversion Reaction	The symbolic expression of an unacceptable idea through body language. Skin color and vital signs may be normal; sometimes with bizarre and purposive movements; occurrence in the presence of other people.	Stressful situation

Predisposing Factors	Prodromal Manifestations	Postural Associations	Recovery
Fatigue, hunger, a hot humid environment	Restlessness, weakness, pallor, nausea, salivation, sweating, yawning	Usually occurs when standing, possibly when sitting	Prompt return of consciousness when lying down, but pallor, weakness, nausea, and slight confusion may persist for a time.
• Peripheral neuropathies and disorders affecting the autonomic nervous system; drugs such as antihypertensives and vasodilators; prolonged bed rest	• Often none	• Occurs soon after the person stands up	• Prompt return to normal when lying down
• Bleeding from the GI tract or trauma, potent diuretics, vomiting, diarrhea, polyuria	• Lightheadedness and palpitations (tachycardia) on standing up	• Usually occurs soon after the person stands up	• Improvement on lying down
Chronic bronchitis in a muscular man	Often none except for cough	May occur in any position	Prompt return to normal
Nocturia, usually in elderly or adult men	Often none	Standing to void	Prompt return to normal
Heart disease and old age decrease tolerance of abnormal rhythms.	Often none	May occur in any position	Prompt return to normal unless brain damage has resulted
Cardiac disorders	Often none. Onset is sudden.	Occurs with or after exercise	Usually a prompt return to normal
Coronary artery disease	Often none	May occur in any position	Variable
Deep vein thrombosis	Often none	May occur in any position	Variable
A predisposition to anxiety attacks and hyperventilation	Dyspnea, palpitations, chest discomfort, numbness and tingling of the hands and around the mouth lasting for several minutes. Consciousness is often maintained.	May occur in any position	Slow improvement as hyperventilation ceases
Insulin therapy and a variety of metabolic disorders	Sweating, tremor, palpitations, hunger, headache, confusion, abnormal behavior, coma	May occur in any position	Variable, depending on severity and treatment
Hysterical personality traits	Variable	A slump to the floor, often from a standing position without injury	Variable, may be prolonged, often with fluctuating responsiveness

TABLE
17-3

Seizure Disorders[15]

Partial Seizures

Partial seizures start with focal manifestations. They are further divided into *simple partial seizures,* which do not impair consciousness, and *complex partial seizures,* which do. *Partial seizures may become generalized*. Partial seizures of all kinds usually indicate a structural lesion in the cerebral cortex, such as a scar, tumor, or infarction. The quality of such seizures helps the clinician to localize the causative lesion in the brain.

Problem	Clinical Manifestations	Postictal *(postseizure)* State
Partial Seizures		
Simple Partial Seizures		
• With motor symptoms		
Jacksonian	Tonic and then clonic movements that start unilaterally in the hand, foot, or face and spread to other body parts on the same side	Normal consciousness
Other motor	Turning of the head and eyes to one side, or tonic and clonic movements of an arm or leg without the Jacksonian spread	Normal consciousness
• With sensory symptoms	Numbness, tingling; simple visual, auditory, or olfactory hallucinations such as flashing lights, buzzing, or odors	Normal consciousness
• With autonomic symptoms	A "funny feeling" in the epigastrium, nausea, pallor, flushing, lightheadedness	Normal consciousness
• With psychiatric symptoms	Anxiety or fear; feelings of familiarity (déjà vu) or unreality; dreamy states; fear or rage; flashback experiences; more complex hallucinations	Normal consciousness
Complex Partial Seizures	The seizure may or may not start with the autonomic or psychic symptoms outlined above. Consciousness is impaired, and the person appears confused. Automatisms include automatic motor behaviors such as chewing, smacking the lips, walking about, and unbuttoning clothes; also more complicated and skilled behaviors such as driving a car.	The patient may remember initial autonomic or psychic symptoms (which are then termed an *aura*), but is amnesic for the rest of the seizure. Temporary confusion and headache may occur.
Partial Seizures That Become Generalized	Partial seizures that become generalized resemble tonic–clonic seizures (see next page). Unfortunately, the patient may not recall the focal onset, and observers may overlook it.	As in a tonic–clonic seizure, described on the next page. Two attributes indicate a partial seizure that has become generalized: (1) the recollection of an *aura*, and (2) a *unilateral* neurologic deficit during the postictal period.

(Source: Commission on Classification and Terminology of the International League Against Epilepsy. Proposal for revised classification of epilepsies and epileptic syndromes. Epilepsia 30:389–399, 1989. See also International League against Epilepsy. A proposed diagnostic scheme for people with epileptic seizures and with epilepsy: report of the ILAE Task Force on Classification and Terminology. Available at: http://www.ilae-epilepsy.org/Visitors/Centre/ctf/overview.cfm#2. Accessed January 10, 2008.)

(table continues on page 719)

Generalized Seizures and Pseudoseizures

Generalized seizures begin with bilateral body movements, impairment of consciousness, or both. They suggest a widespread, bilateral cortical disturbance that may be either hereditary or acquired. When generalized seizures of the tonic–clonic (grand mal) variety start in childhood or young adulthood, they are often hereditary. When tonic–clonic seizures begin after age 30, suspect either a partial seizure that has become generalized or a general seizure caused by a toxic or metabolic disorder. Toxic and metabolic causes include withdrawal from alcohol or other sedative drugs, uremia, hypoglycemia, hyperglycemia, hyponatremia, and bacterial meningitis.

Problem	Clinical Manifestations	Postictal (*postseizure*) State
Generalized Seizures		
Tonic–Clonic Convulsion (grand mal) *	The person loses consciousness suddenly, sometimes with a cry, and the body stiffens into tonic extensor rigidity. Breathing stops, and the person becomes cyanotic. A clonic phase of rhythmic muscular contraction follows. Breathing resumes and is often noisy, with excessive salivation. Injury, tongue biting, and urinary incontinence may occur.	Confusion, drowsiness, fatigue, headache, muscular aching, and sometimes the temporary persistence of bilateral neurologic deficits such as hyperactive reflexes and Babinski responses. The person has amnesia for the seizure and recalls no aura.
Absence	A sudden brief lapse of consciousness, with momentary blinking, staring, or movements of the lips and hands but no falling. Two subtypes are recognized. *Petit mal absences* last less than 10 sec and stop abruptly. *Atypical absences* may last more than 10 sec.	No aura recalled. In petit mal absences, a prompt return to normal; in atypical absences, some postictal confusion
Atonic Seizure, or Drop Attack	Sudden loss of consciousness with falling but no movements. Injury may occur.	Either a prompt return to normal or a brief period of confusion
Myoclonus	Sudden, brief, rapid jerks, involving the trunk or limbs. Associated with a variety of disorders	Variable
Pseudoseizures		
May mimic seizures but are due to a conversion reaction (a psychological disorder)	The movements may have personally symbolic significance and often do not follow a neuroanatomic pattern. Injury is uncommon.	Variable

Febrile convulsions that resemble brief tonic–clonic seizures may occur in infants and young children. They are usually benign but occasionally may be the first manifestation of a seizure disorder.

TABLE
17-4

Tremors and Involuntary Movements[16,17]

Tremors: Tremors are relatively rhythmic oscillatory movements, which may be roughly subdivided into three groups: resting (or static) tremors, postural tremors, and intention tremors.

Resting (Static) Tremors

These tremors are most prominent at rest, and may decrease or disappear with voluntary movement. Illustrated is the common, relatively slow, fine, pill-rolling tremor of parkinsonism, about 5 per second.

Postural (Action) Tremors

These tremors appear when the affected part is actively maintaining a posture. Examples include the fine rapid tremor of hyperthyroidism, the tremors of anxiety and fatigue, and benign essential (and sometimes familial) tremor. Tremor may worsen somewhat with intention.

Intention Tremors

Intention tremors, absent at rest, appear with activity and often get worse as the target is neared. Causes include disorders of cerebellar pathways, as in multiple sclerosis.

Oral–Facial Dyskinesias

Oral–facial dyskinesias are rhythmic, repetitive, bizarre movements that chiefly involve the face, mouth, jaw, and tongue: grimacing, pursing of the lips, protrusions of the tongue, opening and closing of the mouth, and deviations of the jaw. The limbs and trunk are involved less often. These movements may be a late complication of psychotropic drugs such as phenothiazines, termed *tardive* (late) dyskinesias. They also occur in long-standing psychoses, in some elderly individuals, and in some edentulous persons.

(table continues on page 721)

Tics

Tics are brief, repetitive, stereotyped, coordinated movements occurring at irregular intervals. Examples include repetitive winking, grimacing, and shoulder shrugging. Causes include Tourette's syndrome and drugs such as phenothiazines and amphetamines.

Dystonia

Dystonic movements are similar to athetoid movements, but often involve larger portions of the body, including the trunk. Grotesque, twisted postures may result. Causes include drugs such as phenothiazines, primary torsion dystonia, and as illustrated, spasmodic torticollis.

Athetosis

Athetoid movements are slower and more twisting and writhing than choreiform movements, and have a larger amplitude. They most commonly involve the face and the distal extremities. Athetosis is often associated with spasticity. Causes include cerebral palsy.

Chorea

Choreiform movements are brief, rapid, jerky, irregular, and unpredictable. They occur at rest or interrupt normal coordinated movements. Unlike tics, they seldom repeat themselves. The face, head, lower arms, and hands are often involved. Causes include Sydenham's chorea (with rheumatic fever) and Huntington's disease.

Disorders of Speech

Disorders of speech fall into three groups: those affecting (1) the voice, (2) the articulation of words, and (3) the production and comprehension of language.

Aphonia refers to a loss of voice that accompanies disease affecting the larynx or its nerve supply. *Dysphonia* refers to less severe impairment in the volume, quality, or pitch of the voice. For example, a person may be hoarse or only able to speak in a whisper. Causes include laryngitis, laryngeal tumors, and a unilateral vocal cord paralysis (Cranial Nerve X).

Dysarthria refers to a defect in the muscular control of the speech apparatus (lips, tongue, palate, or pharynx). Words may be nasal, slurred, or indistinct, but the central symbolic aspect of language remains intact. Causes include motor lesions of the central or peripheral nervous system, parkinsonism, and cerebellar disease.

Aphasia refers to a disorder in producing or understanding language. It is often caused by lesions in the dominant cerebral hemisphere, usually the left.

Compared below are two common types of aphasia: (1) Wernicke's, a fluent (receptive) aphasia, and (2) Broca's, a nonfluent (or expressive) aphasia. There are other less common kinds of aphasia, which are distinguished by differing responses on the specific tests listed. Neurologic consultation is usually indicated.

	Wernicke's Aphasia	Broca's Aphasia
Qualities of Spontaneous Speech	Fluent; often rapid, voluble, and effortless. Inflection and articulation are good, but sentences lack meaning and words are malformed (paraphasias) or invented (neologisms). Speech may be totally incomprehensible.	Nonfluent; slow, with few words and laborious effort. Inflection and articulation are impaired but words are meaningful, with nouns, transitive verbs, and important adjectives. Small grammatical words are often dropped.
Word Comprehension	Impaired	Fair to good
Repetition	Impaired	Impaired
Naming	Impaired	Impaired, though the patient recognizes objects
Reading Comprehension	Impaired	Fair to good
Writing	Impaired	Impaired
Location of Lesion	Posterior superior temporal lobe	Posterior inferior frontal lobe

Although it is important to recognize aphasia early in your encounter with a patient, its full diagnostic meaning does not become clear until you integrate this information with your neurologic examination.

TABLE
17-6

Nystagmus

Nystagmus is a rhythmic oscillation of the eyes, analogous to a tremor in other parts of the body. Its causes are multiple, including impairment of vision in early life, disorders of the labyrinth and the cerebellar system, and drug toxicity. Nystagmus occurs normally when a person watches a rapidly moving object (e.g., a passing train). Study the three characteristics of nystagmus described in this table so you can correctly identify the type of nystagmus. Then refer to textbooks of neurology for differential diagnoses.

Direction of Gaze in Which Nystagmus Appears

Example: Nystagmus on Right Lateral Gaze

Nystagmus Present (Right Lateral Gaze)

Although nystagmus may be present in all directions of gaze, it may appear or become accentuated only on deviation of the eyes (e.g., to the side or upward). On extreme lateral gaze, the normal person may show a few beats resembling nystagmus. Avoid making assessments in such extreme positions, and *observe for nystagmus only within the field of full binocular vision.*

Nystagmus Not Present (Left Lateral Gaze)

Direction of the Quick and Slow Components

Example: Left-Beating Nystagmus—a Quick Jerk to the Left in Each Eye, Then a Slow Drift to the Right

Nystagmus usually has both slow and fast movements, but *is defined by its fast phase.* For example, if the eyes jerk quickly to the patient's left and drift back slowly to the right, the patient is said to have *left-beating nystagmus.* Occasionally, nystagmus consists only of coarse oscillations without quick and slow components. It is then said to be *pendular.*

(table continues on page 724)

TABLE
17-6

Nystagmus (continued)

Plane of the Movements
Horizontal Nystagmus

The movement of nystagmus mat occur in one or more planes (i.e., horizontal, vertical, or rotary). It is the plane of the movements, not the direction of the gaze, that defines this variable.

Vertical Nystagmus

Rotary Nystagmus

Types of Facial Paralysis

Facial weakness or paralysis may result either (1) from a peripheral lesion of CN VII, the facial nerve, anywhere from its origin in the pons to its periphery in the face, or (2) from a central lesion involving the upper motor neuron system between the cortex and the pons. A peripheral lesion of CN VII, exemplified here by a Bell's palsy, is compared with a central lesion, exemplified by a left hemispheric cerebrovascular accident. These can be distinguished by their different effects on the upper part of the face.

The lower part of the face normally is controlled by upper motor neurons located on only one side of the cortex—the opposite side. *Left-sided damage to these pathways, as in a stroke, paralyzes the right lower face.* The upper face, however, is controlled by pathways from both sides of the cortex. Even though the upper motor neurons on the left are destroyed, others on the right remain, and the right upper face continues to function fairly well.

CN VII—Peripheral Lesion	CN VII—Central Lesion
Peripheral nerve damage to CN VII paralyzes the entire right side of the face, including the forehead.	

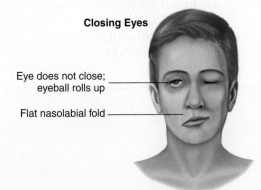

Closing Eyes (left)

Eye does not close; eyeball rolls up

Flat nasolabial fold

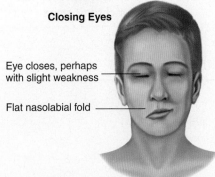

Closing Eyes (right)

Eye closes, perhaps with slight weakness

Flat nasolabial fold

Raising Eyebrows (left)

Forehead not wrinkled; eyebrow not raised

Paralysis of lower face

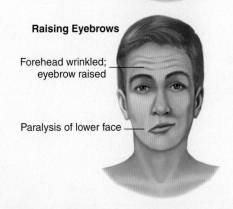

Raising Eyebrows (right)

Forehead wrinkled; eyebrow raised

Paralysis of lower face

TABLE
17-8

Disorders of Muscle Tone

	Spasticity	Rigidity	Flaccidity	Paratonia
Location of Lesion	Upper motor neuron of the corticospinal tract at any point from the cortex to the spinal cord	Basal ganglia system	Lower motor neuron system at any point from the anterior horn cell to the peripheral nerves	Both hemispheres, usually in the frontal lobes
Description	Increased muscle tone (*hypertonia*) that is rate dependent. Tone is greater when passive movement is rapid, and less when passive movement is slow. Tone is also greater at the extremes of the movement arc. During rapid passive movement, initial hypertonia may give way suddenly as the limb relaxes. This spastic "catch" and relaxation is known as "clasp-knife" resistance.	Increased resistance that persists throughout the movement arc, independent of rate of movement, is called *lead-pipe rigidity*. With flexion and extension of the wrist or forearm, a superimposed rachetlike jerkiness is called *cogwheel rigidity*.	Loss of muscle tone (*hypotonia*), causing the limb to be loose or floppy. The affected limbs may be hyperextensible or even flail-like. Flaccid muscles are also weak.	Sudden changes in tone with passive range of motion. Sudden loss of tone that increases the ease of motion is called *mitgehen* (moving with). Sudden increase in tone making motion more difficult is called *gegenhalten* (holding against).
Common Cause	Stroke, especially late or chronic stage	Parkinsonism	Guillain-Barré syndrome; also initial phase of spinal cord injury (spinal shock) or stroke	Dementia

Disorders of the Central and Peripheral Nervous Systems

Central Nervous System Disorders

(table continues on page 728)

Disorders of the Central and Peripheral Nervous Systems (continued)

Central Nervous System Disorders

Location of Lesion	Typical Findings		Deep Tendon Reflexes	Examples of Cause
	Motor	*Sensory*		
Cerebral Cortex (1)	Chronic contralateral corticospinal-type weakness and spasticity. Flexion is stronger than extension in the arm, plantar flexion is stronger than dorsiflexion in the foot, and the leg is externally rotated at the hip.	Contralateral sensory loss in the limbs and trunk on the same side as the motor deficits	↑	Cortical stroke
Brainstem (2)	Weakness and spasticity as above, plus cranial nerve deficits such as diplopia (from weakness of the extraocular muscles) and dysarthria	Variable; no typical sensory findings	↑	Brainstem stroke, acoustic neuroma
Spinal Cord (3)	Weakness and spasticity as above, but often affecting both sides (when cord damage is bilateral), causing paraplegia or quadriplegia depending on the level of injury	Dermatomal sensory deficit on the trunk bilaterally at the level of the lesion, and sensory loss from tract damage below the level of the lesion	↑	Trauma, causing cord compression
Subcortical Gray Matter: Basal Ganglia (4)	Slowness of movement (bradykinesia), rigidity, and tremor	Sensation not affected	Normal or ↓	Parkinsonism
Cerebellar (not illustrated)	Hypotonia, ataxia, and other abnormal movements, including nystagmus, dysdiadochokinesis, and dysmetria	Sensation not affected	Normal or ↓	Cerebellar stroke, brain tumor

(table continues on page 729)

Peripheral Nervous System Disorders

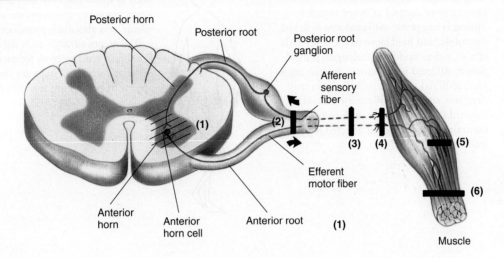

Typical Findings

Location of Lesion	Motor	Sensory	Deep Tendon Reflexes	Examples of Cause
Anterior Horn Cell (1)	Weakness and atrophy in a segmental or focal pattern; fasciculations	Sensation intact	↓	Polio, amyotrophic lateral sclerosis
Spinal Roots and Nerves (2)	Weakness and atrophy in a root-innervated pattern; sometimes with fasciculations	Corresponding dermatomal sensory deficits	↓	Herniated cervical or lumbar disc
Peripheral Nerve— Mononeuropathy (3)	Weakness and atrophy in a peripheral nerve distribution; sometimes with fasciculations	Sensory loss in the pattern of that nerve	↓	Trauma
Peripheral Nerve— Polyneuropathy (4)	Weakness and atrophy more distal than proximal; sometimes with fasciculations	Sensory deficits, commonly in stocking-glove distribution	↓	Peripheral polyneuropathy of alcoholism, diabetes
Neuromuscular Junction (5)	Fatigability more than weakness	Sensation intact	Normal	Myasthenia gravis
Muscle (6)	Weakness usually more proximal than distal; fasciculations rare	Sensation intact	Normal or ↓	Muscular dystrophy

Abnormalities of Gait and Posture

Spastic Hemiparesis

Seen in corticospinal tract lesion in stroke, causing poor control of flexor muscles during swing phase. Affected arm is flexed, immobile, and held close to the side, with elbow, wrists, and interphalangeal joints flexed. Affected leg extensors spastic; ankle plantar-flexed and inverted. Patients may drag toe, circle leg stiffly outward and forward (*circumduction*), or lean trunk to contralateral side to clear affected leg during walking.[38]

Scissors Gait

Seen in spinal cord disease causing bilateral lower extremity spasticity, including adductor spasm, and abnormal proprioception. Gait is stiff. Patients advance each leg slowly, and the thighs tend to cross forward on each other at each step. Steps are short. Patients appear to be walking through water.

Steppage Gait

Seen in foot drop, usually secondary to peripheral motor unit disease. Patients either drag the feet or lift them high, with knees flexed, and bring them down with a slap onto the floor, thus appearing to be walking up stairs. They cannot walk on their heels. The steppage gait may involve one or both legs. Tibialis anterior and toe extensors are weak.

Parkinsonian Gait

Seen in the basal-ganglia defects of Parkinson disease. Posture is stooped, with flexion of head, arms, hips, and knees. Patients are slow getting started. Steps are short and shuffling, with involuntary hastening (*festination*). Arm swings are decreased, and patients turn around stiffly—"all in one piece." Postural control is poor (*retropulsion*).

Cerebellar Ataxia

Seen in disease of the cerebellum or associated tracts. Gait is staggering, unsteady, and wide based, with exaggerated difficulty on turns. Patients cannot stand steadily with feet together, whether eyes are open or closed. Other cerebellar signs are present such as dysmetria, nystagmus, and intention tremor.

Sensory Ataxia

Seen in loss of position sense in the legs (with polyneuropathy or posterior column damage). Gait is unsteady and wide based (with feet wide apart). Patients throw their feet forward and outward and bring them down, first on the heels and then on the toes, with a double tapping sound. They watch the ground for guidance when walking. With eyes closed, they cannot stand steadily with feet together (positive Romberg sign), and the staggering gait worsens.

TABLE
17-11

Metabolic and Structural Coma

Although there are many causes of coma, most can be classified as either *structural* or *metabolic*. Findings vary widely in individual patients; the features listed are general guidelines rather than strict diagnostic criteria. Remember that psychiatric disorders may mimic coma.

	Toxic–Metabolic	Structural
Pathophysiology	Arousal centers poisoned or critical substrates depleted	Lesion destroys or compresses brainstem arousal areas, either directly or secondary to more distant expanding mass lesions.
Clinical Features		
• Respiratory pattern	If regular, may be normal or hyperventilation. If irregular, usually Cheyne-Stokes	Irregular, especially Cheyne-Stokes or ataxic breathing. Also with selected stereotypical patterns like "apneustic" respiration (peak inspiratory arrest) or central hyperventilation
• Pupillary size and reaction	Equal, reactive to light. If *pinpoint* from opiates or cholinergics, you may need a magnifying glass to see the reaction.	Unequal or unreactive to light (fixed) *Midposition, fixed*—suggests midbrain compression
	May be unreactive if *fixed and dilated* from anticholinergics or hypothermia	*Dilated, fixed*—suggests compression of CN III from herniation
• Level of consciousness	Changes *after* pupils change	Changes *before* pupils change
Examples of Cause	Uremia, hyperglycemia	Epidural, subdural, or intracerebral hemorrhage
	Alcohol, drugs, liver failure	
	Hypothyroidism, hypoglycemia	Cerebral infarct or embolus
	Anoxia, ischemia	Tumor, abscess
	Meningitis, encephalitis	Brainstem infarct, tumor, or hemorrhage
	Hyperthermia, hypothermia	Cerebellar infarct, hemorrhage, tumor, or abscess

TABLE
17-12

Pupils in Comatose Patients

Pupillary size, equality, and light reactions help in assessing the cause of coma and in determining the region of the brain that is impaired. Remember that unrelated pupillary abnormalities, including miotic drops for glaucoma or mydriatic drops for a better view of the ocular fundi, may have preceded the coma.

Small or Pinpoint Pupils

Bilaterally small pupils (1–2.5 mm) suggest (1) damage to the sympathetic pathways in the hypothalamus, or (2) metabolic encephalopathy (a diffuse failure of cerebral function that has many causes, including drugs). Light reactions are usually normal.

Pinpoint pupils (< 1 mm) suggest (1) a hemorrhage in the pons, or (2) the effects of morphine, heroin, or other narcotics. The light reactions may be seen with a magnifying glass.

Midposition Fixed Pupils

Pupils that are in the *midposition or slightly dilated* (4–6 mm) and are *fixed to light* suggest structural damage in the midbrain.

Large Pupils

Bilaterally fixed and dilated pupils may be due to severe anoxia and its sympathomimetic effects, as seen after cardiac arrest. They may also result from atropinelike agents, phenothiazines, or tricyclic antidepressants.

Bilaterally large reactive pupils may be due to cocaine, amphetamine, LSD, or other sympathetic nervous system agonists.

One Large Pupil

A pupil that is *fixed and dilated* warns of herniation of the temporal lobe, causing compression of the oculomotor nerve and midbrain.

Abnormal Postures in Comatose Patients

Plantar flexed   Internally rotated   Flexed   Adducted   Flexed

Decorticate Rigidity (Abnormal Flexor Response)

In *decorticate rigidity*, the upper arms are flexed tight to the sides with elbows, wrists, and fingers flexed. The legs are extended and internally rotated. The feet are plantar flexed. This posture implies a destructive lesion of the corticospinal tracts within or very near the cerebral hemispheres. When unilateral, this is the posture of chronic spastic hemiplegia.

Externally rotated   Flaccid

Hemiplegia (Early)

Sudden unilateral brain damage involving the corticospinal tract may produce a *hemiplegia* (one-sided paralysis), which early in its course is flaccid. Spasticity will develop later. The paralyzed arm and leg are slack. They fall loosely and without tone when raised and dropped to the bed. Spontaneous movements or responses to noxious stimuli are limited to the opposite side. The leg may lie externally rotated. One side of the lower face may be paralyzed, and that cheek puffs out on expiration. Both eyes may be turned away from the paralyzed side.

Plantar flexed   Flexed   Pronated   Extended   Adducted

Decerebrate Rigidity (Abnormal Extensor Response)

In *decerebrate rigidity*, the jaws are clenched and the neck is extended. The arms are adducted and stiffly extended at the elbows, with forearms pronated, wrists and fingers flexed. The legs are stiffly *extended at the knees*, with the feet plantar flexed. This posture may occur spontaneously or only in response to external stimuli such as light, noise, or pain. It is caused by a lesion in the diencephalon, midbrain, or pons, although severe metabolic disorders such as hypoxia or hypoglycemia may also produce it.

Special Populations

Assessing Children: Infancy Through Adolescence

Peter G. Szilagyi, MD, MPH

This chapter has been reorganized in this edition to better highlight issues of relevance to each pediatric age group. The content begins with a section on general principles of development and key components of health promotion. It then includes sections on newborns, infants, young and school-aged children, and adolescents, with relevant discussions of development, history taking, health promotion and counseling, and techniques of examination for each. Many new evidence-based citations are woven throughout the chapter as well. The chapter concludes with a detailed sample write-up, an updated Bibliography, and pertinent Tables of Abnormalities.

Guide to Chapter Organization

General Principles of Child Development
Health Promotion and Counseling: Key Components
Assessing the Newborn
    Immediate Assessment at Birth
    Assessment Several Hours After Birth
Assessing the Infant
    Development
    The Health History
    Health Promotion and Counseling
    Techniques of Examination
Assessing Young and School-Aged Children
    Development
    The Health History
    Health Promotion and Counseling
    Techniques of Examination
Assessing Adolescents
    Development: 11 to 20 Years
    The Health History
    Health Promotion and Counseling
    Techniques of Examination
Recording Your Findings

Often, neophyte and even some veteran examiners are intimidated when approaching a tiny baby or a screaming child, especially under the critical eyes of anxious parents. Although it takes courage, you will come to accept the challenge easily and to enjoy almost all such encounters.

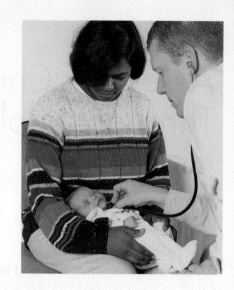

Review Chapter 1, Overview: Physical Examination and History Taking, for the methods and sequence of examining adults. When examining infants and children, the sequence should vary according to the child's age and comfort level. *Perform nondisturbing maneuvers early and potentially distressing maneuvers near the end of the examination.* For example, palpate the head and neck and auscultate the heart and lungs early, and examine the ears and mouth and palpate the abdomen near the end. If the child reports pain in one area, examine that part last.

The format of the pediatric medical record is the same as that of the adult record. Although the sequence of the physical examination may vary, convert your clinical findings back into the traditional written format.

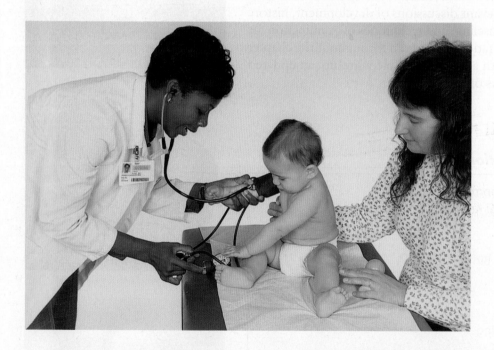

GENERAL PRINCIPLES OF CHILD DEVELOPMENT

Childhood is a period of remarkable physical, cognitive, and social growth—by far the greatest in a person's lifetime. Within a few short years, children physically increase 20-fold, acquire sophisticated language and reasoning, develop complex social interactions, and become mature adults. What a journey!

Understanding the normal physical, cognitive, and social development of children facilitates effective interviews and physical examinations, and helps clinicians to distinguish normal and abnormal findings.

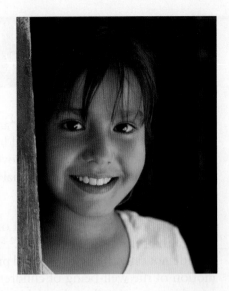

Four Principles of Child Development[1]

- Child development proceeds along a predictable pathway.
- The range of normal development is wide.
- Various physical, social, and environmental factors, as well as diseases, can affect child development and health.
- The child's developmental level affects how you conduct the history and physical examination.

- The first principle of *child development* is that it *proceeds along a predictable pathway* governed by the maturing brain. You can measure age-specific milestones and characterize development as normal or abnormal according to the child's achievement of them. Once the child reaches a milestone, he or she proceeds to the next. Loss of milestones is concerning. Because physical examination takes place at one point in time, you need to determine where the child fits along a developmental trajectory.

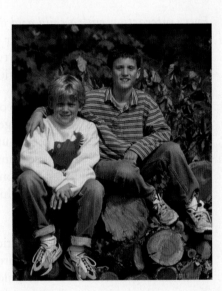

- The second principle is that the *range of normal development is wide*. Children mature at different rates. Each child's physical, cognitive, and social development should fall within a broad developmental range.

- The third principle recognizes that *various physical, social, and environmental factors, as well as diseases, can affect child development and health*. For example, chronic illnesses, child abuse, and poverty can all cause detectable physical abnormalities and alter the rate and course of development. Children with physical or cognitive disabilities may not follow the expected age-specific developmental trajectory. Tailor the physical examination to the child's developmental level.

- A fourth principle, specific to the pediatric examination, is that *the child's developmental level affects how you conduct the medical history and physical examination*. For example, interviewing a 5-year-old is fundamentally different from interviewing an adolescent. The physical examination of a curious toddler who is dismantling the examination room has little in common with that of a shy teenager. Both order and style differ from the examination of an adult. You must adjust your physical examination to the developmental level of the child while simultaneously attempting to ascertain that developmental level. An understanding of normal child development helps you achieve these tasks.

HEALTH PROMOTION AND COUNSELING: KEY COMPONENTS

Benjamin's Franklin's advice that "an ounce of prevention is worth a pound of cure" is particularly true for children and adolescents because prevention at a young age can result in improved health outcomes for decades. Pediatric clinicians dedicate substantial time to health supervision visits and health promotion activities.

Several national and international organizations have identified guidelines for health promotion for children.[2-5] Current concepts of health promotion include not only the detection and prevention of disease but also active promotion of the well-being of children and their families, spanning physical, cognitive, emotional, and social health.

Every interaction with a child and family is an opportunity for health promotion! From your interview to your physical examination, think about your interactions as opportunities for two things: the traditional detection of medical problems and the promotion of health. What a priceless gift!

Capitalize on your examination to offer age-appropriate guidance about the child's development. Provide suggestions about reading, conversing, playing music, and optimizing opportunities for gross and fine motor development. Advise parents about upcoming developmental stages and strategies to encourage their child's development. Remember, parents are the major agents of health promotion for children, and your advice is implemented through them.

The American Academy of Pediatrics (AAP) publishes guidelines for *health supervision visits* and key age-appropriate components of these visits (see www.aap.org). Remember that children and adolescents who have a chronic illness or high-risk family or environmental circumstances will probably require more frequent visits and more intensive health promotion. Key health-promotion issues and strategies, tailored for specific age groups, are found throughout this chapter.

Integrate explanations of your physical findings with health promotion. For example, provide advice about expected maturational changes or how health behaviors can affect physical findings (e.g., exercise may reduce blood pressure and obesity). Be sure to demonstrate the relationship between healthy lifestyles and physical health.

Childhood immunizations are a mainstay for health promotion and have been heralded as the most significant medical achievement of public health worldwide. The childhood immunization schedule changes yearly, and updates are published widely and disseminated on Web sites of the Centers for Disease Control and Prevention and the AAP.[6,7] The figures on the next two pages show the 2008 U.S. Immunization Schedule.

Recommended Immunization Schedule for Persons Aged 0–18 Years—UNITED STATES•2008
For those who fall behind or start late, see the catch-up schedule

Vaccine ▼ Age ►	Birth	1 month	2 months	4 months	6 months	12 months	15 months	18 months	19–23 months	2–3 years	4–6 years
Hepatitis B	HepB	HepB			HepB						
Rotavirus			Rota	Rota	Rota						
Diphtheria, Tetanus, Pertussis			DTaP	DTaP	DTaP		DTaP				DTaP
Haemophilus influenzae type b			Hib	Hib	*Hib*	Hib					
Pneumococcal			PCV	PCV	PCV	PCV				PPV	
Inactivated Poliovirus			IPV	IPV		IPV					IPV
Influenza						Influenza (Yearly)					
Measles, Mumps, Rubella						MMR					MMR
Varicella						Varicella					Varicella
Hepatitis A						HepA (2 doses)				HepA Series	
Meningococcal										MCV4	

Range of recommended ages

Certain high-risk groups

Vaccine ▼ Age ►	7-10 years	11-12 years	13-18 years
Diphtheria, Tetanus, Pertussis		Tdap	Tdap
Human Papillomavirus		HPV (3 doses)	HPV Series
Meningococcal	MCV4	MCV4	MCV4
Pneumococcal	PPV		
Influenza	Influenza (Yearly)		
Hepatitis A	HepA Series		
Hepatitis B	HepB Series		
Inactivated Poliovirus	IPV Series		
Measles, Mumps, Rubella	MMR Series		
Varicella	Varicella Series		

Range of recommended ages

Catch-up immunization

Certain high-risk groups

This schedule indicates the recommended ages for routine administration of currently licensed childhood vaccines, as of December 1, 2007, for children aged 0–18 years. Additional information is available at **www.cdc.gov/vaccines/recs/schedules**. Any dose not administered at the recommended age should be administered at any subsequent visit, when indicated and feasible. Additional vaccines may be licensed and recommended during the year. Licensed combination vaccines may be used whenever any components of the combination are indicated and other components of the vaccine are not contraindicated and if approved by the Food and Drug Administration for that dose of the series. **Providers should consult the respective Advisory Committee on Immunization Practices statement for detailed recommendations, including for high risk conditions:** http://www.cdc.gov/vaccines/pubs/ACIP-list.htm. Clinically significant adverse events that follow immunization should be reported to the Vaccine Adverse Event Reporting System (VAERS). Guidance about how to obtain and complete VAERS form is available at www.vaers.hhs.gov or by telephone, **800-822-7967**.

Catch-up Immunization Schedule

UNITED STATES • 2008

for Persons Aged 4 Months–18 Years Who Start Late or Who Are More Than 1 Month Behind

The table below provides catch-up schedules and minimum intervals between doses for children whose vaccinations have been delayed. A vaccine series does not need to be restarted, regardless of the time that has elapsed between doses. Use the section appropriate for the child's age.

Vaccine	Minimum Age for Dose 1	Minimum Interval Between Doses			
		Dose 1 to Dose 2	Dose 2 to Dose 3	Dose 3 to Dose 4	Dose 4 to Dose 5
CATCH-UP SCHEDULE FOR PERSONS AGED 4 MONTHS–6 YEARS					
Hepatitis B	Birth	4 weeks	**8 weeks** (and 16 weeks after first dose)		
Rotavirus	6 wks	4 weeks	4 weeks		
Diphtheria, Tetanus, Pertussis	6 wks	4 weeks	4 weeks	6 months	6 months
***Haemophilus influenzae* type b**	6 wks	**4 weeks** if first dose administered at younger than 12 months of age / **8 weeks (as final dose)** if first dose administered at age 12-14 months / **No further doses needed** if first dose administered at 15 months of age or older	**4 weeks** if current age is younger than 12 months / **8 weeks (as final dose)** if current age is 12 months or older and second dose administered at younger than 15 months of age / **No further doses needed** if previous dose administered at age 15 months or older	**8 weeks (as final dose)** This dose only necessary for children aged 12 months–5 years who received 3 doses before age 12 months	
Pneumococcal	6 wks	**4 weeks** if first dose administered at younger than 12 months of age / **8 weeks (as final dose)** if first dose administered at age 12 months or older or current age 24–59 months / **No further doses needed** for healthy children if first dose administered at age 24 months or older	**4 weeks** if current age is younger than 12 months / **8 weeks (as final dose)** if current age is 12 months or older / **No further doses needed** for healthy children if previous dose administered at age 24 months or older	**8 weeks (as final dose)** This dose only necessary for children aged 12 months–5 years who received 3 doses before age 12 months	
Inactivated Poliovirus	6 wks	4 weeks	4 weeks	4 weeks	
Measles, Mumps, Rubella	12 mos	4 weeks			
Varicella	12 mos	3 months			
Hepatitis A	12 mos	6 months			
CATCH-UP SCHEDULE FOR PERSONS AGED 7–18 YEARS					
Tetanus, Diphtheria/ Tetanus, Diphtheria, Pertussis	7 yrs	4 weeks	**4 weeks** if first dose administered at younger than 12 months of age / **6 months** if first dose administered at age 12 months or older	**6 months** if first dose administered at younger than 12 months of age	
Human Papillomavirus	9 yrs	4 weeks	12 weeks		
Hepatitis A	12 mos	6 months			
Hepatitis B	Birth	4 weeks	**8 weeks** (and 16 weeks after first dose)		
Inactivated Poliovirus	6 wks	4 weeks	4 weeks	4 weeks	
Measles, Mumps, Rubella	12 mos	4 weeks			
Varicella	12 mos	**4 weeks** if first dose administered at age 13 years or older / **3 months** if first dose administered at younger than 13 years of age			

Screening procedures are performed at certain ages. For all children, these include growth parameters and developmental screening at all ages, blood pressure after infancy, and vision and hearing screening at certain key ages. Screening procedures particularly recommended for high-risk patients include tests for lead poisoning, tuberculosis exposure, anemia, cholesterol, urinary tract infections, and sexually transmitted diseases. There is variation worldwide in recommendations for screening tests; the AAP recommendations are provided at www.aap.org.[2]

Anticipatory guidance is a major component of the pediatric visit. Key areas are shown on the next page and cover a broad range of topics, from purely "medical" to social and emotional health. All these factors affect children's health.

To achieve a healthier world, we *must* emphasize comprehensive and broadly defined health promotion during childhood. Our children's future depends on it.

Key Components of Pediatric Health Promotion

1. Age-appropriate developmental achievement of the child
   - Physical (maturation, growth, puberty)
   - Motor (gross and fine motor skills)
   - Cognitive (achievement of milestones, language, school performance)
   - Emotional (self-efficacy, self-esteem, independence, morality)
   - Social (social competence, self-responsibility, integration with family and community)
2. Health supervision visits
   - Periodic assessment of medical and oral health (per health supervision schedule)
   - Adjustment of frequency for children or families with special needs
3. Integration of physical examination findings with healthy lifestyles
4. Immunizations
5. Screening procedures
6. Anticipatory guidance[9]
   - Healthy habits
   - Nutrition and healthy eating
   - Safety and prevention of injury

   - Sexual development and sexuality
   - Self-responsibility and efficacy
   - Family relationships (interactions, strengths, supports)

   - Emotional and mental health
   - Oral health
   - Prevention or recognition of illness
   - Prevention of risky behaviors
   - School and vocation
   - Peer relationships
   - Community interactions
7. Partnership between health care provider and child, adolescent, and family

ASSESSING THE NEWBORN

The first year of life, infancy, is divided into the neonatal period (the first 28 days) and the postneonatal period (29 days to 1 year).

TIPS FOR EXAMINING NEWBORNS

- Examine the newborn in the presence of the parents.
- Swaddle and then undress the newborn as the examination proceeds.
- Dim the lights and rock the newborn to encourage the eyes to open.

(continued)

TIPS FOR EXAMINING NEWBORNS (CONTINUED)

- Observe feeding if possible, particularly breast-feeding.
- Demonstrate calming maneuvers to parents (e.g., swaddling).
- Observe and teach parents about transitions as the newborn arouses.
- A typical sequence for the examination for minimal disruption of the newborn:
  - Careful observation
  - Head, neck, heart, lungs, abdomen, genitourinary system
  - Lower extremities, back
  - Ears, mouth
  - Eyes, whenever they are spontaneously open
  - Skin, as you go along
  - Neurologic system
  - Hips

Often, the first pediatric examination outside the delivery room is performed in the hospital within 24 hours of birth.

If possible, do the physical examination in front of the parents so that they can interact with you and ask questions. Often parents have specific questions about their baby's physical appearance, so stating normal findings as you go can be quite reassuring. Observe parental bonding with the newborn, and watch how well the breast-feeding baby latches on and sucks. Breast-feeding is physiologically and psychologically optimal, but many mothers will need help and support at first. Early detection of difficulties and anticipatory guidance can promote and sustain breast-feeding.

Newborns are most responsive 1 to 2 hours after a feeding, when they are neither too satiated (becoming less responsive) nor too hungry (and often agitated). Start with the newborn swaddled and comfortable. Then undress the newborn as the examination proceeds, for gradual stimulation and arousal. If the newborn becomes agitated, use a pacifier or a bottle of formula (if not breast-feeding), or allow the baby to suck on your gloved finger. Reswaddle the baby long enough to complete the parts of examination that require a quiet baby.

 ## IMMEDIATE ASSESSMENT AT BIRTH

Examining newborns immediately after birth is important for determining general condition, developmental status, abnormalities in gestational development, and any congenital abnormalities. The examination may reveal diseases of cardiac, respiratory, or neurologic origin. Listen to the anterior thorax with your stethoscope, palpate the abdomen, and inspect the head, face, oral cavity, extremities, genitalia, and perineum.

Apgar Score. The Apgar score is the key assessment of the newborn immediately after birth. It contains five components for classifying the newborn's neurologic recovery from birth and immediate adaptation to extrauterine life. Score each newborn according to the following table, at 1 and 5 minutes after birth. Scoring is based on a 3-point scale (0, 1, or 2) for each component. Total scores may range from 0 to 10. Scoring may continue at 5-minute intervals until the score is greater than 7. If the 5-minute Apgar score is 8 or more, proceed to a more complete examination.[10]

● The Apgar Scoring System[10]

Assigned Score

Clinical Sign	0	1	2
Heart rate	Absent	<100	>100
Respiratory effort	Absent	Slow and irregular	Good; strong
Muscle tone	Flaccid	Some flexion of the arms and legs	Active movement
Reflex irritability*	No responses	Grimace	Crying vigorously, sneeze, or cough
Color	Blue, pale	Pink body, blue extremities	Pink all over

*Reaction to suction of nares with bulb syringe

1-Minute Apgar Score		5-Minute Apgar Score	
8–10	Normal	8–10	Normal
5–7	Some nervous system depression	0–7	High risk for subsequent central nervous system and other organ system dysfunction
0–4	Severe depression, requiring immediate resuscitation		

handwritten note:
* @ 1 min + 5 min
   – cont @ 5 min intervals until score is ≥ 7
   – ≥ 8 cont on w/ more complete/indepth exam

Gestational Age and Birth Weight. *Classify newborns according to their gestational age of maturity and birth weight.* These classifications help predict medical problems and morbidity. Some clinical practice guidelines target infants born before a certain gestational age or below specific birth weight parameters.

Gestational age is based on specific neuromuscular signs and physical characteristics that change with gestational maturity. The *Ballard Scoring System* estimates gestational age to within 2 weeks, even in extremely premature infants. Page 748 includes a complete Ballard Scoring System, with instructions for assessing neuromuscular and physical maturity.[11]

CLASSIFICATION BY GESTATIONAL AGE AND BIRTH WEIGHT

Gestational Age

Classification	Gestational Age
• Preterm	<37 wks (<259th day)
• Term	37–42 wks
• Postterm	>42 wks (>294th day)

Birth Weight

Classification	Weight
• Extremely low birth weight	<1,000 grams
• Very low birth weight	<1,500 grams
• Low birth weight	<2,500 grams
• Normal birth weight	≥2,500 grams

A useful classification, shown below, is derived from the gestational age and birth weight on the intrauterine growth curve.

● Newborn Classifications[10]

Category	Abbreviation	Percentile
Small for gestational age	SGA	<10th
Appropriate for gestational age	AGA	10–90th
Large for gestational age	LGA	>90th

The figure on the next page shows the intrauterine growth curves for the 10th and 90th percentiles and depicts the different categories of maturity for newborns based on gestational age and birth weight.

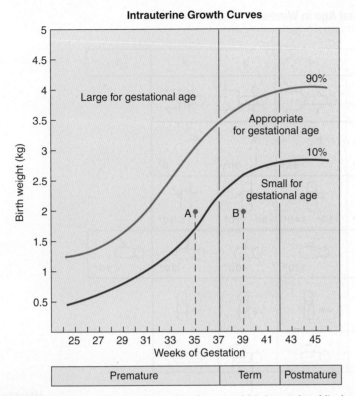

Intrauterine Growth Curves

Large for gestational age

Appropriate for gestational age

90%

10%

Small for gestational age

A

B

Birth weight (kg)

Weeks of Gestation

| Premature | Term | Postmature |

Level of intrauterine growth based on gestational age and birth weight of liveborn, single, white infants. Point A represents a premature infant, while point B indicates an infant of similar birth weight who is mature but SGA; the growth curves are representative of the 10th and 90th percentiles for all of the newborns in the sampling. (Adapted from Sweet YA. Classification of the low-birth-weight infant. In Klaus MH, Fanaroff AA. Care of the High-Risk Neonate, 3rd ed. Philadelphia, WB Saunders, 1986. Reproduced with permission.)

The three babies shown below were all <u>born at 32 weeks'</u> gestational age and weighed 600 g (SGA), 1400 g (AGA), and 2750 g (LGA). Each of these categories has a different mortality rate, highest for <u>preterm</u> SGA and LGA infants, and lowest for term AGA infants.

LGA infants may experience difficulties during birth. Infants of mothers with diabetes are often LGA and may have metabolic abnormalities shortly after birth, as well as congenital anomalies.

— more likely to develop DM2 later in life. [handwritten]

normal-ish [handwritten]

Preterm AGA infants are more prone to respiratory distress syndrome, apnea, patent ductus arteriosus with left-to-right shunt, and infection. *Preterm SGA infants* are more likely to experience asphyxia, hypoglycemia, and hypocalcemia.

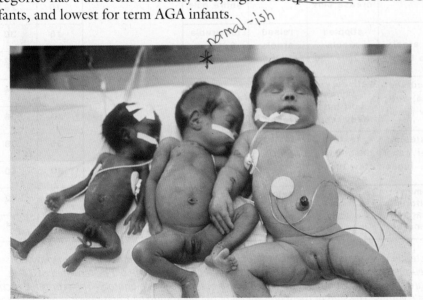

(Reprinted with permission from Korones SB: High-Risk Newborn Infants: The Basis for Intensive Nursing Care, 4th ed. St. Louis, CV Mosby, 1986.)

Ballard Scoring System for Determining Gestational Age in Weeks

Neuromuscular Maturity

	-1	0	1	2	3	4	5
Posture							
Square Window (wrist)	>90°	90°	60°	45°	30°	0°	
Arm Recoil		180°	140°-180°	110°-140°	90-110°	<90°	
Popliteal Angle	180°	160°	140°	120°	100°	90°	<90°
Scarf Sign							
Heel to Ear							

Physical Maturity

								Maturity Rating	
Skin	sticky friable transparent	gelatinous red, translucent	smooth pink, visible veins	superficial peeling &/or rash. few veins	cracking pale areas rare veins	parchment deep cracking no vessels	leathery cracked wrinkled	score	weeks
Lanugo	none	sparse	abundant	thinning	bald areas	mostly bald		-10	20
Plantar Surface	heel-toe 40-50mm: -1 <40mm: -2	>50mm no crease	faint red marks	anterior transverse crease only	creases ant. 2/3	creases over entire sole		-5	22
								0	24
Breast	imperceptible	barely perceptible	flat areola no bud	stippled areola 1-2mm bud	raised areola 3-4mm bud	full areola 5-10mm bud		5	26
								10	28
Eye/Ear	lids fused loosely:-1 tightly:-2	lids open pinna flat stays folded	sl. curved pinna; soft; slow recoil	well-curved pinna; soft but ready recoil	formed &firm instant recoil	thick cartilage ear stiff		15	30
								20	32
Genitals male	scrotum flat, smooth	scrotum empty faint rugae	testes in upper canal rare rugae	testes descending few rugae	testes down good rugae	testes pendulous deep rugae		25	34
								30	36
Genitals female	clitoris prominent labia flat	prominent clitoris small labia minora	prominent clitoris enlarging minora	majora & minora equally prominent	majora large minora small	majora cover clitoris & minora		35	38
								40	40
								45	42
								50	44

The Neuromuscular Maturity Criteria are depicted in the top half of the figure. Asphyxiated neonates or neonates obtunded by anesthetic agents or drugs will score lower on neuromuscular maturity criteria. In such instances, scoring should be repeated at 24 to 48 hours of age. The Physical Maturity Criteria are shown in the bottom half of the figure and are self-explanatory. The scores for each criterion are again the numbers at the top of the columns. The sum of the scores for all of the neuromuscular and physical maturity items provides an estimate of gestational age in weeks, using the maturity rating scale at the lower right portion of the figure. (Figure from Ballard JL, et al. J Pediatr 119:417, 1991.)

ASSESSMENT SEVERAL HOURS AFTER BIRTH

During the first day of life, newborns should have a comprehensive examination. Wait until 1 or 2 hours after a feeding, when the baby is most responsive, and ask the parents to remain in the room. Follow the sequence shown on pp. 743–744.

Observe the undressed newborn. Note the newborn's color, size, body proportions, nutritional status, and posture, as well as respirations and movements of the head and extremities. Most normal, full-term newborns lie in a symmetric position, with the limbs semiflexed and the legs partially abducted at the hip.

In *breech babies*, the legs and head are extended; the legs of a *frank breech baby* are abducted and externally rotated.

Note the baby's spontaneous motor activity, with flexion and extension alternating between the arms and legs. The fingers are usually flexed in a tight fist, but may extend in slow athetoid posturing movements. You will observe brief tremors of the body and extremities during vigorous crying, and even at rest.

By 4 days after birth, tremors at rest signal central nervous system disease from various possible causes, ranging from *asphyxia* to *drug withdrawal.*

Studies by Dr. T. Berry Brazelton and others have demonstrated the wide range of abilities in newborns, which are described below. Parents will be delighted by these abilities.

Asymmetric movements of the arms or legs at any time suggest *central* or *peripheral neurologic deficits, birth injury* (such as a fractured clavicle or brachial plexus injury), or *congenital anomalies.*

WHAT A NEWBORN CAN DO*

Core Elements

- Newborns use all five senses. For example, they prefer to look at human faces and turn to a parent's voice.
- Newborns are unique individuals. Marked differences exist in temperaments, personality, behavior, and learning.
- Newborns interact dynamically with caregivers—a two-way street!

Examples of Complex Newborn Behavior

Habituation	Ability to selectively and progressively shut out negative stimuli (e.g., a repetitive sound)
Attachment	A reciprocal, dynamic process of interacting and bonding with the caregiver
State Regulation	Ability to modulate the level of arousal in response to different degrees of stimulation (e.g., self-consoling)
Perception	Ability to regard faces, turn to voices, quiet in presence of singing, track colorful objects, respond to touch, and recognize familiar scents

*Points from T. Berry Brazelton, MD.[12]

Newborns who cannot perform many of these behaviors may have a neurologic condition, drug withdrawal, or a serious illness.

ASSESSING THE INFANT

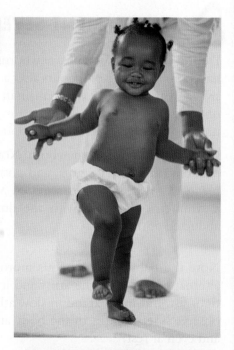

DEVELOPMENT

Physical Development.[13]   Physical growth during infancy is faster than at any other age. By 1 year, the infant's birth weight should have tripled and height increased by 50%.

The figure below shows the amazing developmental progression in infancy. Even newborns have surprising abilities, such as fixing upon and following human faces. Neurologic development progresses centrally to peripherally. Thus, newborns learn head control before trunk control and use of arms and legs before use of hands and fingers.

Activity, exploration, and environmental manipulation contribute to learning. By 3 months, normal infants lift the head and clasp the hands. By 6 months, they roll over, reach for objects, turn to voices, and possibly sit with support. With increasing peripheral coordination, infants reach for objects, transfer them from hand to hand, crawl, stand by holding on, and play with objects by banging and grabbing. A 1-year-old may be standing and putting everything in the mouth.[14]

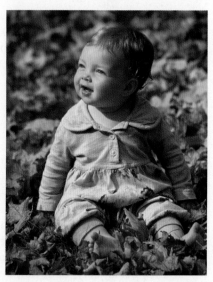

Cognitive and Language Development.   Exploration fosters increased understanding of self and environment. Infants learn cause and effect (e.g., shaking a rattle produces sound), object permanence, and use of tools. By 9 months, they may recognize the examiner as a stranger deserving wary cooperation, seek comfort from parents during examinations, and actively manipulate reachable objects (e.g., equipment). Language development proceeds from cooing at 2 months, to babbling at 6 months, to saying 1 to 3 words by 1 year.[15]

Social and Emotional Development.   Understanding of self and family also matures. Social tasks include bonding, attachment to caregivers, and trust that they will meet needs. Temperaments vary. Some infants are predictable, adaptable, and respond positively to new stimuli; others are less so and respond intensely or negatively. Because environment affects social development, observe the infant's interactions with caregivers.

Developmental Milestones During Infancy[13]

	Birth	1m	2m	3m	4m	5m	6m	7m	8m	9m	10m	11m	12m
Physical	Fixes/follows			Rolls over			Sits		Pulls to stand		Stands		Walks
	Head control			Grasps rattle			Thumb-finger grasp				Crawls		
Cognitive/ Language	Responds to sounds	Squeals		Imitates speech sounds			Dada/Mama specific				2 words		3 words
Social/ Emotional	Smiles				Works for toy						Imitates activities		
	Regards face					Feeds self			Indicates wants			Uses spoon	

THE HEALTH HISTORY

Use developmentally appropriate methods such as *distraction* and *play* to examine the infant. Because infants pay attention to one thing at a time, it is relatively easy to bring the infant's attention to something other than the examination being performed. Distract the infant with a moving object, a flashing light, a game of peek-a-boo, tickling, or any sort of noise.

If you cannot distract the infant or make the awake infant attend to an object, your face, or a sound, consider a possible *visual* or *hearing deficit.*

TIPS FOR EXAMINING INFANTS

- Approach the infant gradually, using a toy or object for distraction.
- Perform much of the examination with the infant in the parent's lap.
- Speak softly to the infant or mimic the infant's sounds to attract attention.
- If the infant is cranky, make sure he or she is well fed before proceeding.
- Ask a parent about the infant's strengths to elicit useful developmental and parenting information.

General Guidelines

Start with the infant sitting or lying in the parent's lap. If the infant is tired, hungry, or ill, ask the parent to hold the baby against the parent's chest. Make sure appropriate toys, a blanket, or other familiar objects are nearby. A hungry infant may need to be fed first.

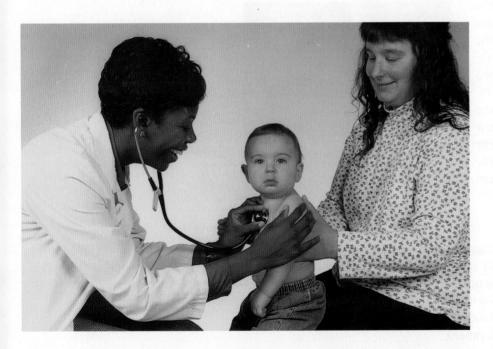

Observe parent–infant interactions. Watch the parent's affect when talking about the infant. Note the parent's manner of holding, moving, dressing, and comforting the infant. Assess and comment on positive interactions, such as the obvious pride in the mother's face above.

Observation of the infant's communication with the parent can reveal abnormalities such as *developmental delay, language delay,*

Infants usually do not object to removal of their clothing. To keep yourself and your surroundings dry, it is wise to leave the diaper in place throughout the examination; remove it only to examine the genitals, rectum, lower spine, and hips.

Testing for Developmental Milestones

Because you'll want to measure the infant's best performance, checking milestones is best at the end of the interview, just before the examination. This "fun and games" interlude also enhances cooperation during the examination. Experienced clinicians can weave the developmental examination into the other parts of the examination. The table on p. 750 shows some key physical or motor, cognitive or language, and social–emotional milestones during the first year.

One standard for measuring developmental milestones throughout infancy and childhood is the Denver Developmental Screening Test (DDST). It is designed to detect developmental delays in four domains of development from birth through 6 years: personal–social, fine motor–adaptive, language, and gross motor.

The DDST form is shown on the following two pages and includes instructions for recording specific observations. Each test item is represented on the form under the age by a bar, which indicates when 25%, 50%, 75%, and 90% of children attain the milestones depicted. The *DDST is a measure of developmental attainment only in the categories indicated. The DDST is not a measure of intelligence.*

The DDST is a highly specific screening test, so that normal children will test as normal. However, the DDST is not very sensitive. Many children with mild developmental delay score as normal. In particular, the language section is sparse and misses children with mild language delay. Although the DDST is useful, other, more sophisticated instruments are available to assess motor, language, and social development.

Use the DDST as an adjunct to a comprehensive developmental examination. Suspected delays from the general examination or DDST warrant further evaluation. For babies born prematurely, adjust expected developmental milestones for the gestational age up to approximately 12 months.

hearing deficits, or *inadequate parental attachment.* Likewise, such observations may identify maladaptive nurturing patterns that may stem from *maternal depression* or *inadequate social support.*

Many disorders cause delays in more than one milestone. For most children with developmental delay, the causes are unknown. Some known causes include *abnormality in embryonic development* (e.g., prenatal insult, chromosomal problem); *hereditary and genetic disorders* (e.g., inborn errors, genetic abnormalities); *environmental and social problems* (e.g., insufficient stimulation); *pregnancy or perinatal problems* (e.g., placental insufficiency, prematurity); and *childhood diseases* (e.g., infection, trauma, chronic illness).

If a cooperative infant fails items on the DDST, developmental delay is possible, necessitating more precise testing and evaluation.

DENVER DEVELOPMENTAL SCREENING TEST

Denver II

Examiner:
Date:

Name:
Birthdate:
ID No.:

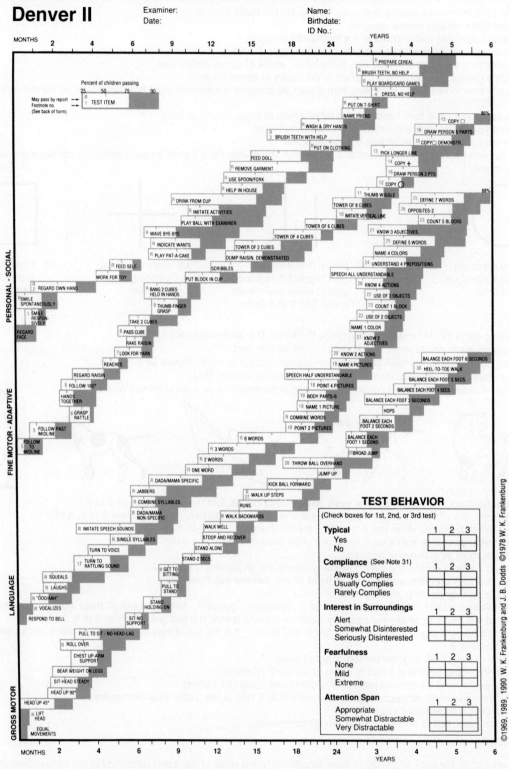

Testing kits, test forms, and reference manuals (which must be used to ensure accuracy in administration of the test) for the DDST may be ordered from Denver Developmental Materials Incorporated, P.O. Box 6919, Denver, CO 80206-0919. (Reprinted with permission from William K. Frankenburg, M.D.)

(figure continues on page 754)

DIRECTIONS FOR ADMINISTRATION

1. Try to get child to smile by smiling, talking or waving. Do not touch him/her.
2. Child must stare at hand several seconds.
3. Parent may help guide toothbrush and put toothpaste on brush.
4. Child does not have to be able to tie shoes or button/zip in the back.
5. Move yarn slowly in an arc from one side to the other, about 8" above child's face.
6. Pass if child grasps rattle when it is touched to the backs or tips of fingers.
7. Pass if child tries to see where yarn went. Yarn should be dropped quickly from sight from tester's hand without arm movement.
8. Child must transfer cube from hand to hand without help of body, mouth, or table.
9. Pass if child picks up raisin with any part of thumb and finger.
10. Line can vary only 30 degrees or less from tester's line.
11. Make a fist with thumb pointing upward and wiggle only the thumb. Pass if child imitates and does not move any fingers other than the thumb.

12. Pass any enclosed form. Fail continuous round motions.
13. Which line is longer? (Not bigger.) Turn paper upside down and repeat. (pass 3 of 3 or 5 of 6)
14. Pass any lines crossing near midpoint.
15. Have child copy first. If failed, demonstrate.

When giving items 12, 14, and 15, do not name the forms. Do not demonstrate 12 and 14.

16. When scoring, each pair (2 arms, 2 legs, etc.) counts as one part.
17. Place one cube in cup and shake gently near child's ear, but out of sight. Repeat for other ear.
18. Point to picture and have child name it. (No credit is given for sounds only.)
    If less than 4 pictures are named correctly, have child point to picture as each is named by tester.

19. Using doll, tell child: Show me the nose, eyes, ears, mouth, hands, feet, tummy, hair. Pass 6 of 8.
20. Using pictures, ask child: Which one flies?... says meow?... talks?... barks?... gallops? Pass 2 of 5, 4 of 5.
21. Ask child: What do you do when you are cold?... tired?... hungry? Pass 2 of 3, 3 of 3.
22. Ask child: What do you do with a cup? What is a chair used for? What is a pencil used for?
    Action words must be included in answers.
23. Pass if child correctly places <u>and</u> says how many blocks are on paper. (1, 5)
24. Tell child: Put block **on** table; **under** table; **in front of** me, **behind** me. Pass 4 of 4.
    (Do not help child by pointing, moving head or eyes.)
25. Ask child: What is a ball?... lake?... desk?... house?... banana?... curtain?... fence?... ceiling? Pass if defined in terms of use, shape, what it is made of, or general category (such as banana is fruit, not just yellow). Pass 5 of 8, 7 of 8.
26. Ask child: If a horse is big, a mouse is __? If fire is hot, ice is __? If the sun shines during the day, the moon shines during the __? Pass 2 of 3.
27. Child may use wall or rail only, not person. May not crawl.
28. Child must throw ball overhand 3 feet to within arm's reach of tester.
29. Child must perform standing broad jump over width of test sheet (8½ inches).
30. Tell child to walk forward, ∞◦∞◦∞◦∞◦➤ heel within 1 inch of toe. Tester may demonstrate.
    Child must walk 4 consecutive steps.
31. In the second year, half of normal children are noncompliant.

OBSERVATIONS:

Instructions printed on the back of the DDST form for administering some of the items contained in the Denver Developmental Screening Test. (Reprinted with permission from William K. Frankenburg, M.D.)

HEALTH PROMOTION AND COUNSELING

The AAP and an expert group, Bright Futures, recommend health supervision visits for infants and their parents when infants are the following ages: birth, within the first week, and 1, 2, 4, 6, 9, and 12 months. This is called the *Infant Periodicity Schedule*. Health supervision visits provide opportunities to answer questions for parents, assess the infant's growth and development, perform a comprehensive physical examination, and provide anticipatory guidance. Age-appropriate anticipatory guidance includes healthy habits and behaviors, social competence of caregivers, family relationships, and community interactions.

Although health supervision visits cover many topics, you will soon learn to enjoy and appreciate them. That infants generally are well during these visits enhances the quality of the experience. Parents usually are receptive to suggestions about health promotion, which can have major, long-term influences on the child and family. Strong interviewing skills are necessary as you discuss with families strategies to optimize the health and well-being of their infants.

Review the critical components of a health supervision visit for a 6-month-old. Adjust the content to the appropriate developmental level of the infant.

COMPONENTS OF A HEALTH SUPERVISION VISIT FOR A 6-MONTH OLD

Discussions with Parents

- Address parents' concerns/questions
- Provide advice
- Perform social history
- Assess development, nutrition, safety, oral health, family relationships, community

Developmental Assessment

- Assess milestones by history (see DDST)
- Measure milestones by examination (see DDST)

Physical Examination

- Perform a careful examination, including growth parameters with percentiles for age

Screening Tests

- Vision and hearing (by exam), possibly hematocrit and lead (if high risk), screen for social risk factors

Immunizations

- See schedule (pp. 741–742)

Anticipatory Guidance

Healthy Habits and Behaviors

- Injury and illness prevention
  Infant seat, rolling walker, poisons, tobacco exposure
- Nutrition
  Breast-feeding or bottle, solids, limit juice, prevent choking, over-feeding
- Oral health
  No bottle in bed, fluoride, brushing teeth

Parent–Infant Interaction

- Promoting development

Family Relationships

- Time for self; babysitters

Community Interaction

- Child care, resources

TECHNIQUES OF EXAMINATION

General Survey and Vital Signs

Measurement of the infant's body size (length, weight, and head circumference) and assessment of vital signs (blood pressure, pulse, respiratory rate, and temperature) are critical. Tables on the accompanying Web site show norms for blood pressure, height, weight, body mass index (BMI), and head circumference. Compare vital signs or body proportions with age-specific norms, because they change dramatically as children grow. Some pediatric practitioners also assess pain regularly, using standardized pain scales.

Generally, measurement deviations beyond two standards for age, or above the 95th percentile or below the 5th percentile, are indications for more detailed evaluation. These deviations may be the first and only indicators of disease (see examples on the Web site tables).

Somatic Growth. Measurement of growth is one of the most important indicators of infant health. Deviations may provide an early indication of an underlying problem. Compare growth parameters with respect to

A common cause of an apparent deviation in somatic growth is *measurement error*, attributed partly to the challenge of measuring a squirming infant or child. Confirm abnormalities by repeat measurement.

● Normal values for age and sex

● Prior readings on the same child, to assess trends

Measure growth parameters carefully, using consistent technique and, optimally, the same scales to measure height and weight.

The most important tools for assessing somatic growth are the growth charts, which are published by the National Center for Health Statistics (see accompanying Web site). All charts include height, weight, and head circumference for age, with one set for children up to 36 months and a second set for 2 to 18 years. Charts plotting weight by length as well as BMI are also available. These growth charts have percentile lines indicating the percentage of normal children above and below the child's measurement by chronologic age. Special growth charts are available for use in infants born prematurely, to correct for this result.

Although many normal infants cross percentiles on growth charts, a sudden or significant change in growth may indicate systemic disease due to various possible organ systems.

Length. For children younger than 2 years, measure body length by placing the child supine on a measuring board or in a measuring tray, as shown on the following page. Direct measurement of the infant using a tape measure is inaccurate unless an assistant holds the child still with hips and knees extended. Velocity growth curves are helpful in older children, especially those who are suspected of having endocrine disorders.

Reduced growth velocity, shown by a drop in height percentile on a growth curve, may signify a chronic condition. Comparison with normal standards is essential, because growth velocity normally is less during the second year than during the first year.

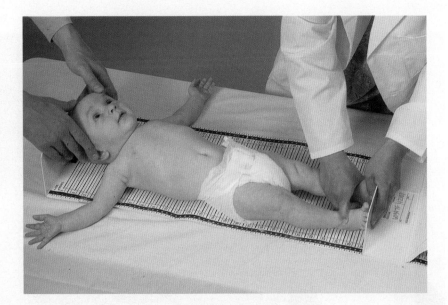

Chronic conditions causing reduced length or height include *neurologic, renal, cardiac*, and *endocrine disorders*.

Weight.   Weigh infants directly with an infant scale; this is more accurate than an indirect method based on weighing the parent and child together and subtracting the weight of the parent from the total weight. Infants should be clothed only in a diaper or weighed naked.

If the infant's weight is unexpectedly and significantly different than anticipated, redo the measurement to ensure accuracy.

Failure to thrive is inadequate weight gain for age. Common scenarios are:

● Growth <5th percentile for age
● Growth drop >2 quartiles in 6 months
● Weight for height <5th percentile

Causes include *environmental* or *psychosocial* factors and a variety of *gastrointestinal, neurologic, cardiac, endocrine, renal,* and other diseases.

Head Circumference.   The head circumference should be measured during the first 2 years of life, but measurement can be useful at any age to assess growth of the head. The head circumference in infants reflects the rate of growth of the cranium and the brain.

A small head size may be from *premature closure of the sutures* or *microcephaly*. Microcephaly may be familial or the result of various *chromosomal abnormalities, congenital infections, maternal metabolic disorders,* and *neurologic insults.*

An abnormally large head size (>97th percentile or 2 standard deviations above the mean) is *macrocephaly,* which may be from *hydrocephalus, subdural hematoma,* or rare causes like *brain tumor* or *inherited syndromes. Familial megaloencephaly* (large head) is a benign familial condition with normal brain growth.

Vital Signs

Blood Pressure.   Although obtaining accurate blood pressure readings in infants is challenging, this measurement is nevertheless important and should be performed at least once during infancy. You will need your skills in distraction or play, as shown in the accompanying photo.

The most easily used measure of systolic blood pressure in infants is the *Doppler method,* which detects arterial blood flow vibrations, converts them to systolic blood pressure levels, and transmits them to a digital read-out device.

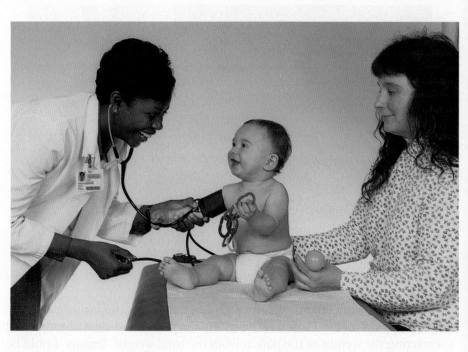

The systolic blood pressure gradually increases throughout childhood. For example, normal systolic pressure in males is about 70 mm Hg at birth, 85 mm Hg at 1 month, and 90 mm Hg at 6 months (see Web site).

Causes of *sustained hypertension* in newborns include renal artery disease (stenosis, thrombosis), congenital renal malformations, and coarctation of the aorta.

Pulse.   The heart rate of infants is more sensitive to the effects of illness, exercise, and emotion than that of adults.

● Heart Rates from Birth to 1 Year

Age	Average Heart Rate	Range
Birth 0–2	140	90–190
0–6 mo	130	80–180
6–12 mo	115	75–155

A pulse rate that is too rapid to count (usually >180–200/min) usually indicates *paroxysmal supraventricular tachycardia.*

Bradycardia may be from *drug ingestion, hypoxia, intracranial* or *neurologic conditions,* or, rarely, *cardiac arrhythmia* such as *heart block.*

You may have trouble obtaining an accurate pulse rate in a squirming infant. The best strategy is to palpate the femoral arteries in the inguinal area or the brachial arteries in the antecubital fossa, or to auscultate the heart.

Respiratory Rate.   As with heart rate, compared with that of adults, the respiratory rate in infants has a greater range and is more responsive to illness, exercise, and emotion. The rate of respirations per minute ranges between 30 and 60 in the newborn.

Extremely rapid and shallow respiratory rates are seen in newborns with *cyanotic cardiac disease* and right-to-left shunting, and metabolic acidosis.

The respiratory rate may vary considerably from moment to moment in the newborn, with alternating periods of rapid and slow breathing. The sleeping respiratory rate is most reliable. Respiratory rates during active sleep compared with quiet sleep may be up to 10 breaths per minute faster. The respiratory pattern should be observed for at least 60 seconds. In infancy and early childhood, diaphragmatic breathing is predominant; thoracic excursion is minimal.

Fever can raise respiratory rates in infants by up to 10 respirations per minute for each degree centigrade of fever.

Commonly accepted cutoffs for defining *tachypnea* are:

Tachypnea and increased respiratory effort in an infant are signs of possible pneumonia.

- Birth–2 months, >60/min

- 2–12 months, >50/min

Temperature. Because fever is so common in children, obtain an accurate body temperature when you suspect infection, collagen vascular disease, or malignancy. The techniques for obtaining rectal, oral, and auditory canal temperatures in adults are described on pages 120 to 121. Axillary and thermal-tape (temporal artery) skin temperature recordings in infants and children are inaccurate. Auditory canal temperatures are accurate.

Fever (>38.0°C or >100.0°F) in infants <2–3 months may be a sign of *serious infection* or disease. These infants should be evaluated promptly.

The technique for obtaining the *rectal temperature* is relatively simple. One method is illustrated below. Place the infant prone, separate the buttocks with the thumb and forefinger on one hand, and with the other hand gently insert a well-lubricated rectal thermometer, to a depth of 2 to 3 centimeters. Keep the thermometer in place for at least 2 minutes.

Body temperature in infants and children is less constant than in adults. The average rectal temperature is higher in infancy and early childhood, usually above 99.0°F (37.2°C) until after age 3 years. Body temperature may fluctuate as much as 3°F during a single day, approaching 101°F (38.3°C) in normal children, particularly in late afternoon and after vigorous activity.

Anxiety may elevate the body temperature of children. *Excessive bundling* of infants may elevate the skin temperature but not the core temperature.

Temperature instability in a newborn may result from sepsis, metabolic abnormality, or other serious conditions. Older infants rarely manifest temperature instability.

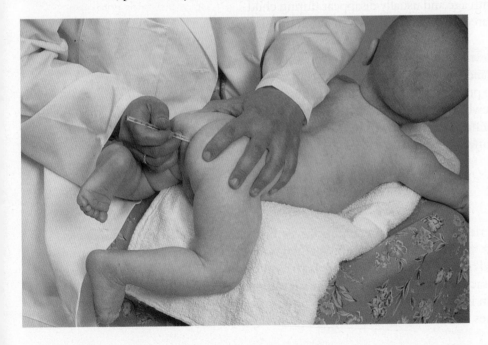

The Skin

Inspection. Examine the skin of the newborn or infant carefully to identify both normal markings and potentially abnormal ones. The photos on pages 762 to 764 demonstrate normal markings. The newborn's skin has a unique characteristic *texture and appearance.* The texture is soft and smooth because it is thinner than the skin of older children. Within the first 10 minutes after birth, a normal newborn progresses from generalized cyanosis to pinkness. In lighter-skinned infants, an erythematous flush, giving the skin the appearance of a "boiled lobster," is common during the first 8 to 24 hours, after which the normal pale pink coloring predominates.

You may be startled to observe the striking effects of vasomotor changes in the newborn's skin. Vasomotor changes in the dermis and subcutaneous tissue—a response to cooling or chronic exposure to radiant heat—can produce a lattice-like, bluish mottled appearance (*cutis marmorata*), particularly on the trunk, arms, and legs. This response to cold may last for months in normal infants. *Acrocyanosis,* a blue cast to the hands and feet when exposed to cold, is very common in newborns for the first few days and may recur throughout early infancy. Occasionally in newborns, a remarkable color change (*harlequin dyschromia*) appears, with transient cyanosis of one half of the body or one extremity, presumably from temporary vascular instability.

Note that the amount of melanin in the skin of newborns varies, affecting *pigmentation.* Black newborns may have a lighter skin color initially than later, except in the nail beds and genitalia, which are dark at birth. A dark or bluish pigmentation over the buttocks and lower lumbar regions is common in newborns of African, Asian, and Mediterranean descent. These areas, formerly called Mongolian spots, result from pigmented cells in the deep layers of the skin; they become less noticeable with age and usually disappear during childhood. Document these pigmented areas to avoid later concern about bruising.

At birth there is a fine, downy growth of hair called *lanugo* over the entire body, but especially the shoulders and back. This hair is shed within the first few weeks. Lanugo is prominent in premature infants. Hair thickness on the head varies considerably among newborns and fortunately is not predictive of later hair growth. All of the original hair is shed within months, replaced with a new crop, sometimes of a different color.

Inspect the newborn closely for a series of common skin conditions. At birth, a cheesy white material called *vernix caseosa,* composed of sebum and desquamated epithelial cells, covers the body. Some newborns have *edema* over their hands, feet, lower legs, pubis, and sacrum; this disappears within a few days. Superficial desquamation of the skin is often noticeable 24 to 36 hours after birth, particularly in post-term babies (>40 weeks' gestation).

Appears as vesicles/blotches all over/under skin surface

Cutis marmorata is prominent in *premature infants* and in infants with *congenital hypothyroidism* and *Down syndrome.*

If acrocyanosis does not disappear within 8 hours or with warming, *cyanotic congenital heart disease* should be considered.

Central cyanosis in a baby or child of any age should raise suspicion of *congenital heart disease.* The best area to look for central cyanosis is the tongue and oral mucosa, not the nail beds or the extremities.

Pigmented light-brown lesions (<1–2 cm at birth) are *café-au-lait spots.* Isolated lesions have no significance, but multiple lesions with smooth borders may suggest *neurofibromatosis* (see Table 18-2, Common Skin Rashes and Skin Findings in Newborns and Infants, p. 857).

Skin desquamation is rarely a sign of placental circulatory insufficiency or *congenital ichthyosis.*

You should be able to identify four common dermatologic conditions in newborns: *miliaria rubra, erythema toxicum, pustular melanosis,* and *milia.* All are found on pp. 762–763. None of these is clinically significant.

Note any signs of trauma from the birth process and the use of forceps or suction; these signs disappear but should prompt a careful neurologic examination.

Jaundice.   Carefully examine and touch the newborn's skin to assess the level of jaundice. Normal "physiologic" *jaundice,* which occurs in half of all newborns, appears on the 2nd or 3rd day, peaks at about the 5th day, and usually disappears within a week. Jaundice can best be appreciated in natural daylight rather than artificial light. Newborn jaundice seems to progress from head to toe, with more intense jaundice on the upper body and less intense yellow color in the lower extremities.

To detect jaundice, apply pressure to the skin (see photos) to press out the normal pink or brown color. A yellowish "blanching" indicates jaundice. Another technique is to press a glass slide against the skin to empty the capillary bed and observe for color contrast.

Pressing the red color from the skin allows better recognition of the yellow of jaundice. The infant on the left has no appreciable jaundice, while the infant on the right has a bilirubin level of 13 mg/dL (222 µmol/L). From Fletcher M. Physical Diagnosis in Neonatology. Philadelphia, Lippincott-Raven, 1998.

Vascular Markings.   A common *vascular marking* is the "salmon patch" (also known as *nevus simplex,* telangiectatic nevus, or capillary hemangioma). These flat, irregular, light pink patches (see p. 764) are most often seen on the nape of the neck ("stork bite"), upper eyelids, forehead, or upper lip ("angel kisses"). They are not true nevi, but result from distended capillaries. They almost all disappear by 1 year of age.

Palpation.   Palpate the newborn or infant's skin to assess the degree of hydration, or *turgor.* Roll a fold of loosely adherent skin on the abdominal wall between your thumb and forefinger to determine its consistency. The skin in well-hydrated infants returns to its normal position immediately upon release. Delay in return is a phenomenon called "tenting" and usually occurs in children with significant *dehydration.*

Both erythema toxicum and pustular melanosis may appear similar to the pathologic vesicular rash of *herpes simplex* or *Staphylococcus aureus* skin infection.

Midline hair tufts over the lumbosacral spine region suggest a *spinal cord defect.*

Jaundice within the first 24 hours of birth may be from *hemolytic disease of the newborn.*

Jaundice that persists beyond 2–3 weeks should raise suspicions of *biliary obstruction* or *liver disease.*

A unilateral dark, purplish lesion, or "port wine stain" over the distribution of the ophthalmic branch of the trigeminal nerve may be a sign of *Sturge-Weber syndrome,* which is associated with seizures, hemiparesis, glaucoma, and mental retardation.

Significant edema of the hands and feet of a newborn girl may be suggestive of *Turner's syndrome.*

Dehydration is a common problem in infants. Usual causes are insufficient intake or excess loss of fluids from diarrhea.

● Newborn Skin Findings

Finding	Description

Common Nonpathologic Conditions

Acrocyanosis

This bluish discoloration usually appears in the palms and soles. *Cyanotic congenital heart disease can present with severe acrocyanosis.*

Jaundice

Physiologic jaundice occurs during days 2 to 5 of life and progresses from head to toe as it peaks. *Extreme jaundice may signify a hemolytic process or biliary or liver disease.*

Common Benign Rashes

Miliaria rubra

Scattered vesicles on an erythematous base, usually on the face and trunk, result from obstruction of the sweat gland ducts; this condition disappears spontaneously within weeks.

(continued)

● **Newborn Skin Findings** (continued)

Finding	Description
Erythema toxicum	Usually appearing on days 2 to 3 of life, this rash consists of erythematous macules with central pinpoint vesicles scattered diffusely over the entire body. They appear similar to flea bites. These lesions are of unknown etiology but disappear within 1 week of birth.
Pustular melanosis	Seen more commonly in black infants, the rash presents at birth as small vesiculopustules over a brown macular base; these can last for several months.
Milia	Pinhead-sized smooth white raised areas without surrounding erythema on the nose, chin, and forehead result from retention of sebum in the openings of the sebaceous glands. Although occasionally present at birth, milia usually appears within the first few weeks and disappears over several weeks.

(continued)

● **Newborn Skin Findings** (continued)

Finding	Description
Benign Birthmarks	
Eyelid patch	This birthmark fades, usually within the first year of life.

| Salmon patch | Also called the "stork bite," this splotchy pink mark fades with age. |

Café-au-lait spots

These light-brown pigmented lesions usually have borders and are uniform. They are noted in more than 10% of black infants.

If more than 5 café-au-lait spots exist, consider the diagnosis of neurofibromatosis See Table 18-2, Common Skin Rashes and Skin Findings in Newborns and Infants (p. 857).

Mongolian spots

These are more common among dark-skinned babies. It is important to note them so that they are not mistaken for bruises.

The Head

At birth, a baby's head may seem relatively large to you. A newborn's head accounts for one fourth of the body length and one third of the body weight; these proportions change, so that by adulthood, the head accounts for one eighth of the body length and about one tenth of the body weight.

Sutures and Fontanelles.   Membranous tissue spaces called *sutures* separate the bones of the skull from one another. The areas where the major sutures intersect in the anterior and posterior portions of the skull are known as *fontanelles*. Examine the *sutures* and *fontanelles* carefully (see the figure below).

On palpation, the sutures feel like ridges and the fontanelles like soft concavities. The *anterior fontanelle* at birth measures 4 cm to 6 cm in diameter and usually closes between 4 and 26 months of age (90% between 7–19 mos). The *posterior fontanelle* measures 1 cm to 2 cm at birth and usually closes by 2 months.

An enlarged posterior fontanelle may be present in *congenital hypothyroidism.*

A bulging, tense fontanelle is observed in infants with *increased intracranial pressure,* which may be caused by *central nervous system infections, neoplastic disease,* or *hydrocephalus* (obstruction of the circulation of cerebrospinal fluid within the ventricles of the brain; see Table 18-5, p. 859).

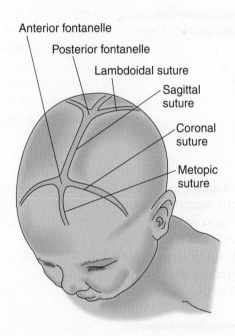

Anterior fontanelle
Posterior fontanelle
Lambdoidal suture
Sagittal suture
Coronal suture
Metopic suture

Carefully examine the fontanelle, because its fullness reflects *intracranial pressure*. Palpate the fontanelle while the baby is sitting quietly or being held upright. Experienced pediatric health care clinicians often palpate the fontanelles at the beginning of the examination. In normal infants, the anterior fontanelle is soft and flat. Increased intracranial pressure produces a bulging, full anterior fontanelle and is seen when a baby cries, vomits, or has underlying pathology. Pulsations of the fontanelle reflect the peripheral pulse.

Inspect the scalp veins carefully to assess for dilatation.

A depressed anterior fontanelle may be a sign of *dehydration.*

Overlap of the cranial bones at the sutures at birth, called *molding,* results from passage of the head through the birth canal; it disappears within 2 days.

Dilated scalp veins are indicative of long-standing *increased intracranial pressure.*

Skull Symmetry and Head Circumference. Assess *skull symmetry*. Various conditions can cause asymmetry; some are benign, while others reflect underlying pathology. Careful inspection of the skull from the front or back of the infant helps you assess its symmetry.

Look for asymmetric head swelling. A newborn's scalp may be swollen over the occipitoparietal region. This is called *caput succedaneum*, from capillary distention and extravasation of blood and fluid resulting from the vacuum effect of rupture of the amniotic sac. This swelling often crosses suture lines and resolves in 1 to 2 days.

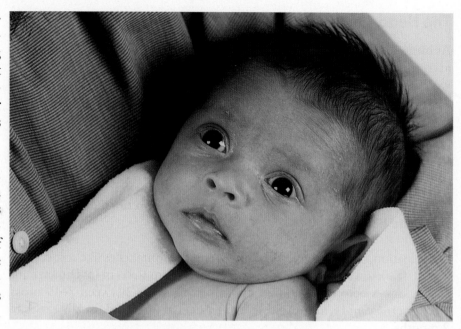

The premature infant's head at birth is relatively long in the occipitofrontal diameter and narrow in the bitemporal diameter (*dolichocephaly*). Usually the skull shape normalizes within 1 to 2 years.

Another type of localized swelling of the scalp is a *cephalohematoma*, caused by subperiosteal hemorrhage from the trauma of birth. This swelling does not cross over suture lines and resolves within 3 weeks. As the hemorrhage resolves and calcifies, there may be a palpable bony rim with a soft center.

Asymmetry of the cranial vault (*plagiocephaly*) occurs when an infant lies mostly on one side, resulting in a flattening of the parieto-occipital region on the dependent side and a prominence of the frontal region on the opposite side. It disappears as the baby becomes more active and spends less time in one position, and symmetry is almost always restored. Interestingly, the current trend to have newborns sleep on their backs to reduce the risk for sudden infant death syndrome has resulted in more cases of plagiocephaly.

Plagiocephaly may also reflect pathology such as *torticollis* from injury to the sternocleidomastoid muscle at birth, or *lack of stimulation* of the infant.

Measure the head circumference (p. 757) to detect abnormally large head size (*macrocephaly*) or small head size (*microcephaly*), which may signify an underlying disorder affecting the brain. Palpate along the suture lines. A raised, bony ridge at a suture line suggests craniosynostosis.

Premature closure of cranial sutures causes *craniosynostosis* (p. 859), with an abnormally shaped skull. *Sagittal suture* synostosis causes a narrow head from lack of growth of the parietal bones.

Palpate the infant's skull with care. The cranial bones usually appear "soft" or pliable; they will normally become firmer with increasing gestational age.

In *craniotabes,* the cranial bones feel springy. Craniotabes can result from increased intracranial pressure, as with *hydrocephaly,* metabolic disturbances such as *rickets,* and infection such as *congenital syphilis.*

Auscultating the skull is not useful in young children because a systolic or continuous bruit may normally be heard over the temporal areas. Older children with significant anemia may have a cranial bruit.

An *arteriovenous fistula* in the brain can produce a loud bruit.

Facial Symmetry.   Check the *face* of infants for symmetry. In utero positioning may result in transient facial asymmetries. If the head is flexed on the sternum, a shortened chin (*micrognathia*) may result. Pressure of the shoulder on the jaw may create a temporary lateral displacement of the mandible.

Micrognathia may also be part of a syndrome, such as the *Pierre Robin syndrome.*

Examine the face for an overall impression of the *facies;* it is helpful to compare with the face of the parents. A systematic assessment of a child with abnormal-appearing facies can identify specific syndromes.[16] The box below describes steps for evaluating facies.

Most developmental and genetic syndromes with abnormal facies also have other abnormalities.

EVALUATING A NEWBORN OR CHILD WITH POSSIBLE ABNORMAL FACIES

Carefully review the history, especially:

- Family history
- Pregnancy
- Perinatal history

Note abnormalities on other parts of the physical examination, especially:

- Growth
- Development
- Other dysmorphic somatic features

Perform measurements (and plot percentiles), especially:

- Head circumference
- Height
- Weight

Consider the three mechanisms of facial dysmorphogenesis:

- Deformations from intrauterine constraint
- Disruptions from amniotic bands or fetal tissue
- Malformations from an intrinsic abnormality in either the face/head or the brain

Examine the parents and siblings:

- Similarity to a parent may be reassuring (e.g., large head) but may also be an indication of a familial disorder.

Try to determine whether the facial features fit a recognizable syndrome, comparing with:

- References (including measurements) and pictures of syndromes
- Tables/databases of combinations of features.

A child with abnormal shape or length of palpebral fissures (see Table 18-6, pp. 860–861):

  Upslanting (Down syndrome)
  Down-slanting (Noonan's
   syndrome)
  Short (fetal alcohol effects)

Chvostek's Sign.   Percuss the cheek to check for *Chvostek's sign,* which is present in some metabolic disturbances and occasionally in normal infants. Percuss at the top of the cheek just below the zygomatic bone in front of the ear, using the tip of your index or middle finger.

A positive Chvostek's sign produces facial grimacing caused by repeated contractions of the facial muscles. A Chvostek sign is noted in cases of *hypocalcemic tetany, tetanus and tetany due to hyperventilation.*

The Eyes

Inspection.   Newborns keep their eyes closed except during brief awake periods. If you attempt to separate their eyelids, they will tighten them even more. Bright light causes infants to blink, so use subdued lighting. If you awaken the baby gently, turn down the lights, and support the baby in a sitting position, you will often find that the eyes open. The eyes of many newborns are edematous from the birth process.

You will have to be clever to examine the eyes of infants and young children and use some tricks to get them to cooperate. Small colorful toys are useful as fixation devices in examining the eyes.

Newborns may look at your face and follow a bright light if you catch them during an alert period. You can get some newborns to follow your face and turn their heads 90° to each side, much to the delight of parents.

Examine infants for *eye movements.* Hold the baby upright, supporting the head. Rotate yourself with the baby slowly in one direction. This usually causes the baby's eyes to open, allowing you to examine the sclerae, pupils, irises, and extraocular movements. The baby's eyes gaze in the direction you are turning. When the rotation stops, the eyes look in the opposite direction, after a few nystagmoid movements.

A newborn who truly cannot open an eye (even when awake and alert) may have *congenital ptosis.* Causes include birth trauma, third cranial nerve palsy, and mechanical problems.

If a newborn fails to gaze at you and follow your face during alert periods, pay particular attention to the rest of the ocular examination. While this may still be a normal child, the newborn may have *visual impairment.*

Nystagmus (wandering or shaking eye movements) persisting after a few days or persisting after the maneuver described on the left may indicate *poor vision* or *central nervous system disease.*

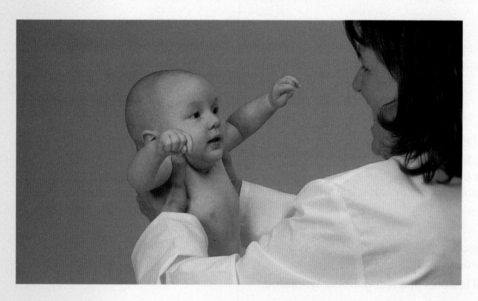

During the first 10 days of life, the eyes may be fixed, staring in one direction if just the head is turned without moving the body (*doll's eye reflex*). During the first few months of life, some infants have intermittent crossed eyes (*intermittent alternating convergent strabismus,* or *esotropia*) or laterally deviated eyes (*intermittent alternating divergent strabismus,* or *exotropia*).

Look for abnormalities or congenital problems in the *sclerae* and *pupils.* Subconjunctival hemorrhages are common in newborns.

Alternating convergent or divergent *strabismus* persisting beyond 3 months, or persistent strabismus of any type, may indicate *ocular motor weakness* or another abnormality in the visual system.

Colobomas may be seen with the naked eye and represent defects in the iris.

Observe pupillary reactions by response to light or by covering each eye with your hand and then uncovering it. Although there may be initial asymmetry in the size of the pupils, over time they should be equal in size and reaction to light.

Inspect the irises carefully for abnormalities.

Brushfield spots are a ring of white specks in the iris (see Table 18-8, p. 862). Although sometimes present in normal children, these strongly suggest *Down syndrome*.

Examine the *conjunctiva* for swelling or redness. You may note chemical conjunctivitis if silver nitrate was used after birth as prophylaxis against gonorrheal conjunctivitis (ophthalmia neonatorum). Most newborn nurseries use erythromycin ointment because it produces less irritation.

Persistent ocular discharge and tearing since birth may be from *dacryocystitis* or *nasolacrimal duct obstruction*.

You will not be able to measure the *visual acuity* of newborns or infants. You can use visual reflexes to indirectly assess vision: direct and consensual pupillary constriction in response to light, blinking in response to bright light (*optic blink reflex*), and blinking in response to quick movement of an object toward the eyes. During the first year of life, visual acuity sharpens as the ability to focus improves. Infants achieve the following visual milestones:

● Visual Milestones of Infancy[17]

Birth	Blinks, may regard face
1 month	Fixes on objects
1½–2 months	Coordinated eye movements
3 months	Eyes converge, baby reaches
12 months	Acuity around 20/50

Failure to progress along these visual developmental milestones may indicate *delayed visual maturation*.

Ophthalmoscopic Examination. For the *ophthalmoscopic examination*, with the newborn awake and eyes open, examine the red retinal (fundus) reflex by setting the ophthalmoscope at 0 diopters and viewing the pupil from about 10 inches. Normally, a red or orange color is reflected from the fundus through the pupil.

Congenital glaucoma may cause cloudiness of the cornea. A dark light reflex can result from *cataracts*, *retinopathy of prematurity*, or other disorders. A white retinal reflex (*leukokoria*) is abnormal, and *cataract*, *retinal detachment*, *chorioretinitis*, or *retinoblastoma* should be suspected.

A thorough ophthalmoscopic examination is difficult in young infants but may be needed if ocular or neurologic abnormalities are noted. The cornea can ordinarily be seen at +20 diopters, the lens at +15 diopters, and the fundus at 0 diopters.

Examine the optic disc area as you would for an adult. In infants, the optic disc is lighter in color, with less macular pigmentation. The foveal light reflection may not be visible. Look carefully for retinal hemorrhages. Papilledema is rare in infants because the fontanelles and open sutures accommodate any increased intracranial pressure, sparing the optic discs.

Small retinal hemorrhages may occur in normal newborns. Extensive hemorrhages may suggest severe *anoxia, subdural hematoma, subarachnoid hemorrhage,* or *trauma*.

Retinal pigment changes can occur in newborns with *congenital toxoplasmosis, cytomegalovirus infection,* or *rubella*.

The Ears

The physical examination of the ears of infants is important because many abnormalities can be detected, including structural problems, otitis media, and hearing loss. This means that you must hone your skills with the otoscope.

The major goals are to determine the *position, shape,* and *features of the ear* and to detect abnormalities. Note ear position in relation to the eyes. An imaginary line drawn across the inner and outer canthi of the eyes should cross the pinna or auricle; if the pinna is below this line, then the infant has low-set ears. Draw this imaginary line across the face of the baby on p. 773; note that it crosses the pinna.

Small, deformed, or low-set auricles may indicate associated *congenital defects,* especially renal disease.

Otoscopic examination of the newborn's ear can detect only patency of the *ear canal* because accumulated vernix caseosa obscures the tympanic membrane for the first few days of life.

A small skin tab, cleft, or pit found just forward of the tragus represents a remnant of the *first branchial cleft* and usually has no significance.

The infant's ear canal is directed downward from the outside; therefore, you may want to pull the auricle gently downward, not upward, for the best view of the eardrum. Once the tympanic membrane is visible, note that the light reflex is diffuse and does not become cone-shaped for several months.

The *acoustic blink reflex* is a blinking of the infant's eyes in response to a sudden sharp sound; you can produce it by snapping your fingers or using a bell, beeper, or other noisemaking device approximately 1 foot from the infant's ear. Be sure you are not producing an airstream that may cause the infant to blink. The reflex may be difficult to elicit during the first 2 to 3 days of life. After it is elicited several times within a brief period, the reflex disappears, a phenomenon known as *habituation*. This crude test of hearing certainly is not diagnostic. A current movement exists toward universal hearing screening for all newborns, not only those at high risk for hearing problems.

Perinatal problems raising the risk for *hearing defects* include birth weight < 1500 grams, anoxia, treatment with potentially ototoxic medications, congenital infections, severe hyperbilirubinemia, and meningitis.

● Signs That an Infant Can Hear

Age	Sign
0–2 mos	Startle response and blink to a sudden noise Calming down with soothing voice or music
2–3 mos	Change in body movements in response to sound Change in facial expression to familiar sounds
3–4 mos	Turning eyes and head to sound
6–7 mos	Turning to listen to voices and conversation

Many children with *hearing deficits* are not diagnosed until as old as 2 years. Clues to hearing deficits include parental concern about hearing, delayed speech, and lack of developmental indicators of hearing.

The Nose and Sinuses

The most important component of the examination of the nose of infants is to test for patency of the nasal passages. You can do this by gently occluding each nostril alternately while holding the infant's mouth closed. This normally will not cause stress because most infants are nasal breathers. Indeed, some infants are *obligate nasal breathers* and have difficulty breathing through their mouths. Do not occlude both nares simultaneously—this will cause considerable distress!

Inspect the nose to ensure that the nasal septum is midline. You can gently insert a wide nasal speculum of the otoscope into the nose.

At birth, only the ethmoid sinuses are developed. Palpation of the sinuses of newborns is not helpful.

The nasal passages in newborns may be obstructed in *choanal atresia*. In severe cases, nasal obstruction can be assessed by attempting to pass a No. 8 feeding tube through each nostril into the posterior pharynx.

The Mouth and Pharynx

Use both inspection with a tongue blade and flashlight and palpation to inspect the mouth and pharynx. The newborn's mouth is edentulous, and the alveolar mucosa is smooth, with finely serrated borders. Occasionally, pearl-like retention cysts are seen along the alveolar ridges and are easily mistaken for teeth—they disappear within 1 or 2 months. Petechiae are commonly found on the soft palate after birth. Palpate the upper hard palate to make sure it is intact. *Epstein's pearls,* tiny white or yellow, rounded mucous retention cysts, are located along the posterior midline of the hard palate. They disappear within months.

Rarely, *supernumerary teeth* are noted. These are usually dysmorphic and are shed within days but are removed to prevent aspiration.

Cysts may be noted on the tongue or mouth. Thyroglossal duct cysts may open under the tongue.

Infants produce little saliva during the first 3 months. Older infants produce lots of saliva and drool frequently.

Inspect the tongue. The frenulum varies, sometimes extending almost to the tip and other times being thick and short, limiting protrusion of the tongue (*ankyloglossia*, or *tongue tie*); these variations rarely interfere with speech or function.

Although unusual, a prominent, protruding tongue may signal *congenital hypothyroidism* or *Down syndrome.*

You will often see a whitish covering on the tongue. If this coating is from milk, it can be easily removed by scraping or wiping it away.

Oral candidiasis (thrush) is common in infants. The lesions are difficult to wipe away and have an erythematous raw base (see Table 18-7, Abnormalities of the Eyes, Ears, and Mouth, p. 862.)

The pharynx of the infant is best seen while the baby is crying. You will likely have difficulty using a tongue blade because it produces a strong gag reflex. Do not expect to be able to visualize the tonsils.

Listen to the quality of the *infant's cry.* Normal infants have a lusty, strong cry. The following box lists some unusual types of infant cries.

Macroglossia is associated with several systemic conditions. If associated with hypoglycemia and omphalocele, the diagnosis is likely Beckwith-Wiedemann's syndrome.

● Abnormal Infant Cries

Type	Possible Abnormality
Shrill or high-pitched	Increased intracranial pressure. Also in newborns born to narcotic-addicted mothers.
Hoarse	Hypocalcemic tetany or congenital hypothyroidism
Continuous inspiratory and expiratory stridor	Upper airway obstruction from various lesions (e.g., a polyp or hemangioma), a relatively small larynx (*infantile laryngeal stridor*), or a delay in the development of the cartilage in the tracheal rings (*tracheomalacia*)
Absence of cry	Severe illness, vocal cord paralysis, or profound brain damage

There is a predictable pattern of tooth eruption and also wide variation. A rule of thumb is that a child will have one tooth for each month of age between 6 and 26 months, up to 20 primary teeth.

The Neck

Palpate the *lymph nodes of the neck* and assess for any additional masses such as *congenital cysts*. Because the necks of infants are short, it is best to palpate the neck while infants are lying supine, whereas older children are best examined while sitting. Check the position of the thyroid cartilage and trachea.

Branchial cleft cysts appear as small dimples or openings anterior to the midportion of the sternocleidomastoid muscle. They may be associated with a sinus tract.

Preauricular cysts and sinuses are common, pinhole-size pits, usually located anterior to the helix of the ear. They are often bilateral and may occasionally be associated with *hearing deficits.*

Thyroglossal duct cysts are located at the midline of the neck, just above the thyroid cartilage. These small, firm, mobile masses move upward with tongue protrusion or with swallowing. They are usually detected after 2 years.

Congenital torticollis, or a "wry neck," is from bleeding into the sternocleidomastoid muscle during the stretching process of birth. A firm fibrous mass is felt within the muscle 2–3 weeks after birth and generally disappears over months.

Parotid nodes
Occipital node
Retroauricular (mastoid) nodes
Superior deep cervical nodes
Middle deep cervical nodes
Posterior cervical nodes
2nd branchial cleft cyst
Supraclavicular node
Inferior deep cervical nodes
Anterior cervical nodes
Epidermoid cyst
Jugulogastric node
Submandibular node
Submental node
Cystic hygroma

In newborns, palpate the *clavicles* and look for evidence of a fracture. If present, you may feel a break in the contour of the bone, tenderness, crepitus at the fracture site, and limited movement of the arm on the affected side.

A *fracture of the clavicle* may occur during birth, particularly during delivery of a difficult arm or shoulder extraction.

The Thorax and Lungs

The infant's *thorax* is more rounded than that of older people. Also, the thin chest wall has little musculature; thus, lung and heart sounds are transmitted quite clearly. The bony and cartilaginous rib cage is soft and pliant. The tip of the xiphoid process often protrudes anteriorly, immediately beneath the skin.

Two types of chest wall abnormalities noted in childhood include *pectus excavatum,* or "funnel chest," and *pectus carinatum,* or "chicken breast deformity."

Inspection. Carefully *assess respirations* and *breathing patterns*. Newborns, especially those born prematurely, show periods of normal rate (30 to 40 per minute) alternating with "periodic breathing," during which respiratory rate slows markedly and may even cease for 5 to 10 seconds.

Do not rush to the stethoscope. Instead, observe the infant carefully as demonstrated on the next page. Inspection is easiest when infants are not crying; thus, work with the parents to settle the child. By observing for perhaps 1 minute, you can note general appearance, respiratory rate, color, nasal component of breathing, audible breath sounds, and work of breathing, as described below.

Because infants are obligate nasal breathers, observe their nose as they breathe. Look for *nasal flaring*. Observe breathing with the infant's mouth closed or during nursing or sucking on a bottle to assess for nasal patency. Listen to the sounds of breathing; note any *grunting, audible wheezing,* or *lack of breath sounds (obstruction)*.

Observe two aspects of the infant's breathing: *audible breath sounds* and *work of breathing*. These are particularly relevant in assessing both upper and lower respiratory illness. Studies in countries with poor access to chest radiographs have found these signs at least as useful as auscultation of both the upper and lower respiratory tracts.

Apnea is cessation of breathing for more than 20 seconds. It is often accompanied by bradycardia and may indicate *respiratory disease, central nervous system disease,* or, rarely, a *cardiopulmonary condition.* Apnea may be a high-risk factor for *sudden infant death syndrome (SIDS).*

In newborns and young infants, nasal flaring may be the result of *upper respiratory infections,* with subsequent obstruction of their small nares, but it may also be caused by pneumonia or other serious respiratory infections.

● Observing Respiration—Before You Touch the Child!

Type of Assessment	Specific Observable Pathology
General appearance	Inability to feed or smile Lack of consolability
Respiratory rate	Tachypnea (see p. 134)
Color	Pallor or cyanosis
Nasal component of breathing	Nasal flaring (enlargement of both nasal openings during inspiration)
Audible breath sounds	Grunting (repetitive, short expiratory sound) Wheezing (musical expiratory sound) Stridor (high-pitched, inspiratory noise) Obstruction (lack of breath sounds)

Work of breathing	Nasal flaring (excessive movement of nares)
	Grunting (expiratory noises)
	Retractions (chest indrawing):
	  Supraclavicular (soft tissue above clavicles)
	  Intercostal (indrawing of the skin between ribs)
	  Subcostal (just below the costal margin)

Any of the abnormalities listed on the left should raise concern about underlying respiratory pathology.

Lower respiratory infections, defined as infections below the vocal cords, are common in infants and include *bronchiolitis* and *pneumonia.*

Acute stridor is a potentially serious condition; causes include *laryngo-tracheo-bronchitis (croup), epiglottitis, bacterial tracheitis, foreign body,* or *a vascular ring.*

In infants, abnormal work of breathing plus abnormal findings on auscultation, are the best findings for ruling in *pneumonia.* The best sign for ruling *out* pneumonia is the absence of tachypnea.

In healthy infants, the ribs do not move much during quiet breathing. Any outward movement is produced by descent of the diaphragm, which compresses the abdominal contents and in turn shifts the lower ribs outward.

Asymmetric chest movement may indicate a space-occupying lesion. Pulmonary disease causes increased

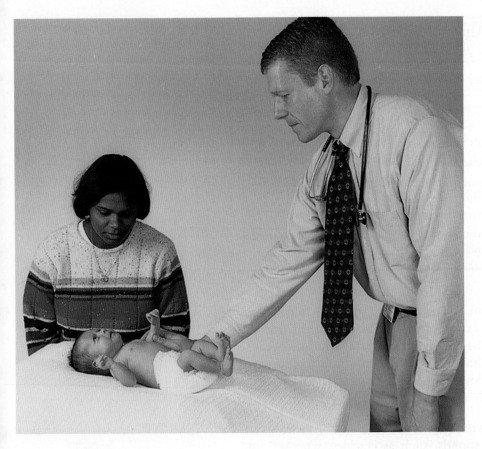

abdominal breathing and can result in *retractions (chest indrawing),* an indicator of pulmonary disease before 2 years of age. Chest indrawing is inward movement of the skin between the ribs during inspiration. Movement of the diaphragm primarily affects breathing, with little assistance from the thoracic muscles. As mentioned in the preceding table, three types of retractions can be noted in infants: supraclavicular, intercostal, and subcostal.

Obstructive respiratory disease in infants can result in the *Hoover sign,* or paradoxical (seesaw), breathing in which the abdomen moves outward while the chest moves inward during inspiration.

Thoracoabdominal paradox, inward movement of the chest and outward movement of the abdomen during inspiration, is a normal finding in newborns. It persists during active, or REM, sleep even when it is no longer seen during wakefulness or quiet sleep because of the decreased muscle tone of active sleep. As muscle strength increases and chest wall compliance decreases with age, paradox is no longer a normal finding.

Children with *muscle weakness* may be noted to have thoracoabdominal paradox at several years of age.

Palpation.   Assess tactile fremitus by *palpation.* Place your hand on the chest when the infant cries or makes noise. Place your hand or fingertips over each side of the chest and feel for symmetry in the transmitted vibrations. Percussion is not helpful in infants except in extreme instances. The infant's chest is hyperresonant throughout, and it is difficult to detect abnormalities on percussion.

Because of the excellent transmission of sounds throughout the chest, any abnormalities of tactile fremitus or on percussion suggest severe pathology, such as a large *pneumonic consolidation.*

Auscultation.   After performing these maneuvers, you are ready for *auscultation.* Breath sounds are louder and harsher than those of adults because the stethoscope is closer to the origin of the sounds. Also, it is often difficult to distinguish transmitted upper airway sounds from sounds originating in the chest. The table that follows has some useful hints. Upper airway sounds tend to be loud, transmitted symmetrically throughout the chest, and loudest as you move your stethoscope toward the neck. They are usually inspiratory, coarse sounds. Lower airway sounds are loudest over the site of pathology, are often asymmetric, and often occur during expiration.

Biphasic sounds imply *severe obstruction from intrathoracic airway narrowing* or *severe obstruction from extrathoracic airway narrowing.*

● Distinguishing Upper Airway From Lower Airway Sounds in Infants

Technique	Upper Airway	Lower Airway
Compare sounds from nose/ stethoscope	Same sounds	Often different sounds
Listen to harshness of sounds	Harsh and loud	Variable
Note symmetry (left/right)	Symmetric	Often asymmetric
Compare sounds at different locations (higher or lower)	Sounds louder as stethoscope is moved up chest	Often sounds louder lower in chest toward abdomen
Inspiratory vs. expiratory	Almost always inspiratory	Often has expiratory phase

Expiratory sounds usually arise from an intrathoracic source, while inspiratory sounds typically arise from an extrathoracic airway such as the trachea. During expiration, the diameter of the intrathoracic airways decreases because radial forces from the surrounding lung do not "tether" the airways open as occurs during inspiration. Higher flow rates during inspiration produce turbulent flow, resulting in appreciable sounds.

The characteristics of the *breath sounds,* such as vesicular and bronchovesicular, and of the adventitious lung sounds, such as crackles, wheezes, and rhonchi, are the same as those for adults, except that they may be more difficult to distinguish in infants and often occur together. Wheezes and rhonchi are common in infants. *Wheezes,* often audible without the stethoscope, occur more frequently because of the smaller size of the tracheobronchial tree. *Rhonchi* reflect obstruction of larger airways, or bronchi. *Crackles* (rales) are discontinuous sounds (see p. 304), near the end of inspiration; they are usually caused by lung disorders, are far less likely to represent cardiac failure in infants than in adults, and tend to be harsher than in adults.

The Heart

Inspection. Before examining the heart itself, *observe* the infant carefully for any cyanosis. Acrocyanosis in the newborn is discussed on p. 762. It is important to detect *central cyanosis* (Table 18-9, Cyanosis in Children, p. 864) because it is always abnormal and because many congenital cardiac abnormalities, as well as respiratory diseases, present with cyanosis (see Table 18-10, Congenital Heart Murmurs, pp. 865–866).[18]

Recognizing minimal degrees of cyanosis requires care. Look inside of the body (i.e., the inside of the mouth, the tongue, or the conjunctivae, instead of peering through the skin). A true strawberry pink is normal, whereas any hint of raspberry red suggests desaturation.

The distribution of the cyanosis should be evaluated. An oxymetry reading will confirm desaturation.

Diminished breath sounds in one side of the chest of a newborn suggest unilateral lesions (e.g., *congenital diaphragmatic hernia*).

Wheezes in infants occur commonly from *asthma* or *bronchiolitis.*

Crackles (rales) can be heard with *pneumonia* and *bronchiolitis.*

Central cyanosis without acute respiratory symptoms suggests cardiac disease.

● Cardiac Causes of Central Cyanosis in Infants and Children

Age of Onset	Potential Cardiac Cause
Immediately at birth	Transposition of the great arteries Pulmonary valve atresia Severe pulmonary valve stenosis Possibly Ebstein's malformation
Within a few days after birth	All of the above plus: 　Total anomalous pulmonary venous return 　Hypoplastic left heart syndrome 　Truncus arteriosus (sometimes) 　Single ventricle variants
Weeks, months, or years of life	All of the above plus: 　Pulmonary vascular disease with atrial, 　　ventricular, or great vessel shunting

Observe the infant for *general signs of health*. The infant's nutritional status, responsiveness, happiness, and irritability are all clues that may be useful in evaluating cardiac disease. Note that noncardiac findings can be present in infants with cardiac disease.

Tachypnea, tachycardia, and hepatomegaly in infants suggest *congestive heart failure*.

Common Noncardiac Findings in Infants with Cardiac Disease

Poor feeding	Tachypnea	Poor overall appearance
Failure to thrive	Hepatomegaly	Weakness
Irritability	Clubbing	

Observe the respiratory rate and pattern to help distinguish the degree of illness and cardiac versus pulmonary diseases. An increase in respiratory effort is expected from pulmonary diseases, whereas in cardiac disease there may be tachypnea but not increased work of breathing until congestive heart failure becomes significant.

A diffuse bulge outward of the left side of the chest suggests longstanding *cardiomegaly*.

Palpation.　The major branches of the aorta can be assessed by evaluation of the *peripheral pulses*. All neonates should have an evaluation of all pulses at the time of their newborn examination. In neonates and infants, the brachial artery pulse in the antecubital fossa is easier to feel than the radial artery pulse at the wrist. Both temporal arteries should be felt just in front of the ear.

Feel the femoral pulses. They lie in the midline just below the inguinal crease, between the iliac crest and the symphysis pubis. Take your time and search for femoral pulses; they are difficult to detect in chubby, squirming infants. If you first flex the infant's thighs on the abdomen, this may overcome the reflex flexion that occurs when you then extend the legs.

The absence or diminution of femoral pulses is indicative of *coarctation of the aorta*. If you can't detect femoral pulses, measure blood pressures of the lower and upper extremities. If they are equal or lower in the legs, coarctation is likely to be present.

The dorsalis pedis and posterior tibial pulses (see figure) may be difficult to feel unless there is an abnormality involving aortic run-off. Normal pulses should have a sharp rise and should be firm and well localized.

A weak or thready, difficult-to-feel pulse may reflect *myocardial dysfunction* and *congestive heart failure*, particularly if associated with an unusual degree of tachycardia.

Although the pulses in the feet of neonates and infants are often faint, several conditions can cause full pulses, such as *patent ductus arteriosus* or *truncus arteriosus*.

As discussed on p. 758, carefully measure the *blood pressure* of infants and children as part of the cardiac examination.

The *point of maximal impulse*, or *PMI*, is not always palpable in infants and is affected by respiratory patterns, a full stomach, and the infant's positioning. It is usually an interspace higher than in adults during the first few years of life because the heart lies more horizontally within the chest.

A *"rolling" heave* at the left sternal border suggests an *increase in right ventricular work*, whereas the same kind of motion closer to the apex suggests the same thing for the left ventricle.

Palpation of the chest wall will allow you to assess volume changes within the heart. For example, a hyperdynamic precordium reflects a big volume change.

Thrills are palpable when turbulence within the heart or great vessels is transmitted to the surface. Knowledge of the structures of the precordium helps pinpoint the origin of the thrill. Thrills are easiest to feel with your palm or the base of your fingers rather than your fingertips. Thrills have a somewhat rough, vibrating quality. The figure below shows locations of thrills from various cardiac abnormalities that occur in infants and children.

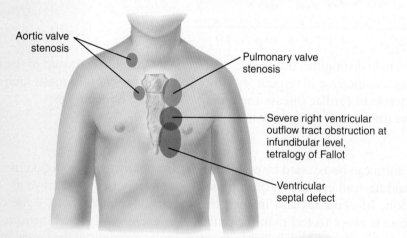

Aortic valve stenosis

Pulmonary valve stenosis

Severe right ventricular outflow tract obstruction at infundibular level, tetralogy of Fallot

Ventricular septal defect

LOCATION OF THRILLS IN INFANTS AND CHILDREN

Visible and palpable chest pulsations suggest a hyperdynamic state from either increased metabolic rate or inefficient pumping as a result of an underlying cardiac effect.

Auscultation. You can evaluate the *heart rhythm* more easily in infants by listening to the heart than by feeling the peripheral pulses; in older children it can be done either way. Infants and children commonly have a normal sinus dysrhythmia, with the heart rate increasing on inspiration and decreasing on expiration, sometimes quite abruptly. This normal finding can be

The most common dysrhythmia in infants is *paroxysmal supraventricular tachycardia*, or *paroxysmal atrial tachycardia (PSVT, or PAT)*. It can occur at any age, including in utero.

identified by its repetitive nature, its correlation with respiration, and its involvement of several beats rather than a single beat.

Many neonates and some older children have premature atrial or ventricular beats that are often appreciated as "skipped" beats. You can usually eradicate them by increasing their intrinsic sinus rate by exercise through crying in an infant or jumping in an older child, although they may also be more frequent in the postexercise period. In a completely healthy child, they are usually benign and rarely persist.

It is remarkably well tolerated by some infants and children and is found on examination when the child looks perfectly healthy, may be mildly pale or has tachypnea, but has a rapid, sustained, completely regular heart rate of 240 beats per minute or more. Other children, particularly neonates, appear very ill. In older children, this dysrhythmia is more likely to be truly paroxysmal, with episodes of varying duration and frequency.

Heart Sounds. Evaluate the S_1 and S_2 *heart sounds* carefully. They are normally crisp. You can usually hear the second sounds (S_2) at the base separately, but they should fuse into a single sound in deep expiration. In the neonate, you should be able to detect a split S_2 if you examine the infant when the infant is completely quiet or asleep. Detecting this split eliminates many, but not all, of the more serious congenital cardiac defects.

Pathologic arrhythmias in children can be from *structural cardiac lesions* but also from other causes such as *drug ingestion, metabolic abnormalities, endocrine disorders, serious infections,* and *postinfectious states,* or conduction disturbances without structural heart disease.

● Characteristics of Normal Variants of Heart Rhythms in Children

Characteristics	Atrial Premature Contractions (APCs) or Ventricular Premature Contractions (VPCs)	Normal Sinus Arrhythmias
Most common age	Neonates (may occur at any time)	After infancy Throughout childhood (less common in adults)
Correlation with respiration	No	Yes: Increases on inspiration Decreases on expiration
Effect of exercise on tachycardia	Eradicated by exercise May be more frequent postexercise	Disappears
Characteristic of rhythm	Skipped or missed beat Irregularly occurring	Gradually faster with inspiration Often suddenly slower on expiration
Number of beats	Usually single abnormal beats	Several beats, usually in repetitive cycles
Severity	Usually benign	Benign (by definition)

Although VPCs generally occur in otherwise healthy infants, they can occur with underlying cardiac disease, particularly *cardiomyopathies* and *congenital heart disorders.* Electrolyte or metabolic disturbances are additional causes.

Distant heart tones suggest *pericardial effusion;* mushy, less distinct heart sounds suggest *myocardial dysfunction.*

In addition to trying to detect splitting of the S_2, listen for the intensity of A_2 and P_2. The aortic, or first component of the second sound at the base, is normally louder than the pulmonic, or second component.

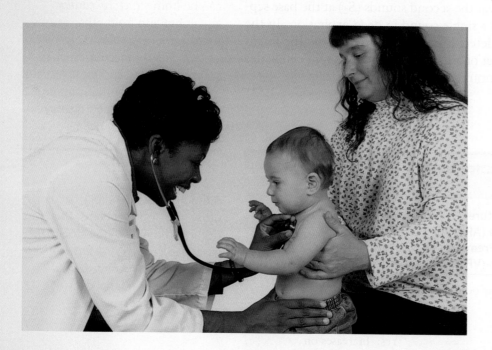

You may detect *third heart sounds*, which are low-pitched, early diastolic sounds best heard at the lower left sternal border, or apex. These are frequently heard in children and are normal. They reflect rapid ventricular filling.

Fourth heart sounds (S_4), which are not often heard in children, are low-frequency, late diastolic sounds, occurring just before the first heart sound.

You may also detect an *apparent gallop* (widely split S_2 that varies), in the presence of a normal heart rate and rhythm. This frequent finding in normal children does not represent pathology.

Heart Murmurs. One of the most challenging aspects of cardiac examination in children is the evaluation of *heart murmurs*. In addition to trying to

A louder-than-normal pulmonic component, particularly when louder than the aortic sound, suggests *pulmonary hypertension*.

Persistent splitting of S_2 may indicate a right ventricular volume load such as *atrial septal defect, anomalies of pulmonary venous return,* or *chronic anemia*.

The third heart sound (S_3) should be differentiated from the higher-intensity third heart sound gallop, which is a sign of underlying pathology.

Fourth heart sounds represent decreased ventricular compliance, suggesting *congestive heart failure*.

A *gallop rhythm*—tachycardia plus a loud S_3, S_4, or both—is pathologic and indicates *congestive heart failure (poor ventricular function)*.

listen to a squirming, perhaps uncooperative child, a major challenge is to distinguish common benign murmurs from unusual or pathologic ones. Characterize heart murmurs in infants and children by noting their specific location (e.g., left upper sternal border, not just left sternal border), timing, intensity, and quality. If each murmur is delineated that completely, the diagnosis is usually made, and all that is needed is confirmation and amplification with laboratory tools such as ECG, chest x-ray, and echocardiography.

An important rule of thumb is that, by definition, *benign murmurs in children have no associated abnormal findings.* Many (but not all) children with serious cardiac malformations have signs and symptoms other than a heart murmur obtainable on careful history or examination. Many have other noncardiac signs and symptoms, including evidence of genetic defects that may offer helpful diagnostic clues.

Most children (indeed, some say nearly all) will have one or more *functional, or benign, heart murmurs* before reaching adulthood.[19] It is important to identify functional murmurs by their specific qualities rather than by their intensity. With practice, you will be able to recognize the common functional murmurs of infancy and childhood, which under most circumstances do not require evaluation.

The figure below characterizes two *benign* heart murmurs in infants according to their locations and key characteristics.

Any of the *noncardiac findings* that frequently accompany cardiac disease in children markedly raises the possibility that a murmur that appears benign is really pathologic.

Many *pathologic murmurs of congenital heart disease* are present at birth. Others are not apparent until later, depending on their severity, drop in pulmonary vascular resistance following birth, or changes associated with growth of the child. Table 18-10, on pp. 865–866, shows examples of pathologic murmurs of childhood.

Two Common Benign Murmurs in Infants

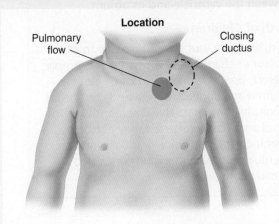

Typical Age	Name	Characteristics	Description and Location
Newborn	*Closing ductus*		Transient, soft, ejection Upper left sternal border
Newborn to 1 year	*Peripheral pulmonary flow murmur*	S₁ S₂	Soft, slightly ejectile, systolic To left of upper left sternal border and in lung fields and axillae

In some infants, you will detect a soft, somewhat ejectile murmur, not over the precordium but over the lung fields, particularly in the axillae. This represents peripheral pulmonary artery flow and is partly the result of inadequate pulmonary artery growth in utero (when there is little pulmonary blood flow) and the sharp angle at which the pulmonary artery curves backward. In the absence of any physical findings to suggest additional underlying diseases, this *peripheral pulmonary flow murmur* can be considered benign and usually disappears by 1 year.

A pulmonary flow murmur in the newborn with other signs of disease is more likely to be pathologic. Diseases may include *Williams syndrome, congenital rubella syndrome,* and *Alagille syndrome.*

A newborn with a heart murmur and central cyanosis likely has congenital heart disease and requires urgent cardiac evaluation.

PHYSIOLOGIC BASIS FOR SOME PATHOLOGIC HEART MURMURS

Change in Pulmonary Vascular Resistance

Heart murmurs that are dependent on a postnatal drop in pulmonary vascular resistance, allowing turbulent flow from the high-pressure systemic circuit to the lower-pressure pulmonary circuit, are not audible until such a drop has occurred. Therefore, except in premature infants, murmurs of a *ventricular septal defect* or *patent ductus arteriosus* are not expected in the first few days of life and usually become audible after a week to 10 days.

Obstructive Lesions

Obstructive lesions, such as *pulmonic and aortic stenosis,* are caused by normal blood flow through two small valves and, therefore, are not dependent on a drop in pulmonary vascular resistance and are audible at birth.

Pressure Gradient Differences

Murmurs of *atrioventricular valve regurgitation* are audible at birth because of the high pressure gradient between the ventricle and its atrium.

Changes Associated With Growth of Children

Some murmurs do not follow the rules above, but are audible due to alterations in normal blood flow and occur or change with growth. For example, even though it is an obstructive defect, *aortic stenosis* may not be audible until considerable growth has occurred and, indeed, is frequently not heard until adulthood, although a congenitally abnormal valve is responsible. Similarly, the pulmonary flow murmur of an *atrial septal defect* may not be heard for a year or more because right ventricular compliance gradually increases and the shunt becomes larger, eventually producing a murmur caused by too much blood flow across a normal pulmonic valve.

When you detect any murmur in children, note all of the qualities as described in Chapter 9, The Cardiovascular System, to help you distinguish *pathologic murmurs* from the benign murmurs just described. Heart murmurs that reflect underlying structural heart disease are easier to evaluate if you have a good knowledge of intrathoracic anatomy and the functional cardiac changes following birth and if you understand the physiologic basis for heart murmurs. Understanding these physiologic changes can help you to distinguish pathologic murmurs from benign heart murmurs in children.

Characteristics of specific pathologic heart murmurs in children are described in Table 18-10 on pp. 865–866.

The Breasts

The breasts of the newborn in both males and females are often enlarged from maternal estrogen effect; this may last several months. The breasts may also be engorged with a white liquid, sometimes colloquially called "witch's milk," which may last 1 or 2 weeks.

In *premature thelarche*, breast development occurs, most often between 6 months and 2 years. Other signs of puberty or hormonal abnormalities are not present.

The Abdomen

Inspection.   *Inspect* the abdomen with the infant lying supine (and, optimally, asleep). The infant's abdomen is protuberant as a result of poorly developed abdominal musculature. You will easily notice abdominal wall blood vessels and intestinal peristalsis.

Inspect the newborn's *umbilical cord* to detect abnormalities. Normally, there are two thick-walled umbilical arteries and one larger but thin-walled umbilical vein, which is usually located at the 12-o'clock position.

A *single umbilical artery* may be associated with congenital anomalies or as an isolated anomaly.

The umbilicus in the newborn may have a long cutaneous portion (*umbilicus cutis*), which is covered with skin, or an amniotic portion (*umbilicus amnioticus*), which is covered by a firm gelatinous substance. The amniotic portion dries up and falls off within 2 weeks, whereas the cutaneous portion retracts to be flush with the abdominal wall.

An *umbilical granuloma* at the base of the navel is the development of pink granulation tissue formed during the healing process.

Inspect the area around the umbilicus for redness or swelling. *Umbilical hernias* are detectable at a few weeks of age. Most disappear by 1 year, nearly all by 5 years.

Umbilical hernias in infants are caused by a defect in the abdominal wall and can be up to 6 cm in diameter and quite protuberant with intra-abdominal pressure.

In some normal infants, you will notice a *diastasis recti*. This involves separation of the two rectus abdominis muscles, causing a midline ridge, most apparent when the infant contracts the abdominal muscles. A benign condition in most cases, it resolves during early childhood. Chronic abdominal distention may also predispose to this condition.

Auscultation.   *Auscultation* of a quiet infant's abdomen is easy. Don't be surprised if you hear an orchestra of musical tinkling bowel sounds upon placement of your stethoscope on the infant's abdomen.

An increase in pitch or frequency of bowel sounds is heard with *gastroenteritis* or, rarely, with *intestinal obstruction*.

Percussion and Palpation.   You can *percuss* an infant's abdomen as you would an adult's, but be prepared to note greater tympanitic sounds because of the infant's propensity to swallow air. Percussion is useful for determining the size of organs and abdominal masses.

A silent, tympanic, distended and tender abdomen suggests *peritonitis*.

You will find it easy to *palpate* an infant's abdomen because infants like being touched. A useful technique to relax the infant, shown here, is to hold the legs flexed at the knees and hips with one hand and palpate the abdomen with the other. You may also want to use a pacifier to quiet the infant in this position.

Start gently palpating the liver of infants low in the abdomen, moving upward with your fingers. This technique helps you avoid missing an extremely enlarged liver that extends down into the pelvis. With a careful examination, you can feel the liver edge in most infants, 1 to 2 cm below the right costal margin.

An enlarged, tender liver may be due to *congestive heart failure* or to *storage diseases*. Among newborns, causes of hepatomegaly include *hepatitis, storage diseases, vascular congestion, and biliary obstruction.*

One technique for assessing liver size in infants is simultaneous percussion and auscultation.[20] Percuss and simultaneously auscultate, noting a change in sound as you percuss over the liver or beyond it.

The *spleen*, like the liver, is felt easily in most infants. It too is soft with a sharp edge, and it projects downward like a tongue from under the left costal margin. The spleen is moveable and rarely extends more than 1 cm to 2 cm below the left costal margin.

Several diseases can cause splenomegaly, including *infections, hemolytic anemias, infiltrative disorders, inflammatory* or *autoimmune diseases,* and *portal hypertension.*

Palpate the *other abdominal structures.* You will commonly note pulsations in the epigastrium caused by the aorta. This is felt on deep palpation to the left of the midline.

In fact, you may be able to palpate the kidneys of infants by carefully placing the fingers of one hand in front of and those of the other behind each kidney. The descending colon is a sausage-like mass in the left lower quadrant.

Abnormal abdominal masses in infants can be associated with the kidney (e.g., *hydronephrosis*), bladder (e.g., *urethral obstruction*), bowel (e.g., *Hirschsprung's disease,* or *intussusception*), and tumors.

Once you have identified the normal structures in the infant's abdomen, use palpation to identify abnormal masses.

In *pyloric stenosis,* deep palpation in the right upper quadrant or midline can reveal an "olive," or a 2-cm firm pyloric mass. While feeding, some infants with this condition will have visible peristaltic waves pass across their abdomen, followed by projectile vomiting.

● Liver Size in Healthy Term Newborns[21]

By palpation and percussion	Mean, 5.9 ± 0.7 cm
Projection below right costal margin	Mean, 2.5 ± 1.0 cm

Male Genitalia

Inspect the male genitalia with the infant supine, noting the appearance of the penis, testes, and scrotum. The *foreskin* completely covers the *glans penis.* It is nonretractable at birth, though you may be able to retract it

A *hypospadias* is present when the urethral orifice appears at some point along the ventral surface of enough to visualize the external urethral meatus. Retraction of the foreskin in the uncircumcised male occurs months to years later. The rate of circumcision has declined recently in North America and varies worldwide, depending on cultural practices.

Inspect the *shaft of the penis*, noting any abnormalities on the ventral surface. Make sure the penis appears straight.

Scrotal edema may be present for several days following birth because of the effect of maternal estrogen.

Inspect the *scrotum*, noting rugae, which should be present by 40 weeks' gestation. Palpate the testes in the scrotal sacs, proceeding downward from the external inguinal ring to the scrotum. If you feel a testis up in the inguinal canal, gently milk it downward into the scrotum. The newborn's testes should be about 10 mm in width and 15 mm in length and should lie in the scrotal sacs most of the time.

In 3% of neonates, one or both *testes* cannot be felt in the scrotum or inguinal canal. This raises concern of *cryptorchidism*. In two thirds of these cases, both testes are descended by 1 year of age.

Examine the testes for swelling within the scrotal sac and over the inguinal ring. If you detect swelling in the scrotal sac, try to differentiate it from the testis. Note whether the size changes when the infant increases abdominal pressure by crying. See if your fingers can get above the mass, trapping it in the scrotal sac. Apply gentle pressure to try to reduce the size of the mass and note any tenderness. Note whether it transilluminates.

TRANSILLUMINATION OF A HYDROCELE

From Fletcher M. Physical Diagnosis in Neonatology. Philadelphia, Lippincott-Raven, 1998.

Female Genitalia

Although it is challenging, you should become familiar with the anatomy of an infant's female genitalia. Anatomical structures are depicted on the next page on both a figure of newborn female genitalia and a close-up photograph.

In the newborn female, the genitalia will be prominent from the effects of maternal estrogen. The labia majora and minora have a dull pink color in light-skinned infants and may be hyperpigmented in dark-skinned infants. During the first few weeks of life, there is often a milky white discharge that may be blood tinged. This estrogenized appearance of the genitalia decreases during the first year of life.

Examine the female genitalia with the infant supine.

the glans or shaft of the penis (see Table 18-12, The Male Genitourinary System, p. 868). The foreskin is incompletely formed ventrally.

A fixed, downward bowing of the penis is a *chordee;* this may accompany a hypospadias.

In newborns with an *undescended testicle* (*cryptorchidism*), the scrotum often appears underdeveloped and tight, and palpation reveals an absence of scrotal contents (see Table 18-12, The Male Genitourinary System, p. 868).

Two common scrotal masses in newborns are *hydroceles* and *inguinal hernias;* frequently both coexist, and both are more common on the right side. Hydroceles overlie the testes and the spermatic cord, are not reducible, and can be transilluminated (see photo at left). Most resolve by 18 months. Hernias are separate from the testes, are usually reducible, and often do not transilluminate. They do not resolve. Sometimes a thickened spermatic cord (called the *silk sign*) is noted.

Ambiguous genitalia, involving masculinization of the female external genitalia, is a rare condition caused by endocrine disorders such as *congenital adrenal hyperplasia.*

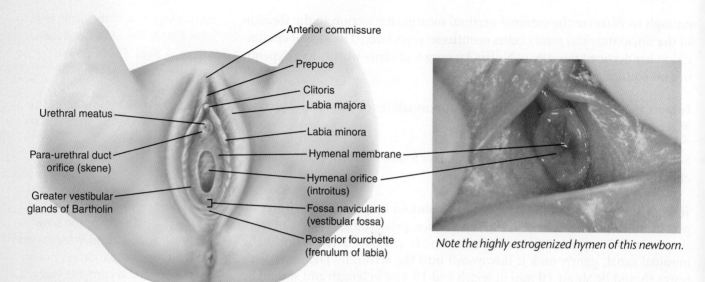

This figure depicts the anatomy of a young female to best demonstrate anatomic structures.

Note the highly estrogenized hymen of this newborn.

Examine the different structures systematically, including the size of the clitoris, the color and size of the labia majora, and any rashes, bruises, or external lesions. Next, separate the labia majora at their midpoint with the thumb of each hand for young infants, or as shown in the diagrams on p. 827 for early and late childhood. Infants will not mind the examination because they are used to having their diapers changed and their bodies washed.

Labial adhesions occur not infrequently, tend to be paper thin, and often disappear without treatment.

Inspect the urethral orifice and the labia minora. Assess the hymen, which in newborns and infants is a thickened, avascular structure with a central orifice, covering the vaginal opening. You should note a vaginal opening, although the hymen will be thickened and redundant. Note any discharge.

An imperforate hymen may be noted at birth.

Rectal Examination

The rectal examination generally is not performed for infants or children unless there is question of patency of the anus or an abdominal mass. In such cases, flex the infant's hips and fold the legs to the head. Use your lubricated and gloved pinky.

The Musculoskeletal System

Enormous changes in the musculoskeletal system occur during infancy. Much of the examination focuses on detection of congenital abnormalities, particularly in the hands, spine, hips, legs, and feet. With a little practice, you will be able to combine the musculoskeletal examination with the neurologic and developmental examination.

Careful inspection can reveal gross deformities such as dwarfism, congenital abnormalities of the extremities or digits, and annular bands that constrict an extremity.

The *newborn's hands* are clenched. Because of the palmar grasp reflex (see the discussion on the nervous system), you will need to help the infant extend the fingers. Inspect the fingers carefully, noting any defects.

Skin tags, remnants of digits, polydactyly (extra fingers), or *syndactyly* (webbed fingers) are congenital defects noted at birth.

Palpate along the *clavicle*, noting any lumps, tenderness, or crepitus; these may indicate a fracture.

Inspect the *spine* carefully. Although major defects of the spine such as *meningomyelocele* are obvious and often detected by ultrasound before birth, subtle abnormalities may include pigmented spots, hairy patches, or deep pits. These abnormalities, if present within 1 cm or so of the midline, may overlie external openings of sinus tracts that extend to the spinal canal. Do not probe sinus tracts because of the potential risk for introducing infection. Palpate the spine in the lumbosacral region, noting any deformities of the vertebrae.

Examine the newborn and infant's *hips* carefully at each examination for signs of dislocation.[22] The following photos and subsequent page demonstrate the two major techniques, one to test for the presence of a posteriorly dislocated hip (*Ortolani test*) and another to test for the ability to sublux or dislocate an intact but unstable hip (*Barlow test*).[22]

A *fracture of the clavicle* can occur during a difficult birth.

Spina bifida occulta (a defect of the vertebral bodies) may be associated with defects of the spinal cord, which can cause severe neurologic dysfunction.

A soft audible "click" heard with these maneuvers does not prove a dislocated hip, but should prompt a careful examination.

ORTOLANI TEST

BARLOW TEST

Make sure the baby is relaxed for these two techniques. For the *Ortolani test*, place the baby supine with the legs pointing toward you. Flex the legs to form right angles at the hips and knees, placing your index fingers over the greater trochanter of each femur and your thumbs over the lesser trochanters. Abduct both hips simultaneously until the lateral aspect of each knee touches the examining table.

With a *hip dysplasia,* you feel a "clunk" as the femoral head, which lies posterior to the acetabulum, enters the acetabulum. A palpable movement of the femoral head back into place constitutes a *positive Ortolani sign*.

Congenital hip dysplasia is important to detect: Early appropriate treatment has excellent outcomes.

For the *Barlow test*, place your hands in the same position as for the Ortolani test. This time, press in the opposite direction with your thumbs moving down toward the table and outward. Feel for any movement of the head of the femur laterally. Normally there is no movement and the hip feels "stable."

A positive Barlow sign is not diagnostic of a *dysplastic hip*, but it indicates laxity and a dislocatable hip progressively, and the baby needs to be reexamined in the future. If you feel the head of the femur slipping out onto the posterior lip of the acetabulum, this constitutes a *positive Barlow sign*. If you do feel this dislocation movement, abduct the hip by pressing with your index and middle fingers back inward and feel for the movement of the femoral head as it returns to the hip socket.

Children older than 3 months may have a negative Ortolani or Barlow sign and still have a *dislocated hip* due to tightening of the hip muscles and ligaments.

In addition to examining the hips, it is important to examine a newborn or infant's *legs and feet* to detect developmental abnormalities. Assess symmetry, bowing, and torsion of the legs. There should be no discrepancy in leg length. It is common for normal infants to have asymmetric thigh skin folds, but if you do detect asymmetry, make sure you perform the instability tests because dislocated hips are commonly associated with this finding.

Most newborns are *bowlegged*, reflecting their curled-up intrauterine position.

Another finding after 3 months of age is apparent femoral shortening (*positive Galeazzi* or *Alice test*). This picture demonstrates the technique. Place the feet together and note any difference in knee heights.

Some normal infants exhibit twisting or *torsion of the tibia* inwardly or outwardly on its longitudinal axis. Parents may be concerned about a toeing in or toeing out of the foot and an awkward gait, all of which are usually normal. Tibial torsion corrects itself during the second year of life after months of weight bearing.

Pathologic tibial torsion occurs only in association with *deformities of the feet or hips.*

Now examine the feet of newborns and infants. At birth, the feet may appear deformed from retaining their intrauterine positioning, often turned inward as shown on the next page. You should be able to correct the feet to the neutral and even to an overcorrected position. You can also scratch or stroke along the outer edge to see if the foot assumes a normal position.

True *deformities of the feet* do not return to the neutral position even with manipulation.

The normal newborn's foot has several benign features that may initially concern you. The newborn's foot appears flat because of a plantar fat pad. There is often inversion of the foot, elevating the medial margin. Other babies will have adduction of the forefoot without inversion, called *metatarsus adductus.* Still others will have adduction of the entire foot. Finally, most toddlers have some pronation during early stages of weight bearing, with eversion of the foot. In all of these normal variants, the abnormal position can be easily overcorrected past midline. They all tend to resolve within 1 or 2 years.

The most common severe congenital foot deformity is talipes equinovarus (talipes calcaneovalgus), or *clubfoot.*

The Nervous System

The examination of the nervous system in infants includes techniques that are highly specific to this particular age. Further, unlike many neurologic abnormalities in adults that produce asymmetric localized findings, neurologic abnormalities in infants often present as developmental abnormalities such as failure to do age-appropriate tasks. Therefore, the neurologic and developmental examinations need to proceed hand in hand. Finding a developmental abnormality should prompt you to pay particular attention to the neurologic examination.

The neurologic screening examination of all newborns should include assessment of mental status, gross and fine motor function, tone, cry, deep tendon reflexes, and primitive reflexes. More detailed examination of cranial nerve function, sensory function, and less common primitive reflexes are indicated if you suspect any abnormalities from the history or screening.[23]

The neurologic examination can reveal extensive disease but will not pinpoint specific functional deficits or minute lesions.

Mental Status.   Assess the *mental status* of newborns by observing many of the newborn activities discussed on p. 749 ("What newborns can do"). Make sure you test the newborn during alert periods.

Motor Function and Tone.   Assess the *motor tone* of newborns and infants, first by carefully watching their position at rest and testing their resistance to passive movement.

Then assess *tone* as you move each major joint through its range of motion, noting any spasticity or flaccidity. Hold the baby in your hands, as shown on the next page, to determine whether the tone is normal, increased, or decreased. Either increased or decreased tone may indicate intracranial disease, although such disease is usually accompanied by a number of other signs.

Sensory Function.   You can test for *sensory function* of the newborn in only a limited way. Test for pain sensation by flicking the infant's palm or

---

Signs of severe neurologic disease include *extreme irritability; persistent asymmetry of posture; persistent extension of extremities; constant turning of the head to one side; marked extension of the head, neck,* and *extremities (opisthotonus); severe flaccidity;* and *limited response to pain.*

Persistent irritability in the newborn may be a sign of neurologic insult or may reflect a variety of metabolic, infectious, or other constitutional abnormalities, or environmental conditions such as drug withdrawal.

Newborns with hypotonia often lie in a frog-leg position, with arms flexed and hands near the ears. Hypotonia can be caused by a variety of central nervous system abnormalities and disorders of the motor unit.

If changes in facial expression or cry follow a painful stimulus but no sole with your finger. Observe for withdrawal, arousal, and change in facial expression. Do not use a pin to test for pain.

Cranial Nerves. The *cranial nerves* of the newborn or infant can be tested, although you will have to open your bag of tricks for methods that differ from those used for the older child or adult. The following table provides useful strategies.

withdrawal occurs, *paralysis* may be present.

● Strategies to Assess Cranial Nerves in Newborns and Infants

Cranial Nerve		Strategy
I	Olfactory	Difficult to test
II	Visual acuity	Have baby regard your face and look for facial response and tracking.
II, III	Response to light	Darken room, raise baby to sitting position to open eyes. Use light and test for *optic blink reflex* (blinking in response to light). Use the otoscope (no speculum) to assess papillary responses.
III, IV, VI	Extraocular movements	Observe how well the baby tracks your smiling face. Use light if needed.
V	Motor	Test rooting reflex. Test sucking reflex (watch baby suck breast, bottle, or pacifier).
VII	Facial	Observe baby crying and smiling; note symmetry of face and forehead.
VIII	Acoustic	Test acoustic blink reflex (blinking of both eyes in response to loud noise). Observe tracking in response to sound.
IX, X	Swallow	Observe coordination during swallowing.
	Gag	Test for gag reflex.
XI	Spinal accessory	Observe symmetry of shoulders.

(continued)

Abnormalities in the cranial nerves suggest an intracranial lesion such as hemorrhage or a congenital malformation.

● Strategies to Assess Cranial Nerves in Newborns and Infants (continued)

Cranial Nerve		Strategy
XII	Hypoglossal	Observe coordination of sucking, swallowing, and tongue thrusting. Pinch nostrils; observe reflex opening of mouth with tip of tongue to midline.

Deep Tendon Reflexes. The *deep tendon reflexes* are variable in newborns and infants because the corticospinal pathways are not fully developed. Thus, their exaggerated presence or their absence has little diagnostic significance, unless this response is different from results of previous testing or extreme responses are observed.

A progressive increase in deep tendon reflexes during the first year of life may indicate central nervous system disease such as *cerebral palsy,* especially if it is coupled with increased tone.

Use the same techniques to elicit deep tendon reflexes as you would for an adult. You can substitute your index or middle finger for the neurologic hammer, as shown below.

As in adults, asymmetric reflexes suggest a lesion of the peripheral nerves or spinal segment.

The triceps, brachioradialis, and abdominal reflexes are difficult to elicit before 6 months of age. The *anal reflex* is present at birth and important to elicit if a spinal cord lesion is suspected.

Although a normal flexion plantar response is obtained in 90% of infants, a *positive Babinski response* to plantar stimulation (dorsiflexion of big toe and fanning of other toes) can be elicited in some normal babies until 2 years of age.

You can try to elicit the ankle reflex as for adults by tapping on the Achilles tendon but often will not get a response. Another method, shown next, is

An absent anal reflex suggests loss of innervation of the external sphincter muscle caused by a spinal cord abnormality such as a congenital anomaly (e.g., *spina bifida*), *tumor,* or *injury.*

When the contractions are continuous (*sustained ankle clonus*), to grasp the infant's malleolus with one hand and abruptly dorsiflex the ankle. Don't be surprised if you note rapid, rhythmic plantar flexion of the newborn's foot (*ankle clonus*) in response to this maneuver. Up to 10 beats are normal in newborns and young infants; this is *unsustained ankle clonus*.

Primitive Reflexes.   Evaluate the newborn and infant's developing central nervous system by assessing *infantile automatisms*, called *primitive reflexes*. These develop during gestation, are generally demonstrable at birth, and disappear at defined ages. Abnormalities in these primitive reflexes suggest neurologic disease and merit more intensive investigation.[24] The most important primitive reflexes are illustrated on the next page.

Additional primitive reflexes shown on p. 795 are not usually used in the general examination but are helpful in a more extensive evaluation of an infant with abnormal neurologic findings.

Development.   Refer to the developmental milestones on page 750 and to the DDST on pages 753–754 to learn which age-specific developmental tasks to evaluate. By observation and play with the infant, you can do both a developmental screening examination and an assessment for gross and fine motor achievement. Specifically, look for *weakness* by observing sitting, standing, and transitions. Note *station*, or the posture of sitting or standing. Carefully observe the *gait* of the toddler, including balance and fluidity of movements. Fine motor development can be assessed in a similar way, combining the neurologic and developmental exam. Key milestones include the development of the pincer grasp, ability to manipulate objects with the hands, and more precise tasks, such as building a tower of cubes or scribbling, as fine motor development progresses in a proximal to distal direction.

Assess the infant's cognitive and social–emotional development as you proceed with the comprehensive neurologic and developmental examination. Some neurologic abnormalities produce deficits or slowing in cognitive and

A *neurologic* or *developmental abnormality* is suspected if primitive reflexes are
- Absent at appropriate age
- Present longer than normal
- Asymmetric
- Associated with posturing or twitching

● Primitive Reflex

Primitive Reflex		Maneuver	Ages
Palmar Grasp Reflex		Place your fingers into the baby's hands and press against the palmar surfaces. The baby will flex all fingers to grasp your fingers.	Birth to 3–4 mos
Plantar Grasp Reflex		Touch the sole at the base of the toes. The toes curl.	Birth to 6–8 mos
Moro Reflex (Startle Reflex)		Hold the baby supine, supporting the head, back, and legs. Abruptly lower the entire body about 2 feet. The arms abduct and extend, hands open, and legs flex. Baby may cry.	Birth to 4 mos
Asymmetric Tonic Neck Reflex		With baby supine, turn head to one side, holding jaw over shoulder. The arms/legs on side to which head is turned extend while the opposite arm/leg flex. Repeat on other side.	Birth to 2 mos
Positive Support Reflex		Hold the baby around the trunk and lower until the feet touch a flat surface. The hips, knees, and ankles extend, the baby stands up, partially bearing weight, sags after 20–30 seconds.	Birth or 2 mos until 6 mos

Palmar Grasp Reflex

Persistence beyond 4 mos suggests pyramidal tract dysfunction.

Persistence of clenched hand beyond 2 mos suggests central nervous system damage, especially if fingers overlap thumb.

Plantar Grasp Reflex

Persistence beyond 8 mos suggests pyramidal tract dysfunction.

Moro Reflex

Persistence beyond 4 mos suggests neurologic disease (e.g., cerebral palsy); beyond 6 mos strongly suggests it.

Asymmetric response suggests fracture of clavicle or humerus or brachial plexus injury.

Asymmetric Tonic Neck Reflex

Persistence beyond 2 mos suggests asymmetric central nervous system development and sometimes predicts the development of cerebral palsy.

Positive Support Reflex

Lack of reflex suggests hypotonia or flaccidity.

Fixed extension and adduction of legs (scissoring) suggests spasticity from neurologic disease, such as cerebral palsy.

● Primitive Reflex (continued)

Primitive Reflex		Maneuver	Ages	
Rooting Reflex		Stroke the perioral skin at the corners of the mouth. The mouth will open and baby will turn the head toward the stimulated side and suck.	Birth to 3–4 mos	Absence of rooting indicates severe generalized or central nervous system disease.
Trunk Incurvation (Galant's) Reflex		Support the baby prone with one hand, and stroke one side of the back 1 cm from midline, from shoulder to buttocks. The spine will curve toward the stimulated side.	Birth to 2 mos	Absence suggests a transverse spinal cord lesion or injury. Persistence may indicate delayed development.
Placing and Stepping Reflexes		Hold baby upright from behind as in positive support reflex. Have one sole touch the tabletop. The hip and knee of that foot will flex and the other foot will step forward. Alternate stepping will occur.	Birth (best after 4 days). Variable age to disappear	Absence of placing may indicate paralysis. Babies born by breech delivery may not have placing reflex.
Landau Reflex		Suspend the baby prone with one hand. The head will lift up, and the spine will straighten.	Birth to 6 mos	Persistence may indicate delayed development.
Parachute Reflex		Suspend the baby prone and slowly lower the head toward a surface. The arms and legs will extend in a protective fashion.	4–6 mos and does not disappear	Delay in appearance may predict future delays in voluntary motor development.

social development. As stated, infants who have developmental delay may have abnormalities found on the neurologic examination because much of the examination is based on age-specific norms.

A normative measure of development is the developmental quotient,[25] which is shown here:

$$\text{Development quotient} = \frac{\text{Developmental age}}{\text{Chronologic age}} \times 100$$

Assess the development of an infant or child using standard scales such as the DDST for each type of development. For example, you can assign to a child a gross motor developmental quotient, a fine motor developmental quotient, a cognitive developmental quotient, and so forth.

DEVELOPMENTAL QUOTIENTS

>85	Normal
70–85	Possibly delayed; follow-up needed
<70	Delayed

CASE EXAMPLES OF GROSS AND FINE MOTOR DEVELOPMENT

Gross Motor Development

A 12-month-old child who is just pulling to stand (gross motor developmental age of 9 mos), cruising (10 mos), and walking when both hands are held (10 mos) has a gross motor developmental age of 10 months. This child's gross motor developmental quotient is:

$$\left(\tfrac{10}{12} \times 100\right) = 83$$

This child is in the gray zone, is likely to do well without intervention, but requires close follow-up.

Fine Motor Development

A 12-month-old child can transfer objects from hand to hand (a fine motor developmental age of 6 mos), rake objects into his palm (7 mos), and pull things (7 mos). He cannot hold blocks in each hand and does not have thumb and finger grasp (8–9 mos).

He has normal primitive reflexes (most absent), increased tone, scissoring of legs when held, spasticity, and delays on the gross motor part of the DDST.

This child's fine motor developmental quotient is:

$$\left(\tfrac{7}{12} \times 100\right) = 58$$

This child is delayed in fine motor development and has signs of *cerebral palsy*.

ASSESSING YOUNG AND SCHOOL-AGED CHILDREN

 ## DEVELOPMENT

Early Childhood: 1 to 4 Years

Physical Development. After infancy, the rate of physical growth slows by approximately half. After 2 years, toddlers gain about 2 to 3 kg and grow 5 cm per year. Physical changes are impressive. Chubby, clumsy toddlers transform into leaner, more muscular preschoolers.

Gross motor skills also develop quickly. Most children walk by 15 months, run well by 2 years, and pedal a tricycle and jump by 4 years. Fine motor skills develop through neurologic maturation and environmental manipulation. The 18-month-old who scribbles becomes a 2-year-old who draws lines and then a 4-year-old who makes circles.

Cognitive and Language Development. Toddlers move from sensorimotor learning (through touching and looking) to symbolic thinking, solving simple problems, remembering songs, and engaging in imitative play. Language develops with extraordinary speed. An 18-month-old with 10 to 20 words becomes a 2-year-old with three-word sentences, and then a 3-year-old who converses well. By 4 years, preschoolers form complex sentences. They remain preoperational, however, without sustained logical thought processes.

Social and Emotional Development. New intellectual pursuits are surpassed only by an emerging drive for independence. Because toddlers are impulsive, temper tantrums are common.

Developmental Milestones During Early Childhood

	1 yr	2 yr	3 yr	4 yr	5 yr
Physical/ Motor	Walks	Throws	Jumps in place Balances on 1 foot	Hops Pedals tricycle	Skips Balances well
Cognitive/ Language	2-3 words	2-3 word phrases	Sentences	Speech all understandable	Copies figures Defines words
Social/ Emotional	Plays games (peek-a-boo)	Imitates activities	Feeds self	Imaginative Sings	Dresses self Plays games

Middle Childhood: 5 to 10 Years

Despite Freud's view, middle childhood certainly is not a latent period. Goal-directed exploration, increased physical and cognitive abilities, and achievements by trial and error mark this stage. Physical examination is more straightforward, but always consider the developmental stages and tasks that school-age children are facing.

Physical Development. Children grow steadily but more slowly. Nevertheless, strength and coordination improve dramatically, with more participation in activities. This is also when children with physical disabilities or chronic illnesses become more aware of their limitations.

Cognitive and Language Development. Children become "concrete operational"—capable of limited logic and more complex learning. They remain rooted in the present, with little ability to understand consequences or abstractions. School, family, and environment greatly influence learning. A major developmental task is self-efficacy, or the ability to thrive in different situations. Language becomes increasingly complex.

Social and Emotional Development. Children become progressively more independent, initiating activities and enjoying accomplishments. Achievements are critical for self-esteem and developing a "fit" within major social structures—family, school, and peer activity groups. Guilt and poor self-esteem also may emerge. Family and environment contribute enormously to the child's self-image. Moral development remains simple and concrete, with a clear sense of "right and wrong."

● Developmental Tasks During Middle Childhood

Task	Characteristic	Health Care Needs
Physical	Enhanced strength and coordination	Screening for strengths, assessing problems
	Competence in various tasks and activities	Involving parents
		Support for disabilities
		Anticipatory guidance: safety
Cognitive	"Concrete operational": focus on the present	Emphasis on short-term consequences
	Achievement of knowledge and skills, self-efficacy	Support; screening about skills and school performance
Social	Achieving good "fit" with family, friends, school	Assessment, support, advice about interactions
	Sustained self-esteem	Support, emphasis on strengths
	Evolving self-identity	Understanding, advice, support

THE HEALTH HISTORY

An important and unique aspect of examining children is that parents are usually watching and taking part in the interaction, providing you the opportunity to observe the parent–child interaction. Note whether the child displays age-appropriate behaviors. Assess the "goodness of fit" between parents and child. Although some abnormal interactions may result from the unnatural setting of the examination room, others may be a consequence of interactional problems. Careful *observation* of the child's interactions with parents and the child's unstructured play in the examination room can reveal *abnormalities in physical, cognitive, and social development.*

Normal toddlers are occasionally terrified or angry at the examiner. Often, they are completely uncooperative. Most eventually warm up to you. If this behavior continues or is not developmentally appropriate, there may be an *underlying behavioral or developmental abnormality.* Older, school-aged children have more self-control and prior experience with clinicians and are generally cooperative with the examination. You can detect a surprising amount by using observation.

ABNORMALITIES DETECTED WHILE OBSERVING PLAY

Behavioral Problems*

Poor parent–child interactions
Sibling rivalry
Inappropriate parental discipline
"Difficult temperament"

Developmental Delay (see DDST)

Gross motor delay
Fine motor delay
Language delay (expressive, receptive)
Delay in social or emotional tasks

Social or Environmental Problems

Parental problem, e.g., stress, depression
Risk for abuse or neglect

Neurologic Problems

Weakness
Abnormal posture
Spasticity
Clumsiness
Attentional problems and hyperactivity
Autistic features
Musculoskeletal abnormalities
  Foot deformities
  Gait problems

*Note: The child's behavior during the visit may not represent typical behavior, but your observations may serve as a springboard for discussion with parents.

Assessing Younger Children

One of the most difficult challenges you will face in examining children in this age group is avoiding a physical struggle, a crying child, or a distraught parent. Accomplishing this successfully is immensely satisfying and is one aspect of the "art of medicine" in the practice of pediatrics.

Begin to gain the child's confidence and allay the child's fears from the start of the encounter. Your approach will vary with the circumstances of the visit. A health supervision visit for a well child allows greater rapport than a visit when the child is acutely ill.

Let the child remain dressed during the interview to minimize the child's apprehension. It also allows you to interact more naturally and observe the child playing, interacting with the parents, and undressing and dressing.

Toddlers who are 9 to 15 months may have *stranger anxiety,* a fear of strangers that is developmentally normal. It signals the toddler's growing awareness that the stranger is "new." You should not approach these toddlers quickly. Make sure they remain solidly in their parent's lap throughout much of the examination.

The following are useful tips in examining young children.

SOME TIPS FOR EXAMINING YOUNG CHILDREN (1–4-YEAR-OLDS)

Useful Strategies for Examination	Useful Toys and Aids
Examine a child sitting on parent's lap. Try to be at the child's eye level.	"Blow out" the otoscope light.
First examine the child's toy or teddy bear, then the child.	"Beep" the stethoscope on your nose.
Let the child do some of the exam (e.g., move the stethoscope). Then go back and "get the places we missed."	Make tongue-depressor puppets.
Ask the toddler who keeps pushing you away to "hold your hand." Then have the toddler "help you" with the exam.	Use the child's own toys for play.
Some toddlers believe that if they can't see you, then you aren't there. Perform the exam while the child stands on the parent's lap, facing the parent.	Jingle your keys to test for hearing.
If 2-year-olds are holding something in each hand (such as tongue depressors), they can't fight or resist!	Shine the otoscope through the tip of your finger, "lighting it up," and then examine the child's ears with it.

Engage children in age-appropriate conversation. Ask simple questions about their illness or toys. Compliment their appearance or behavior, tell a story, or play a simple game to "break the ice." If a child is shy, turn your attention to the parent to allow the child to warm up gradually.

With certain exceptions, physical examination does not require use of the examining table—it can be done on the floor or with the child in a parent's lap. The key is to engage the child's cooperation. For young children who resist undressing, expose only the body part being examined. When examining siblings, begin with the oldest child, who is more likely to cooperate and set a good example. Approach the child pleasantly. Explain each step as you perform it. Continue conversing with the family to provide distraction.

Plan the examination to start with the least distressing procedures and end with the most distressing (usually involving the throat and ears). Begin with parts that can be done with the child sitting, such as examining the eyes or palpating the neck. Lying down may make a child feel vulnerable, so change positions with care. Once a child is supine, start with the abdomen, saving throat and ears or genitalia for last. You may need a parent's help to restrain the child for examination of the ears or throat; however, use of formal restraints is inappropriate. Patience, distraction, play, flexibility in the order of the examination, and a caring but firm and gentle approach are all key to successfully examining the young child.

More Tips for Examining the Young Child

Use a reassuring voice throughout the examination.
Let the child see and touch the examination tools you will be using.
Avoid asking permission to examine a body part because you will do the examination anyway. Instead, ask the child which ear or which part of the body he or she would like you to examine "first."
Examine the child in the parent's lap. Let the parent undress the child.
If unable to console the child, give the child a short break.
Make a game out of the examination! For example, "Let's see how big your tongue is!" or "Is Barney in your ear? Let's see!"

Reassure parents that resistance to examination is developmentally appropriate. Some embarrassed parents scold the child, compounding the problem. Involve parents in the examination. Learn which techniques and approaches work best and are most comfortable for you.

Assessing Older Children

Examining children after they reach school age usually poses few difficulties. Although some have unpleasant memories of previous clinical encounters, most children respond well when the examiner is attuned to developmental level.

Many children at this age are modest. Providing gowns and leaving underwear in place as long as possible are wise approaches. Suggest that children disrobe behind a curtain. Consider leaving the room while they change with parents' help. Some children may prefer opposite-sex siblings to leave, but most prefer a parent of either sex to remain in the room. Parents of children younger than 11 years should stay with them.

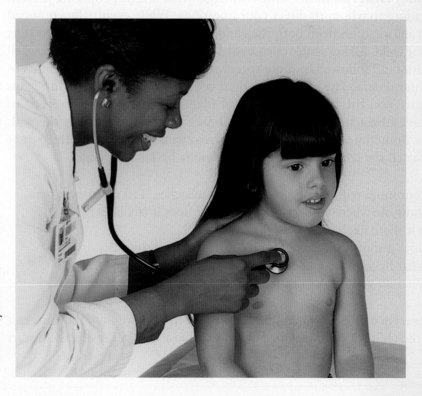

Children usually are accompanied by a parent or caregiver. Even when alone, they are often seeking health care at the request of their parents—indeed, the parent is usually sitting in the waiting room. When interviewing a child, you need to consider the needs and perspectives of both the child and the caregivers.

Establishing Rapport. Begin the interview by greeting and establishing rapport with each person present. Refer to the child by name rather than by "him" or "her." Clarify the role or relationship of all of the adults and children. "Now, are you Jimmy's grandmother?" "Please help me by telling me Jimmy's relationship to everyone here." Address the parents as "Mr. Smith" and "Ms. Smith" rather than by their first names or "Mom" or "Dad." When the family structure is not immediately clear, you may avoid embarrassment by asking directly about other members. "Who else lives in the home?" "Who is Jimmy's father?" "Do you live together?" Do not assume that just because parents are separated, only one parent is actively involved in the child's life.

To establish rapport, meet children on their own level. Use your personal experiences with children to guide how you interact in a health care setting. Eye contact on their level, participating in playful engagement, and talking about what interests them are always good strategies. Ask children about their clothes, one of their toys, what book or TV show they like, or their adult companion in an enthusiastic but gentle style. Spending time at the beginning of the interview to calm down and connect with an anxious child can put both the child and the caregiver at ease.

Working With Families. One challenge when several people are present is deciding to whom to direct your questions. While eventually you need to get information from both the child and the parent, it is useful to start with the child. Asking simple open-ended questions like "Are you sick? . . . Tell me about it," followed by more specific questions, often provides much of the clinical data. The parents can then verify the information, add details that give you the larger context, and identify other issues you need to address. Characterize symptom attributes the same way you do with adults. Sometimes children are embarrassed to begin, but once the parent has started the conversation, direct questions back to the child:

> Your mom tells me that you get stomachaches. Tell me about them.
> Show me where you get the pain. What does it feel like?
> Is it sharp like a pin prick, or does it ache?
> Does it stay in the same spot, or does it move around?
> What helps make it go away? What makes it worse?
> What do you think causes it?

The presence of family members allows you to observe how they interact with the child. A child may be able to sit still or may get restless and start fidgeting. Watch how the parents set limits or fail to set limits when needed.

Multiple Agendas.   Each individual in the room, including the clinician, may have a different idea about the nature of the problem and what needs to be done about it. It is your job to discover as many of these perspectives and agendas as possible. Family members who are not present (e.g., the absent parent or grandparent) may also have concerns. Ask about those concerns, too. "If Suzie's father were here today, what questions or concerns would he have?" "Have you, Mrs. Jones, discussed this with your mother or anyone else?" "What does she think?" For example, Mrs. Jones brings Suzie in for abdominal pain because she is worried that Suzie may have an ulcer and is also worried about Suzie's eating habits. Suzie is not worried about the belly pain, but is uneasy about the changes in her body and about getting fat. Mr. Jones thinks that Suzie's school work is not getting enough attention. You, as the clinician, need to balance these concerns with what you see as a healthy 12-year-old girl in early puberty with some mild functional abdominal pain. Your goals need to include helping the family to be realistic about the range of "normal" and uncovering the concerns of Mr. and Mrs. Jones and Suzie.

The Family as a Resource.   In general, family members provide most of the care and are your natural allies in promoting the child's health. Being open to a wide range of parenting behaviors helps to make this alliance. Raising a child reflects cultural, socioeconomic, and family practices. It is important to respect the tremendous variation in these practices. A good strategy is to view the parents as experts in the care of their child and yourself as their consultant. This demonstrates respect for the parents' care and minimizes their likelihood of discounting or ignoring your advice. Parents face many challenges raising children, so practitioners need to be supportive, not judgmental. Comments like, "Why didn't you bring him in sooner?" or "What did you do that for!" do not improve your rapport with the parent. Statements acknowledging the hard work of parenting and praising successes are always appreciated. "Mr. Smith, you are doing such a wonderful job with Bobby. Being a parent takes so much work and Bobby's behavior here today clearly shows your efforts." Or to the child, "Bobby you are so lucky to have such a wonderful Dad."

Hidden Agendas.   Finally, as with adults, the chief complaint may not relate to the real reason the parent has brought the child to see you. The complaint may be a "ticket to care" or bridge to concerns that may not seem quite legitimate as a reason to go to the doctor. Try to create a trusting atmosphere that allows parents to be open about all their concerns. Ask facilitating questions like:

Do you have any other concerns about Randy?
Was there anything else that you wanted to tell/ask me today?

HEALTH PROMOTION AND COUNSELING

Children 1 to 4 Years

The AAP and Bright Futures periodicity schedules for children include health supervision visits at 12, 15, 18, and 24 months, followed by annual visits when the child is 3 and 4 years old.[8] An additional visit at 30 months is also recommended to assess the child's development.

During these health supervision visits, clinicians address concerns and questions from parents, evaluate the child's growth and development, perform a comprehensive physical examination, and provide anticipatory guidance about healthy habits and behaviors, social competence of caregivers, family relationships, and community interactions.

This is a critical age for preventing childhood obesity: many children begin their trajectory toward obesity between ages 3 and 4. It is also important to adequately assess the child's development. Standardized developmental screening instruments are increasingly being recommended to measure the different dimensions of a child's development. Similarly, it is important to differentiate normal (but potentially challenging) childhood behavior from abnormal behavioral or mental health problems.

The following box demonstrates the major components of a health supervision visit for a 3-year-old, stressing health promotion. You don't have to wait for a health supervision visit to address many of these health promotion issues—they can be addressed during other types of visits, even when the child is mildly ill.

COMPONENTS OF A HEALTH SUPERVISION VISIT FOR A 3-YEAR-OLD

Discussions with Parents

- Address parent concerns
- Provide advice
- Childcare, school, social
- Assess major topic areas: development, nutrition, safety, oral health, family relationships, community

Developmental Assessment

- Assess milestones (DDST): gross and fine motor, social–personal, language

Physical Examination

- Perform a careful examination, including growth parameters with percentiles for age.

Screening Tests

- Vision and hearing (formal testing at age 4), hematocrit and lead

(if high risk or at ages 1–3), screen for social risk factors

Immunizations

- See schedule (pages 741–742)

Anticipatory Guidance

Healthy Habits and Behaviors
- Injury & illness prevention
  Car seat, poisons, tobacco exposure, supervision
- Nutrition
  Obesity assessment; healthy meals and snacks
- Oral health
  Brushing teeth; dentist

Parent–Infant Interaction
- Reading and fun times, TV

Family Relationships
- Activities, babysitters

Community Interaction
- Childcare, resources

Children 5 to 10 Years

The AAP and Bright Futures periodicity schedules for children recommend annual health supervision visits during this period.[8] As for prior ages, these visits present wonderful opportunities to assess the child's physical, mental, and developmental health and the parent–child relationship. Once again, health promotion should be incorporated into all interactions with children and families—take advantage of any opportunity to promote optimal health and development!

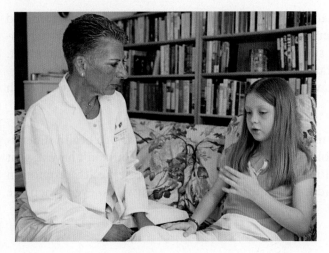

One of the most satisfying components of health promotion for the older child involves talking directly with the child. In addition to discussing issues of health, safety, development, and anticipatory guidance with parents, you should be including the child in these conversations, using age-appropriate language and concepts. For example, the child's major environment beyond the family involves school. Discuss the child's experience and perceptions of school, as well as other cognitive and social activities. During these discussions, focus on healthy habits such as good nutrition, exercise, reading, stimulating activities, and safety.

About 12% to 20% of children have some type of chronic physical, developmental, or mental condition.[26] Also, some behaviors that become established at this age can lead to or exacerbate chronic conditions such as obesity or eating disorders. Therefore, health promotion is critical to optimize healthy habits and minimize unhealthy ones. Further, helping families and children with chronic diseases deal most effectively with these disorders is a key part of health promotion. For all children, the well-being of the family is critical to the child's health; thus, health promotion involves assessing and promoting the family's overall health.

The specific components of the health supervision visit for older children are the same as the components for younger children, shown in the box on the previous page. Emphasize school performance and experiences, as well as appropriate and safe sports and activities.

 ## TECHNIQUES OF EXAMINATION

The order of the examination now begins to follow that used for adults. Examine painful areas last, and forewarn children about areas you are going to examine. If a child resists part of the examination, you can return to it at the end.

General Survey and Vital Signs

Somatic Growth

The figures on the next page demonstrate somatic growth patterns of various systems in children.

Height.   For children older than 2 years, measure standing height, optimally using wall-mounted stadiometers. Have the child stand with heels, back, and head against a wall or the back of the stadiometer. If using a wall

Short stature, defined as subnormal height for age, can be a normal variant or caused by endocrine or

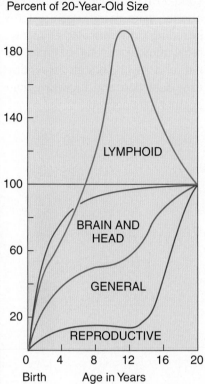

Growth Patterns of Various Systems

Percent of 20-Year-Old Size

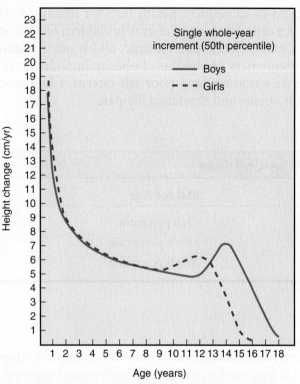

Velocity curves for length and height for boys and girls based on intervals of 1 year. (From Lowrey GH. Growth and development of children, 8th ed. Chicago, Mosby, 1986.)

with a marked ruler, make sure to place a flat board or surface against the top of the child's head and at right angles to the ruler. Stand-up weight scales with a height attachment are not very accurate.

Rule of thumb on height: After age 2 years, children should grow at least 5 centimeters per year.

Weight.   Young children who can stand and school-age children should be weighed in their underpants or in a gown on a stand-up scale. Although initially nervous, most young children can be coaxed onto such scales. Use the same scales if possible.

Head Circumference.   In general, head circumference is measured until the child reaches 24 months. Afterward, head circumference measurement may be helpful if you suspect a genetic or central nervous system disorder.

Body Mass Index for Age.   Age- and sex-specific charts are now available to assess BMI in children (see the following table). BMI in children is asso-

other diseases. Normal variants include *familial short stature* and *constitutional delay.* Chronic diseases include *growth hormone deficiency,* other endocrine diseases, *gastrointestinal disease, renal* or *metabolic disease,* and *genetic syndromes.*

Young children can have inadequate weight and height gain if caloric intake is insufficient. Etiologies of failure to thrive include *psychosocial, interactional, gastrointestinal,* and *endocrine disorders.*

Most children with exogenous obesity are also tall for their age. Children with endocrine causes of obesity tend to be short.

Childhood obesity is a major epidemic: 36% of U.S. children have a ciated with body fat, related to subsequent health risks for obesity. BMI measurements are helpful for early detection of obesity in children older than 2 years. Obesity is now a major childhood epidemic, and it often begins before 6 to 8 years. Consequences of childhood obesity include hypertension, diabetes, metabolic syndrome, and poor self-esteem. Childhood obesity often leads to adult obesity and shortened lifespan.

BMI > the 85th percentile, and 16% have a BMI ≥ the 95th percentile.[27] Long-term morbidity from childhood obesity spans many organ systems, including cardiovascular, endocrine, renal, musculoskeletal, gastrointestinal, and psychological. Prevention, early detection, and aggressive management are needed.

● Interpreting BMI in Children

Group	BMI-for-Age
Underweight	<5th percentile
At risk of overweight	≥85th percentile
Overweight	≥95th percentile

Vital Signs

Blood Pressure.   Hypertension during childhood is more common than previously thought, and it is important to recognize, confirm, and appropriately manage it. Thus, you must learn to accurately measure blood pressure in children.

Children have elevated blood pressure during exercise, crying, and anxiety. Although young children may be anxious at first, when the procedure is explained and demonstrated beforehand, most children are cooperative. If the blood pressure is initially elevated, you can perform blood pressure readings again at the end of the examination; one trick is to leave the cuff on the arm (deflated) and repeat the reading later. Elevated readings must always be confirmed by subsequent measurements.

The most frequent "cause" of an elevated blood pressure in children is probably an *improperly performed examination,* often due to an incorrect cuff size.

Select the blood pressure cuff as you would for adults. It should be wide enough to cover two thirds of the upper arm or leg. A narrower cuff falsely elevates the blood pressure reading, whereas a wider cuff lowers it and may interfere with proper placement of the stethoscope diaphragm over the artery. *Thus, a proper cuff size is essential for accurate determinations of blood pressure in children.*

In children, as in adults, blood pressure readings from the thigh are approximately 10 mm Hg higher than those from the upper arm. If they are the same or lower, *coarctation of the aorta* should be suspected.

With children, as with adults, the point at which the Korotkoff sounds disappear constitutes the diastolic pressure. At times, especially among chubby young children, the Korotkoff sounds are not easily heard. In such instances, you can use palpation to determine the systolic blood pressure, remembering that the systolic pressure is approximately 10 mm Hg lower by palpation than by auscultation.

A relatively inaccurate means is to use "inspection." Watch for the needle to bounce about 10 mm Hg higher than it does in auscultation. Although this technique is suboptimal, in squirming children it is sometimes all you can get.

Transient hypertension in children can be caused by some common childhood medications, including those to treat asthma (e.g., prednisone) and ADHD (e.g., ritalin).

In 2004, the National Heart, Lung, and Blood Institute's National High Blood Pressure Working Group on Hypertension Control in Children and Adolescents defined normal, high-normal, and high blood pressure as follows, with measurements on at least three separate occasions[28]:

Causes of *sustained hypertension* in childhood include renal parenchymal or artery disease, coarctation of the aorta, and primary hypertension.

● Blood Pressure

Blood Pressure Category	Average Systolic and/or Diastolic Blood Pressure for Age, Sex, and Height
Normal	<90th percentile
Prehypertensive	90th–95th percentile
Hypertensive	≥95th percentile

Children who have hypertension should be evaluated extensively to determine the cause. For infants and young children, a specific cause can usually be found. An increasing proportion of older children and adolescents, however, have essential or primary hypertension. In all cases, it is important to repeat measurements to reduce the possibility that the elevation reflects anxiety. Sometimes repeating measurements in school is a way to obtain readings in a more relaxed environment. Hypertension and obesity often co-exist in children.

It is also important not to *falsely label* a child or adolescent as having hypertension, because of the stigma of labeling, potential limitations to activities, and possible side effects of treatment.

Pulse.   Average heart rates and ranges of normal are shown in the table below. Measure the heart rate over a 90- or 60-second interval.

● Average Heart Rate of Children at Rest		
Age	Average Rate	Range (Two Standard Deviations)
1–2 years	110	70–150
2–6 years	103	68–138
6–10 years	95	65–125

Sinus bradycardia is a heart rate <100 beats per minute in children younger than 3 years, and <60 beats per minute in children 3 to 9 years.

Respiratory Rate.   The rate of respirations per minute ranges from 20 to 40 during early childhood, and 15 to 25 during late childhood, reaching adult levels at around 15 years of age.

For young children, observe the movements of the chest wall for two 30-second intervals or over 1 minute, preferably before stimulating them. Direct auscultation of the chest or placing the stethoscope in front of the mouth is also useful for counting respirations, but the measurement may be falsely elevated if the child becomes agitated. For older children, use the same technique as that used for adults.

Children with respiratory diseases such as *bronchiolitis* or *pneumonia* have rapid respirations (up to 80–90/min) but *also* increased work of breathing such as grunting, nasal flaring, or use of accessory muscles.

The commonly accepted cutoff for tachypnea in children older than 1 year is a respiratory rate greater than 40 breaths per minute.

The best single physical finding for ruling out *pneumonia* is an absence of tachypnea

Temperature.   In children, auditory canal temperature recordings are preferable because they can be obtained quickly with essentially no discomfort.

Young children with infections can have extremely high fevers (up to 104°F or 40°C). Children younger than 3 years, who appear very ill with a fever, should be evaluated for possible sepsis, urinary tract infection, pneumonia, or other infectious etiology.

The Skin

After a child's first year of life, the techniques of examination are the same as those for the adult (see Chapter 6, The Skin, Hair, and Nails.)

The Head

In examining the head and neck, tailor your examination to the child's stage of growth and development.

Even before touching the child, carefully observe the shape of the head, its symmetry, and the presence of abnormal facies. Abnormal facies may not be apparent until later in childhood; therefore, carefully examine the face as well as the head of all children.

There are diagnostic facies in childhood (Table 18-6, Diagnostic Facies in Infancy and Childhood, pp. 860–861, shows several) that reflect chromosomal abnormalities, endocrine defects, chronic illness, and other disorders.

The Eyes

The two most important components of the eye examination for young children are to determine whether the gaze is conjugate or symmetric and to test visual acuity in each eye.

Strabismus (see Table 18-7, Abnormalities of the Eyes, Ears, and Mouth, p. 862) in children requires treatment by an ophthalmologist.

Conjugate Gaze. Use the methods described in Chapter 7 for adults to assess *conjugate gaze*, or the *position and alignment of the eyes*, and the function of the extraocular muscles. The corneal light reflex test and the cover–uncover test are particularly useful in young children.

You can perform the cover–uncover test as a game by having the young child watch your nose or tell you if you are smiling or not, while you cover one of the child's eyes.

Both *ocular strabismus* and *anisometropia* (eyes with significantly different refractive errors) can result in *amblyopia*, or reduced vision in an otherwise normal eye. *Amblyopia* can lead to a "lazy eye," with permanently reduced visual acuity if not corrected early (generally by 6 years).

Visual Acuity. It may not be possible to measure the *visual acuity* of children younger than 3 years who cannot identify pictures on an eye chart. For these children, the simplest examination is to assess for fixation preference by alternately covering one eye; the child with normal vision will not object, but a child with poor vision in one eye will object to having the good eye covered. In all tests of visual acuity, it is important that both eyes show the same result.

Reduced visual acuity is more likely among children who were born prematurely, and among those with other neurologic or developmental disorders.

● Visual Acuity

Age	Acuity
3 months	Eyes converge, baby reaches
12 months	~20/200
Less than 4 years	20/40
4 years and older	20/30

Any difference in visual acuity between the eyes (e.g., 20/20 on the left and 20/30 on the right) is abnormal, and the patient should be referred to an ophthalmologist.

As shown below, visual acuity in children 3 years and older can usually be formally tested using an eye chart with one of a variety of optotypes (characters or symbols).[29] A child who does not know letters or numbers reliably can be tested using pictures, symbols, or the "E" chart. Using the "E" chart, most children will cooperate by telling you in which direction the "E" is pointing.

Visual Fields.   The *visual fields* can be examined in infants and young children with the child sitting on the parent's lap. One eye should be tested at a time with the other eye covered. Hold the child's head in the midline while bringing an object such as a toy into the field of vision from behind the child. The overall method is the same as that for adults, except that you will have to make this into a game for your patient.

The most common visual disorder of childhood is *myopia,* which can be easily detected using this examination technique.

The Ears

You may feel as if you need 10 hands and a bag of tricks to examine the *ear canal and drum* of young children, who are sensitive and fearful because they cannot observe the procedure. With a little practice you can master this technique. Unfortunately, many young children need to be briefly restrained during this examination, which is why you may want to leave it for the end.

If the child is not too fearful, you may examine the ears with the child sitting on a parent's lap. It is helpful to make a game out of the otoscopic examination, such as finding an imaginary object in the child's ear, or talking playfully to allay fears. It may help to place the otoscopic speculum gently into the external auditory canal of one ear and then withdraw it so the child gets used to the procedure, before the actual examination.

Ask the parent for a preference regarding the positioning of the child for the examination. There are two common positions—the child lying down and restrained, and the child sitting in the parent's lap. If the child is held supine, have the parent hold the arms either extended or close to the sides to limit motions. Hold the head and retract the tragus with one hand while you hold the otoscope with your other hand. If the child is on the parent's lap, the child's legs should be between the parent's legs. The parent could help by placing one arm around the child's body and using the second arm to steady the head.

Tympanic Membranes. Many students have difficulty even visualizing a child's tympanic membrane. In young children, the external auditory canal is directed upward and backward from the outside, and the auricle must be pulled upward, outward, and backward to afford the best view. Hold the child's head with one hand (your left hand if you are right-handed), and with that same hand pull up on the auricle. With your other hand, position the otoscope.

TIPS FOR CONDUCTING THE OTOSCOPIC EXAMINATION

Use the best angle of the otoscope.
Use the largest possible speculum.
 A larger speculum allows you to better visualize the tympanic membrane.
 A small speculum may not provide a seal for pneumatic otoscopy.
Don't apply too much pressure, which will cause the child to cry and may
 cause false-positive results on pneumatic otoscopy.
Insert the speculum ¼ to ½ inch into the canal.
First find the landmarks.
 Sometimes the ear canal resembles the tympanic membrane—don't be
 fooled!
Note whether the tympanic membrane is abnormal.
Remove cerumen if it is blocking your view, using
 Special plastic curettes
 A moistened microtipped cotton swab
 Flushing of ears for older children
 Special instruments that can also be purchased.

Not only are there two positions for the child (lying down or sitting), but also there are two ways to hold the otoscope, as illustrated by the following photos:

● The first is the method generally used in adults, with the otoscope handle pointing upward or laterally while you pull up on the auricle. Hold the lateral aspect of your hand that has the otoscope against the child's head to provide a buffer against sudden movements by the patient.

- The second technique is used by many pediatricians because of the different angle of the auditory canal in children. Hold the otoscope with the handle pointing down toward the child's feet, while you pull up on the auricle. Hold the head and pull up on the auricle with one hand, while you hold the otoscope with the other hand.

Acute otitis media is a common condition of childhood. A symptomatic child typically has a red, bulging tympanic membrane, with a dull or absent light reflex and diminished movement on pneumatic otoscopy. Purulent material may also be seen behind the tympanic membrane. See Table 18-7, Abnormalities of the Eyes, Ears, and Mouth, p. 862. The most useful symptom in making the diagnosis is ear pain, if combined with the above signs.[30,31]

Learn to use a *pneumatic otoscope* to improve your accuracy of diagnosis of otitis media in children. This allows you to assess the mobility of the tympanic membrane as you increase or decrease the pressure in the external auditory canal by squeezing the rubber bulb of the pneumatic otoscope.

First, check the pneumatic otoscope for leaks by placing your finger over the tip of the speculum and squeezing the bulb. Note the pressure on the bulb. Then insert the speculum, obtaining a proper seal; this is critical because failure to obtain a seal can produce a false-positive finding (lack of movement of the tympanic membrane).

Sometimes during acute otitis media the tympanic membrane ruptures, leading to pus in the auditory canal. In these cases you won't generally visualize the tympanic membrane.

When air is introduced into the normal ear canal, the tympanic membrane and its light reflex move inward. When air is removed, the tympanic membrane moves outward, toward you. This to-and-fro movement of the tympanic membrane has been likened to the luffing of a sail. If the tympanic membrane fails to move perceptibly as you introduce positive or negative pressure, then the child is likely to have a middle ear effusion. A child with acute otitis media may flinch because of pain due to the air pressure.

Movement of the tympanic membrane is absent in middle ear effusion (*otitis media with effusion*).

Significant, temporary hearing loss for several months can accompany otitis media with effusion.

Gently move and pull on the *pinna* before or during your otoscopic examination. Carefully inspect the area behind the pinna, over the mastoid bone.

With *otitis externa* (but not otitis media), movement of the pinna elicits pain.

With acute *mastoiditis,* the auricle may protrude forward, and the area over the mastoid bone is red, swollen, and tender.

Formal Hearing Testing. Although formal hearing testing is necessary for accurate detection of hearing deficits in young children, you can grossly test for hearing by using the whispered voice test. To do this, stand behind the child (so that the child cannot read your lips), cover one of the child's ear canals, and rub the tragus, using a circular motion. Whisper letters, numbers, or a word and have the child repeat it, then test the other ear. This technique has relatively high sensitivity and specificity compared with formal testing.[32]

Younger children who fail these screening maneuvers or who have speech delay should have audiometric testing. These children may have *hearing deficits.*

Up to 15% of school-aged children have at least mild hearing loss, emphasizing the importance of screening for hearing prior to school age.[32]

The American Academy of Pediatrics recommends that all children older than 4 years have a full-scale acoustic screening test using standardized equipment. Some other expert groups do not recommend formal hearing screening in asymptomatic children. If you do use an acoustic screening test, be sure to test the entire acoustic range, including the speaking range (500 to 6,000 Hz). The table below shows one classification of hearing ranges.

● **Hearing Ranges on Formal Acoustic Screening Tests**	
Normal hearing	0–20 dB
Mild hearing loss	21–40 dB
Moderate hearing loss	41–60 dB
Severe hearing loss	61–90 dB
Profound hearing loss	>90 dB

The Nose and Sinuses

Inspect the anterior portion of the nose by using a large speculum on your otoscope. Inspect the nasal mucous membranes, noting their color and condition. Look for nasal septal deviation and the presence of polyps.

Pale, boggy nasal mucous membranes are found in children with *chronic (perennial) allergic rhinitis.*

Maxillary sinuses are noted on x-rays by age 4 years, sphenoid sinuses by age 6, and frontal sinuses by age 6 to 7. The sinuses of older children can be palpated as in adults, looking for tenderness.[33] Transillumination of the paranasal sinuses of younger children has poor sensitivity and specificity for diagnosing sinusitis or fluid in the sinuses.

The Mouth and Pharynx

For anxious or young children, you may want to leave this part of the examination toward the end, because it may require parental restraint. The young, cooperative child may be more comfortable sitting in the parent's lap, as shown on the next page.

The accompanying figure demonstrates some tricks to getting children to open their mouths. The child who can say "ahhh" will usually offer a sufficient (albeit brief) view of the posterior pharynx so that a tongue blade is unnecessary. Healthy children are more likely to cooperate with this examination than sick children, especially if the sick child sees the tongue blade or has had previous experience with throat cultures.

If you need to use the tongue blade, push down and pull slightly forward toward yourself while the child says "ahhh," being careful not to place the blade too far posteriorly, eliciting a gag reflex. Sometimes young and anxious children will need to be restrained and will clamp their teeth and purse their lips. In these cases, carefully slip the tongue depressor between the teeth and onto the tongue. This will either allow you to push down on the tongue or elicit a gag reflex, which should permit a brief look at the posterior pharynx and tonsils. Remember, an unplanned, direct frontal assault on the front teeth will only meet with failure and a splintered tongue blade; careful planning and parental help are needed.

Examine the *teeth* for the timing and sequence of eruption, number, character, condition, and position. Abnormalities of the enamel may reflect local or general disease.

HOW TO GET CHILDREN TO OPEN THEIR MOUTHS (AKA, "WOULD YOU *PLEASE* SAY 'AHHH'?")

- Turn it into a game.
  - "Now let's see what's in your mouth."
  - "Can you stick out your *whole tongue*?"
  - "I bet you can't open your mouth *really wide*!"
  - "Let me see the inside of your teeth."
  - "Is Barney stuck in there?"
- Don't show a tongue blade unless really necessary.
- Demonstrate first on an older sibling (or even the parent).
- Offer enthusiastic praise for opening their mouths a little, and encourage them to open even wider!

Dental caries are the most common health problem in children. They are particularly prevalent in impoverished populations and can cause both short-term and long-term problems.[34] Caries are highly treatable.

Carefully inspect the upper teeth, as shown in the photo. This is a common location for *nursing-bottle caries*. The technique shown in the photo, called "lift the lip," can facilitate visualization of dental caries. Visualize the inside of the upper teeth by having the child look up at the ceiling with the mouth wide open.

Dental caries are caused by bacterial activity. Caries are more likely among young children who have prolonged bottle-feeding ("nursing-bottle caries"). See Table 18-8, Abnormalities of the Teeth, Pharynx, and Neck, p. 863, for different stages of caries.

The table below displays a common pattern of teeth eruption. In general, lower teeth erupt a bit earlier than upper teeth.

Staining of the teeth may be intrinsic or extrinsic. Intrinsic stains may be from tetracycline use before 8 years (yellow, gray, or brown stain). Iron preparation (black stain) is an example of extrinsic stain. Extrinsic stains can be polished off; intrinsic stains cannot (see Table 18-8, Abnormalities of the Teeth, Pharynx, and Neck, p. 863).

● Tooth Types and Age of Eruption[35]

	Approximate Age of Eruption	
Tooth Type	Primary (mos)	Permanent (yrs)
Central incisor	5–8	6–8
Lateral incisor	5–11	7–9
Cuspids	24–30	11–12
First bicuspids	—	10–12
Second bicuspids	—	10–12
First molars	16–20	6–7
Second molars	24–30	11–13
Third molars	—	17–22

Look for abnormalities of the position of the teeth. These include malocclusion, maxillary protrusion (*overbite*), and mandibular protrusion (*underbite*). You can demonstrate the latter two by asking the child to bite down hard while either you or the child parts the lips. Observe the true bite. In normal children, the lower teeth are contained within the arch formed by the upper teeth.

Malocclusion and misalignment of teeth are often from excessive thumb sucking and are reversible if the habit is arrested by 6 or 7 years. Malocclusion can also be a hereditary condition or from premature loss of primary teeth.

Carefully inspect the *tongue,* including the underside. Most children will happily stick their tongue out at you, move it from side to side, and demonstrate its color (the blue tongue below is from eating candy!).

Common abnormalities include *coated tongue* in viral infections, *congenital geographic tongue,* and *strawberry tongue,* found in scarlet fever.

Some young children have a tight frenulum. Children who are severely "tongue-tied" might have a speech impediment. Have the child touch the tongue to the roof of the mouth to diagnose this condition, which is easily treated.

Note the size, position, symmetry, and appearance of the *tonsils.* The peak growth of tonsillar tissue is between 8 and 16 years (see figure on p. 863). The size of the tonsils varies considerably in children and is often categorized on a scale of 1+ to 4+, with 1+ being easy visibility of the gap between the tonsils, and 4+ being tonsils that touch in the midline with the mouth wide open. The tonsils in children often appear more obstructive than they really are.

Streptococcal pharyngitis typically produces a strawberry tongue, white or yellow exudates on the tonsils or posterior pharynx, a beefy-red uvula, and palatal petechiae. Together with these signs, the most helpful historical information is exposure to strep throat infection within 2 weeks.[36]

Tonsils in children usually have deep crypts on their surfaces, which often have white concretions or food particles protruding from their depths. This does not indicate disease.

A *peritonsillar abscess* is suggested by asymmetric enlargement of the tonsils and lateral displacement of the uvula.

Look for clues of a submucosal cleft palate, such as notching of the posterior margin of the hard palate or a bifid *uvula*. Because the mucosa is intact, the underlying defect is easily missed.

Extremely rarely, you may encounter a child who has a sore throat and has difficulty swallowing saliva, who is sitting up stiffly in a "tripod" position because of throat obstruction. Do not open this child's mouth because he may have acute epiglottitis.

Note the quality of the child's voice. Certain abnormalities can change the pitch and quality of the voice.

Acute epiglottitis is now rare in the United States because of immunization against *Haemophilus influenzae* type B. This is a contra-indication to examination of the throat because of potential gagging and laryngeal obstruction.

Tonsillitis can be caused by bacteria, such as *Streptococcus,* or viruses. The "rocks in the mouth" voice is accompanied by enlarged tonsils with exudates.

● **Voice Changes—Clues to Underlying Abnormalities**	
Voice Change	**Possible Abnormality**
Hypernasal speech	Submucosal cleft palate
Nasal voice plus snoring	Adenoidal hypertrophy
Hoarse voice plus cough	Viral infection (croup)
"Rocks in mouth"	Tonsillitis

The epidemic of childhood obesity has resulted in many children who snore and have *sleep apnea.*

You may note an abnormal breath odor, which may help lead to a specific diagnosis.

Halitosis in a child can be caused by upper respiratory, pharyngeal, or mouth infection; foreign body in the nose; dental disease; and gastroesophageal reflux.

The Neck

Beyond infancy, the techniques for examining the neck are the same as for adults. Lymphadenopathy is unusual during infancy but very common during childhood. The child's lymphatic system reaches its zenith of growth at 12 years, and cervical or tonsillar lymph nodes reach their peak size between 8 and 16 years.

The vast majority of enlarged lymph nodes in children are due to infections (mostly viral but frequently bacterial) and not to malignant disease, even though the latter is a concern for many parents. It is important to differentiate normal lymph nodes from abnormal ones or from congenital cysts of the neck.

The figure on page 773 demonstrates the typical anatomical locations of lymph nodes and congenital cysts of the neck.

Check for *neck mobility*. It is important to ensure that the neck of all children is supple and easily mobile in all directions. This is particularly impor-

Lymphadenopathy is usually from viral or bacterial infections (see Table 18-8, Abnormalities of the Teeth, Pharynx, and Neck, p. 863).

Malignancy is more likely if the node is greater than 2 cm, is hard, or is fixed to the skin or underlying tissues (i.e., not mobile), is accompanied by serious systemic signs such as weight loss, and, in the case of cervical lymph nodes, if the chest x-ray findings are abnormal.

In young children with small necks, it may be difficult to differentiate tant when the patient is holding the head in an asymmetric manner, and when central nervous system disease such as meningitis is suspected.

In children, the presence of nuchal rigidity is a more reliable indicator of meningeal irritation than *Brudzinski's sign* or *Kernig's sign*. To detect nuchal rigidity in older children, ask the child to sit with legs extended on the examining table. Normally, children should be able to sit upright and touch their chins to their chests. Younger children can be persuaded to flex their necks by having them follow a small toy or light beam. You also can test for nuchal rigidity with the child lying on the examining table, as shown below. Nearly all children with nuchal rigidity will be extremely sick, irritable, and difficult to examine. In developed countries, the incidence of bacterial meningitis has plummeted because of vaccinations.

low posterior cervical lymph nodes from *supraclavicular lymph nodes* (which are always abnormal and raise suspicion for malignancy).

Nuchal rigidity is marked resistance to movement of the head in any direction. It suggests meningeal irritation due to *meningitis, bleeding, tumor,* or *other causes.* These children are extremely irritable and difficult to console and may have "paradoxical irritability"—increased irritability when being held.

When meningeal irritation is present, the child assumes the *tripod position* and is unable to assume a full upright position to perform the chin-to-chest maneuver.

The Thorax and Lungs

As children age, lung examination becomes similar to that for adults. Cooperation is critical. Auscultation usually is easiest when a child barely notices (as when in a parent's lap). Let a toddler who seems fearful of the stethoscope play with it before touching the child's chest.

Assess the relative proportion of time spent on inspiration versus expiration. The normal ratio is about 1:1. Prolonged inspirations or expirations are a clue to disease location. Degree of prolongation and effort or "work of breathing," are related to disease severity.

With upper airway obstruction such as croup, inspiration is prolonged and accompanied by other signs such as stridor, cough, or rhonchi. With lower airway obstruction such as asthma, expiration is prolonged and often accompanied by wheezing.

Young children asked to "take deep breaths" often hold their breath, further complicating auscultation. It is easier to let preschoolers breathe normally. Demonstrate to older children how to take nice, quiet, deep breaths. Make it a game. To accomplish a forced expiratory maneuver, ask the child to blow out candles on an imaginary birthday cake.

Older children will be cooperative for the respiratory examination and can even go through the maneuvers of assessing fremitus or listening to "E to A" changes (see pp. 304–305). As children grow, the evaluation by observation discussed on the previous page, such as assessing the work of breathing, nasal flaring, and grunting, becomes less helpful in assessing for respiratory pathology. Palpation, percussion, and auscultation achieve greater importance in a careful examination of the thorax and lungs.

The Heart

The examination of the heart and vascular systems in infants and children is similar to that in adults, but recognition of their fear, their inability to cooperate, and in many instances, their desire to play, will make the examination easier and more productive. Use your knowledge of the developmental stage of each child. A 2-year-old may be easiest to examine while standing or

Pneumonia in young children generally is manifested by fever, tachypnea, dyspnea, and increased work of breathing.

While *upper respiratory infections* due to viruses can cause young infants to appear quite ill, upper respiratory infections in children present with the same signs as in adults, and children can appear well, without lower respiratory signs.

Childhood asthma is an extremely common condition throughout the world. Children with acute asthma present with varying severity and often have increased work of breathing. Expiratory wheezing and a prolonged expiratory phase, caused by reversible bronchospasm, can be heard without the stethoscope and are apparent on auscultation. Wheezes are often accompanied by inspiratory rhonchi caused by viruses that triggered the asthma.[37]

General abnormalities may suggest increased likelihood of congenital cardiac disease, as exemplified by Down syndrome or Turner's syndrome.

sitting on the mother's lap, facing her shoulder, or being held, as shown on the previous page. Give young children something to hold in each hand. They cannot figure out how to drop the object and therefore have no hand free to push you away. Endless chatter to small children will hold their attention and they will forget you are examining them. Let children move the stethoscope themselves, going back to listen properly. Use your imagination to make the examination work!

Blood Pressure.   Measure the blood pressure in both arms and one leg at one time around age 3 to 4 years to check for possible *coarctation of the aorta*. Thereafter, only the right arm blood pressure needs to be measured.

In *coarctation of the aorta,* the blood pressure is lower in the legs than in the arms.

Benign Murmurs.   Preschool and school-aged children often have benign murmurs (see figure on next page). The most common (*Still's murmur*) is a grade I–II/VI, musical, vibratory, early and midsystolic murmur with multiple overtones, located over the mid or lower left sternal border, but also frequently heard over the carotid arteries. Carotid artery compression will usually cause the precordial murmur to disappear. This murmur may be extremely variable and may be accentuated when cardiac output is increased, as occurs with fever or exercise.

Also in preschool or school-age children, you may detect a *venous hum*. This is a soft, hollow, continuous sound, louder in diastole, heard just below the right clavicle. It can be completely eliminated by maneuvers that affect venous return, such as lying supine, changing head position, or jugular venous compression. It has the same quality as breath sounds and therefore is frequently overlooked.

Among young children, murmurs without the recognizable features of the three common benign murmurs on the next page may signify underlying heart disease and should be evaluated thoroughly by a pediatric cardiologist.

Pathologic murmurs that signify cardiac disease can first appear after infancy and during childhood. Examples include aortic stenosis and mitral valve disease.

The murmur heard in the carotid area or just above the clavicles is known as a *carotid bruit*. It is early and midsystolic, with a slightly harsh quality. It is usually louder on the left and may be heard alone or in combination with the Still's murmur, as noted above. It may be completely eradicated by carotid artery compression.

Location and Characteristics of Benign Heart Murmurs in Children

Location

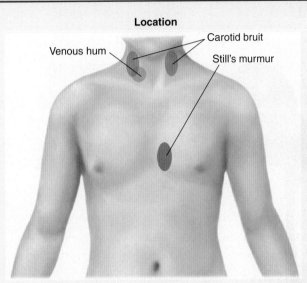

Typical Age	Name	Characteristics	Description and Location
Preschool or early school age	*Still's murmur*		Grade I–II/VI, musical, vibratory Multiple overtones Early and midsystolic Mid/lower left sternal border Frequently also a carotid bruit
Preschool or early school age	*Venous hum*		Soft, hollow, continuous Louder in diastole Under clavicle Can be eliminated by maneuvers
Preschool and later	*Carotid bruit*	S_1 S_2 S_1	Early and midsystolic Usually louder on left Eliminated by carotid compression

The Abdomen

Toddlers and young children commonly have protuberant abdomens, most apparent when they are upright. The examination can follow the same order as for adults, except that you may need to open your bag of tricks to distract the child during the examination.

Most children are ticklish when you first place your hand on their abdomens for *palpation*. This reaction tends to disappear, particularly if you distract the child with conversation and place your whole hand flush on the abdominal surface for a few moments without probing. For children who are particularly sensitive and who tighten their abdominal muscles, you can start by placing the child's hand under yours. Eventually you will be able to remove the child's hand and palpate the abdomen freely.

An exaggerated "pot-belly appearance" may indicate malabsorption from *celiac disease, cystic fibrosis,* or *constipation* or *aerophagia.*

A common condition of childhood that can occasionally cause a protuberant abdomen is constipation. The abdomen is often tympanitic on percussion, and stool is often felt on palpation.

You can also try flexing the knees and hips to relax the child's abdominal wall, as shown below. Palpate lightly in all areas, then deeply, leaving the site of potential pathology to the end.

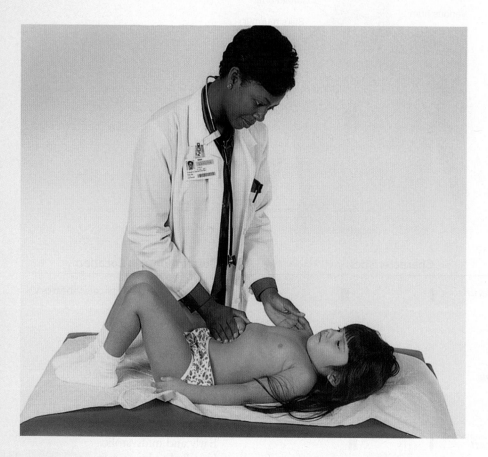

Many children present with abdominal pain from *acute gastroenteritis*. Despite pain, their physical examination is relatively normal except for increased bowel sounds on auscultation and mild tenderness on palpation.

The childhood obesity epidemic has resulted in many children who have extremely *obese abdomens*. While it is difficult to accurately examine these children, the steps to the examination are the same as for normal children.

● Expected Liver Span of Children by Percussion

Age in Years	Mean Estimated Liver Span (cm)	
	Males	Females
2	3.5	3.6
3	4.0	4.0
4	4.4	4.3
5	4.8	4.5
6	5.1	4.8
8	5.6	5.1
10	6.1	5.4

One method to determine the lower border of the liver involves the *scratch test*, shown next. Place the diaphragm of your stethoscope just above the right costal margin at the midclavicular line. With your fingernail, lightly scratch the skin of the abdomen along the midclavicular line, moving from

Hepatomegaly in young children is unusual. It can be caused by cystic fibrosis, protein malabsorption, parasites, and tumors.

below the umbilicus toward the costal margin. When your scratching finger reaches the liver's edge, you will hear a change in the scratching sound as it passes through the liver to your stethoscope.[38]

If hepatomegaly is accompanied by splenomegaly, *portal hypertension, storage diseases, chronic infections, and malignancy* should be considered.

Various diseases can cause splenomegaly, including *infections, hematologic disorders* such as *hemolytic anemias, infiltrative disorders,* and *inflammatory* or *autoimmune diseases,* as well as congestion from *portal hypertension.*

The *spleen*, like the liver, is felt easily in most children. It too is soft with a sharp edge, and it projects downward like a tongue from under the left costal margin. The spleen is moveable and rarely extends more than 1 cm to 2 cm below the costal margin.

Palpate the *other abdominal structures.* You will commonly note pulsations in the epigastrium caused by the aorta. This is felt most easily to the left of the midline, on deep palpation.

Palpating for abdominal tenderness in an older child is the same as for the adult; however, the causes of abdominal pain are often different, encompassing a wide spectrum of acute and chronic diseases. Localization of tenderness may help you pinpoint the abdominal structures most likely to be causing the abdominal pain.

In a child with an acute abdomen, as in *acute appendicitis,* special techniques are helpful, such as checking for involuntary rigidity, rebound tenderness, a Rovsing's sign, or a positive psoas or obturator sign (see p. 450).[39] *Gastroenteritis, constipation,* and *gastrointestinal obstruction* may be the causes.

Male Genitalia

Inspect the penis. The size in prepubertal children has little significance unless it is abnormally large. In obese boys, the fat pad over the symphysis pubis may obscure the penis.

There is an art to *palpation* of the young boy's scrotum and testes because many have an extremely active cremasteric reflex that may cause the testis to retract upward into the inguinal canal and thereby appear to be undescended. Examine the child when he is relaxed because anxiety stimulates the cremasteric reflex. With warm hands, palpate the lower abdomen, working your way downward toward the scrotum along the inguinal canal. This will minimize retraction of the testes into the canal.

In *precocious puberty,* the penis and testes are enlarged, with signs of pubertal changes. This is caused by a variety of conditions associated with excess androgens, including *adrenal or pituitary tumors.* Other pubertal changes also occur.

A useful technique is to have the boy sit cross-legged on the examining table, as shown here. You can also give him a balloon to inflate or an object to lift to increase intra-abdominal pressure. If you can detect the testis in the scrotum, it is descended even if it spends much time in the inguinal canal.

Cryptorchidism may be noted at this age. It requires surgical correction. It should be differentiated from a retractible testis.

The cremasteric reflex can be tested by scratching the medial aspect of the thigh. The testis on the side being scratched will move upward.

A painful testicle requires rapid treatment; common causes include infection such as *epididymitis* or *orchitis, torsion of the testicle*, or *torsion of the appendix testis*.

Examine the inguinal canal as you would for adults, noting any swelling that may reflect an *inguinal hernia*. Have the boy increase abdominal pressure as described above and note whether a bulge in the inguinal canal increases.

Inguinal hernias in older boys present as they do in adult men, with swelling in the inguinal canal, particularly following a Valsalva maneuver.

Female Genitalia

The genital examination can be anxiety provoking for the older child and adolescent (especially if you are of the opposite sex), for parents, and for you; however, if not performed, a significant finding may be missed. Depending on the child's developmental stage, explain what parts of the body you will check, and that this is part of the routine examination.

The appearance of pubic hair before 7 years should be considered *precocious puberty* and requires evaluation to determine the cause.

After infancy, the labia majora and minora flatten out, and the hymenal membrane becomes thin, translucent, and vascular, with the edges easily identified.

Rashes on the external genitals can be from various causes such as physical irritation, sweating, and candidal or bacterial infections.

The genital examination is the same for all ages of children, from late infancy until adolescence. Use a calm, gentle approach, including a developmentally appropriate explanation as you do the examination. A bright light source is essential. Most children can be examined in the supine, frog-leg position.

If the child seems reluctant, it may be helpful to have the parent sit on the examination table with the child; alternatively, the examination may be performed while the child sits in the parent's lap. Do not use stirrups, as these may frighten the child. The following diagram demonstrates a 5-year-old child sitting on her parent's lap with the parent holding her knees outstretched.

Examine the genitalia in an efficient and systematic manner. Inspect the external genitalia for pubic hair, the size of the clitoris, the color and size of the labia majora, and the presence of rashes, bruises, or other lesions.

Next, visualize the structures by separating the labia with your fingers as shown on the left below. You can also apply gentle traction by grasping the labia between your thumb and index finger of each hand, and separating the labia majora laterally and posteriorly to examine the inner structures, as shown below on the right. *Labial adhesions,* or fusion of the labia minora, may be noted in prepubertal children and can obscure the vaginal and urethral orifices. They may be a normal variant.

A *vaginal discharge* in early childhood can be from *perineal irritation* (e.g., bubble baths or soaps), *foreign body, vaginitis,* or a *sexually transmitted disease* from sexual abuse.

Vaginal bleeding is always concerning. Etiologies include *vaginal irritation, accidental trauma, sexual abuse, foreign body,* and *tumors. Precocious puberty* from many causes can induce menses in a young girl.

Purulent, profuse, malodorous, and blood-tinged discharge should be evaluated for the presence of *infiltration, foreign body,* or *trauma.*

Note the condition of the labia minora, urethra, hymen, and proximal vagina. If you are unable to visualize the edges of the hymen, ask the child to take a deep breath to relax the abdominal muscles. Another useful technique is to position her in the knee-chest position, as shown on the right and below. These maneuvers will often open the hymen. You can also use saline drops to make the edges of the hymen less sticky.

Sexual abuse is unfortunately far too common throughout the world. Up to 25% of women report some history of sexual abuse; while many of these do not involve severe physical trauma, some do.

Avoid touching the hymenal edges because the hymen is exquisitely tender without the protective effects of hormones. Examine for discharge, labial adhesions, lesions, estrogenization (indicating onset of puberty), hymenal variations (such as imperforate or septate hymen, which is rare), and hygiene. A thin, white discharge (leukorrhea) is often present. A speculum examination of the vagina and cervix is not necessary in a prepubertal child unless there is suspicion of severe trauma or foreign body.

Abrasions or signs of trauma of the external genitalia can be from benign causes such as masturbation, irritants, or accidental trauma, but should also raise the possibility of *sexual abuse*. See Table 18-11, Physical Signs of Sexual Abuse, p. 867.

The normal hymen in infants and young children can have various configurations, as shown on the next page.

The physical examination may reveal signs that suggest *sexual abuse*, and the exam is particularly important if there are suspicious clues in the history. Bear in mind that, even with known abuse, the great majority of examinations will be unremarkable; thus, a normal genital examination does not rule out sexual abuse. Mounds, notches, and tags on the hymen may all be normal variants. The size of the orifice can vary with age and the examination technique. If the hymenal edges are smooth and without interruption in the inferior half, the hymen is probably normal. Certain physical findings, however, suggest the possibility of sexual abuse and require more complete evaluation by an expert in the field. See Table 18-11, Physical Signs of Sexual Abuse, p. 867.

NORMAL CONFIGURATIONS OF THE HYMEN IN PREPUBERTAL AND ADOLESCENT FEMALES

7-year-old girl with a crescent-shaped hymenal orifice

2-year-old girl with an annular orifice, located off-center, visible with labial traction

6-year-old girl with a septate hymen causing two orifices. Traction is needed to visualize the two openings.

9-year-old girl with redundant labial tissue. Greater traction or a knee–chest position would reveal a normal orifice.

12-year-old girl with annular-shaped orifice and hormonal influence of puberty, causing thickened, pink tissue

(Source of photos: Reece R, Ludwig S (eds). Child Abuse: Medical Diagnosis and Management, 2nd ed. Philadelphia, Lippincott Williams & Wilkins, 2001.)

The Rectal Examination

The rectal examination is not routine but should be done whenever intra-abdominal, pelvic, or perirectal disease is suspected.

The rectal examination of the young child can be performed with the child in either the side-lying or lithotomy position. For many young children, the lithotomy position is less threatening and easier to perform. Have the child lie on the back with the knees and hips flexed and the legs abducted. Drape the child from the waist down. Provide frequent reassurance during the examination, and ask the child to breathe in and out through the mouth to relax. Spread the buttocks and observe the anus. You can use your lubricated gloved index finger, even in small children. Palpate the abdomen with your other hand, both to distract the child and to note the abdominal structures between your hands. The prostate gland is not palpable in young boys.

Anal skin tags are present in *inflammatory bowel disease* but are more often an incidental finding.

Tenderness noted on rectal examination of a child usually indicates an infectious or inflammatory cause, such as an *abscess,* or *appendicitis.*

The Musculoskeletal System

In older children, abnormalities of the upper extremities are rare in the absence of injury.

Toddlers may acquire *nursemaid's elbow* or subluxation of the radial head from a tugging injury.

The normal young child has increased lumbar concavity and decreased thoracic convexity compared with the adult, and often a protuberant abdomen.

Observe the child standing and walking barefoot. You can also ask the child to touch the toes, rise from sitting, run a short distance, and pick up objects. You will detect most abnormalities by watching carefully from both front and behind. To indirectly assess the child's gait pattern, you can also note the soles of the shoes to see which side of the soles is worn down.

During early infancy, there is a common and normal progression of increased bowlegged growth (see below left), which begins to disappear at about 18 months of age, often followed by transition toward knock-knees. The *knock-knee pattern* (as shown below right), is usually maximal by age 3 to 4 years and gradually corrects by age 9 or 10 years.

Severe bowing of the legs (genu varum) may still be physiologic bowing and will spontaneously resolve. Extreme bowing or unilateral bowing may be from pathologic causes such as *rickets* or *tibia vara (Blount's disease)*.

The presence of tibial torsion can be assessed in several ways[41]; one method is shown here. Have the toddler lie prone on the examination table, with the knees flexed to 90°, as shown. Note the thigh–foot axis. Usually there is ±10° of internal or external rotation noted by a foot pointing off in a direction.

Children may *toe in* when they begin to walk. This may increase up to 4 years of age and then gradually disappear by about 10 years of age.

Inspect any child who can stand for *scoliosis,* using techniques described under "Adolescents."

Determine any *leg shortening* that may accompany hip disease, by comparing the distance from the anterior superior spine of the ilium with the medial malleolus on each side. First, straighten out the child by pulling gently on the legs, and then compare the levels of the medial with each other. Put a small ink dot over the prominent malleoli and touch them together for a direct measure.

Also, have the child stand straight and place your hands horizontally over the iliac crests from behind. Small discrepancies can be appreciated. If such a discrepancy is noted and you suspect leg length discrepancy, with one iliac crest higher than the other, a clever trick is to place a book under the shorter leg; this should eliminate the discrepancy.

Test for severe hip disease, with its associated weakness of the gluteus medius muscle. Observe from behind as the child shifts weight from one leg to the other. A pelvis that remains level when weight is borne on the unaffected side is a *negative Trendelenburg's sign.*[42] With an abnormal positive sign in *severe hip disease,* the pelvis tilts toward the unaffected hip during weight-bearing on the affected side (positive Trendelenburg sign).

The most common lower-extremity pathology in childhood is injury from accidents. Joint injuries, fractures, sprains, strains, and serious ligament injuries such as ACL tears of the knee are all too common in children.

Normal hip abductors

Weak hip abductors

NEGATIVE TRENDELENBURG'S SIGN

POSITIVE TRENDELENBURG'S SIGN

The Nervous System

Beyond infancy, the neurologic examination includes the components evaluated in adults. Again, you should combine the neurologic and developmental assessment and will need to turn this into a game with the child to assess optimal development and neurologic performance.

Perform the DDST as shown on pp. 753–754. Children usually enjoy this component, and you can too. Remember that the DDST is better at detecting delays in motor skills than in language or cognitive milestones. Many practitioners now use other standardized developmental instruments.

Sensation.   The sensory examination can be performed by using a cotton ball or tickling the child. This is best performed with the child's eyes closed. Do not use pin pricks, or you will have a very uncooperative patient!

Gait, Strength, and Coordination.   Observe the child's gait while the child is walking and, optimally, running. Note any asymmetries, weakness, undue tripping, or clumsiness. Follow the DDST examination milestones to test for appropriate maneuvers such as heel-to-toe walking (photo below), hopping, and jumping. Use a toy to test for coordination and strength of the upper extremities.

If you are concerned about the child's strength, have the child lie on the floor and then stand up, and closely observe the stages. Most normal children will first sit up, then flex the knees and extend the arms to the side to push off from the floor and stand up.

Hand preference is demonstrated in most children by age 2. If a younger child has clear hand preference, check for weakness in the nonpreferred upper extremity.

Deep Tendon Reflexes.   Deep tendon reflexes can be tested as in adults. First demonstrate the use of the reflex hammer on the child's hand, assuring the child that it will not hurt. Children love to feel their legs bounce when you test their patellar reflexes. You will need to have the child cooperate and keep the eyes closed during some of this examination because tensing will disrupt the results. One trick is to ask the child to pretend the arms or legs "are dead."

Children with *spastic diplegias* will often have hypotonia as infants and then excessive tone with spasticity, scissoring, and perhaps clenched fists as toddlers and young children.

In children with uncoordinated gait, be sure to distinguish *orthopedic causes* such as positional deformities of the hip, knee, or foot from *neurologic abnormalities* such as *cerebral palsy, ataxia,* or *neuromuscular conditions.*

In certain forms of *muscular dystrophy* with weakness of the pelvic girdle muscles, children will rise to standing by rolling over prone and pushing off the floor with the arms while the legs remain extended (*Gower's sign*).

Children with mild cerebral palsy may have both slightly increased tone and hyperreflexia.

You can ask children older than 3 years to draw a picture, copy objects as is done in the DDST, and then discuss their pictures to test simultaneously for fine motor coordination, cognition, and language.

The cerebellar examination can be tested using finger-to-nose and rapid alternating movements of the hands or fingers. Children enjoy this game. Children older than 5 years should be able to tell right from left, so you can assign them right–left discrimination tasks, as is done in the adult patient.

Distinguish between isolated delays in one aspect of development (e.g., coordination or language) and more generalized delays that occur in several components. The latter is more likely to reflect global neurologic disorders such as *mental retardation* that can be caused by many etiologies.

Some children with *attention deficit disorder with hyperactivity (ADHD)* will have great difficulty cooperating with your neurologic and developmental examination because of problems focusing. These children often have high energy levels, cannot stay still for extended periods, and have a history of difficulty in school or structured situations.

Cranial Nerves. The cranial nerves can be assessed quite well using developmentally appropriate strategies, as shown in the following table:

● Strategies to Assess Cranial Nerves in Young Children

Localizing neurologic signs are rare in children but can be caused by trauma, brain tumor, intracranial bleed, or infection.

Cranial Nerve		Strategy
I	Olfactory	Testable in older children.
II	Visual acuity	Use Snellen chart after age 3 years. Test visual fields as for an adult. A parent may need to hold the child's head.
III, IV, VI	Extraocular movements	Have the child track a light or an object (a toy is preferable). A parent may need to hold the child's head.
V	Motor	Play a game with a soft cotton ball to test sensation. Have the child clench the teeth and chew or swallow some food.

(continued)

● Strategies to Assess Cranial Nerves in Young Children (continued)

Cranial Nerve		Strategy
VII	Facial	Have the child "make faces" or imitate you as you make faces (including moving your eyebrows), and observe symmetry and facial movements.
VIII	Acoustic	Perform auditory testing after age 4 years. Whisper a word or command behind the child's back and have the child repeat it.
IX, X	Swallow and gag	Have the child stick the "whole tongue out" or "say 'ah'." Observe movement of the uvula and soft palate. Test the gag reflex.
XI	Spinal accessory	Have the child push your hand away with his head. Have the child shrug his shoulders while you push down with your hands to "see how strong you are."
XII	Hypoglossal	Ask the child to "stick out your tongue all the way."

ASSESSING ADOLESCENTS

● DEVELOPMENT: 11 TO 20 YEARS

Adolescence can be divided into three stages: early, middle, and late, as shown in the table on the next page. Your interview and examination techniques will vary widely depending on the adolescent's physical, cognitive, and social–emotional levels of development.

Physical Development.   Adolescence is the period of transition from childhood to adulthood. The physical transformation generally occurs over a period of years, beginning at an average age of 10 in girls and 11 in boys. On average, girls end pubertal development with a growth spurt by age 14 and boys by age 16. The age of onset and duration of puberty vary widely, although the stages follow the same sequence in all adolescents. Early adolescents are preoccupied with these physical changes.

Cognitive Development. Although less obvious, cognitive changes during adolescence are as dramatic as changes in physique. Most adolescents progress from concrete to formal operational thinking, acquiring an ability to reason logically and abstractly and to consider future implications of current actions. Although the interview and examination resemble those of adults, keep in mind the wide variability in cognitive development of adolescents and their often erratic and still limited ability to see beyond simple solutions. Moral thinking becomes sophisticated, with lots of time spent debating issues.

Social and Emotional Development. Adolescence is a tumultuous time, marked by the transition from family-dominated influences to increasing autonomy and peer influence. The struggle for identity, independence, and eventually intimacy leads to much stress, many health-related problems, and, often, high-risk behaviors. This struggle also provides you with an important opportunity for health promotion.

● Developmental Tasks of Adolescence

Task	Characteristic	Health Care Approaches
Early Adolescence (10–14-year-olds)		
Physical	Puberty (F: 10–14; M: 11–16) variable	Confidentiality; privacy
Cognitive	"Concrete operational"	Emphasis on short-term
Social		
Identity	Am I normal? Peers increasingly important	Reassurance and positive attitude
Independence	Ambivalence (family, self, peers)	Support for growing autonomy
Middle Adolescence (15–16-year-olds)		
Physical	Females more comfortable, males awkward	Support if patient varies from "normal"
Cognitive	Transition; many ideas	Problem solving; decision making

(continued)

● Developmental Tasks of Adolescence (continued)

Task	Characteristic	Health Care Approaches
Social		
Identity	Who am I? Much intro-spection; global issues	Nonjudgmental acceptance
Independence	Limit testing; "experimental" behaviors; dating	Consistency; limit setting
Late Adolescence (17–20-year-olds)		
Physical	Adult appearance illness	Minimal unless chronic
Cognitive	"Formal operational"	Approach as an adult
Social		
Identity	Role with respect to others; sexuality; future	Encouragement of identity to allow growth
Independence	Separation from family; toward real independence	Support, anticipatory guidance

THE HEALTH HISTORY

The key to successfully examining adolescents is a comfortable, confidential environment. This makes the examination more relaxed and informative. Consider the teen's cognitive and social development when deciding issues of privacy, parental involvement, and confidentiality.

Like most people, adolescents usually respond positively to anyone demonstrating a genuine interest in them. Show such interest early and then sustain the connection for effective communication.

Adolescents are more likely to open up when the interview focuses on them rather than on their problems. In contrast to most other interviews, *start with specific questions* to build trust and rapport and get the conversation going. You may have to do more talking than usual, at the beginning. A good way to start is to chat informally about friends, school, hobbies, and family. Using silence in an attempt to get adolescents to talk or asking about feelings directly is usually not a good idea.

It is particularly important to use summarization and transitional statements and to explain what you are going to do during the physical examination. The physical examination can also be an opportunity to engage young persons. Once you have established rapport, return to more openended questions. At that point, make sure to ask what concerns or questions the adolescent may have. Because adolescents are often reluctant to ask their most important questions (which are sometimes about sensitive topics), ask if the adolescent has anything else to discuss. A useful phrase to use is "tell me what other questions you have."

Remember also that adolescents' behavior is related to their developmental stage, and not necessarily to chronologic age or physical maturation. Their age and appearance may fool you into assuming that they are functioning on a more future-oriented and realistic level. This is particularly true regarding "early bloomers," who look older than their age. The reverse can also be true, especially in teens with delayed puberty or chronic illness.

Issues of *confidentiality* are important in adolescence. Explain to both parents and adolescents that the best health care allows adolescents some degree of independence and confidentiality. It helps if the clinician starts asking the parent to leave the room for part of the interview when the child is age 10 or 11 years. This prepares both parents and teens for future visits when the patient spends time alone with the clinician.

Before the parent leaves, obtain relevant medical history from him or her, such as certain elements of past history, and clarify the parent's agenda for the visit. Also discuss the need for confidentiality. Explain that the purpose of confidentiality is to improve health care, not to keep secrets. Adolescents need to know that you will hold in confidence what they discuss with you. However, never make confidentiality unlimited. Always state explicitly that you may need to act on information that makes you concerned about safety: "I will not tell your parents what we talk about unless you give me permission or I am concerned about your safety—for example, if you were to talk to me about killing yourself and I thought that you really were at risk to follow through, I would need to discuss it with others in order to help you."

Your goal is to help adolescents bring their concerns or questions to their parents. Encourage adolescents to discuss sensitive issues with their parents and offer to be present or help. Although young people may believe that their parents would "kill them if they only knew," you may be able to promote more open dialogue. This entails a careful assessment of the parents' perspective and the full and explicit consent of the young person.

As in middle childhood, modesty is important. The patient should remain dressed until the examination begins, and you should leave the room while the patient puts on a gown. Most adolescents older than 13 years prefer to be examined without a parent in the room, but this depends on the patient's developmental level, familiarity with the examiner, relationship with the parent, and cultural medical issues. For younger adolescents, ask the adolescent and parent their preferences. While the examination of the adolescent can be anxiety-provoking for the novice clinician, with practice these interactions can be very rewarding for both the adolescent and the clinician.

The sequence and content of the physical examination of the adolescent are similar to those in the adult. Keep in mind, however, particular issues unique to adolescents, such as puberty, growth, development, family and peer relationships, sexuality, decision making, and high-risk behaviors.

 HEALTH PROMOTION AND COUNSELING

The AAP recommends annual health supervision visits for adolescents.[43] Because adolescents tend to be seen less frequently than do younger children for any health care visit, be sure to include health promotion during all health encounters with youth. In addition, adolescents with chronic problems or high-risk behaviors may require additional visits for health promotion and anticipatory guidance.

Most chronic diseases of adults have their antecedents in childhood or adolescence. For example, obesity, cardiovascular disease, addiction (to drugs, tobacco, or alcohol), and depression are all influenced by childhood and teen experiences and by behaviors established during adolescence. More specifically, most obese adults were obese as adolescents or had abnormal indicators such as elevated BMI scores. Almost all adults who are addicted to tobacco began their tobacco habits before 18 years. Therefore, a major component of health promotion for adolescents includes discussions about health behaviors or habits. Effective health promotion can help patients develop healthy habits and lifestyles and avoid several chronic health problems.

Because some health promotion topics involve confidential issues such as mental health, addiction, sexual behavior, and eating disorders, you will want to speak to adolescents (particularly older youth) privately during part of a visit that involves health supervision.

COMPONENTS OF A HEALTH SUPERVISION VISIT FOR ADOLESCENTS 11–18 YEARS

Discussions with Parents

- Address parent concerns
- Provide advice
- School, activities, social interactions
- Youth's behaviors and habits, mental health

Discussions with Adolescent

- *Social and Emotional Development:* mental health, friends, family
- *Physical Development:* puberty, self-concept
- *Behaviors and Habits:* nutrition, exercise, TV or computer screen time, drug/alcohol
- *Relationships and Sexuality:* dating, sexual activity, forced sex
- *Family Functioning:* relations with parents and siblings
- *School Performance:* activities, strengths

Physical Examination

- Perform a careful examination; note growth parameters, sexual maturity ratings

Screening Tests

- Vision and hearing, blood pressure; consider hematocrit; assess emotional health and risk factors

Immunizations

- See schedule (pp. 741–742)

Anticipatory Guidance—Teen

Promote Healthy Habits and Behaviors:

- Injury & illness prevention
  Seat belts, drunk driving, helmets, sun, weapons
- Nutrition
  Healthy meals/snacks, obesity prevention
- Oral health: dentist, brushing

Sexuality:

- Confidentiality, sexual behaviors, safer sex, contraception if needed

Substance Abuse:

- Prevention strategies; treatment if appropriate
- Parent–teen interaction
- Communication, rules

Social Achievement:

- Activities, school, future

Community Interaction

- Resources, involvement

Anticipatory Guidance—Parent

Positive interactions, support, safety, limit setting, family values, modeling behaviors

TECHNIQUES OF EXAMINATION

General Survey and Vital Signs

Somatic Growth. Adolescents should wear gowns to be weighed. This is particularly important for adolescent girls being evaluated for underweight problems. Ideally, serial weights (and heights) should use the same scales.

Both obesity and eating disorders among adolescent girls are major public health problems, requiring frequent assessments of weight.

Vital Signs. Ongoing evaluations of blood pressure are important for adolescent[28]. The average heart rate from age 10 to 14 years is 85 beats per minute, with a range of 55 to 115 beats per minute considered normal. Average heart rate for those 15 years and older is 60 to 100 beats per minute.

Causes of sustained hypertension for this age group include *primary hypertension, renal parenchymal disease,* and *drug use.*

The Skin

Examine the adolescent's skin carefully. Many teens will have concerns about various skin lesions, such as acne, dimples, blemishes, and moles.

Adolescent acne, a very common skin condition, tends to resolve eventually but often benefits from proper treatment. It tends to begin during middle to late puberty.

Many adolescents spend considerable time in the sun and at tanning salons. You may detect this during a comprehensive health history or by noticing signs of tanning during the physical examination. This is a good opportunity to counsel adolescents about the dangers of excessive ultraviolet exposure, the need for sunscreen, and the risks of tanning salons.

Counsel adolescents to begin performing a regular self-examination of the skin, as shown on pp. 170–171.

Head, Ears, Eyes, Throat, and Neck

The examination of these body parts is generally the same as for adults.

The methods used to examine the eye, including testing for visual acuity, are the same as those for adults. Refractive errors become common, and it is important to test visual acuity monocularly at regular intervals, such as during the annual health supervision visit.

The ease and techniques of examining the ears and testing the hearing approach the methods used for adults. There are no ear abnormalities or variations of normal unique to this age group. Of course, parents of older children routinely refer to the normal condition of "selective deafness," defined as choosing to hear what the adolescent wishes to hear.

The Heart

The technique and sequence of examination are the same as those for adults. Murmurs are a continued cardiovascular issue for evaluation.

Moles or benign nevi may appear during adolescence. Their characteristics differentiate them from atypical nevi, described on pp. 857–858.

● Location and Characteristics of Benign Heart Murmurs in Adolescents

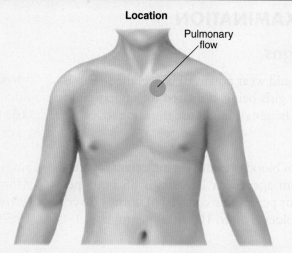

Location

Pulmonary flow

Typical Age	Name	Characteristics		Description and Location
Adolescence and later	*Pulmonary flow murmur*	S_1	S_2	Grade I–II/VI soft, nonharsh Ejection in timing Upper left sternal border Normal P_2

The benign *pulmonary flow murmur* is a grade I–II/VI soft, nonharsh murmur with the timing characteristics of an ejection murmur, beginning after the first sound and ending before the second sound but without the marked crescendo–decrescendo quality of an organic ejection murmur. If you hear this murmur, make sure to evaluate whether the pulmonary closure sound is of normal intensity and whether splitting of the second heart sound is eliminated during expiration. An adolescent with a benign pulmonary ejection murmur will have normal intensity and normally split second heart sounds.

A pulmonary flow murmur accompanied by a fixed split-second heart sound suggests right-heart volume load such as an *atrial septal defect.*

This pulmonary flow murmur may also be heard in the presence of volume overload from any cause such as chronic anemia, and following exercise. It may persist into adulthood.

The Breasts

Physical changes in a young girl's breasts are one of the first signs of puberty. As in most developmental changes, there is a systematic progression. Generally, over a 4-year period, the breasts progress through five stages, called Tanner stages or Tanner sex maturity rating (SMR) stages, as shown on the next page. Breast buds in the preadolescent stage progress to subsequent enlargement and change in the contour of the breasts and areola. These stages are accompanied by the development of pubic hair and other secondary sexual characteristics, as shown on page 845. Menarche usually occurs when a girl is in breast stage 3 or 4, and by then she has passed her peak growth spurt (see the figure on p. 846).

Masses or nodules in the breasts of adolescent girls should be examined carefully. They are usually *benign fibroadenomas* or *cysts;* less likely etiologies include *abscesses* or *lipomas.* Breast carcinoma is extremely rare in adolescence and nearly always occurs in families with a strong history of the disease.[44]

For years, the normal range for onset of breast development was 8 to 13 years (average, 11 years), with earlier onset considered abnormal.[45] Some studies suggest that the lower age cutoff should be 7 years for white girls and 6 years for African-American and Hispanic girls. Controversy over the exact age remains. Breasts develop at different rates in approximately 10% of girls, with resultant asymmetry of size or Tanner stage. Reassurance that this generally resolves is helpful to the patient.

Older adolescent girls should undergo a comprehensive breast examination with instructions for self-examination (see p. 410). A chaperone (parent or nurse) should assist male clinicians.

Breasts in boys consist of a small nipple and areola. During puberty about one third of boys develop a firm button of tissue 2 cm or more in diameter, usually in one breast. Obese boys may develop substantial breast tissue.

Many adolescent boys develop *gynecomastia* (enlarged breasts) on one or both sides. Although usually slight, it can be embarrassing. It generally resolves in a few years.

SEX MATURITY RATINGS IN GIRLS: BREASTS

Stage 1

Preadolescent. Elevation of nipple only

Stage 2

Breast bud stage. Elevation of breast and nipple as a small mound; enlargement of areolar diameter

Stage 3

Further enlargement of elevation of breast and areola, with no separation of their contours

Stage 4

Projection of areola and nipple to form a secondary mound above the level of breast

Stage 5

Mature stage; projection of nipple only. Areola has receded to general contour of the breast (although in some normal individuals, the areola continues to form a secondary mound).

(Photos used with permission of the American Academy of Pediatrics, *Assessment of Sexual Maturity Stages in Girls,* 1995.)

The Abdomen

Techniques of abdominal examination are the same as for adults. The size of the liver approaches the adult size as the teen progresses through puberty, and is related to the adolescent's overall height. Although data are lacking about the usefulness of different techniques to assess liver size, it is likely that evidence from adult studies apply, particularly for older adolescents. Thus, palpate the liver. If it is nonpalpable, hepatomegaly is highly unlikely. If you can palpate the lower edge, use light percussion to assess liver span.

Hepatomegaly in teens may be from *infections* such as hepatitis or infectious mononucleosis, inflammatory bowel disease, or tumors.

Male Genitalia

The genital examination of the adolescent boy proceeds like the examination of the adult male. Be particularly aware of the embarrassment of many boys regarding this aspect of the examination.

Important anatomical changes in the male genitalia accompany puberty and help to define its progress. The first reliable sign of puberty, starting between ages 9 and 13.5 years, is an increase in the size of the testes. Next, pubic hair appears, along with progressive enlargement of the penis. The complete change from preadolescent to adult anatomy requires about 3 years, with a range of 1.8 to 5 years.

Delayed puberty is suspected in boys who have no signs of pubertal development by 14 years of age.

When examining the adolescent male, assign a sexual maturity rating. The five stages of sexual development, first described by Tanner, are outlined and illustrated below.[20] These involve changes in the penis, testes, and scrotum. In addition, in about 80% of men, pubic hair spreads farther up the abdomen in a triangular pattern pointing toward the umbilicus; this phase is not completed until the 20s.

The most common cause of delayed puberty in males is *constitutional delay,* frequently a familial condition involving delayed bone and physical maturation but normal hormonal levels.

● Sex Maturity Ratings in Boys

In assigning SMRs in boys, observe each of the three characteristics separately because they may develop at different rates. Record two separate ratings: pubic hair and genital. If the penis and testes differ in their stages, average the two into a single figure for the genital rating.

	Pubic Hair	Penis	Testes and Scrotum
Stage 1	Preadolescent—no pubic hair except for the fine body hair (vellus hair) similar to that on the abdomen	Preadolescent—same size and proportions as in childhood	Preadolescent—same size and proportions as in childhood
Stage 2	Sparse growth of long, slightly pigmented, downy hair, straight or only slightly curled, chiefly at the base of the penis	Slight or no enlargement	Testes larger; scrotum larger, somewhat reddened, and altered in texture
Stage 3	Darker, coarser, curlier hair spreading sparsely over the pubic symphysis	Larger, especially in length	Further enlarged
Stage 4	Coarse and curly hair, as in the adult; area covered greater than in stage 3 but not as great as in the adult and not yet including the thighs	Further enlarged in length and breadth, with development of the glans	Further enlarged; scrotal skin darkened

(continued)

● Sex Maturity Ratings in Boys (continued)

		Pubic Hair	Penis	Testes and Scrotum
Stage 5	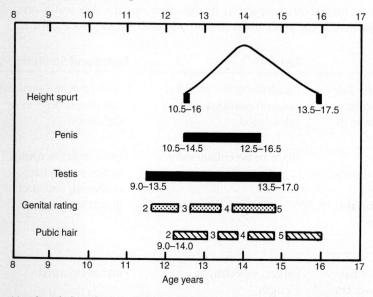	Hair adult in quantity and quality, spread to the medial surfaces of the thighs but not up over the abdomen	Adult in size and shape	Adult in size and shape

(Photos reprinted from *Pediatric Endocrinology and Growth,* 2nd ed., Wales & Wit, 2003, with permission from Elsevier.)

An important developmental principle is that physical pubertal changes progress along a well-established sequence (below). Although age ranges for start and completion are wide, the sequence for each boy is nevertheless the same. This is helpful in counseling an anxious adolescent regarding his current and future maturation, and regarding the normality of pubertal changes along a wide age range. It is also helpful for detecting abnormal physical changes.

Although nocturnal or daytime ejaculation tends to begin around Sexual Maturity Rating 3, a finding on either history or physical examination of penile discharge may indicate a *sexually transmitted disease.*

Height spurt
10.5–16   13.5–17.5

Penis
10.5–14.5   12.5–16.5

Testis
9.0–13.5   13.5–17.0

Genital rating
2 3 4 5

Pubic hair
2 3 4 5
9.0–14.0

Age years

Numbers below the bars indicate the ranges in age within which certain changes occur. (Redrawn from Marshall WA, Tanner JM. Variations in the patterns of pubertal changes in boys. Arch Dis Child 45:22, 1970.)

Female Genitalia

The external examination of adolescent female genitalia proceeds in the same manner as for school-age children. If it is necessary to complete a full pelvic examination on an adolescent, the actual technique is the same as that used for an adult, including the rectal examination. A full explanation of the steps of the examination, demonstration of the instruments, and a gentle, reassuring approach are necessary because the adolescent is usually quite anxious. A chaperone (parent or nurse) must be present. An adolescent's first pelvic examination should be performed by an experienced health care provider.

Vaginal discharge in a young adolescent should be treated as in the adult. Causes include *physiologic leukorrhea, sexually transmitted diseases* from consensual sexual activity or *sexual abuse, bacterial vaginosis, foreign body,* and *external irritants.*

A girl's initial signs of puberty are hymenal changes secondary to estrogen, widening of the hips, and beginning of a height spurt, although these changes are difficult to detect. The first easily detectable sign of puberty is usually the appearance of breast buds, although pubic hair sometimes appears earlier. The average age of the appearance of pubic hair has decreased in recent years, and current consensus is that the appearance of pubic hair as early as 7 years can be normal, particularly in dark-skinned girls who develop secondary sexual characteristics at an earlier age.

Assign a sexual maturity rating to every female, irrespective of chronologic age. The assessment of sexual maturity in girls is based on both growth of pubic hair and the development of breasts.[45] The assessment (Tanner staging) of pubic hair growth is shown in the figure below. See page 842 for breast development assessment. Counsel girls about this sequence and their current stage.

Pubertal development prior to the normal age ranges may signify *precocious puberty*, which has a variety of endocrine and central nervous system causes.

SEX MATURITY RATINGS IN GIRLS: PUBIC HAIR

Stage 1

Preadolescent—no pubic hair except for the fine body hair (vellus hair) similar to that on the abdomen

Stage 2	Stage 3
Sparse growth of long, slightly pigmented, downy hair, straight or only slightly curled, chiefly along the labia	Darker, coarser, curlier hair, spreading sparsely over the pubic symphysis

Stage 4	Stage 5
Coarse and curly hair as in adults; area covered greater than in stage 3 but not as great as in the adult and not yet including the thighs	Hair adult in quantity and quality, spread on the medial surfaces of the thighs but not up over the abdomen

(Photos used with permission of the American Academy of Pediatrics, *Assessment of Sexual Maturity Stages in Girls*, 1995.)

Although there is a wide variation in the age of onset and completion of puberty, remember that the stages occur in a predictable sequence, as shown next.

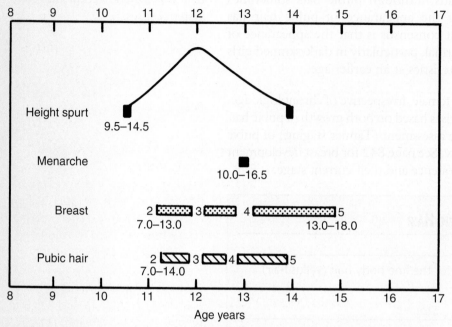

Numbers below the bars indicate the ranges in age within which certain changes occur. (Redrawn from Marshall WA, Tanner JM. Variations in the pattern of pubertal changes in girls. Arch Dis Child 45:22, 1970.)

The Musculoskeletal System

Evaluations for scoliosis and screening for participation in sports (pp. 847–849) remain common components of examination in adolescents. Other segments of the musculoskeletal examination are the same as for adults.

Assessing for Scoliosis. Make sure the child bends forward with the knees straight (*Adams' bend test*). Evaluate any asymmetry in positioning or gait. Scoliosis in a young child is unusual and abnormal; mild scoliosis in an older child is not uncommon.

If you detect scoliosis, use a *scoliometer* to test for the degree of scoliosis. With the patient standing, look for asymmetry of the shoulder blades or gluteal folds. Have the teen bend forward as described. Look for prominence of the posterior ribs. Place the scoliometer over the spine at a point of maximum prominence, making sure that the spine is parallel to the floor at that point, as shown above. Have the teen bend fully forward to assess lumbar scoliosis, and less so to assess thoracic scoliosis.

Delayed puberty in an adolescent female below the 3rd percentile in height may be from Turner's syndrome or chronic disease. The two most common causes of delayed sexual development in an extremely thin adolescent girl are anorexia nervosa and chronic disease.

Several types of *scoliosis* may present during childhood. Idiopathic scoliosis (75% of cases), seen mostly in girls, is usually detected in early adolescence.

You can also use a *plumb line*, a string with a weight attached, to assess symmetry of the back. Place the top of the plumb line at C-7 and have the child stand straight. The plumb line should extend to the gluteal crease (not shown here).

Apparent scoliosis, including an abnormal plumb line test, can be caused by a *leg-length discrepancy* (see p. 831)

The Sports Preparticipation Screening Musculoskeletal Examination. More than 25 million children and adolescents in the United States and several other countries participate in organized sports and often require "medical clearance." Start the examination with a thorough medical history, focusing on cardiovascular risk factors, prior surgeries, prior injuries, other medical problems, and a family history. The preparticipation physical examination is often the only time a healthy adolescent will see a medical professional, so it is important to include some screening questions and anticipatory guidance (see the discussion in Health Promotion and Counseling). Finally, perform a general physical, with special attention to the heart and lungs and a vision and hearing screening. Include a focused, thorough musculoskeletal examination, looking for weakness, limited range of motion, and evidence of previous injury.

A 2-minute preparticipation screening musculoskeletal examination has been recommended.[46,47] See an illustrated version of this examination below.

Important risk factors for sudden cardiovascular death during sports include episodes of *dizziness or palpitations, prior syncope* (particularly if associated with exercise), or family history of *sudden death* in young or middle-aged relatives.

During the preparticipation sports physical, assess carefully for *cardiac murmurs* and *wheezing* in the lungs.

● Screening Musculoskeletal Examination for Sports

Position and Instruction to Patient		Common Abnormalities from Prior Injury
Step 1: Stand straight, facing forward.	**Step 2:** Move neck in all directions	**Step 1:** Asymmetry, swelling of joints **Step 2:** Loss of range of motion

(continued)

● Screening Musculoskeletal Examination for Sports (continued)

Position and Instruction to Patient	Common Abnormalities from Prior Injury

Step 3: Shrug shoulders against resistance.

Step 4: Hold arms out to the side against resistance.

Step 3: Weakness of shoulder, neck or, trapezius muscles

Step 4: Loss of strength of deltoid muscle

Step 5: Hold arms out to side with elbows bent 90°; raise and lower arms.

Step 6: Hold arms out, completely bend, and straighten elbows.

Step 5: Loss of external rotation and injury of glenohumeral joint.

Step 6: Reduced range of motion of elbow.

(continued)

● Screening Musculoskeletal Examination for Sports (continued)

Position and Instruction to Patient		Common Abnormalities from Prior Injury

Step 7: Hold arms down, bend elbows 90°, and pronate and sulpinate forearms.

Step 8: Make a fist, clench, and then spread fingers.

Step 7: Reduced range of motion from injury to forearm, elbow, or wrist

Step 8: Protruding knuckle, reduced range of motion of fingers from prior sprain or fracture

Step 9: Squat and duck-walk for four steps forward.

Step 10: Stand straight with arms at sides, facing back.

Step 9: Inability to fully flex knees and difficulty standing up from prior knee or ankle injury

Step 10: Asymmetry from scoliosis, leg-length discrepancy, or weakness from injury

Step 11: Bend forward with knees straight and touch toes.

Step 12: Stand on heels and rise to the toes.

Step 11: Asymmetry from scoliosis and twisting of back from low back pain

Step 12: Wasting of calf muscles from ankle or Achilles tendon injury

The Nervous System

The neurologic examination of the adolescent and the adult is the same. Still, assess the adolescent's developmental achievement according to age-specific milestones, as described on pages 834–836.

RECORDING YOUR FINDINGS

Note that initially you may use sentences to describe your findings; later you will use phrases. The style here contains phrases appropriate for most write-ups. As you read through this write-up, you will notice some atypical findings. Try to test yourself. See if you can interpret these findings in the context of all you have learned about the examination of children. You also will note the modifications necessary to accommodate reports from the small child's parent, rather than from the child.

Recording the Examination: The Pediatric Patient

2/1/09
Brian is an active, 26-month-old boy accompanied by his mother for concern about his development and behavior.
Referral. None
Source and Reliability. Mother (Mom).

Chief Complaint: Slow development and difficult behavior.

Present Illness: Brian appears to be developing more slowly than his older sister did. He uses only single words and simple phrases, rarely combines words, and appears frustrated with not being able to communicate. People understand approximately 25% of his speech. Physical development seems normal; he can throw a ball, kick, scribble, and dress himself well. He has had no head trauma, chronic illnesses, seizures, or regression in his milestones.

Mom also is concerned about his behavior. Brian is extremely stubborn, frequently has tantrums, gets angry easily (especially with his older sister), throws objects, bites, and physically strikes others when he doesn't get his way. His behavior seems worse around Mom, who reports that he is "fine" at his childcare center. He moves from one activity to another with an inability to sit still to read or play a game.

Brian is an extremely picky eater who eats a large quantity of junk food and little else. He will not eat fruits or vegetables and drinks enormous quantities of juice and soda. His mother has tried everything to get him to eat healthy food, to no avail.

The family has been under substantial stress during the past year from Brian's father being unemployed. Although Brian now has Medicaid insurance, the parents are uninsured.
Medications. One multivitamin daily.

(continued)

Past History

Pregnancy. Uneventful. Mom reduced tobacco intake to a half-pack a day and drank alcohol at times. She denies use of other drugs or having infections.

Newborn Period. Born vaginally at 40 weeks; left the hospital in 2 days. Birth weight 2.5 kg (5 lbs, 8 oz). Mom does not know why Brian was small at birth.

Illnesses. Only minor illnesses; no hospitalizations.

Accidents. Required sutures last year for a facial laceration secondary to a fall on the road.

Preventive Care. Brian has had regular preventive check-ups. At the last appointment 6 months ago, his regular physician said that Brian was a bit behind on some developmental milestones and suggested a childcare center that he knew was excellent, as well as increased parental attention to reading, speaking, playing, and stimulation. Immunizations are up-to-date. His lead level was elevated mildly last year, and Mom reports that he had "low blood." His physician recommended iron supplements and foods high in iron, but Brian really won't eat these foods.

Family History

Strong family history of diabetes (two grandparents, none with diabetes as children) and hypertension. No family history of childhood developmental, psychiatric, or chronic illnesses.

Developmental History: Sat up at 6 months, crawled at 9 months, and walked at 13 months. First words ("mama" and "car") said at approximately 1 year.

Personal and Social History: Parents are married and live with the two children in a rented apartment. Dad has not had a steady job for 1 year but has worked intermittently in construction. Mom works as a waitress part-time while Brian is in childcare.

Mom had depression during Brian's first year and attended some counseling sessions, but stopped because she could not pay for them or medications. She gets support from her mother who lives 30 minutes away, and many friends, some of whom babysit occasionally.

Despite substantial family stress, Mom describes a loving and intact family. They try to eat dinner together daily, limit television, read to both children (although Brian won't sit still), and go to the nearby park regularly to play.
Environmental Exposures. Both parents smoke, although generally outside the house.
Safety. Mom reports this as a major concern: she can barely leave Brian out of her sight without him getting into something. She fears he will run under a car; the family is thinking of fencing in their small yard. Brian sits in his car seat most of the time; smoke detectors work in the home. Dad's guns are locked; medications are in a cabinet in the parents' bedroom.

Review of Systems

General. No major illnesses.

Skin. Dry and itchy. Last year he was prescribed hydrocortisone for it.

(continued)

Head, Eyes, Ears, Nose, and Throat (HEENT). *Head:* No trauma. *Eyes:* Vision fine. *Ears:* Multiple infections in the past year. Frequently ignores parents' requests; they can't tell if this is purposeful or if he can't hear well. *Nose:* Often runny; Mom wonders about allergies. *Mouth:* No dentist visit yet. Brushes teeth sometimes (a frequent source of dispute).

Neck. No lumps. Glands in neck seem large.

Respiratory. Frequent cough and whistle in chest. Mom cannot identify trigger; it tends to go away. He can run around all day without seeming to get tired.

Cardiovascular. No known heart disease. He had a murmur when younger, but it went away.

Gastrointestinal. Appetite and eating habits described above. Regular bowel movements. He is in the process of toilet training and wears pull-ups at night, but not at childcare.

Urinary. Good stream. No prior urinary tract infections.

Genital. Normal.

Musculoskeletal. He is "all boy" and never gets tired. Minor bumps and bruises occasionally.

Neurologic. Walks and runs well; seems coordinated for age. No stiffness, seizures, or fainting. Mom says his memory seems great, but his attention span is poor.

Psychiatric. Generally seems happy. Cries easily; bounces back and forth from trying to be independent to needing cuddling and comforting.

Physical Examination

Brian is active, and energetic toddler. He plays with the reflex hammer, pretending it is a truck. He appears closely bonded with his mother, looking at her occasionally for comfort. She seems concerned that Brian will break something. His clothes are clean.

Vital Signs. Ht 90 cm (90th percentile). Wt 16 kg (>95th percentile). BMI 19.8 (>95th percentile). Head circumference 50 cm (75th percentile). BP 108/58. Heart rate 90 and regular. Respiratory rate 30; varies with activity. Temperature (ear) 37.5°C. Obviously no pain.

Skin. Normal except for bruises on legs, and patchy, dry skin over external surface of elbows.

HEENT. *Head:* Normocephalic; no lesions. *Eyes:* Difficult to examine because he won't sit still. Symmetric with normal extraocular movements. Pupils 4 to 5 mm constricting. Discs difficult to visualize; no hemorrhages noted. *Ears:* Normal pinna; no external abnormalities. Normal external canals and tympanic membranes (TMs). *Nose:* Normal nares; septum midline. *Mouth:* Several darkened teeth (inside surface of upper incisors). One clear cavity on upper right incisor. Tongue normal. Cobblestoning of posterior pharynx; no exudates. Tonsils large but adequate gap (1.5 cm) between them.

(continued)

Neck. Supple, midline trachea, no thyroid palpable.

Lymph Nodes. Easily palpable (1.5 to 2 cm) tonsillar lymph nodes bilaterally. Small (0.5 cm) nodes in inguinal canal bilaterally. All lymph nodes mobile and nontender.

Lungs. Good expansion. No tachypnea or dyspnea. Congestion audible, but seems to be upper airway (louder near mouth, symmetric). No rhonchi, rales, or wheezes. Clear to auscultation.

Cardiovascular. PMI in 4th or 5th interspace and midsternal line. Normal S_1 and S_2. No murmurs or abnormal heart sounds. Normal femoral pulses; dorsalis pedis pulses palpable bilaterally.

Breasts. Normal, with some fat under both.

Abdomen. Protuberant but soft; no masses or tenderness. Liver span 2 cm below right costal margin (RCM) and not tender. Spleen and kidneys not palpable.

Genitalia. Tanner I circumcised penis; no pubic hair, lesions, or discharge. Testes descended, difficult to palpate because of active cremasteric reflex. Normal scrotum both sides.

Musculoskeletal. Normal range of motion of upper and lower extremities and all joints. Spine straight. Gait normal.

Neurologic. *Mental Status:* Happy, cooperative child. *Developmental (DDST):* Gross motor—Jumps and throws objects. Fine motor—Imitates vertical line. Language—Does not combine words; single words only, three to four noted during examination. Personal-social—Washes face, brushes teeth, and puts on shirt. Overall—Normal, except for language, which appears delayed. *Cranial Nerves:* Intact, although several difficult to elicit. *Cerebellar:* Normal gait; good balance. *Deep tendon reflexes (DTRs):* Normal and symmetric throughout with downgoing toes. *Sensory:* Deferred.

B I B L I O G R A P H Y

CITATIONS

1. Levine MD, Carey WB, Crocker AC. Developmental–Behavioral Pediatrics, 3rd ed. Philadelphia: WB Saunders, 2002.
2. American Academy of Pediatrics. Guidelines for Health Supervision III, revised ed. Elk Grove Village, IL: Author, 2002.
3. American Academy of Pediatrics. Bright Futures. Available at: http://brightfutures.aap.org/web/aboutBrightFutures.asp. Accessed February 19, 2008.
4. American Medical Association. Guidelines for Adolescent Preventive Services (GAPS). Available at: http://www.ama-assn.org/ama/upload/mm/39/gapsmono.pdf. Accessed February 19, 2008.
5. United States Department of Health and Human Services. U.S. Preventive Services Task Force (USPSTF). Available at: http://www.ahrq.gov/clinic/uspstfix.htm. Accessed February 19, 2008.

6. Centers for Disease Control and Prevention. Recommendations and Guidelines: 2008 Child & Adolescent Immunization Schedules. Available at: http://www.cdc.gov/vaccines/recs/schedules/child-schedule.htm. Accessed February 19, 2008.

7. American Academy of Pediatrics Committee on Infectious Diseases. Recommended Immunization Schedules for Children and Adolescents—United States, 2007. Pediatrics 119(1): 207–208, 2007.

8. AHRA Guide to Clinical Preventive Services. Available at: http://www.ahra.gov/clinic/cps3dix.htm. Accessed July 10, 2008.

9. American Academy of Pediatrics and American College of Obstetricians and Gynecologists. Guidelines for Perinatal Care, 4th ed. Washington, DC: American Academy of Pediatrics, 1997.

10. Fuloria M, Kreiter S. The newborn examination: part 1. Emergencies and common abnormalities involving the skin, head, neck, chest, and respiratory and cardiovascular system. Am Fam Phys 65(1):61–68.

11. Ballard JL, Khoury JC, Wedig K. Ballard scoring system for determining gestational age in weeks. J Pediatr 119:417, 1991.

12. Brazelton TB. Working with families: opportunities for early intervention. Pediatr Clin North Am 42(1):1–9, 1995.

13. Johnson CP, Blasco PA. Infant growth and development. Pediatr Rev 18(7):224–242, 1997.

14. Colson ER, Dworkin PH. Toddler development. Pediatr Rev 18(8):255–259, 1997.

15. Copelan J. Normal speech and development. Pediatr Rev 18:91–100, 1995.

16. Fong CT. Clinical diagnosis of genetic diseases. Pediatr Ann 22(5):277–281, 1993.

17. Hyvarinen L. Assessment of visually impaired infants. Ophthalm Clin North Am 7:219, 1994.

18. Lees MH. Cyanosis of the newborn infant: recognition and clinical evaluation. J Pediatr 77:484, 1970.

19. Gessner IH. What makes a heart murmur innocent? Pediatr Ann 26(2):82–84, 87–88, 90–91, 1997.

20. Callahan CW Jr, Alpert B. Simultaneous percussion auscultation technique for the determination of liver span. Arch Pediatr Adolesc Med 148(8):873–875, 1994.

21. Reiff MI, Osborn LM. Clinical estimation of liver size in newborn infants. Pediatrics 71:46–48, 1983.

22. Burger BJ, Burger JD, Bos CF, et al. Neonatal screening and staggered early treatment for congenital dislocation or dysplasia of the hip. Lancet 336(8730):1549–1553, 1990.

23. Zafeiriou DI. Primitive reflexes and postural reactions in the neurodevelopmental examination. Pediatr Neurol 31(1):1–8, 2004.

24. Schott JM, Rossor MN. The grasp and other primitive reflexes. J Neurol Neurosurg Psychiatry 74(5):558–560, 2003.

25. Luiz DM, Foxcroft CD, Stewart R. The construct validity of the Griffiths Scales of Mental Development. Child Care Health Dev 27:73–83, 2001.

26. Newacheck PW, Strickland B, Shonkoff JP, et al. An epidemiologic profile of children with special health care needs. Pediatrics 102:117–123, 1998.

27. Ogden CL, Carroll MD, Curtin LR, et al. Prevalence of overweight and obesity in the United States, 1999–2004. JAMA 295:1549–1555, 2006.

28. National High Blood Pressure Education Program Working Group on High Blood Pressure in Children and Adolescents. The Fourth Report on the Diagnosis, Evaluation, and Treatment of High Blood Pressure in Children and Adolescents. Pediatrics 114:555–576, 2004.

29. Shamis, DI. Collecting the "facts": vision assessment techniques: perils and pitfalls. Am Orthop J 46:7, 1996.

30. Rothman R, Owens T, Simel DL. Does this child have acute otitis media? JAMA 290:1633–1640, 2003.

31. Blomgren K, Pitkaranta A. Current challenges in diagnosis of acute otitis media. Intl J Ped Otorhinolaryn 69(3):295–299, 2005.

32. Pirozzo S, Papinczak T, Glasziou P. Whispered voice test for screening for hearing impairment in adults and children: systematic review. BMJ 327(7421):967, 2003.

33. Wolf G, Anderhuber W, Kuhn F. Development of the paranasal sinuses in children: implications for paranasal sinus surgery. Ann Otol Rhinol Laryngol 102(9):705–711, 1993.

34. Selwitz RH, Ismail AI, Pitts NB. Dental caries. Lancet 369(9555):51–59, 2007.

35. Lunt RC, Law DB. A review of the chronology of eruption of deciduous teeth. J Am Dent Assoc 89:872, 1974.

36. Ebell MH, Smith MA, Barry HC, et al. Does this patient have strep throat? JAMA 284:2912–2918, 2000.

37. Centers for Disease Control and Prevention. National Surveillance for Asthma—United States, 1980–2004. MMWR Morb Mortal Wkly Rep 56:1–60, 2007.

38. Tucker WN, Saab S, Leland SR, et al. The scratch test is unreliable for determining the liver edge. J Clin Gastroenterol 25:410–414, 1997.

39. Ashcraft KW. Consultation with the specialist: acute abdominal pain. Pediatr Rev 21:363–367, 2000.

40. Hymel KP, Jenny C. Child sexual abuse. Pediatr Rev 17(7): 236–249; quiz, 249–250, 1996.

41. Scherl S. Common lower extremity problems in children. Pediatr Rev 25:43–75, 2004.

42. Bruce RW. Torsional and angular deformities. Pediatr Clin North Am 43:867–881, 1996.

43. Elster AB, Kuznets MJ. AMA Guidelines for Adolescent Preventive Services (GAPS): Recommendations and Rationale. Baltimore, MD: Williams & Wilkins, 1993.

44. ACOG Committee. Opinion no. 350, November 2006: Breast concerns in the adolescent. Obstet Gynecol 108(5):1329–1336, 2006.

45. Herman-Giddens ME, Slora EJ, Wasserman RC, et al. Secondary sexual characteristics and menses in young girls seen in office practice: a study from the Pediatric Research in Office Settings Network. Pediatrics 99(4): 505–512, 1997.

46. Metzl JD. Preparticipation examination of the adolescent athlete: part 1. Pediatr Rev 22(6):119–204, 2001.

47. Metzl JD. Preparticipation examination of the adolescent athlete: part 2. Pediatr Rev 22(7):227–239, 2001.

ADDITIONAL REFERENCES

American Academy of Pediatrics. Bright Futures: Guidelines for Health Supervision of Infants, Children, and Adolescents, 3rd ed. Elk Grove Village, IL: American Academy of Pediatrics, 2008.

Bergen D. Human Development: Traditional and Contemporary Theories. Upper Saddle River, NJ: Pearson/Prentice Hall, 2008.

Burns CE, Dunn AM, Brady MA, et al. Pediatric Primary Care: A Handbook for Nurse Practitioners, 3rd ed. St. Louis: Saunders, 2004.

Colyar MR. Well-child Assessment for Primary Care Providers. Philadelphia: FA Davis, 2003.

Cote P, Kreitz BG, Cassidy JD, et al. A study of the diagnostic accuracy and reliability of the scoliometer and Adam's forward bend test. Spine 23:796–802; discussion, 803, 1998.

Dixon SD, Stein MT. Encounters with children: pediatric behavior and development, 4th ed. Philadelphia: Mosby, 2006.

Dubowitz LMS, Dubowitz V, Mercuri E. The neurological assessment of the preterm and full-term newborn infant, 2nd ed. Clinics in Developmental Medicine, no. 148. London: Cambridge University Press, 1999:1–155.

Emans SJ, Laufer MR, Goldstein DP. Pediatric and Adolescent Gynecology, 5th ed. Philadelphia: Lippincott Williams & Wilkins, 2004.

Fenichel G. Clinical Pediatric Neurology: A Signs and Symptoms Approach, 5th ed. Philadelphia: Saunders, 2005.

Fuloria M, Kreiter S. The newborn examination: Part 2. Emergencies and common abnormalities involving the abdomen, pelvis, extremities, genitalia, and spine. Am Fam Phys 65(2):265–270, 2002.

Korovessis PG, Stamatakis MV. Prediction of scoliotic Cobb angle with the use of the scoliometer. Spine 21:1661–1666, 1996.

Naylor CD. The rational clinical examination: physical examination of the liver. JAMA 271:1859–1865, 1994.

Neinstein LS. Adolescent Health Care: A Practical Guide, 4th ed. Philadelphia: Lippincott Williams & Wilkins, 2002.

Sass P, Hassan G. Lower extremity abnormalities in children. Am Fam Phys 68:661–668, 2003.

Stellwagen L, Boies E. Care of the well newborn. Pediatr Rev 27(3):89–98, 2006.

Swaiman KF, Ashwal S, Ferriero DM. Neurologic examination of the term and preterm infant. In: Pediatric Neurology: Principles & Practice, 4th ed. Philadelphia: Mosby Elsevier, 2006:47–64.

Viviani GR, Budgell L, Dok C, et al. Assessment of accuracy of the scoliosis school screening examination. Am J Public Health 74:497–498, 1984.

Wallace GB, Newton RW. Gowers' sign revisited. Arch Dis Child 64:1317–1319, 1989.

Zitelli BJ, Davis HW. Atlas of Pediatric Physical Diagnosis, 4th ed. St. Louis: Mosby, 2002.

The Bates' suite offers these additional resources to enhance learning and facilitate understanding of this chapter:

- Bates' Pocket Guide to Physical Examination and History Taking, 6th edition
- Bates' Nursing Online
- Bates' Visual Guide to Physical Examination, 4th edition
- thePoint online resources, http://thepoint.lww.com
- Student CD-ROM included with the book

Abnormalities in Heart Rhythm and Blood Pressure

Supraventricular Tachycardia

Paroxysmal supraventricular tachycardia (SVT) is the most common dysrhythmia in children. Some infants with SVT look well or may be somewhat pale with tachypnea, but have a heart rate of 240 beats per minute or greater. Others are ill and in cardiovascular collapse.

SVT in infants is usually sustained, requiring medical therapy for conversion to a normal rate and rhythm. In older children, it is more likely to be truly paroxysmal, with episodes of varying duration and frequency.

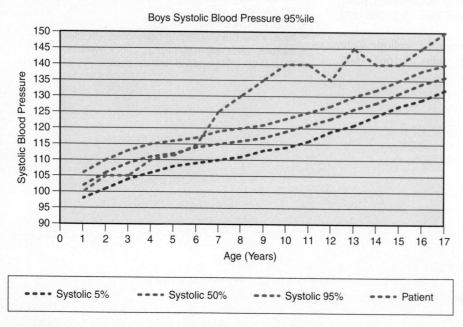

Hypertension in Childhood—A Typical Example[28]

Hypertension can start in childhood. While elevated blood pressure in young children is more likely to have a renal, cardiac, or endocrine cause, adolescents with hypertension are most likely to have primary or essential hypertension.

This child developed hypertension and it "tracked" into adulthood. Children tend to remain in the same percentile for blood pressure as they grow. This tracking of blood pressure continues into adulthood, supporting the concept that adult essential hypertension often begins during childhood.

The consequences of untreated hypertension can be severe.

Common Skin Rashes and Skin Findings in Newborns and Infants

Erythema Toxicum
These common yellow or white pustules are surrounded by a red base.

Neonatal Acne
Red pustules and papules are most prominent over the cheeks and nose of some normal newborns.

Seborrhea
The salmon red, scaly eruption often involves the face, neck, axilla, diaper area, and behind the ears.

Body and Extremities

Atopic Dermatitis (Eczema)
Erythema, scaling, dry skin, and intense itching characterize this condition.

Neurofibromatosis
Characteristic features include more than 5 café-au-lait spots and axillary freckling, both shown above. Later findings include neurofibromas and Lish nodules (not shown).

Diaper Region

Candidal Diaper Dermatitis
This bright red rash involves the intertriginous folds, with small "satellite lesions" along the edges.

Contact Diaper Dermatitis
This irritant rash is secondary to diarrhea or irritation and is noted along contact areas (here, the area touching the diaper).

Impetigo
This infection is due to bacteria and can appear bullous or crusty and yellowed with some pus.

Warts, Lesions That Resemble Warts, and Other Raised Lesions

Verruca Vulgaris
Dry, rough warts on hands

Verruca Plana
Small, flat warts

Plantar Warts
Tender warts on feet

Molluscum Contagiosum
Dome-shaped, fleshy lesions

Adolescent Acne
Acne in adolescents involves open comedones (blackheads) and closed comedones (whiteheads) shown at the left, and inflamed pustules (right).

Common Skin Lesions During Childhood

Insect Bites
Intensely pruritic, red, distinct papules characterize these lesions.

Urticaria (Hives)
This pruritic, allergic sensitivity reaction changes shape quickly.

Tinea Capitis
Scaling, crusting, and hair loss are seen in the scalp, along with a painful plaque (kerion) and occipital lymph node (*arrow*).

Tinea Corporis
This annular lesion has central clearing and papules along the border.

(Source of all photos except *Urticaria*—Goodheart H. A Photoguide of Common Skin Disorders. Baltimore, Williams & Wilkins, 1999.)

Cephalohematoma

Although not present at birth, cephalohematomas appear within the first 24 hours from subperiosteal hemorrhage involving the outer table of one of the cranial bones. The swelling, as above, does not extend across a suture, though it is occasionally bilateral following a difficult birth. The swelling is initially soft, then develops a raised bony margin within a few days from calcium deposits at the edge of the periosteum. It tends to resolve within several weeks.

Hydrocephalus

In hydrocephaly, the anterior fontanelle is bulging, and the eyes may be deviated downward, revealing the upper scleras and creating the *setting sun* sign, as shown above. The setting sun sign is also seen briefly in some normal newborns. (From Zitelli BJ, Davis HW. Atlas of Pediatric Physical Diagnosis, 3rd ed. St. Louis, Mosby–Year Book, 1997. Courtesy of Dr. Albert Briglan, Children's Hospital of Pittsburgh.)

Anterior

Normal

Posterior

Scaphocephaly
(sagittal)

Frontal plagiocephaly
(unilateral coronal)

Trigonocephaly
(metopic)

Brachycephaly
(coronal, metopic)

Occipital plagiocephaly
(unilateral lambdoid)

Craniosynostosis

Craniosynostosis is a condition of premature closure of one or more sutures of the skull. This results in an abnormal growth and shape of the skull because growth will occur across sutures that are not affected but not across sutures that are affected. The figures demonstrate different skull shapes associated with the various types of craniosynostosis. The prematurely closed suture line is noted by the absence of a suture line in each figure. Scaphocephaly and frontal plagiocephaly are most common. The *blue shading* shows areas of maximal flattening. The *red arrows* show the direction of continued growth across the sutures, which is normal.

Fetal Alcohol Syndrome

Babies born to women with chronic alcoholism are at increased risk for growth deficiency, microcephaly, and mental retardation. Facial characteristics include short palpebral fissures, a wide and flattened philtrum (the vertical groove in the midline of the upper lip), and thin lips.

Congenital Syphilis

In utero infection by *Treponema pallidum* usually occurs after the 16th week of gestation and affects virtually all fetal organs. If it is not treated, 25% of infected babies die before birth and another 30% shortly thereafter. Signs of illness appear in survivors within the first month of life. Facial stigmata shown here include bulging of the frontal bones and nasal bridge depression (*saddle nose*), both from periostitis; rhinitis from weeping nasal mucosal lesions (*snuffles*); and a circumoral rash. Mucocutaneous inflammation and fissuring of the mouth and lips (*rhagades*), not shown here, may also occur as stigmata of congenital syphilis, as may craniotabes tibial periostitis (*saber shins*) and dental dysplasia (*Hutchinson's teeth*—see p. 278).

Congenital Hypothyroidism

The child with congenital hypothyroidism (*cretinism*) has coarse facial features, a low-set hair line, sparse eyebrows, and an enlarged tongue. Associated features include a hoarse cry, umbilical hernia, dry and cold extremities, myxedema, mottled skin, and mental retardation. Most infants with congenital hypothyroidism have no physical stigmata; this has led to screening of all newborns in the United States and most other developed countries for congenital hypothyroidism.

Facial Nerve Palsy

Peripheral (lower motor neuron) paralysis of the facial nerve may be from (1) an injury to the nerve from pressure during labor and birth, (2) inflammation of the middle ear branch of the nerve during episodes of acute or chronic otitis media, or (3) unknown causes (Bell's palsy). The nasolabial fold on the affected left side is flattened, and the eye does not close. This is accentuated during crying, as shown here. Full recovery occurs in ≥ 90% of those affected.

(table continues on page 861)

Down Syndrome

The child with Down syndrome (trisomy 21) usually has a small, rounded head, a flattened nasal bridge, oblique palpebral fissures, prominent epicanthal folds, small, low-set, shell-like ears, and a relatively large tongue. Associated features include generalized hypotonia, transverse palmar creases (*simian lines*), shortening and incurving of the 5th fingers (*clinodactyly*), Brushfield's spots (see p. 862), and mental retardation.

Battered Child Syndrome

The child who has been physically abused (battered) may have old *and* fresh bruises on the head and face and may either look sad and forlorn or be actively seeking to please, sometimes even particularly involved with and attentive to the abusing parent. Other stigmata include bruises in areas (axilla and groin) not usually subject to injury rather than the bony prominences; x-ray evidence of fractures of the skull, ribs, and long bones in various stages of healing; and skin lesions that are morphologically similar to implements used to inflict trauma (hand, belt buckle, strap, rope, coat hanger, or lighted cigarette).

Perennial Allergic Rhinitis

The child suffering from perennial allergic rhinitis has an open mouth (cannot breathe through the nose) and edema and discoloration of the lower orbitopalpebral grooves ("allergic shiners"). Such a child is often seen to push the nose upward and backward with a hand ("allergic salute") and to grimace (wrinkle the nose and mouth) to relieve nasal itching and obstruction. (Photograph reproduced with permission from Marks MB. Allergic shiners: dark circles under the eyes in children. Clin Pediatr 5:656, 1966.)

Hyperthyroidism

Thyrotoxicosis (*Graves' disease*) occurs in approximately 2 per 1,000 children younger than 10 years. Affected children exhibit hypermetabolism and accelerated linear growth. Facial characteristics shown in this 6-year-old girl are "staring" eyes (not true exophthalmos, which is rare in children) and an enlarged thyroid gland (*goiter*). See p. 281.

Abnormalities of the Eyes, Ears, and Mouth

Eye Abnormalities

Brushfield's Spots

These abnormal speckling spots on the iris suggest Down syndrome.

Strabismus

Strabismus, or misalignment of the eyes, can lead to visual impairment. Esotropia, shown here, is an inward deviation.

Ear Abnormalities

A　　　　　　　　**B**　　　　　　　　**C**

Otitis Media

Otitis media is one of the most common conditions in young children. The spectrum of otitis media is shown here. (**A**) Typical acute otitis media with a red, distorted, bulging tympanic membrane in a highly symptomatic child. (**B**) Acute otitis media with bullae formation and fluid visible behind the tympanic membrane. (**C**) Otitis media with effusion, showing a yellowish fluid behind a retracted and thickened tympanic membrane.

(Source of photos: *Otitis Media*—Courtesy of Alejandro Hoberman, Children's Hospital of Pittsburgh, University of Pittsburgh.)

Mouth Abnormalities

Oral Candidiasis ("thrush")

This infection is common in infants. The white plaques do not rub off.

Herpetic Stomatitis

Tender ulcerations on the oral mucosa are surrounded by erythema.

Dental Abnormalities

Dental Caries

Dental caries is a major global health and pediatric problem. The photographs below show different characteristics of caries.

Nursing-bottle caries

Erosion of teeth

Severe erosion

Staining of the Teeth

Various causes can lead to staining of the teeth of children, including intrinsic stains such as tetracycline (right) or extrinsic stains such as poor oral hygiene (not shown). Extrinsic stains can be removed.

Streptococcal Pharyngitis ("strep throat")

This common childhood infection has a classic presentation of erythema of the posterior pharynx and palatal petechiae (*left*). A foul-smelling exudate (*right*) is also commonly noted.

Lymphadenopathy

Enlarged and tender cervical lymph nodes are common in children. The most likely causes are viral and bacterial infections. Lymph node enlargement can be bilateral, as shown above.

TABLE
18-9

Cyanosis in Children

It is important to recognize cyanosis. The best location to examine is the mucous membranes. Cyanosis is a "raspberry" color, whereas normal mucous membranes should have a "strawberry" color. Try to identify the cyanosis in these photographs before reading the captions.

Generalized Cyanosis
This baby has total anomalous pulmonary venous return and an oxygen saturation level of 80%.

Perioral Cyanosis
This baby has mild cyanosis above the lips, but the mucous membranes remain pink.

Bluish Lips, Giving Appearance of Cyanosis
Normal pigment deposition in the vermilion border of the lips gives them a bluish hue, but the mucous membranes are pink.

Acrocyanosis
This commonly appears on the feet and hands of babies shortly after birth. This infant is a 32-week newborn.

(Source of photos: Fletcher M. Physical Diagnosis in Neonatology. Philadelphia, Lippincott-Raven, 1998.)

Congenital Heart Murmurs

Some heart murmurs reflect underlying heart disease. If you understand their physiologic causes, you will more readily be able to identify and distinguish them from innocent heart murmurs. Obstructive lesions result when blood flows through valves that are too small. Because this problem does not depend on the drop in pulmonary vascular resistance following birth, these murmurs are audible at birth. Defects with left-to-right shunts, on the other hand, depend on the drop in pulmonary vascular resistance. High-pressured shunts such as ventricular septal defect, patent ductus arteriosus, and persistent truncus arteriosus are not heard until 1 week or more after birth. Low-pressured left-to-right shunts, such as in atrial septal defects, may not be heard for considerably longer, usually first being noted at 1 year or more. Many children with congenital cardiac defects have combinations of defects or variations of abnormalities, so findings on cardiac examination may not follow these classic patterns. This table shows a limited selection of the more common defects.

Congenital Defect and Mechanism	Characteristics of the Murmur	Associated Findings
Pulmonary Valve Stenosis Usually a normal valve anulus with fusion of some or most of the valve leaflets, restricting flow across the valve *Mild* *Severe* 	*Location.* Upper left sternal border *Radiation.* In mild degrees of stenosis, the murmur may be heard over the course of the pulmonary arteries in the lung fields. *Intensity.* Increases in intensity and duration as the degree of obstruction increases *Quality.* Ejection, peaking later in systole as the obstruction increases	Usually a prominent ejection click in early systole Pulmonary component of the second sounds at the base (P₂) becomes delayed and softer, disappearing as obstruction increases. Inspiration may increase murmur; expiration may increase click. Growth is usually normal. Newborns with severe stenosis may be cyanotic from right-to-left atrial shunting and rapidly develop congestive heart failure.
Aortic Valve Stenosis Usually a bicuspid valve with progressive obstruction, but there may be a dysplastic valve or damage from rheumatic fever or degenerative disease 	*Location.* Midsternum, upper right sternal border *Radiation.* To the carotid arteries and suprasternal notch; may also be a thrill *Intensity.* Varies, louder with increasingly severe obstruction *Quality.* An ejection, often harsh, systolic murmur	May be an associated ejection click The aortic closure sound may be increased in intensity. There may be a diastolic murmur of aortic valve regurgitation. Newborns with severe stenosis may have weak or absent pulses and severe congestive heart failure. May not be audible until adulthood even though the valve is congenitally abnormal
Tetralogy of Fallot Complex defect with ventricular septal defect, infundibular and usually valvular right ventricular outflow obstruction, malrotation of the aorta, and right-to-left shunting at ventricular septal level *With Pulmonic Stenosis* *With Pulmonic Atresia* 	*General.* Variable cyanosis, increasing with activity *Location.* Mid-to-upper left sternal border. If pulmonary atresia, there is no systolic murmur but the continuous murmur of ductus arteriosus flow at upper left sternal border or in the back. *Radiation.* Little, to upper left sternal border, occasionally to lung fields *Intensity.* Usually grade III–IV *Quality.* Midpeaking, systolic ejection murmur	Normal pulses The pulmonary closure sound is usually not heard. May have abrupt hypercyanotic spells with sudden increase in cyanosis, air hunger, altered level of awareness Failure to gain weight with persistent and increasingly severe cyanosis Long-term persistence of cyanosis accompanied by clubbing of fingers and toes Persistent hypoxemia leads to polycythemia, which will accentuate the cyanosis..

(table continues on page 866)

TABLE
18-10

Congenital Heart Murmurs (continued)

Congenital Defect and Mechanism	Characteristics of the Murmur	Associated Findings
Transposition of the Great Arteries A severe defect with failure of rotation of the great vessels, leaving the aorta to arise from the right ventricle and the pulmonary artery from the left ventricle	*General.* Intense generalized cyanosis *Location.* No characteristic murmur. If present, it may reflect an associated defect such as VSD. *Radiation and Quality.* Depends on associated abnormalities	Single loud second sound of the anterior aortic valve Frequent rapid development of congestive heart failure Frequent associated defects as described at the left
Ventricular Septal Defect Blood going from a high-pressured left ventricle through a defect in the septum to the lower-pressured right ventricle creates turbulence, usually throughout systole. *Small to Moderate* 	*Location.* Lower left sternal border *Radiation.* Little *Intensity.* Variable, only partially determined by the size of the shunt. Small shunts with a high pressure gradient may have very loud murmurs. Large defects with elevated pulmonary vascular resistance may have no murmur. Grade II–IV/VI with a thrill if grade IV/VI or higher. *Quality.* Pansystolic, usually harsh, may obscure S_1 and S_2 if loud enough	With large shunts, there may be a low-pitched middiastolic murmur of relative mitral stenosis at the apex. As pulmonary artery pressure increases, the pulmonic component of the second sounds at the base increases in intensity. When pulmonary artery pressure equals aortic pressure, there may be no murmur, and P_2 will be very loud. In low-volume shunts, growth is normal. In larger shunts, congestive heart failure may occur by 6–8 weeks; poor weight gain. Associated defects are frequent.
Patent Ductus Arteriosus Continuous flow from aorta to pulmonary artery throughout the cardiac cycle when ductus arteriosus does not close after birth *Small to Moderate* 	*Location.* Upper left sternal border and to left *Radiation.* Sometimes to the back *Intensity.* Varies depending on size of the shunt, usually grade II–III/VI. *Quality.* A rather hollow, sometimes machinery-like murmur that is continuous throughout the cardiac cycle, although occasionally almost inaudible in late diastole, uninterrupted by the heart sounds, louder in systole	Full to bounding pulses Noticed at birth in the premature infant who may have bounding pulses, a hyperdynamic precordium, and an atypical murmur Noticed later in the full-term infant as pulmonary vascular resistance falls May develop congestive heart failure at 4–6 weeks if large shunt Poor weight gain related to size of shunt Pulmonary hypertension affects murmur as above.
Atrial Septal Defect Left-to-right shunt through an opening in the atrial septum, possible at various levels 	*Location.* Upper left sternal border *Radiation.* To the back *Intensity.* Variable, usually grade II–III/VI *Quality.* Ejection but without the harsh quality	Widely split second sounds throughout all phases of respiration, normal intensity Usually not heard until after age of 1 year Gradual decrease in weight gain as shunt increases Decreased exercise tolerance, subtle, not dramatic Congestive heart failure is rare.

TABLE 18-11

Physical Signs of Sexual Abuse

Possible Indications

1. Marked and immediate dilatation of the anus in knee–chest position, with no constipation, stool in the vault, or neurologic disorders
2. Hymenal notch or cleft that extends greater than 50% of the inferior hymenal rim (confirmed in knee–chest position)
3. Condyloma acuminata in a child older than 3 years
4. Bruising, abrasions, lacerations, or bite marks of labia or perihymenal tissue
5. Herpes of the anogenital area beyond the neonatal period
6. Purulent or malodorous vaginal discharge in a young girl (culture and view all discharges under a microscope for evidence of a sexually transmitted disease)

Strong Indications

1. Lacerations, ecchymoses, and newly healed scars of the hymen or the posterior fourchette
2. No hymenal tissue from 3 to 9 o'clock (confirmed in various positions)
3. Healed hymenal transections, especially between 3 and 9 o'clock (complete cleft)
4. Perianal lacerations extending to external sphincter

A child with concerning physical signs must be evaluated by a sexual abuse expert for a complete history and sexual abuse examination.

Any physical sign must be evaluated in light of the entire history, other parts of the physical examination, and laboratory data.

Key to Photos

(**A**) Acute hemorrhage and ecchymoses of tissues (10-mo-old)

(**B**) Erythema and superficial abrasions to the labia minora (5-yr-old)

(**C**) Healed interruption of hymenal membrane at 9 o'clock (4-yr-old)

(**D**) Narrowed posterior ring continuous with floor of vagina (12-yr-old)

(**E**) Copious vaginal discharge and erythema (9-yr-old)

(**F**) Extensive condylomata around the anus (2-yr-old)

Source: Reece R, Ludwig S, eds. Child Abuse Medical Diagnosis and Management, 2nd ed. Philadelphia, Lippincott Williams & Wilkins, 2001.)

TABLE
18-12

The Male Genitourinary System

Hypospadius

Hypospadius is the most common congenital penile abnormality. The urethral meatus opens abnormally on the ventral surface of the penis. One form is shown above; more severe forms involve openings on the lower shaft or scrotum.

Undescended Testicle

You should distinguish between undescended testes, shown above (with testes in the inguinal canals), from highly retractile testes from an active cremasteric reflex.

(Sources of photos: *Hypospadius*—Courtesy of Warren Snodgrass, MD, UT–Southwestern Medical Center at Dallas; *Undescended Testicle*—Fletcher M. Physical Diagnosis in Neonatology. Philadelphia, Lippincott-Raven, 1998.)

TABLE
18-13

Common Musculoskeletal Findings in Young Children

Flat feet or *pes planus* from laxity of the soft-tissue structures of the foot

Inversion of the foot (*varus*)

Metatarsus adductus in a child. The forefoot is adducted and not inverted.

A

B

Pronation in a toddler. (**A**) When viewed from behind, the hindfoot is everted. (**B**) When viewed from the front, the forefoot is everted and abducted.

TABLE
18-14

The Power of Prevention:
Vaccine-Preventable Diseases

This table shows photographs of children with vaccine-preventable diseases. Childhood vaccines have been named the single most important medical intervention in the world in terms of influence on public health. Because of vaccinations, we hope you will never see many of these conditions, but you should be able to identify them. Try to identify the diseases before reading the captions.

Polio
The deformed leg of this child is from polio.

Measles
Characteristic rash of measles

Rubella
Infant born with congenital rubella syndrome

Tetanus
Rigid newborn with neonatal tetanus

Haemophilus influenzae
Type b
Periorbital cellulitis from this
invasive bacterial disease

Varicella
An infant with a severe form of varicella

(Sources of photos: *Polio*—Courtesy of World Health Organization; *Haemophilus influenzae*—Courtesy of American Academy of Pediatrics; *Varicella*—Courtesy of Barbara Watson, MD, Albert Einstein Medical Center and Division of Disease Control, Philadelphia Department of Health; all others courtesy of Centers for Disease Control and Prevention.)

The Pregnant Woman

This chapter focuses on history taking and physical examination of the healthy adult woman during pregnancy. The techniques of examination are similar to those of the nonpregnant woman; however, the clinician must distinguish the changes in anatomy and physiology arising from pregnancy from abnormal findings. This chapter emphasizes common changes in anatomy and physiology that evolve throughout pregnancy; special concerns when eliciting the health history; and recommendations for nutrition, exercise, and screening for domestic violence. Then follow techniques of examination basic to prenatal care.

ANATOMY AND PHYSIOLOGY

Hormonal Changes. During pregnancy, hormonal changes lead to extensive anatomical and physiologic changes in every major body system. Increasing levels of estradiol and progesterone and the placental hormones, especially human chorionic gonadotropin (HCG), drive many of the pregnancy-related endocrine and metabolic changes. These many complex changes can only be summarized here in brief:

- Estradiol appears to stimulate lactotrophs in the *anterior lobe of the pituitary gland*. These cells may triple in size as increasing prolactin output readies the breast tissue for lactation.[1]

- The *posterior pituitary gland* stores oxytocin and antidiuretic hormone (ADH)—HCG appears to reset the receptors for thirst and ADH release, leading to decreases in serum sodium concentration and, in some women, polyuria.

- The *thyroid gland* remains normal in size; however, the effects of estrogen on thyroxine-binding globulin and the stimulation of the thyrotropin (TSH) receptor by HCG lead to fluctuations in free T4 and T3 levels and in TSH, usually within the normal range.[2]

- *Placental hormones* contribute to increased *insulin resistance* in later pregnancy and a shift from carbohydrate to fat metabolism. Insulin resistance is linked to transient hyperglycemia after meals; however, between meals, fasting glucose levels fall, partly because of the demands of fetal growth and increased peripheral use of glucose.[3]

- At the end of pregnancy, increases in placental corticotrophin-releasing hormone (CRH) and adrenal adrenocorticotropic hormone (ACTH) produce a "state of *relative hypercortisolism*" that may be a trigger for labor. Placental production of CRH suggests that a placental clock determines the timing of birth.[4]

- Rising *progesterone* levels have several effects. Although respiratory rate does not change, tidal volume and minute ventilation increase, sometimes leading to complaints of dyspnea. Progesterone and estradiol lower esophageal sphincter tone, contributing to symptoms of reflux and heartburn. Progesterone also relaxes tone and contraction in the ureters, causing hydronephrosis, and in the bladder, increasing risk for bacteriuria.

- *Cardiovascular changes* in pregnancy are significant. To meet the circulatory demands of an enlarging uterus, both erythrocyte mass and plasma volume increase. The latter increases more, causing relative hemodilution and physiologic anemia, which can protect against blood loss during childbirth. Cardiac output increases, and systemic vascular resistance and blood pressure fall.

- Finally, *musculoskeletal changes* ensue from weight gain and *relaxin,* a hormone secreted in the corpus luteum and placenta: lumbar lordosis as the gravid uterus enlarges, contributing to mechanical low back discomfort, and ligamentous laxity in the sacroiliac joints and the pubic symphysis, to ease passage of the baby through the birth canal.

Changes in the Breasts and Pelvis.   Changes in the breasts and uterus are the most visible signs of pregnancy. To refresh your understanding of basic anatomy and physiology of the breasts and pelvis, review those sections of Chapter 10, The Breasts and Axillae, and Chapter 14, Female Genitalia.

Breasts.   The breasts enlarge moderately as a result of hormone stimulation, increased vascularity, and hyperplasia of glandular tissue. Tenderness and tingling in the breasts may make them more sensitive during examination. By the third month of gestation, the breasts become more nodular. Palpate carefully to avoid discomfort as you examine for any breast masses. The nipples become larger and more erectile. From mid- to late pregnancy, *colostrum,* a thick, yellowish secretion rich in nutrients, may be expressed from the nipples. The areolae darken, and Montgomery's glands are more pronounced. The venous pattern over the breasts becomes increasingly visible as pregnancy progresses.

EXPECTED HEIGHT OF THE UTERINE FUNDUS BY WEEKS OF PREGNANCY

36 wks
32 wks
28 wks
24 wks
20 wks
16 wks
12-14 wks

Uterus and Vagina. The abdomen becomes increasingly prominent to accommodate the growing fetus and enlarging uterus. The pregnant uterus is most easily palpable beyond 12 to 14 weeks as it expands cephalad to the pelvic brim. Expected growth patterns of the gravid uterus are shown on the left. The standing contours of the primigravid abdomen in each trimester appear on the right.[5]

FIRST TRIMESTER

The early diagnosis of pregnancy is based in part on changes in the vagina and uterus. With increased vascularity throughout the pelvic region, the vagina takes on a bluish or violet color, known as *Chadwick's sign*. The vaginal walls appear thicker and deeply rugated because of increased thickness of the mucosa, loosening of the connective tissue, and hypertrophy of smooth muscle cells. Vaginal secretions are thick, white, and more profuse. Vaginal pH often becomes more acidic from the action of *Lactobacillus acidophilus* on the increased levels of glycogen stored in the vaginal epithelium.[6] This change in pH helps protect the woman against some vaginal infections, but increased glycogen may contribute to higher rates of vaginal candidiasis (see p. 550).

Softened isthmus

HEGAR'S SIGN

Early in pregnancy, the uterus loses the firmness and resistance of the nonpregnant organ. The palpable softening at the isthmus, called *Hegar's sign*, is an early diagnostic sign of pregnancy, and is illustrated on the left.

SECOND TRIMESTER

With advancing pregnancy, uterine weight increases from 50 to 70 grams to 800 to 1200 grams, and its volume expands from approximately 10 ml to 5 liters. Contributing to these changes are muscle cell hypertrophy, more extensive fibrous and elastic tissue, and considerable increases in the size and number of blood vessels and lymphatics.

The growing uterus changes shape and position. The nongravid uterus may be anteverted, retroverted, or retroflexed. Until up to 12 weeks of gestation, the gravid uterus is still a pelvic organ. Regardless of its initial positioning, the enlarging uterus becomes anteverted and quickly fills space usually occupied by the bladder, triggering frequent voiding. By 12 weeks' gestation, the uterus straightens and rises out of the pelvis and can be felt when palpating the abdomen.

The enlarging uterus pushes intestinal contents laterally and superiorly and stretches its supporting ligaments, sometimes causing "round ligament pain" in the lower quadrants, more typically on the right. The uterus adapts to fetal growth and positions, and tends to rotate to the right to accommodate to the rectosigmoid structures on the left side of the pelvis.

THIRD TRIMESTER

Cervix and Ovaries. The cervix also looks and feels quite different. *Chadwick's sign,* the early softening and cyanosis of the cervix, continues throughout pregnancy. The cervical canal fills with a tenacious *mucous plug,* thought to protect the developing fetus from infection. Red velvety mucosa, termed *cervical erosion* or *eversion,* also commonly appears on the cervix and is considered normal.

The ovaries and fallopian tubes undergo changes as well, but few are noticeable during physical examination. Early in pregnancy, the *corpus luteum,* the ovarian follicle that has discharged its ovum, may be sufficiently prominent to be felt on the affected ovary as a small nodule, but it disappears by midpregnancy.

Abdomen. As the skin over the abdomen stretches to adapt to the growing fetus, purplish striae may appear. A *linea nigra,* a brownish-black pigmented line along the midline, may become visible.

As muscle tone diminishes with advancing pregnancy, the rectus abdominis muscles may separate at the midline, termed *diastasis recti.* If diastasis is severe, as in some multiparous women, only a layer of skin, fascia, and peritoneum covers most of the anterior uterine wall. The fetus is easily palpable through this muscular gap.[7, 8]

The anatomy and physiology of common concerns in pregnancy are provided in the adjacent table.

STRIAE AND LINEA NIGRA

● Common Concerns During Pregnancy and Their Explanations

Common Concerns	Trimester	Explanation
No menses (*amenorrhea*)	All	Continued high levels of estrogen, progesterone, and HCG following fertilization build up the supportive endometrium, averting menses and shedding of the endometrial lining.
Nausea with or without vomiting	First	Possible causes include hormonal changes leading to slowed peristalsis throughout the GI tract, changes in taste and smell, the growing uterus, or emotional factors. Women may have a modest (2–5 lb) weight loss in the first trimester.[9]
Breast tenderness, tingling	First	Pregnancy hormones stimulate growth of breast tissue. As the breasts enlarge, women may experience upper backache. Blood flow throughout the breasts increases, and delicate veins become visible beneath the skin.
Weight loss	First	If a woman experiences nausea and vomiting, she may not be eating normally in early pregnancy (see nausea, above).
Fatigue	First/third	Rapid change in energy requirements; hormonal changes (progesterone has a sedative effect); in the third trimester, weight gain, changes in mechanics of movement, and sleep disturbances contribute.
Groin/lower abdominal pain	Second (14–20 weeks)	Rapid uterine growth early in second trimester causes tension and stretching of round ligaments, causing spasm with sudden movement or change of position.
Abdominal striae	Late second or third	Ninety percent of pregnant women have *striae distensae,* thin and usually pink bands on the abdomen, breasts, or thighs. These reflect tearing of the collagen in the dermis and stretching of the skin.
Contractions	Third	The uterus might contract irregularly and unpredictably, sometimes called "Braxton Hicks contractions." They are rarely associated with labor. If they become regular, painful, or both, evaluate for possible onset of labor.
Loss of mucous plug	Third	Although most women have vaginal passage of mucus during labor, some pass mucus late in pregnancy but prior to labor. As long as there are no accompanying contractions, bleeding, or loss of fluid, there is no cause for concern.
Edema	Third	There is increased venous pressure in the legs, obstruction of lymphatic flow, and reduced plasma colloid osmotic pressure.
Heartburn, constipation	All	Relaxation of the lower esophageal sphincter allows stomach contents to back up into the lower esophagus. The decreased GI motility caused by pregnancy hormones slows peristalsis. Subsequent constipation may cause or aggravate existing hemorrhoids.
Backache	All	Hormonally induced relaxation of joints and ligaments and the minor lordosis required to balance the growing uterus sometimes result in a lower backache. Pathologic causes must be ruled out.
Urinary frequency	All	There are increases in blood volume, filtration rate in the kidneys, and urine production. As a result of less space for the bladder from pressure from the growing uterus (first trimester) or from the descent of the fetal head (third trimester), the woman needs to empty her bladder more frequently.
Leukorrhea	All	Increased secretions from the cervix and the vaginal epithelium, from the hormones and vasocongestion of pregnancy, result in an asymptomatic milky white vaginal discharge.

THE HEALTH HISTORY

Common Concerns

- Symptoms of pregnancy
- Maternal attitudes about pregnancy
- Current health: Smoking, alcohol, use of illicit drugs, domestic violence
- Prior complications of pregnancy
- Chronic illnesses and family history
- Determining weeks of gestation by date and expected date of delivery

Focus your prenatal care on optimal health for the mother and fetus, while minimizing risk to the mother. She will value an empathic relationship at this momentous time as she adjusts other family and work responsibilities to accommodate the arrival of a new child.

The Initial Prenatal Visit. Goals of the initial prenatal visit are three-fold: confirming the pregnancy, assessing the health status of the mother and any risks for complications, and counseling to ensure birth of a healthy baby.

- Ask about *symptoms of pregnancy:* absence of menses, breast fullness or tenderness, nausea or vomiting, fatigue, and urinary frequency (see table on p. 885). Explain that urine testing for beta HCG offers the best confirmation of pregnancy. Serum testing for beta HCG is rarely needed for confirmation.

- Ask about the mother's *concerns and attitudes about the pregnancy.* How does she feel about the pregnancy? Was it planned? Is it desired? Does she plan to continue to term? Is the father of the baby or any current partner supportive? Does she have a broader support network? Is she excited, concerned, or scared? If she has fears, what are they? Ask these questions in an open-ended fashion, without conveying a judgmental response.

- Assess the *current state of health* and any risk factors that could adversely affect the mother or fetus or cause any complications. Ask about her eating patterns and assess the quality of her nutrition. Does she smoke, drink alcohol, or use any illicit drugs? Does she take any medications? Or have any toxic exposures? What about her income and social support network? Are there any sources of unusual stress at home or work? Is there any history of physical abuse or domestic violence?

- Assess the *past obstetric history.* What about prior pregnancies? (Past obstetric problems tend to recur.) Has she had any complications during labor and birth? Were her babies delivered vaginally, with the assistance of forceps or vacuum, or by cesarean section? Ask about the birth weights of prior children. Has she had a premature or growth-retarded infant, or a baby large for gestational age? Also, has there been a prior fetal demise? Is there any history of postpartum depression?

● Ask about the *past medical history*. A thorough inquiry into acute or chronic illnesses in the major systems is in order. Ask especially about hypertension, diabetes, cardiac conditions, asthma, systemic lupus erythematosis (SLE), seizures, any history of sexually transmitted diseases, exposure to diethylstilbestrol in utero, or HIV infection.

● Also review any *family history* of chronic illnesses or genetically transmitted diseases such as sickle cell anemia, cystic fibrosis, or muscular dystrophy.

Weeks of Gestation and Expected Date of Delivery.

You will need to elicit features of the current pregnancy that enable you to calculate the *expected weeks of gestation by dates* and the *expected date of delivery* (EDD).

● To establish *expected weeks of gestation,* count in weeks from either (1) the first day of the last menstrual period (LMP), known as *menstrual age;* or (2) the date of conception (if this is known), or *conception age.* Menstrual age is the most frequently used method of calculation. The expected weeks of gestation can help with later assessment of uterine size, but this assumes that the LMP was normal and the dates are remembered accurately. During the examination, compare your estimate of expected uterine size with the palpable size of the uterus if still within the pelvic cavity, or by the height of the fundus if above the symphysis pubis. Investigate possible causes for any discrepancies.

● The first day of the LMP is also used to calculate the *expected date of delivery,* or the time projected to term labor and delivery, assuming regular 28- to 30-day menstrual cycles. Using *Naegele's rule,* estimate the EDD by adding 7 days to the first day of the LMP, subtract 3 months, and add 1 year. This date may be one of the first questions the mother asks you.

Accurate dating of the pregnancy is best done early and improves decision making in the event of later delays in fetal growth, preterm labor, or pregnancy beyond 42 weeks of gestation. If the patient cannot remember her LMP or has irregular menstrual cycles, or if the dating is uncertain, vaginal probe ultrasound is used to confirm dating in the first trimester.

Establish the desired frequency of *follow-up visits* based on the patient's needs. These visits will include measurement of blood pressure and weight, palpation of the uterine fundus to assess fetal growth, verification of fetal heart tones, and determination of fetal presentation and activity. Many clinicians also check for urinary protein and glucose. Additional laboratory tests will be needed in the second and third trimesters.

HEALTH PROMOTION AND COUNSELING

Important Topics for Health Promotion and Counseling

- Nutrition
- Weight gain
- Exercise
- Smoking, alcohol, and illicit drugs
- Screening for domestic violence
- Immunizations

Nutrition. Counseling about *nutrition* and *weight gain* helps protect the health of the pregnant woman and fetus. Evaluate the nutritional status of the mother during the first prenatal visit, including a diet history; measure height, weight, and body mass index (BMI); and obtain a hematocrit to screen for anemia. Be sure to explore the mother's habits and attitudes about eating and weight gain, as well as her use of needed vitamin and mineral supplements.

- Develop a meal plan appropriate to the woman's cultural preferences. Three meals each day consisting of a balanced diet with increased intake of calories and protein are generally sufficient. Advise the pregnant woman to increase her diet each day by the following amounts: 300 additional kilocalories; 5 to 10 grams of protein; 15 milligrams of iron; 250 milligrams of calcium; and 400 to 800 micrograms of folic acid.[10]

- Prescribe a multivitamin with at least 400 micrograms of folic acid per day. Prescribing multivitamins during pregnancy, regardless of diet, is common practice. No one brand has been shown to be clinically superior.

- Caution the pregnant woman about ingesting unpasteurized dairy products, undercooked meats, and excess amounts of vitamin A, which can become toxic.[11] Consumption of seafood during pregnancy is controversial. Intake of trace minerals may benefit verbal intelligence in maternal offspring; however, higher levels of mercury in some fish and shellfish may harm development of the nervous system in the fetus or infant.[12] The Food and Drug Administration and the Environmental Protection Agency recommend avoiding fish with higher levels of mercury such as shark, swordfish, king mackerel, and canned albacore tuna.[13]

Weight Gain. Ideal weight gain during pregnancy follows a pattern: very little increase in the first trimester, rapid increase in the second trimester, and mild slowing of the increase in the third trimester. Average weight gain is approximately 28 pounds, or approximately 10 kilograms. Women should be weighed at each visit, with the results plotted on a graph for the patient and provider to review and discuss. Recommended weight gain ranges from the Institute of Medicine (1992), displayed next, are still current.

● Recommended Total Weight Gain Ranges for Pregnant Women

Prepregnancy Weight-for-Height Category	Recommended Total Gain	
	lbs	kg
Low—BMI <19.8	28–40	12.5–18
Normal—BMI 19.8 to 26.0	25–35	11.5–16
High—BMI 26.0 to 29.0	15–25	7.0–11.5
Obese—BMI >29.0	~15	~7.0

Figures are for single pregnancies. The range for women carrying twins is 35 to 45 lb (16 to 20 kg). Young adolescents (<2 years after menarche) should strive for gains at the upper end of the range. Short women (<62 in or <157 cm) should strive for gains at the lower end of the range.

(Source: Institute of Medicine. Nutrition During Pregnancy and Lactation: An Implementation Guideline. Washington, DC, National Academy Press, 1992.)

Exercise. *Exercise* is important to the health and lifestyle of pregnant women. The 2002 guidelines from the American College of Obstetricians and Gynecologists (ACOG) recommend that in conjunction with their physician, and in the absence of contraindications, pregnant women should engage in moderate exercise for 30 minutes or more on most days of the week.[14] Women exercising regularly before pregnancy can continue mild to moderate exercise, preferably for short periods three times a week. Women initiating exercise during pregnancy should be more cautious and consider programs developed specifically for pregnant women. After the first trimester, women should avoid exercise in the supine position, which can compress the inferior vena cava and decrease blood flow to the placenta. The pregnant woman should stop exercise when she feels fatigued or uncomfortable and avoid overheating and dehydration. Because the center of gravity shifts in the third trimester, advise her that exercises that could cause loss of balance or result in abdominal trauma, such as contact sports, are unwise.

Smoking, Alcohol, and Illicit Drugs. Any *smoking* should be discontinued. Smoking has been linked to complications of labor such as placental abruption and placenta previa, and to preterm births, low-birth-weight babies, and even perinatal death.

Pregnant women with *addictions to alcohol or using illicit drugs* should be referred for treatment. The use of alcohol and illicit drugs can have serious consequences for the neonate, including adverse neurodevelopmental outcomes.[15]

Screening for Domestic Violence. Pregnancy may be a time when women are more likely to be abused by an intimate partner or when patterns of abuse may intensify, increasing the risk for delayed prenatal care, miscarriage, and low-birth-weight babies. The prevalence of abuse during pregnancy ranges from 7% to 20%, depending on the setting, and may result in femicide, or murder of the mother and child.[16,17] The ACOG recommends universal assessment of all women for any history of *domestic violence* that may escalate during the pregnancy.[18] Clues to domestic violence include frequent changes in appointments at the last minute, behavior during the interview, chronic headache or abdominal pain, and bruises or other signs of injury.

Clinicians can overcome barriers to screening by adopting direct, nonjudgmental questioning in a private setting at each prenatal visit.[19,20] For example, you may ask "Since you've been pregnant, have you been hit or slapped or otherwise physically hurt by anyone?" Women may need multiple opportunities to discuss abuse because of fears about safety and reprisal. Validate positive responses and mark the area of injury on a body diagram. Above all, in situations of admitted abuse, ask the woman how you might help her. Offer information on safe shelters, counseling centers, hotline telephone numbers, and other sources of assistance when she is ready to pursue these. Assess the patient's safety and make any necessary referrals. Learn about any requirements for mandatory reporting.

NATIONAL DOMESTIC VIOLENCE HOTLINE

- Web site: www.ndvh.org/index.html
- 1-800-799-SAFE (7233)
- TTY for hearing impaired: 1-800-787-3224

Immunizations. Review the patient's immunization history. All pregnant women should be up to date on their tetanus and influenza vaccines. These can be administered in any trimester. If indicated, pneumococcal, meningococcal, and hepatitis B vaccines are also safe in pregnancy.[21]

TECHNIQUES OF EXAMINATION

As you begin the examination, show respect for the patient's comfort and need for privacy and for her individual needs and sensitivities. If this is a first visit, take the history before asking her to change into a gown. Ask if she has ever had a complete pelvic examination. If not, take the time to explain what is involved and seek her cooperation with each of its components. This will strengthen rapport and help her understand the changes in her body in response to pregnancy. Note that if she has ever experienced a sexual assault, she may resist the examination of the pelvis.

Now ask your patient to put on the gown with the opening in the front. This will ease examination of the breasts and the pregnant abdomen. Have the needed equipment readily at hand.

Positioning. Take a few minutes to adjust the positioning of the pregnant woman. You will need to give added time and attention to palpating the uterus and listening to the fetal heart. The semi-sitting position with the knees bent, as shown below, affords the greatest comfort and reduces the weight of the gravid uterus on the abdominal organs and vessels, especially in the later trimesters.

Avoid asking the pregnant woman to spend prolonged periods lying on her back. In this position, the uterus lies directly on the woman's vertebral column and may compress the descending aorta and inferior vena cava, interfering with the return of venous blood from the lower extremities and the pelvic vessels. Therefore, make your abdominal palpation efficient in time and results.

Encourage the woman to sit again briefly before proceeding to the pelvic evaluation. This pause also provides time for the woman to empty her bladder again. However, make sure that she is acclimated to sitting before allow-

Supine hypotensive syndrome after approximately 20 weeks is a form of diminished circulation and may lead the woman to feel dizzy and faint, especially when lying down.

ing her to stand up. The pelvic examination should likewise be relatively quick. All other examination procedures should be done in the sitting or left-side–lying position.

Equipment. The examiner's hands are the primary means of examination. They should be warm and firm, yet gentle in palpation. Whenever possible the fingers should be together and flat against the abdominal or pelvic tissue to minimize discomfort. Likewise, all touching and palpation should be done with smooth, continuous contact against the skin rather than kneading or abrupt motion. The palmar surfaces of the ends of the fingers are the most sensitive.

The gynecologic speculum is used for inspecting the cervix and the vagina before taking specimens for cytologic or bacteriologic study. Because the vaginal walls are relaxed during pregnancy and may fall medially, obscuring your view, a speculum of larger than expected size may be needed. The relaxation of perineal and vulvar structures minimizes any discomfort. Because of the increased vascularity of the vaginal and cervical structures, insert and open the speculum gently. This will help avoid tissue trauma and bleeding, which interfere with the interpretation of Pap smears.

The Ayre wooden spatula or "broom" sampling device is generally used to obtain the Pap smear. In pregnant women, the cervical brush may cause bleeding.

Review Chapter 14 for instruments and techniques used to take cervical smears (pp. 533–546).

GENERAL INSPECTION

Observe overall health, emotional state, nutritional status, and neuromuscular coordination as the woman walks into the room and climbs on the examination table. Discussion of her priorities for the examination, responses to pregnancy, and general health provide useful information and help to put your patient at ease.

VITAL SIGNS, HEIGHT, AND WEIGHT

Take the blood pressure. A baseline reading helps to determine the woman's usual range. In midpregnancy, blood pressure is normally lower than in the nonpregnant state.

Gestational hypertension is systolic blood pressure (SBP) ≥140 and diastolic blood pressure (DBP) ≥90, first occurring after week 20 and *without proteinuria.*

Chronic hypertension is SBP ≥140 and DBP ≥90 before pregnancy, before week 20, and after 12 weeks postpartum.

Preeclampsia is SBP ≥140 and DBP ≥90 after week 20 and *with proteinuria.*[22]

Measure the height and weight. Calculate the BMI with standard tables, using 19 to 25 as normal for the prepregnant state (see p. 113).

Note that first-trimester weight loss related to nausea and vomiting is common but should not exceed 5% of prepartum weight.

Weight loss of more than 5% during the first trimester may be from excessive vomiting, or *hyperemesis.*

 ## HEAD AND NECK

Stand facing the seated woman and observe the head and neck, including the following features:

- *Face.* The mask of pregnancy, *chloasma*, is common, though not present in all pregnancies. It consists of irregular brownish patches around the forehead and cheeks, across the nose, or along the jaw.

Facial edema after 24 weeks of gestation may suggest *gestational hypertension.*

- *Hair,* including texture, moisture, and distribution. Dryness, oiliness, and sometimes minor generalized hair loss may be noted. Mild degrees of hirsutism on the face, abdomen, or extremities are common.

Localized patches of hair loss should not be attributed to pregnancy (though hair loss is common postpartum).

- *Eyes.* Note the conjunctival color.

Anemia of pregnancy may cause pallor.

- *Nose,* including the mucous membranes and the septum. Nasal congestion is common during pregnancy.

Nosebleeds are more common during pregnancy. The nasal septum can show any signs of cocaine use.

- *Mouth,* especially the gums and teeth.

Gingival enlargement with bleeding (p. 277) is common during pregnancy.

- *Thyroid gland.* Inspect and palpate the gland. Modest symmetric enlargement is expected.[23]

Significant enlargement is abnormal and should be investigated.

 ## THORAX AND LUNGS

Inspect the thorax for contours and pattern of breathing. Elevation of the diaphragm and increased chest diameter may be seen as early as the first trimester. Tidal volume and alveolar minute ventilation increase, but respiratory rate remains constant. These changes sometimes lead to subjective complaints of shortness of breath. Expect respiratory alkalosis.[24]

Pursue complaints of dyspnea accompanied by cough or respiratory distress for possible infection, *asthma,* or *pulmonary embolus.*

HEART

Palpate the apical impulse. In advanced pregnancy, it may be slightly higher than normal in the 4th intercostal space, because of transverse and leftward rotation of the heart from the higher diaphragm.

Auscultate the heart. A venous hum and systolic or continuous mammary souffle (see p. 387) are common during pregnancy, reflecting increased blood flow in normal vessels.[25] Listen for a mammary souffle (pronounced *soo-fl*), late in pregnancy and during lactation. It is most easily heard in the second or third interspace in the parasternal areas and is typically both systolic and diastolic. Only the systolic component may be audible.

Murmurs may also accompany anemia. New diastolic murmurs and dyspnea with exertion should be investigated.

 BREASTS

Inspect the breasts and nipples for symmetry and color. The venous pattern may be marked, the nipples and areolae are dark, and Montgomery's glands are prominent.

An inverted nipple needs attention if breast-feeding is planned.

Palpate for masses. During pregnancy, breasts are tender and nodular.

A pathologic mass may be difficult to isolate.

Compress each nipple between your index finger and thumb. This maneuver may express colostrum from the nipples.

A bloody or purulent discharge should not be attributed to pregnancy.

 ABDOMEN

Help the pregnant woman into a semi-sitting position with her knees flexed (see p. 881).

Inspect any scars or striae, the shape and contour of the abdomen, and the fundal height. Purplish striae and linea nigra are normal in pregnancy. The shape and contour may indicate pregnancy size (see figure on p. 874).

Scars may confirm the type of prior surgery, especially cesarean section.

Palpate the abdomen for:

● *Organs or masses.* The mass of pregnancy is expected.

● *Fetal movements.* The examiner can usually feel these after 24 weeks (the mother, at 18–20 weeks).

If movements cannot be felt after 24 weeks, consider error in calculating gestation, fetal death or morbidity, or false pregnancy.

● *Uterine contractility.* Irregular uterine contractions occur after 12 weeks, and often in response to palpation during the third trimester. The abdomen then feels tense or firm to the examiner, and it is difficult to feel fetal parts. If the hand is left resting on the fundal portion of the uterus, the fingers will sense the relaxation of the uterine muscle.

Before 37 weeks, regular uterine contractions with or without pain or bleeding are abnormal, suggesting *preterm labor.*

Measure the fundal height with a paper tape measure if the woman is more than 20 weeks pregnant. Holding the tape as illustrated and following the midline of the abdomen, measure from the top of the symphysis pubis to the top of the uterine fundus. Although subject to error, for weeks 20 to 32, measurement in centimeters should roughly equal the weeks of gestation.[26,27]

If fundal height is more than 4 cm higher than expected, consider *multiple gestation,* a large fetus, extra amniotic fluid, or *uterine leiomyoma.* If it is lower than expected by more than 4 cm, consider missed abortion, transverse lie, growth retardation, or false pregnancy.

Auscultate the fetal heart, noting its rate (FHR), location, and rhythm. A doptone will detect the FHR after approximately 10 weeks. The FHR is audible with a fetoscope after approximately 18 weeks, although this instrument is now used less commonly.

Lack of an audible fetal heart may indicate pregnancy of fewer weeks than expected, fetal demise, or false pregnancy.

The *location* of the audible FHR is in the midline of the lower abdomen from 12 to 18 weeks of gestation. After 28 weeks, the fetal heart is heard best over the fetal back or chest. The location of the FHR then depends on how the fetus is positioned. Palpating the fetal head and back helps you

DOPTONE (LEFT) AND FETOSCOPE (RIGHT)

identify where to listen. (See Modified Leopold's Maneuvers, pp. 888–890.) If the fetus is head down with its back on the woman's left side, the FHR is heard best in the lower left quadrant. If the fetal head is under the xiphoid process (*breech presentation*) with its back on the right, the FHR is heard in the upper right quadrant.

After 24 weeks, auscultation of more than one FHR with varying rates in different locations suggests more than one fetus.

The *rate* is usually in the 160s during early pregnancy and then slows to the 120s to 140s near term. After 32 to 34 weeks, the FHR should increase with fetal movement.

An FHR that drops noticeably near term with fetal movement could indicate poor placental circulation or decreased amniotic fluid volume.

Rhythm becomes important in the third trimester. Expect a variance of 10 to 15 beats per minute (BPM) over 1 to 2 minutes.

Lack of beat-to-beat variability late in pregnancy warrants investigation with an FHR monitor.

 ## GENITALIA, ANUS, AND RECTUM

Inspect the *external genitalia,* noting the hair distribution, the color, and any scars. Parous relaxation of the introitus and noticeable enlargement of the labia and clitoris are normal. Scars from an *episiotomy,* a perineal incision to facilitate delivery of an infant, or from perineal lacerations may be present in multiparous women.

Some women have labial varicosities that become tortuous and painful.

Inspect the *anus* for *hemorrhoids.* If these are present, note their size and location.

Hemorrhoids often engorge later in pregnancy. They may be painful and bleed.

Palpate *Bartholin's* and *Skene's glands*. No discharge or tenderness should be present.

Check for a *cystocele* or *rectocele*.

May be pronounced from the muscle relaxation of pregnancy

Speculum Examination.   Inspect the *cervix* for color, shape, and healed lacerations. A parous cervix may look irregular because of lacerations (see p. 549).

A pink cervix suggests a non-pregnant state.

Take *Pap smears* and, if indicated, other vaginal or cervical specimens. The cervix may bleed more easily when touched because of the vasocongestion of pregnancy.

Specimens may be needed for diagnosis if vaginal or cervical infection is present.

Inspect the *vaginal walls* for color, discharge, rugae, and relaxation. A bluish or violet color, deep rugae, and an increased milky white discharge, *leukorrhea,* are normal.

A pink vagina suggests a non-pregnant state. Vaginal irritation and itching with discharge suggest infection.

Bimanual Examination.   Insert two lubricated fingers into the introitus, palmar side down, with slight pressure downward on the perineum. Slide the fingers into the posterior vaginal vault. Maintaining downward pressure, gently turn the fingers palmar side up. Avoid the sensitive urethral structures at all times. With the relaxation of pregnancy, the bimanual examination is usually easier to accomplish. Tissues are soft, and the vaginal walls usually close in on the examining fingers. It may be difficult to distinguish the cervix at first because of its softer texture.

Place your finger gently in the os, then sweep it around the *surface of the cervix*. A nulliparous cervix should be closed, whereas a multiparous cervix may admit a fingertip through the *external os*. The *internal os*—the narrow passage between the endocervical canal and the uterine cavity—should be closed regardless of parity. The surface of a normal multiparous cervix may feel irregular because of the healed lacerations from a previous birth.

A shortened effaced cervix before 32 weeks may indicate preterm labor.

Estimate the *length of the cervix* by palpating the lateral surface of the cervix from the cervical tip to the lateral fornix. Prior to 34 to 36 weeks, the cervix should retain its usual length of about 1.5 to 2 cm.

Palpate the *uterus* for size, shape, consistency, and position. These depend on the weeks of gestation. Early softening of the isthmus, *Hegar's sign,* is characteristic of pregnancy. The uterus is shaped like an inverted pear until 8 weeks, with slight enlargement in the fundal portion. The uterus becomes globular by 10 to 12 weeks. Anteflexion or retroflexion is lost by 12 weeks, with the fundal portion measuring about 8 cm in diameter.

With your internal fingers placed at either side of the cervix, palmar surfaces upward, gently lift the uterus toward the abdominal hand. Capture the fundal portion of the uterus between your two hands and gently estimate uterine size.

An irregularly shaped uterus suggests uterine myomata or a *bicornuate uterus,* which has two distinct uterine cavities separated by a septum.

Palpate the *left and right adnexa*. The corpus luteum may feel like a small nodule on the affected ovary during the first few weeks after conception. Late in pregnancy, adnexal masses may be difficult to feel.

Palpate for *pelvic muscle strength* as you withdraw your examining fingers.

Currently, use of the *rectovaginal examination* is limited to conditions needing confirmation of the integrity of the rectovaginal septum or investigation of symptoms such as rectal bleeding that are suggestive of rectal pathology. This examination may assist in determining the size of the retroverted or retroflexed uterus, but a transvaginal ultrasound may be preferable.

Early in pregnancy, it is important to rule out a tubal (*ectopic*) pregnancy. See Table 14-9, Adnexal Masses, p. 553.

EXTREMITIES

General inspection may be done with the woman seated or lying on her left side.

Inspect the legs for *varicose veins*.

Varicose veins may begin or worsen during pregnancy.

Inspect the hands and legs for *edema*. Palpate for pretibial, ankle, and pedal edema. Edema is rated on a 0 to 4+ scale. Physiologic edema is more common in advanced pregnancy, during hot weather, and in women who stand for long periods.

Check *knee and ankle reflexes*.

SPECIAL TECHNIQUES

Modified Leopold's Maneuvers

These maneuvers are important adjuncts to palpation of the pregnant abdomen, beginning at 28 weeks of gestation. They help determine where the fetus is lying in relation to the woman's back (longitudinal or transverse), which end of the fetus is presenting at the pelvic inlet (head or buttocks), where the fetal back is located, how far the presenting part of the fetus has descended into the maternal pelvis, and the estimated weight of the fetus. This information is necessary to assess the adequacy of fetal growth and the probability of successful vaginal birth.

Common deviations include *breech presentation* (the fetal buttocks presenting at the outlet of the maternal pelvis) and absence of the presenting part well down into the maternal pelvis at term. Neither situation necessarily precludes vaginal birth. The most serious findings are a *transverse lie* close to term and slowed fetal growth that could represent *intrauterine growth restriction (IUGR)*.

First Maneuver (Upper Pole). Stand at the woman's side, facing her head. Keeping the fingers of both examining hands together, palpate gently with the fingertips to determine what part of the fetus is in the upper pole of the uterine fundus.

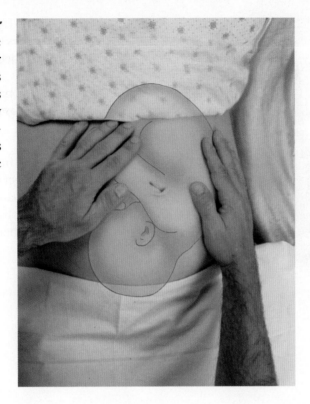

The fetal buttocks are usually at the upper pole. They feel firm but irregular, and less globular than the head. The fetal head feels firm, round, and smooth.

Second Maneuver (Sides of the Maternal Abdomen). Place one hand on each side of the woman's abdomen, aiming to capture the body of the fetus between them. Use one hand to steady the uterus and the other to palpate the fetus.

The hand on the fetal back feels a smooth, firm surface the length of the hand (or longer) by 32 weeks of gestation. The hand on the fetal arms and legs feels irregular bumps, and also perhaps kicking if the fetus is awake and active.

Third Maneuver (Lower Pole). Turn and face the woman's feet. Using the flat palmar surfaces of the fingers of both hands and, at the start, touching the fingertips together, palpate the area just above the symphysis pubis. Note whether the hands diverge with downward pressure or stay together. This tells you whether or not the presenting part of the fetus—head or buttocks—is descending into the pelvic inlet.

If the fetal head is presenting, the fingers feel a smooth, firm, rounded surface on both sides.

If the hands diverge, the presenting part is descending into the pelvic inlet, as illustrated.

If the hands stay together and you can gently depress the tissue over the bladder without touching the fetus, the presenting part is above your hands.

If the presenting fetal part is descending, palpate its texture and firmness. If not, gently move your hands up the lower abdomen and capture the presenting part between your hands.

The fetal head feels smooth, firm, and rounded; the buttocks, firm but irregular.

Fourth Maneuver (Confirmation of the Presenting Part). With your dominant hand, grasp the part of the fetus in the lower pole, and with your nondominant hand, the part of the fetus in the upper pole. With this maneuver, you may be able to distinguish between the head and the buttocks.

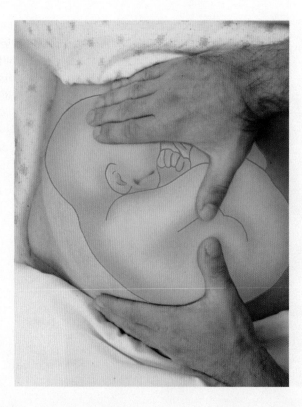

The head is usually in the lower pole, and the fetal buttocks are in the upper pole. If the head is above the pelvic inlet, it moves somewhat independently of the rest of the fetal body.

CONCLUDING THE VISIT

Once your examination is completed and your patient has dressed, affirm your commitment to her health and concerns during pregnancy. Ask for any further questions and review your findings. If further data are necessary to confirm the pregnancy, discuss any next steps. Reinforce the importance of regular prenatal care and review the sequence of future visits. Record your findings in the prenatal record.

RECORDING YOUR FINDINGS

Note that initially you may use sentences to describe your findings; later you will use phrases. The style below contains phrases appropriate for most write-ups.

Recording the Physical Examination—The Pregnant Woman

"*Abdomen*: Low transverse surgical scar. Active bowel sounds. Soft, nontender; no palpable hepatosplenomegaly or masses. Fundus: barely palpable above symphysis pubis. Fetal heart rate not heard. No inguinal adenopathy. *Bimanual examination*: cervix midline, soft, internal os closed. No pain on movement of cervix. Right and left ovaries nonpalpable; no other adnexal masses. Fundus anteverted, enlarged to 14–16 weeks' size; moderate vaginal tone."	Describes examination of healthy pregnant woman at 16 weeks' gestation.
OR	
"*Abdomen*: No surgical scars. Active bowel sounds. Soft, nontender; no palpable hepatosplenomegaly or masses. Fundus palpable 2 fingerbreadths below the umbilicus; shape is ovoid and smooth. Fetal heart rate 144. No inguinal adenopathy. *External genitalia*: midline episiotomy scar present. No lesions, discharge, or signs of infection. *Bimanual examination:* cervix midline, soft 4 cm in length; external os admits fingertip, internal os closed. No pain elicited on movement of cervix; no adnexal masses. Fundus enlarged to 20 weeks' size, midline, smooth; vaginal tone reduced."	Describes examination of healthy pregnant woman at 20 weeks' gestation.

BIBLIOGRAPHY

CITATIONS

1. Cunningham FG, Leveno KL, Bloom SL, et al. (eds). Williams Obstetrics, 22nd ed. New York, McGraw Hill, Medical Publishers Division, 2005.
2. Berghout A, Wiersinga W. Thyroid size and function during pregnancy: an analysis. Eur J Endocrinol 138:536–542, 1998.
3. Boden G. Fuel metabolism in pregnancy and in gestational diabetes mellitus. Obstet Gynecol Clin North Am 23:1–10, 1996.
4. Smith R. Parturition. N Engl J Med 356(3):271–283, 2007.
5. Andersen HF, Johnson TR, Barclay ML, et al. Gestational age assessment. I. Analysis of individual clinical observations. Am J Obstet Gynecol 139(2):173–177, 1981.
6. Hillier SL, Krohn MA, Rabe LK, et al. The normal vaginal flora, H202-producing lactobacilli, and bacterial vaginosis in pregnant women. Clin Infect Dis 16(Suppl 4):S273–S281, 1994.

7. Boisonnault JS, Blaschak MJ. Incidence of diastasis rectus abdominis during the childbearing year. Phys Ther 68(7): 1082–1086, 1988.

8. Gilleard WL, Brown JMM. Structure and function of the abdominal muscles in primigravid subjects during pregnancy and the immediate postbirth period. Phys Ther 76(7):750–762, 1996.

9. American College of Obstetricians and Gynecologists (ACOG). Nausea and vomiting of pregnancy. Practice Bulletin No. 52. Obstet Gynecol 104(4):803–814, 2004.

10. Institute of Medicine. Nutrition during Pregnancy and Lactation: An Implementation Guideline, p. 14. Washington, DC: National Academy Press, 1992.

11. Kaiser L, Allen LH, American Dietetic Association. Position of American Dietetic Association: nutrition and life style for a healthy pregnancy outcome. JAM Diet Assoc 108(3):553–561, 2008.

12. Hibbeln JR, Davis JM, Steer C, et al. Maternal seafood consumption in pregnancy and neurodevelopmental outcomes in childhood (ALSPAC study): an observational cohort study. Lancet 369(9561):578–585, 2007.

13. Food and Drug Administration. Mercury and seafood advice still current. FDA Consumer Magazine 40(5):2–3, 2006. Also What you need to know about mercury in fish and shellfish. 2004 EPA and FDA advice for: women who might become pregnant, women who are pregnant, nursing mothers, young children. EPA-823-R-04-005, March 2004.

14. American College of Obstetricians and Gynecologists (ACOG). Exercise during pregnancy and the postpartum period. ACOG Committee Opinion, No. 267, January 2002.

15. American College of Obstetricians and Gynecologists (ACOG). At-risk drinking and illicit drug use: ethical issues in obstetric and gynecologic practice. ACOG Committee Opinion, No. 294, January 2004.

16. Gazmararian JA, Lazorick S, Spitz AM, et al. Prevalence of violence against pregnant women. JAMA 275(24):1915–1920, 1996.

17. Martin SL, Mackie L, Kupper LL, et al. Physical abuse of women before, during, and after pregnancy. JAMA 85(12): 1581–1584, 2001.

18. American College of Obstetricians and Gynecologists (ACOG). Psychosocial risk factors: perinatal screening and intervention. ACOG Committee Opinion, No. 255, 1999.

19. Elliott L, Nerney M, Jones T, et al. Barriers to screening for domestic violence. J Gen Intern Med 17:112–116, 2002.

20. Friedman LS, Samet JH, Roberts MS, et al. Inquiry about victimization experiences: a survey of patient preferences and physician practices. Arch Intern Med 152:1186–1190, 1992.

21. American College of Obstetricians and Gynecologists (ACOG). Guidelines for Women's Health Care, 2nd ed. Washington, DC, ACOG, 2002.

22. American College of Obstetricians and Gynecologists (ACOG). Chronic hypertension in pregnancy. ACOG Committee Opinion, No. 29. Obstet Gynecol 98(1):S177–S185, 2001.

23. American College of Obstetricians and Gynecologists (ACOG). Guidelines for Women's Health Care, 2nd ed. Washington, DC, 2002.

24. Periera A, Kreiger BP. Pulmonary complications of pregnancy. Clin Chest Med 25(2):299–310, 2004.

25. Gei AF, Hankins CD. Cardiac disease and pregnancy. Obstet Gynecol Clin N Am 28(3):465–512, 2001.

26. Belizan JM, Villar J, Nardin JC, et al. Diagnosis of intrauterine growth retardation by a simple clinical method: measurement of uterine height. Am J Obstet Gynecol 131(6):643–646, 1978.

27. Persson B, Stangenberg M, Lunell NO, et al. Prediction of size of infants at birth by measurement of symphysis fundus height. Br J Obstet Gynaecol 93(3):206–211, 1986.

ADDITIONAL REFERENCES

American College of Obstetricians and Gynecologists, Committee on Health Care for Underserved Women. ACOG Committee Opinion No. 361. Breastfeeding: maternal and infant aspects. Obstet Gynecol 109(2 Pt 1):479–480, 2007.

American Diabetes Association. Preconception care of women with diabetes. Diabetes Care 26(Suppl 1):S91–S93, 2003.

Bell R, Bailey K, Cresswell T, et al. Northern Diabetic Pregnancy Survey Steering Group. Trends in prevalence and outcomes of pregnancy in women with pre-existing type I and type II diabetes. BJOG 115(4):445–452, 2008.

Blenning CE, Paladine H. An approach to the postpartum office visit. Am Fam Phys 72(12):2491–2496, 2005.

Cunningham FG, Williams JW. Williams Obstetrics, 22nd ed. New York, McGraw-Hill, Medical Pub Division, 2005.

Fraser DC, Cooper MA, Myles MF. Myles Textbook for Midwives, 14th ed. New York, Churchill Livingstone, 2003.

Gavin NI, Gaynes BN, Lohr KN, et al. Perinatal depression: a systematic review of prevalence and incidence. Obstet Gynecol 106 (5 Pt 1):1071–1083, 2005.

Kirkham C, Harris S, Grzybowski S. Evidence-based prenatal care: Part I. General prenatal care and counseling issues. Am Fam Physician 71(7):1307–1316, 2005.

Pick ME, Edwards M, Moreau D, et al. Assessment of diet quality in pregnant women using the Healthy Eating Index. J Am Diet Assoc 105(2):240–246, 2005.

Read JS, American Academy of Pediatrics Committee on Pediatric AIDS. Human milk, breastfeeding, and transmission of human immunodeficiency virus type 1 in the United States. American Academy of Pediatrics Committee on Pediatric AIDS. Pediatrics 112(5):1196–1205, 2003.

Turok DK, Ratcliffe SD, Baxley EG. Management of gestational diabetes mellitus. Am Fam Phys 68(9):1767–1772, 2003.

U.S. Preventive Services Task Force. Screening for family and intimate partner violence: recommendation statement. Ann Intern Med 140(5):382–386, 2004.

Varney, HK, Kriebs JM, Gegor CL. Varney's Midwifery, 4th ed. Sudbury, MA, Jones and Bartlett Publishers, 2004.

Yang J, Cummings EA, O'Connell C, et al. Fetal and neonatal outcomes of diabetic pregnancies. Obstet Gynecol 108(3 Pt 1): 644–650, 2006.

Wisner KL, Parry BL, Piontek CM. Postpartum depression. N Engl J Med 347(3):194–199, 2002.

The Bates' suite offers these additional resources to enhance learning and facilitate understanding of this chapter:

- Bates' Pocket Guide to Physical Examination and History Taking, 6th edition
- Bates' Nursing Online
- Bates' Visual Guide to Physical Examination, 4th edition
- thePoint online resources, http://thepoint.lww.com
- Student CD-ROM included with the book

The Older Adult

Older adults now number more than 37 million in the United States and are expected to reach 86 million by 2050.[1] These seniors will live longer than previous generations: life span at birth is currently 79 years for women and 74 years for men. Those older than 85 years are projected to increase to 5% of the U.S. population within 40 years. Hence, the "demographic imperative" is to maximize not only the life span but also the "health span" of our older population, so that seniors maintain full function for as long as possible, enjoying rich and active lives in their homes and communities.

Clinicians now recognize frailty as one of society's common myths about aging—more than 95% of Americans older than 65 years live in the community, and only 5% reside in long-term care facilities.[1,2] Over the past 20 years, seniors actually have become more active and less disabled. These changes call for new goals for clinical care—"an informed activated patient interacting with a prepared proactive team, resulting in high quality satisfying encounters and improved outcomes"—and a distinct set of clinical attitudes and skills.[3,4]

Assessing the older adult presents special opportunities and special challenges. Many of these are quite different from the disease-oriented approach of history taking and physical examination for younger patients: the focus on healthy or "successful" aging; the need to understand and mobilize family, social, and community supports; the importance of skills directed to functional assessment, "the sixth vital sign"; and the opportunities for promoting the older adult's long-term health and safety.

See Table 20-1, Minimum Geriatrics Competencies, p. 930.

Chapter Overview: The Aging Adult

- Anatomy and Physiology: Changes of Aging
- The Health History
  - Approach to the Patient: adjusting the office environment; shaping the content and pace of the visit; eliciting symptoms; responsiveness to the cultural dimensions of aging
  - Special Areas of Concern: activities of daily living; instrumental activities of daily living; medications; nutrition; acute and chronic pain; smoking and alcohol; advance directives and palliative care
- Health Promotion and Counseling
  - Includes when to screen, vision and hearing, exercise, immunizations, household safety, cancer screening, depression, dementia, and elder mistreatment
- Techniques of Examination
  - Functional Assessment, including The 10-Minute Geriatric Screener and assessing for falls
  - Physical Examination of the Older Adult
- Recording your findings

ANATOMY AND PHYSIOLOGY

Primary aging reflects changes in physiologic reserves over time that are independent of and not induced by any disease. These changes are especially likely to appear during periods of stress, such as exposure to fluctuating temperatures, dehydration, or even shock. Decreased cutaneous vasoconstriction and sweat production can impair responses to heat; declines in thirst may delay recovery from dehydration; and the physiologic drops in maximum cardiac output, left ventricular filling, and maximum heart rate seen with aging may impair the response to shock.

At the same time, the aging population displays marked heterogeneity. Investigators have identified vast differences in how people age and have distinguished "usual" aging, with its complex of diseases and impairments, from "optimal" aging. Optimal aging occurs in those people who escape debilitating disease entirely and maintain healthy lives late into their 80s and

90s. Studies of centenarians show that genes account for approximately 20% of the probability of living to 100, with healthy lifestyles accounting for approximately 20% to 30%.[5–7]

These findings provide compelling evidence for promoting optimal nutrition, strength training and exercise, and daily function for older adults to delay unnecessary depletion of physiologic reserves.

Vital Signs

Blood Pressure.   In Western societies, systolic blood pressure tends to rise from childhood through old age. The aorta and large arteries stiffen and become atherosclerotic. As the aorta becomes less distensible, a given stroke volume causes a greater rise in systolic blood pressure; *systolic hypertension* with a *widened pulse pressure* often ensues. Diastolic blood pressure stops rising at approximately the sixth decade. At the other extreme, some elderly people develop a tendency toward *postural (orthostatic) hypotension*—a sudden drop in blood pressure when they rise to standing.

Heart Rate and Rhythm.   In older adults, resting heart rate remains unchanged, but pacemaker cells decline in the sinoatrial node, as does maximal heart rate, affecting response to physiologic stress.[8]

Elderly people are more likely to have abnormal heart rhythms such as atrial or ventricular ectopy. Asymptomatic rhythm changes are generally benign. Like postural hypotension, however, they may cause *syncope,* or temporary loss of consciousness.

Respiratory Rate and Temperature.   Respiratory rate is unchanged, but changes in temperature regulation lead to susceptibility to *hypothermia.*

Skin, Nails, and Hair.   With age, the skin wrinkles, becomes lax, and loses turgor. The vascularity of the dermis decreases, causing lighter skin to look paler and more opaque. Skin on the backs of the hands and forearms appears thin, fragile, loose, and transparent. There may be purple patches or macules, termed *actinic purpura,* that fade over time. These spots and patches come from blood that has leaked through poorly supported capillaries and spread within the dermis.

Nails lose luster with age and may yellow and thicken, especially on the toes.

Hair undergoes a series of changes. Scalp hair loses its pigment, producing the well-known graying. Hair loss on the scalp is genetically determined. As early as 20 years, a man's hairline may start to recede at the temples; hair loss at the vertex follows. In women, hair loss follows a similar but less severe pattern. In both sexes, the number of scalp hairs decreases in a generalized pattern, and the diameter of each hair gets smaller. Less familiar, but probably more important clinically, is normal hair loss elsewhere on the body: the trunk, pubic areas, axillae, and limbs. As women reach age 55 years, coarse facial hairs appear on the chin and upper lip but do not increase further thereafter.

Many of the changes described here pertain to lighter-skinned people and do not necessarily apply to those with darker skin tones. For example, Native American men have relatively little facial and body hair compared with lighter-skinned men and should be evaluated according to their own norms.

Head and Neck. The eyes, ears, and mouth bear the brunt of old age. The fat that surrounds and cushions the eye within the bony orbit may atrophy, allowing the eyeball to recede somewhat. The skin of the eyelids becomes wrinkled, occasionally hanging in loose folds. Fat may push the fascia of the eyelids forward, creating soft bulges, especially in the lower lids and the inner third of the upper lids. Because their eyes produce fewer lacrimal secretions, aging patients may complain of dry eyes. The corneas lose some of their luster.

The pupils become smaller, which makes it more difficult to examine the ocular fundi. The pupils may also become slightly irregular but should continue to respond to light and near effort.

Visual acuity remains fairly constant between 20 and 50 years. It diminishes gradually until approximately 70 years and then more rapidly. Nevertheless, most elderly people retain good to adequate vision (20/20 to 20/70 as measured by standard charts). Near vision, however, begins to blur noticeably for virtually everyone. From childhood on, the lens gradually loses its elasticity, and the eye grows progressively less able to accommodate and focus on nearby objects. Ensuing *presbyopia* usually becomes noticeable during the fifth decade.

Aging affects the lenses and increases risk for *cataracts, glaucoma,* and *macular degeneration.* Thickening and yellowing of the lenses impair the pas-

See Chapter 7, Head and Neck, pp. 257–259.

sage of light to the retinas, requiring more light for reading and doing fine work. Cataracts affect 1 in 10 people in their 60s and 1 in 3 people in their 80s. Because the lens continues to grow over the years, it may push the iris forward, narrowing the angle between iris and cornea and increasing the risk of *narrow-angle glaucoma.*

Acuity of hearing, like that of vision, usually diminishes with age. Early losses, which start in young adulthood, involve primarily the high-pitched sounds beyond the range of human speech and have relatively little functional significance. Gradually, loss extends to sounds in the middle and lower ranges. When a person fails to catch the upper tones of words while hearing the lower ones, words sound distorted and are difficult to understand, especially in noisy environments. Hearing loss associated with aging, known as *presbycusis,* becomes increasingly evident, usually after 50 years.

Diminished salivary secretions and a decreased sense of taste accompany aging, but medications or various diseases probably contribute considerably to such changes. Decreased olfaction and increased sensitivity to bitterness and saltiness also affect taste. Teeth may wear down, become abraded, or be lost to dental caries or other conditions over time. Periodontal disease is the chief cause of tooth loss in most adults. If a person has no teeth, the lower portion of the face looks small and sunken, with accentuated "purse-string" wrinkles radiating from the mouth. Overclosure of the mouth may lead to maceration of the skin at the corners, a condition known as *angular cheilitis.* The bony ridges of the jaws that once surrounded the tooth sockets are gradually resorbed, especially in the lower jaw.

See Chapter 7, The Head and Neck, pp. 231–236.

The frequency of palpable cervical nodes gradually diminishes with age and, according to one study, falls below 50% between 50 and 60 years. In contrast to the lymph nodes, the submandibular glands become easier to feel.

Thorax and Lungs.   As people age, their capacity for exercise decreases. The chest wall becomes stiffer and harder to move, respiratory muscles may weaken, and the lungs lose some of their elastic recoil. Lung mass declines, and residual volume increases. The speed of breathing out with maximal effort gradually diminishes, and cough becomes less effective.

Skeletal changes associated with aging may accentuate the dorsal curve of the thoracic spine, producing kyphosis from osteoporotic vertebral collapse and increasing the anteroposterior diameter of the chest. The resulting "barrel chest," however, has little effect on function.

Cardiovascular System.   Cardiovascular findings vary significantly with age. Aging also affects vascular sounds in the neck and adds to the significance of extra heart sounds like S_3 and S_4 and of selected systolic murmurs.

Review the effects of aging on blood pressure and heart rate described on pp. 336–337.

Neck Vessels.   Lengthening and tortuosity of the aorta and its branches occasionally result in kinking or buckling of the carotid artery low in the neck, especially on the right. The resulting pulsatile mass, occurring chiefly in women with hypertension, may be mistaken for a carotid aneurysm—a true dilatation of the artery. A tortuous aorta occasionally raises the pressure in the jugular veins on the left side of the neck by impairing their drainage within the thorax.

In older adults, systolic bruits heard in the middle or upper portions of the carotid arteries suggest, but do not prove, partial arterial obstruction from atherosclerosis. In contrast, cervical bruits in younger people are usually innocent.

Extra Heart Sounds—S_3 and S_4. A physiologic *third heart sound,* commonly heard in children and young adults, may persist as late as age 40 years, especially in women. After age 40, however, an S_3 strongly suggests congestive heart failure from volume overload of the left ventricle, as in coronary artery disease or valvular heart disease (e.g., mitral regurgitation). In contrast, a *fourth heart sound* is seldom heard in young adults other than well-conditioned athletes. An S_4 can be heard in otherwise healthy older people, but often suggests decreased ventricular compliance and impaired ventricular filling.

See Table 9-8, Extra Heart Sounds in Diastole, p. 382.

Cardiac Murmurs.   Middle-aged and older adults commonly have a *systolic aortic murmur.* This murmur is detected in approximately one third of people close to 60 years, and in well more than half of those reaching 85 years. Aging thickens the bases of the aortic cusps with fibrous tissue. Calcification follows, resulting in audible vibrations. Turbulence produced by blood flow into a dilated aorta may further augment this murmur. In most people, the process of fibrosis and calcification—known as *aortic sclerosis*—does not impede blood flow. In some, the aortic valve leaflets become calcified and immobile, resulting in *aortic stenosis* and outflow obstruction. A brisk carotid upstroke may help distinguish aortic sclerosis from aortic stenosis, with its delayed upstroke, but clinical differentiation between aortic sclerosis and aortic stenosis may be difficult. Both carry increased risk for cardiovascular morbidity and mortality.

Similar changes alter the mitral valve, usually approximately one decade later than aortic sclerosis. Calcification of the mitral valve annulus, or valve ring, impedes normal valve closure during systole, causing the systolic murmur of *mitral regurgitation.* This murmur may become pathologic as volume overload increases in the left ventricle.

Peripheral Vascular System.   Aging itself confers relatively few clinically important changes for the peripheral vascular system. Although arterial and venous disorders, especially atherosclerosis, do affect older people more frequently, they probably cannot be considered part of normal aging. Peripheral arteries tend to lengthen, become tortuous, and feel harder and less resilient. These changes do not necessarily indicate atherosclerosis, however, or pathologic changes in the coronary or cerebral vessels.

The common changes in skin, nails, and hair discussed earlier are not specific for arterial insufficiency, even though they are classically associated with it. Loss of arterial pulsations is not typical, however, and demands careful evaluation. Rarely, in those older than 50 years, the temporal arteries may become subject to giant cell, or temporal arteritis, leading to loss of vision in 15% of those affected, and to complaints of headache and jaw claudication. Mean age of onset is 72 years. An important concern is possible aneurysm in the abdominal aorta in older adults with abdominal or back pain, especially those who are male, smoke, and have coronary disease.

Breasts and Axillae. The normal adult breast may be soft, but also granular, nodular, or lumpy. This uneven texture represents physiologic nodularity. It may be bilateral and palpable throughout or only in parts of the breast. With aging, the female breasts tend to diminish as glandular tissue atrophies and is replaced by fat. Although the proportion of fat increases, its total amount may decrease. The breasts often become flaccid and more pendulous. The ducts surrounding the nipple may become more easily palpable as firm, stringy strands. Axillary hair diminishes.

Abdomen. During the middle and later years, fat tends to accumulate in the lower abdomen and near the hips, even when total body weight is stable. This accumulation, together with weakening of the abdominal muscles, often produces a soft, more protruding abdomen. Occasionally a person notes this change with alarm and interprets it as fluid or evidence of disease.

Aging may blunt the manifestations of acute abdominal disease. Pain may be less severe, fever is often less pronounced, and signs of peritoneal inflammation, such as muscular guarding and rebound tenderness, may be diminished or even absent.

See Chapter 11, The Abdomen, pp. 415–470.

Male and Female Genitalia, Anus, Rectum, and Prostate. As men age, sexual interest appears to remain intact, although frequency of intercourse declines. Several physiologic changes accompany decreasing testosterone levels. Erections become more dependent on tactile stimulation and less responsive to erotic cues. The penis decreases in size, and the testicles drop lower in the scrotum. Protracted illnesses, more than aging, lead to decreased testicular size. Pubic hair may decrease and become gray. Erectile dysfunction, or the inability to have an erection, affects approximately 50% of older men. Usual causes include hypogastric-cavernous arterial insufficiency or venous leakage through the subtunical venules.[9]

In women, ovarian function usually starts to diminish during the fifth decade; on average, menstrual periods cease between 45 and 52 years. As estrogen stimulation falls, many women experience hot flashes, sometimes for up to 5 years. Symptoms range from flushing, sweating, and palpitations to chills and anxiety. Sleep disruption and mood changes are common. Women may report vaginal dryness, urge incontinence, or dyspareunia. Several vulvovaginal changes occur: pubic hair becomes sparse as well as gray; the labia and clitoris become smaller. The vagina narrows and shortens, and the vaginal mucosa becomes thin, pale, and dry, with loss of lubrication. The uterus and ovaries diminish in size. Within 10 years after menopause, the ovaries are usually no longer palpable. The suspensory ligaments of the adnexa, uterus, and bladder may also relax. Sexuality and sexual interest are often unchanged, particularly in the absence of partner issues, partner loss, or unusual work or life stress.[10]

In men, proliferation of prostate epithelial and stromal tissue, termed benign prostatic hyperplasia (BPH), begins in the third decade, yet prostate enlargement results in only about half, and symptoms occur in only about half of men with enlargement.[11] Symptoms of urinary hesitancy, dribbling, and incomplete emptying can often be traced to causes other than BPH, such as coexisting disease, use of medication, and lower tract abnormalities. Hyperplasia continues to increase prostate volume until the seventh decade then appears to plateau. These changes are androgen dependent.

Musculoskeletal System.   Musculoskeletal changes continue throughout the adult years. Soon after maturity, subtle losses in height begin; significant shortening is obvious by old age. Most loss of height occurs in the trunk as intervertebral discs become thinner and the vertebral bodies shorten or even collapse from osteoporosis. Flexion at the knees and hips may also contribute to shortened stature. Alterations in the discs and vertebrae also contribute to the kyphosis of aging and increase the anteroposterior diameter of the chest, especially in women. For these reasons, the limbs of an elderly person tend to look long in proportion to the trunk.

With aging, skeletal muscles decrease in bulk and power, and ligaments lose some of their tensile strength. Range of motion diminishes, partly because of osteoarthritis.

Nervous System.   Aging may affect all aspects of the nervous system, from mental status to motor and sensory function and reflexes. Age-related losses can exact a heavy toll. Older adults experience the death of loved ones and friends, retirement from valued employment, diminution in income, decreased physical capacities including impairments in vision and hearing, and often growing social isolation. Moreover, the aging brain experiences biologic changes. Brain volume and the number of cortical brain cells decrease, and both microanatomical and biochemical changes have been identified. Nevertheless, most adults adapt well to getting older. They maintain self-esteem, adapt to their changing capacities and circumstances, and eventually prepare themselves for death.

Most elderly people do well on the mental status examination, but selected impairments may become evident, especially at advanced ages. Many older people complain about their memories. "Benign forgetfulness" is the usual explanation and may occur at any age. This term refers to difficulty recalling the names of people or objects or certain details of specific events. Identifying this common phenomenon, when appropriate, may assuage worries about Alzheimer's disease. In addition to this circumscribed forgetfulness, elderly people retrieve and process data more slowly, and they take more time to learn new material. Their motor responses may slow, and their ability to perform complex tasks may become impaired.

Frequently, the clinician must try to distinguish these age-related changes in the nervous system from manifestations of specific mental disorders whose prevalence increases with aging, such as depression and dementia. Sorting out these ailments may be difficult, because both mood disturbances and cognitive changes can alter the patient's ability to recognize or report symptoms. Older patients are also more susceptible to delirium, a temporary state of confusion that may be the first clue to infection or problems with medications. The clinician must learn to recognize these conditions promptly and to protect the patient from harm. Some findings that would be abnormal in younger people, however, occur so often in the elderly that they can be attributed to aging alone, such as the changes in hearing, vision, extraocular movements, and pupillary size, shape, and reactivity described earlier.

Changes in the motor system are common. Older adults move and react with less speed and agility than younger ones, and skeletal muscles decrease in bulk. The hands of an aged person often look thin and bony as a result of atrophy of the interosseous muscles, causing muscle wasting in the backs of the hands that leaves concavities or grooves. As illustrated on pp. 678–679, this change may first appear between the thumb and the hand (1st and 2nd metacarpals) but may also be seen between the other metacarpals. Small muscle wasting may also flatten the thenar and hypothenar eminences of the palms. Arm and leg muscles can also show signs of atrophy, exaggerating the apparent size of adjacent joints. Muscle strength, though diminished, is relatively well maintained.

Occasionally, an older person develops a benign essential tremor in the head, jaw, lips, or hands that may be confused with parkinsonism (pp. 720–721). Unlike parkinsonian tremors, however, benign tremors are slightly faster and disappear at rest, and there is no associated muscle rigidity.

Aging may also affect vibratory sense and reflexes. Older adults frequently lose some or all vibration sense in the feet and ankles (but not in the fingers or over the shins). Less commonly, position sense may diminish or disappear. The gag reflex may be diminished or absent. Abdominal reflexes may diminish or disappear. Ankle reflexes may be symmetrically decreased or absent, even when reinforced. Less commonly, knee reflexes are similarly affected. Partly because of musculoskeletal changes in the feet, the plantar responses become less obvious and more difficult to interpret. If other neurologic abnormalities accompany these changes, or if atrophy and reflex changes are asymmetric, you should search for an explanation other than age alone.

Review Chapter 5, Behavior and Mental Status. The Mental Status Examination, pp. 145–152, and Table 20-2, Delirium and Dementia, p. 931.

See Chapter 17, The Nervous System, Table 17-4, Tremors and Involuntary Movement, pp. 720–721.

THE HEALTH HISTORY

 APPROACH TO THE PATIENT

As you talk with older adults, begin to refine your usual techniques for obtaining the Health History. Your demeanor should convey respect, patience, and cultural awareness. Be sure to address patients by an appropriate title and their last name.

Approach to the Older Adult Patient

- Adjusting the office environment
- Shaping the content and pace of the visit
- Eliciting symptoms
- Addressing the cultural dimensions of aging

Adjusting the Office Environment. First, take the time to adapt the environment of the office, hospital, or nursing home to put your patient at ease. Recall the physiologic changes in temperature regulation, and make sure the office is neither too cool nor too warm. Brighter lighting helps compensate for changes in lens proteins—a well-lit room allows the older adult to see your facial expressions and gestures. Face the patient directly, sitting at eye level.

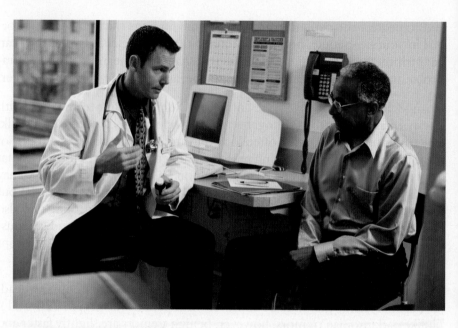

More than 50% of older adults have hearing deficits, especially loss of high-tone discrimination, so a quiet room, free of distractions or noise, is most conducive to good communication. In the hospital setting, turn off the radio or television before starting your discussions. If appropriate, consider using a "pocket talker," a microphone that amplifies your voice and connects to an earpiece inserted by the patient. Adopt low speaking tones, and make sure the patient is using glasses, hearing aids, and dentures when needed to assist with communication. Patients with quadriceps weakness benefit from chairs with higher seating and a wide stool with a handrail leading up to the examining table.[12]

Shaping the Content and Pace of the Visit. With older adults, plan to alter the traditional format of the initial or follow-up visit. From middle age on, people begin to measure their lives in terms of years left rather than years lived. Older people often reminisce about the past and reflect on previous experiences. Listening to this process of life review provides important insights and helps you support patients as they work through painful feelings or recapture joys and accomplishments.

At the same time, it is important to balance the need to assess complex problems with the patient's endurance and possible fatigue. To provide enough time to fully listen to the patient but prevent him or her from becoming exhausted, make ample use of brief screening tools, information from home visits and the medical record, and reports from family members, caregivers, and allied health disciplines. Consider dividing the initial assessment into two visits. Two or more shorter visits may be less fatiguing and more productive because older patients frequently need more time to respond to questions, and their explanations may be slow and lengthy.

See brief screening tools, p. 914.

Eliciting Symptoms in the Older Adult. Eliciting the history from older adults calls for an astute clinician: patients may accidentally or purposefully underreport symptoms; the presentation of acute illnesses may be different; common symptoms may mask a geriatric syndrome; patients may have cognitive impairment.

Older patients tend to overestimate their health when affected by increasing disease and disability.[12] It is best to start the visit with open-ended questions like "How can I help you today?" Older patients may be reluctant to report their symptoms. Some are afraid or embarrassed; others try to avoid medical expenses or the discomforts of diagnosis and treatment. Still others overlook their symptoms, thinking them to be merely part of aging, and simply forget about them. To reduce the risk for late recognition and delayed intervention, you may need to adopt more directed questions or health screening tools, as well as consult with family members and caregivers.

Acute illnesses present differently in older adults. Older patients with infections are less likely to have fever. In those with myocardial infarction, reports of chest pain fall with increasing age, and complaints of shortness of breath, syncope, stroke, and acute confusion become more common.[13] Older patients with hyperthyroidism and hypothyroidism present with fewer symptoms and signs. In hyperthyroidism, fatigue, weight loss, and tachycardia comprise the most common symptom triad in patients age 50 or older.[14] Older patients are more likely to have anorexia and atrial fibrillation; heat intolerance, increased sweating, and hyperreflexia are considerably rarer. In hypothyroidism, fatigue and weakness are common but notably nonspecific; the usual chilliness, paresthesias, weight gain, and cramps found in younger patients are uncommon.[15]

Managing an increasing number of interrelated conditions calls for recognizing the symptom clusters typical of different *geriatric syndromes*. These are understood to have the following features: multifactorial origin; typically in older, often frail adults; often precipitated by an acute event; episodic; and often followed by functional decline. Because consensus on the definition is still in flux, some prefer the term *geriatric conditions*, or "a collection of symptoms and signs common in older adults not necessarily related to a specific disease."[16] Examples of geriatric syndromes or conditions include delirium, cognitive impairment, falls, dizziness, depression, urinary incontinence, and functional impairment.[16,17] Student clinicians need to learn about these syndromes because one symptom may relate to several others in a pattern unfamiliar to the patient. Searching for the usual "unifying diagnosis" may pertain to fewer than 50% of older adults.[18]

Finally, the student must be knowledgeable about how cognitive impairment affects the patient's history. Evidence suggests that when older patients do report symptoms, their reports are reliable and contain more symptoms than reports from family or collateral sources.[19–21] When compared with unimpaired counterparts, even elders with mild cognitive impairment provide sufficient history to reveal concurrent disorders.[9] Use simple sentences with prompts about necessary information. For patients with more severe impairments, confirm key symptoms with family members or caregivers in the patient's presence and with his or her consent.

Learn to recognize and avoid stereotypes that distort your appreciation of each patient as unique, with a treasure of life experiences. Discover how older patients see themselves and their situations. Listen for their priorities, goals, and coping skills. Such knowledge strengthens your alliance with older patients as you plan for their care and treatment.

> ### TIPS FOR COMMUNICATING EFFECTIVELY WITH OLDER ADULTS
>
> - Provide a well-lit, moderately warm setting with minimal background noise and safe chairs and access to the examining table.
> - Face the patient and speak in low tones; make sure the patient is using glasses, hearing devices, and dentures if needed.
> - Adjust the pace and content of the interview to the stamina of the patient; consider two visits for initial evaluations when indicated.
> - Allow time for open-ended questions and reminiscing; include family and caregivers when needed, especially if the patient has cognitive impairment.
> - Make use of brief screening instruments, the medical record, and reports from allied disciplines.
> - Carefully assess symptoms, especially fatigue, loss of appetite, dizziness, and pain, for clues to underlying disorders.
> - Make sure written instructions are in large print and easy to read.

Addressing Cultural Dimensions of Aging. Clinicians must acquire new knowledge and awareness about the health beliefs and culture that shape the older adult's response to illness and the health care system.[23] Between 1990 and 2000, Hispanics, African-Americans, Native Americans, and other ethnic groups accounted for approximately 43% of the total growth of the population.[24] By 2050, the overall older adult population will increase by 230%, with the minority older adult population growing by 510%.[25] The broad categories used for federal reporting no longer capture the wide array of cultural differences that affect how older adults understand suffering, illness, and decisions about care, ranging from use of alternative therapies to timing of health care visits. Immigrant and refugee groups in the United States with particular health care needs include Vietnamese, Laotians, Haitians, Somalis, Russians and Eastern Europeans, Afghans, and Bosnians.

Cultural differences affect the epidemiology of illness and mental health, the process of acculturation, the specific concerns of the elderly, the potential for misdiagnosis, and disparities in health outcomes.[25–28] Take a few minutes to review the components of self-awareness needed for cultural competency discussed in Chapter 3 (pp. 87–91). Learn culturally specific ways to show respect to elders and use appropriate nonverbal communication styles. Direct eye contact or handshaking, for example, may not be culturally syntonic. Identify critical experiences that affect the patient's outlook and psyche arising from the country of origin or migration history. Ask about spiritual advisors and native healers.

Cultural values particularly affect decisions about the end of life. Elders, family, and even an extended community group may make these decisions with or for the older patient. Such group decision making is in contrast to the patient autonomy and informed consent that many contemporary health care providers value, expect, and automatically assume to be desired by all.[24] Being sensitive to the stresses of migration and acculturation, using translators effectively, enlisting "patient navigators" from the family and community, and accessing culturally validated assessment tools like the Geriatric Depression Scale are important for empathic care of older adults.[26]

See Chapter 3, Interviewing and the Health History, on working with translators, pp. 78–79.

SPECIAL AREAS OF CONCERN WHEN ASSESSING COMMON OR CONCERNING SYMPTOMS

Common Concerns

> - Activities of daily living
> - Instrumental activities of daily living
> - Medications
> - Nutrition
> - Acute and persistent pain
> - Smoking and alcohol
> - Advance directives and palliative care

Symptoms in the older adult can have many meanings and interconnections, as we have seen in the geriatric syndromes. Explore the meaning of these symptoms as you would with all patients, and review the Common or Concerning Symptoms sections in previous chapters. For older adults, be sure to place these symptoms in the context of your overall functional assessment. Several areas warrant special attention as you gather the health history. Approach the following areas with extra thoroughness and sensitivity, always focusing on helping the older adult to maintain optimal well-being and level of function.

Activities of Daily Living. Learning how older adults, especially those with chronic illness, function in terms of daily activities is essential and provides an important baseline for the future. First, ask about his or her capacity to perform the *Activities of Daily Living (ADLs)*—these consist of basic self-care abilities—and then move on to inquiries about capacity for higher level functions, the *Instrumental Activities of Daily Living (IADLs)* listed on the next page. Can the patient perform these activities independently, does he or she need some help, or is the patient entirely dependent on others?

You may wish to start with an open-ended request like "Tell me about your typical day" or "Tell me about your day yesterday." Then move to a greater level of detail . . . You got up at 8 AM? How is it getting out of bed? . . . "What did you do next?" Ask how things have changed, who is available for help, and what helpers actually do. Remember that assessing the patient's safety is one of your priorities.

Medications. Prescription drug statistics expose the dramatic rationale for obtaining a complete drug history.[3] Approximately 80% of older adults have at least one chronic disease and take at least one prescription drug each

ACTIVITIES OF DAILY LIVING AND INSTRUMENTAL ACTIVITIES OF DAILY LIVING	
Physical Activities of Daily Living (ADLs)	*Instrumental Activities of Daily Living (IADLs)*
Bathing	Using the telephone
Dressing	Shopping
Toileting	Preparing food
Transferring	Housekeeping
Continence	Laundry
Feeding	Transportation
Managing money	Taking medicine

day. Those older than 65 years receive approximately 30% of all prescriptions. Roughly 30% take more than eight prescribed drugs each day! Older adults have more than 50% of all reported adverse drug reactions causing hospital admission, reflecting pharmacodynamic changes in the distribution, metabolism, and elimination of drugs that place them at increased risk.

Take a thorough medication history, including name, dose, frequency, and indication for each drug. Be sure to explore all components of polypharmacy, including suboptimal prescribing, concurrent use of multiple drugs, underuse, inappropriate use, and nonadherence. Ask about use of over-the-counter medications, vitamin and nutritional supplements, and mood-altering drugs such as narcotics, benzodiazepines, and recreational substances. Assess medications for drug interactions. Be particularly careful when treating insomnia, estimated to occur in approximately 40% of older adults. Increased exercise may be the best remedy. Recall that medications are the most common modifiable risk factor associated with falls. Review strategies for avoiding polypharmacy with your instructors. It is wise to keep the number of drugs prescribed to a minimum. Learn about drug–drug interactions and drugs contraindicated in older adults.[29,30]

Nutrition. Taking a diet history and using the Rapid Screen for Dietary Intake and the Nutrition Screening Checklist are especially important in older adults. Prevalence of undernutrition increases with age, affecting 5% to 10% of elderly outpatients and 30% to 50% of hospitalized elders.[31] Those with chronic disease are particularly at risk, especially those with poor dentition, oral or gastrointestinal disorders, depression or other psychiatric illness, and drug regimens that affect appetite and oral secretions. For underweight elders, the serum albumin is an independent risk factor for all-cause mortality.[32]

Acute and Persistent Pain. Pain and associated complaints account for 80% of clinician visits. Prevalence of pain may reach 25% to 50% in community-dwelling adults and 40% to 80% in nursing home residents. Pain usually arises from musculoskeletal complaints like back and joint pain.[33] Headache, neuralgias from diabetes and herpes zoster, nighttime leg pain, and cancer pain are also common. Older patients are less likely to report pain, leading to undue suffering, depression, social isolation, physical disability, and loss of function. The American Geriatrics Society favors the term *persistent pain,* because chronic pain is associated with negative stereotypes.[34]

Pain is subjective, so some view pain as a spectrum disorder rather than "the fifth vital sign."[35] See discussion, pp. 121–124.

● Characteristics of Acute and Persistent Pain

Acute Pain	Persistent Pain
Distinct onset	Lasts more than 3 months
Obvious pathology	Often associated with psychological or functional impairment
Short duration	Can fluctuate in character and intensity over time
Common causes: postsurgical, trauma, headache	Common causes: arthritis, cancer, claudication, leg cramps, neuropathy, radiculopathy

(Source: Reuben DB, Herr KA, Pacala JT, et al. Geriatrics at Your Fingertips: 2004, 6th ed., p. 119. Malden, MA: Blackwell Publishing, Inc., for the American Geriatrics Society, 2004.)

Inquire about pain *each time* you meet with an older patient. Assessing pain in older adults is challenging. Patients may not want to report symptoms because of fears of additional testing, costs, or progression of disease.[35] There may be cognitive or verbal impairments or barriers of trust, language, or cultural understanding. Or the patient may report multiple conditions that complicate assessment. Nonetheless, evidence shows that pain-reporting by patients with even mild to moderate cognitive impairment is reliable. Ask specifically, "Are you having any pain right now? How about during the past week?" Be alert for red flags of untreated pain, such as use of the terms "burning," "discomfort," or "soreness," depressed affect, and nonverbal change in posture or gait. Many multidimensional and unidimensional pain scales are available. Unidimensional scales such as the Visual Analog Scale, graphic pictures, and the Verbal 0–10 Scale have all been validated and are easiest to use.[33,36] Recruit caregivers or family members for relevant history in patients with severe cognitive deficits.

Learn to distinguish acute pain from chronic pain and thoroughly investigate its cause. In older adults, confusion, restlessness, fatigue, or irritability may all arise from conditions causing pain. Assessing pain includes comprehensive evaluation of its effects on quality of life, social interactions, and functional level. Multidisciplinary assessment is warranted if the cause cannot be identified and risks of disability and comorbidity are high. Study the many modalities of pain relief, ranging from analgesics to the full range of nonpharmacologic therapies, especially those that engage patients directly and actively in their treatment plan and build self-reliance. Patient education

See the *10-Minute Geriatric Screener* for functional assessment, on p. 914.

alone has been shown effective.[34] Relaxation techniques, tai chi, acupuncture, massage, and biofeedback can avert adding more medications.

Smoking and Alcohol.
Smoking is harmful at all ages. At each visit, advise elderly smokers to quit. The commitment to stop smoking may take time, but quitting is an important step in reducing risk for heart disease, pulmonary disease, malignancy, and loss of daily function.

An estimated 5% to 10% of adults older than 65 years have alcohol-related problems.[37] Lifelong prevalence of alcohol abuse or dependency among community residents older than 65 years ranges from 4% to 8%.[38] Rates of alcoholism in older patients in hospital, emergency room, and clinic settings have been reported to reach 21%, 24%, and 36% respectively, and account for approximately 1% of hospital admissions for this age group.[38] The number of older people with problem drinking is expected to rise as the population ages over the coming decades.

Despite the prevalence of alcohol problems among the elderly, rates of detection and treatment are low. Detection is especially important, because as many as 100 medications have adverse interactions with alcohol, and up to 30% of older adult drinkers exacerbate chronic ailments like cirrhosis, gastrointestinal bleeding or reflux disease, gout, hypertension, diabetes, insomnia, gait disorders, and depression.[39] Look for the clues shown in the accompanying box, especially in elders with recent bereavement or losses, pain, disability or depression, or a family history of alcohol disorders.

DETECTING ALCOHOL USE DISORDERS IN OLDER ADULTS: CLINICAL CLUES

- Memory loss, cognitive impairment
- Depression, anxiety
- Neglect of hygiene, appearance
- Poor appetite, nutritional deficits
- Sleep disruption
- Hypertension refractory to therapy
- Blood sugar control problems
- Seizures refractory to therapy
- Impaired balance and gait, falls
- Recurrent gastritis and esophagitis
- Difficulty managing warfarin dosing

(Source: American Geriatrics Society. Screening recommendation: clinical guidelines for alcohol use disorders in older adults. Available at: http://www.americangeriatrics.org/products/positionpapers/alcohol.shtml. Accessed February 23, 2008.)

Use the CAGE questions to uncover problem drinking. Although symptoms and signs are subtler in older adults, making early detection more difficult, the four CAGE questions remain sensitive and specific in this age group, using the conventional cutoff score of 2 or more.[38,39]

See Chapter 3, Interviewing and the Health History, Alcohol and Illicit Drugs, pp. 84–85.

Advance Directives and Palliative Care. Many older patients are interested in expressing their wishes about end-of-life decisions and would like providers to initiate these discussions before any serious illness develops.[40] Advance care planning involves several tasks—providing information, invoking the patient's preferences, identifying proxy decision makers, and conveying empathy and support. Use clear and simple language. You can often begin the discussion by relating these decisions to a current illness or experiences with relatives or friends. Ask about preferences relating to written "Do Not Resuscitate" orders specifying life support measures "if the heart or lungs were to stop or give out." Second, encourage the patient to establish in writing a health care proxy or durable power of attorney for health care, "someone who can make decisions reflecting your wishes in case of confusion or emergency." These conversations, although difficult at first, convey your respect and concern for patients and help them and their families prepare openly and in advance for a peaceful death.[41] Plan to include these discussions in an office setting rather than in the uncertain and stressful environment of emergency or acute care.

For patients with advanced or terminal illnesses, include these discussions in an overall plan for palliative care. The goal of palliative care is "to relieve suffering and improve the quality of life for patients with advanced illnesses and their families through specific knowledge and skills, including communication with patients and family members; management of pain and other symptoms; psychosocial, spiritual, and bereavement support; and coordination of an array of medical and social services."[42] To ease patient and family distress, accent your communication skills: make good eye contact; ask open-ended questions; respond to anxiety, depression, or changes in the patient's affect; and show empathy.

See also Chapter 3, The Patient With Altered Capacity, pp. 76–77, and Death and the Dying Patient, pp. 86–87.

HEALTH PROMOTION AND COUNSELING

Important Topics for Health Promotion and Counseling in the Older Adult

- When to screen
- Vision and hearing
- Exercise
- Immunizations
- Household safety

- Cancer screening
- Depression
- Dementia and mild cognitive impairment
- Elder mistreatment

When to Screen. As the life span for older adults extends into the 80s, new issues for screening emerge. Given the heterogeneity of the aging population, guiding principles for deciding who might benefit from screening and when screening might be stopped are helpful, especially because evidence for making screening decisions is not always available. In general, base screening decisions on each older person's particular circumstances, rather than age alone. Three factors should be considered: life expectancy, time interval until benefit from screening accrues, and patient preference.[43] The American Geriatrics Society recommends that if life expectancy is short, give priority to treatment that will benefit the patient in the time that remains. Consider deferring screening if it places added burdens on the older adult with multiple medical problems, a shortened life expectancy, or dementia. Tests that help with prognosis and planning, however, are still warranted even if the patient would not pursue treatment.[44]

Vision and Hearing.   Screening for age-related changes in *vision* and *hearing* is important in helping older adults maintain optimal function, and is included in the 10-Minute Geriatric Screener.[45] Test *vision* objectively using an eye chart. Asking the patient about any *hearing* loss may be adequate, followed by the whisper test and more formal testing if indicated.

See 10-Minute Geriatric Screener, p. 914.

See Chapter 7, The Head and Neck, techniques for assessing hearing, pp. 225–227.

Exercise.   Recommend regular aerobic exercise to improve strength and aerobic capacity, increase physiologic reserve, improve energy level for doing ADLs, and slow onset of disability.

The American College of Sports Medicine and the American Heart Association Recommendations on Physical Activity and Public Health for Older Adults in 2007 advocate a physically active lifestyle and target intensity of aerobic activity based on the older adult's degree of aerobic fitness, activities that increase muscle strength and flexibility, balance exercises for those at risk of falls, and therapeutic plans that integrate both treatment and prevention, including at the community level. Older adults are advised to perform moderate-intensity aerobic activities for at least 30 minutes five days each week, or vigorous-intensity activity for at least 20 minutes three days each week.[46]

Immunizations.   Advise your patients to have the pneumococcal vaccine, the influenza vaccine, and the zoster vaccine.[47,48]

See also Chapter 8, The Thorax and Lungs, Immunizations, pp. 294–295.

● *Influenza vaccine.* The following groups should receive the *influenza vaccine* each year: people 50 years or older; any older adult with chronic disorders of the cardiovascular or pulmonary systems, diabetes, renal or hepatic dysfunction, immunosuppression, or HIV/AIDS; residents and health care personnel of nursing homes and long-term care facilities; caregivers of children; or anyone requesting vaccination.[49]

● *Pneumococcal vaccine.* The *pneumococcal vaccine* should be given every 5 years to adults 65 years or older with chronic disorders of the cardiovascular or pulmonary systems, diabetes, renal or hepatic dysfunction, asplenia, chronic alcoholism, immunosuppression, cerebrospinal fluid leak, or HIV/AIDS; residents of nursing homes or long-term care facilities; and Alaska Natives and selected American Indian populations, such as the Navajo and Apache.

● *Zoster vaccine.* *Zoster vaccine* is recommended at age 60 years, regardless of whether the patient reports a prior episode of herpes zoster. Studies show that vaccination reduces incidence of herpes zoster by approximately 50% and incidence of postherpetic neuralgia by more than 65%.[50]

Household Safety. Emergency room visits for household injuries are increasing at a rapid rate, particularly for adults older than 75 years. In a special report in 2002, the U.S. Consumer Product Safety Commission estimated that almost 1.5 million adults older than 65 years were treated for injuries related to household products, including more than 60% of those with falls.[51] ER visits and deaths were most likely to involve yard and garden equipment, ladders and stepstools, personal use items like hair dryers and flammable clothing, and bathroom and sports injuries. Encourage older adults to adopt corrective measures for poor lighting, chairs at awkward heights, slippery or irregular surfaces, and environmental hazards.

See also Assessing and Preventing Falls, pp. 913–916.

HOME SAFETY TIPS FOR OLDER ADULTS

- Handrails on both sides of any stairway
- Well-lit stairways, paths, and walkways
- Rugs secured by non-slip backing or adhesive tape
- Grab bars and non-slip mat or safety strips in the bath or shower
- Smoke alarms and plan for escaping fire

Cancer Screening. Cancer screening for selected conditions can be controversial because of limited evidence supporting its use for adults older than 70 to 80 years. The American Geriatrics Society recommends annual or biennial mammography for breast cancer screening up to age 75 years, then every 2 to 3 years if life expectancy remains more than 4 years. Although the prevalence of cervical cancer has declined in the United States, 40% to 50% of deaths from cervical cancer are in women older than 65 years. Provide Pap smears every 1 to 3 years until age 65 to 70 years when there is no history of cervical pathology. Colonoscopy is recommended for colon cancer screening every 10 years beginning at 50 years. This examination is difficult for many older patients, who may decline despite encouragement. Review the discussion about colonoscopy, fecal occult blood tests, and the pitfalls of the prostate-specific antigen test and the digital rectal examination on pages 558–560. Screening for lung cancer and ovarian cancer is not recommended. Check for skin cancer and oral cancer in high-risk patients.[52]

Depression. *Depression* affects 10% of older adults but is both underdiagnosed and undertreated.[53] A positive response to asking "Do you often feel sad or depressed?" is approximately 80% sensitive and specific and should prompt further investigation, possibly with the Geriatric Depression Scale. Depressed men older than 65 years are at increased risk for suicide; they require particularly careful evaluation.

See Chapter 5, Behavior and Mental Status, Depression, p. 143.

Dementia and Mild Cognitive Impairment. *Dementia,* "an acquired syndrome of decline in memory and at least one other cognitive domain such as language, visuospatial, or executive function sufficient to interfere with social or occupational functioning in an alert person," affects 11% of Americans older than 65 years, or roughly 4.5 million people.[54,55] Prominent features include short- and long-term memory deficits and impaired judgment.

See Table 20-2, Delirium and Dementia, p. 931, and Table 20-3, Screening for Dementia: The Mini-Cog, p. 932.

Thought processes are impoverished; speech may be hesitant as a result of difficulty in finding words. Loss of orientation to place may make navigating by foot or car problematic or even dangerous. Most dementias represent Alzheimer's disease (50% to 85%) or vascular multi-infarct dementia (10% to 20%). Watch for Alzheimer's disease in patients with a positive family history, because their risk is three times higher than the risk in the general population.

Dementia often has a slow, insidious onset and may escape detection by both families and clinicians, especially in the early stages of *mild cognitive impairment (MCI)*. MCI refers to a milder syndrome of cognitive loss compared with dementia; specifically, the impairment is not of such magnitude as to interfere with social or vocational function. The person may or may not complain of cognitive deterioration, but standardized cognitive testing reveals reasonable evidence of significant decline in at least one cognitive domain. When the domain affected is memory, the disorder is called *amnestic MCI*; when the domain affected is not memory but language or visuospatial function, for example, the disorder is called *non-amnestic MCI*. A significant percentage, but not all, of these people progress to a clinical diagnosis of Alzheimer's disease. There are syndromes of even milder cognitive change later in the life cycle, such as *age-associated cognitive impairment (AACI)*. People with this syndrome complain of age-associated cognitive loss, but such deterioration cannot be documented on cognitive testing. The clinical significance of AACI and related mild cognitive loss syndromes is not yet known. Current research seeks to identify the clinical features of these various syndromes.[56-61]

In Alzheimer's dementia, look for amnestic memory impairment, deterioration of language, and visuospatial deficits. Initial loss of higher-level ADLs such as check-writing and use of public transportation progresses to eventual loss of basic activities like eating and grooming. Mood change and apathy often appear early; psychosis and agitation emerge in the later stages.[55] Watch for family complaints of new or unusual behaviors. Testing with the Mini-Mental State Examination may be helpful, although level of education and cultural variables such as language may affect scores. If you identify cognitive changes, investigate contributing factors such as medications, depression, metabolic abnormalities, or other medical and psychiatric conditions. In patients with dementia, counsel families about the potential for disruptive behavior, accidents, falls, and termination of driving privileges. Foster discussion of legal arrangements such as power of attorney and advance directives while the patient can still contribute to decision making.

Elder Mistreatment. Finally, consider screening all older patients for possible *elder mistreatment*, which includes abuse, neglect, exploitation, and abandonment. Depression, dementia, and malnutrition are independent risk factors. Prevalence of elder mistreatment is approximately 1% to 5% of the older population; however, that statistic is based solely on self-reported cases of elder mistreatment, and many more cases may remain undetected. Self-neglect is a growing national concern and represents more than 50% of adult protective service referrals.[62] Although several screening instruments are available, no single instrument has emerged for rapid yet accurate assessment and diagnosis of these important problems.[62-64]

As you have seen, assessment of the older adult does not follow the traditional format of the history and physical examination. It calls for enhanced techniques of interviewing, special emphasis on daily function and key topics related to elder health, and a focus on functional assessment during the physical examination. Because of its importance to the health of older adults and the order of your assessment, this section begins with Assessing Functional Status: The "Sixth Vital Sign." This segment includes how to evaluate risk for falls, one of the greatest threats to health and well-being in elders. Next, follow features of the traditional "head-to-toe" examination tailored to the older adult.

ASSESSING FUNCTIONAL STATUS: THE "SIXTH VITAL SIGN"

During assessment of older adults, the clinician places a special premium on maintaining the patient's health and well-being. In a sense, all visits are opportunities to promote the patient's independence and optimal level of function. Although the specific goals of care may vary, a primary focus is preserving the patient's functional status, the "sixth vital sign." Functional status specifically means the ability to perform tasks and fulfill social roles associated with daily living across a wide range of complexity.[65] Your assessment of functional status begins when the patient enters the room. Several well-validated and time-efficient assessment tools can help maintain focus on these observations and assist with this approach.

Assessing Functional Ability. Deficits in function are now recognized as better predictors of mortality and patient outcomes after hospitalization than admitting diagnoses.[66] Several performance-based assessment instruments are available. The 10-minute Geriatric Screener is brief, has high inter-rater agreement, and can be used easily by office staff. It also covers the three important domains of geriatric assessment: physical, cognitive, and psycho-social function. Note that it addresses vision and hearing, key sensory modalities, and includes questions about urinary incontinence, an often unreported problem that greatly affects social interactions and self-esteem in the elderly.

These mnemonics help students assess incontinence: **DIAPERS**—**D**elerium, **I**nfection, **A**trophic urethritis/vaginitis, **P**harmaceuticals, **E**xcess urine output from conditions like hyperglycemia or congestive heart failure, **R**estricted mobility, and **S**tool impaction; and **DDRRIIPP**—**D**elerium, **D**rug side effects, **R**etention of feces, **R**estricted mobility, **I**nfection of urine, **I**nflammation, **P**olyuria, and **P**sychogenic.[67,68]

Further Assessment of Falls. A veritable avalanche of evidence links falls to morbidity and mortality in our older population. Each year approximately 35% to 40% of healthy community-dwelling older adults experience falls. Incidence rates in nursing homes and hospitals are almost three times higher, with related injuries in approximately 25%. Loss of confidence from fear of falling and postfall anxiety further impair full recovery.[67,68]

● 10-Minute Geriatric Screener

Problem	Screening Measure	Positive Screen
Vision	2 Parts: Ask: "Do you have difficulty driving, or watching television, or reading, or doing any of your daily activities because of your eyesight?" If yes, then: Test each eye with Snellen chart while patient wears corrective lenses (if applicable).	Yes to question and inability to read greater than 20/40 on Snellen chart
Hearing	Use audioscope set at 40 dB. Test hearing using 1,000 and 2,000 Hz.	Inability to hear 1,000 or 2,000 Hz in both ears or either of these frequencies in one ear
Leg mobility	Time the patient after asking: "Rise from the chair. Walk 20 feet briskly, turn, walk back to the chair and sit down."	Unable to complete task in 15 seconds
Urinary incontinence	2 Parts: Ask: "In the last year, have you ever lost your urine and gotten wet?" If yes, then ask: "Have you lost urine on at least 6 separate dates?"	Yes to both questions
Nutrition/weight loss	2 Parts: Ask: "Have you lost 10 lbs over the past 6 months without trying to do so?" Weigh the patient.	Yes to the question or weight <100 lbs
Memory	Three-item recall	Unable to remember all three items after 1 minute
Depression	Ask: "Do you often feel sad or depressed?"	Yes to the question
Physical disability	Six questions: "Are you able to . . . : "Do strenuous activities like fast walking or bicycling?" "Do heavy work around the house like washing windows, walls, or floors?" "Go shopping for groceries or clothes?" "Get to places out of walking distance?" "Bathe, either a sponge bath, tub bath, or shower?" "Dress, like putting on a shirt, buttoning and zipping, or putting on shoes?"	Yes to any of the questions

(Source: Moore AA, Siu AL. Screening for common problems in ambulatory elderly: clinical confirmation of a screening instrument. Am J Med 100:438–440, 1996.)

The American Geriatrics Society recommends risk factor assessment for falls during routine primary care visits, with more intensive assessment in high-risk groups—those with first or recurrent falls, nursing home residents, and those prone to fall-related injuries.[68] Fall-related assessments should include details about the how the fall occurred, especially from witnesses, and identification of risk factors, medical comorbidities, functional status, and environmental risks—coupled with interventions for prevention.[69]

Gait velocity is also emerging as a significant predictor of falls and related adverse events.[70] Effective single interventions include gait and balance training and exercise to strengthen muscles, reduction of home hazards, discontinuation of psychotropic medication, and multifactorial assessment with targeted interventions. Additional useful strategies include addressing change in postural blood pressure, attention to concurrent acute illness, reduction in medications to fewer than four, detection of sensory neuropathy and impairment of proprioception, investigation of any episodes of syncope, patient and family education, treatment of osteoporosis, and possible use of hip protectors.[71] Study the following algorithm from the American Geriatrics Society on Prevention of Falls in Older Adults.

PREVENTION OF FALLS IN OLDER ADULTS

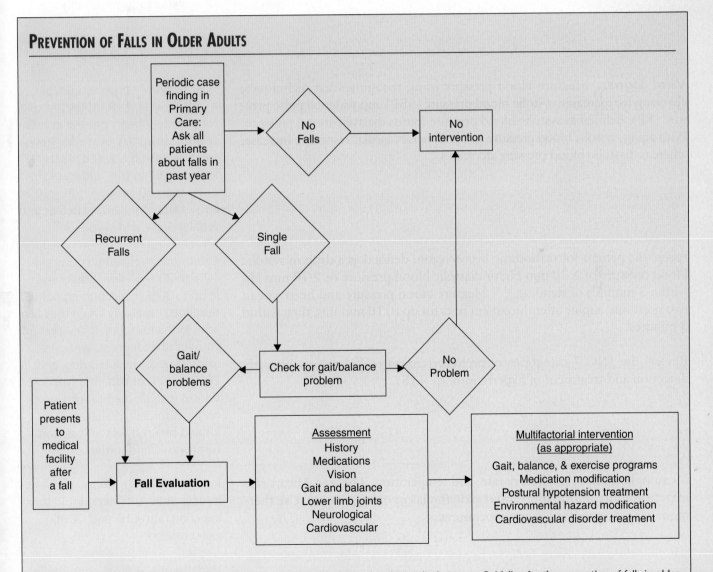

(Source: American Society, British Geriatrics Society, American Academy of Orthopaedic Surgeons. Guideline for the prevention of falls in older persons. J Am Geriatr Soc. 49(5):664–672, 2001.)

PHYSICAL EXAMINATION OF THE OLDER ADULT

General Survey. Deepen the observations about the patient that you have been compiling since the visit began. What is the patient's apparent state of health and degree of vitality? What about mood and affect? Is screening for cognitive changes needed? Note the patient's hygiene and how the patient is dressed. How does the patient walk into the room? Move onto the examining table? Are there changes in posture or involuntary movements?

Flag or impoverished affect in *depression, Parkinson's disease,* or *Alzheimer's disease.*

See Table 20-3, Screening for Dementia: The Mini-Cog, p. 932, for a brief and well-validated screening tool for dementia.[72,73]

Undernutrition, slowed motor performance, loss of muscle mass, or weakness suggests frailty.

Kyphosis or abnormal gait can impair balance and increase risk of falls.

Vital Signs. Measure blood pressure using recommended techniques, checking for increased systolic blood pressure (SBP) and widened pulse pressure (PP), defined as systolic blood pressure minus diastolic blood pressure. With aging, systolic blood pressure and peripheral vascular resistance increase, whereas diastolic blood pressure decreases.

Isolated systolic hypertension (SBP ≥140) after age 50 triples the risk for coronary heart disease in men and increases risk of stroke; however, caution is advised when lowering BP in the "oldest old" older than 80 years.[74–76] PP ≥60 is a risk factor for cardiovascular and renal disease and stroke.[77–80]

Assess the patient for orthostatic hypotension, defined as a drop in systolic blood pressure of ≥ 20 mm Hg or diastolic blood pressure of ≥ 10 mm Hg within 3 minutes of standing.[81,82] Measure blood pressure and heart rate in two positions: supine after the patient rests for up to 10 minutes, then within 3 minutes.

Review the JNC 7 categories of prehypertension to help you with early detection and treatment of hypertension (p. 118).

Orthostatic hypotension occurs in 10% to 20% of older adults and in up to 30% of frail nursing home residents, especially when they first arise in the morning. It can present with lightheadedness, weakness, unsteadiness, visual blurring, and, in 20% to 30% of patients, syncope. Causes include medications, autonomic disorders, diabetes, prolonged bed rest, blood loss, and cardiovascular disorders.[77,83–85]

Measure heart rate, respiratory rate, and temperature. The apical heart rate may yield more information about arrhythmias in older patients. Use thermometers accurate for lower temperatures.

Respiratory rate ≥ 25 breaths per minute indicates lower respiratory infection; also CHF and COPD exacerbation.

Hypothermia is more common in elderly patients.[12]

Weight and height are especially important in the elderly and needed for calculation of the body mass index. Weight should be measured at every visit.

Low weight is a key indicator of poor nutrition.

Undernutrition is seen with depression, alcoholism, cognitive impairment, malignancy, chronic organ failure (cardiac, renal, pulmonary), medication use, social isolation, and poverty.

Skin.   Note physiologic changes of aging, such as thinning, loss of elastic tissue and turgor, and wrinkling. Skin may be dry, flaky, rough, and often itchy (*asteatosis*), with a latticework of shallow fissures that creates a mosaic of small polygons, especially on the legs.

Observe any patchy changes in color. Check the extensor surface of the hands and forearms for white depigmented patches, or *pseudoscars*, and for well-demarcated vividly purple macules or patches that may fade after several weeks (*actinic purpura*).

ACTINIC PURPURA—FOREARM

Look for changes from sun exposure. Areas of skin may appear weather beaten, thickened, yellowed, and deeply furrowed; there may be *actinic lentigines*, or "liver spots," and *actinic keratoses*, superficial flattened papules covered by a dry scale.

Inspect for the benign lesions of aging, namely *comedones*, or blackheads, on the cheeks or around the eyes; *cherry angiomas*, which often appear early in adulthood; and *seborrheic keratoses*, raised yellowish lesions that feel greasy and velvety or warty.

Distinguish such lesions from a *basal cell carcinoma*, initially a translucent nodule that spreads and leaves a depressed center with a firm elevated border, and from a *squamous cell carcinoma*, a firm reddish-appearing lesion often emerging in a sun-exposed area. A dark raised asymmetric lesion with irregular borders may be a *melanoma*. See Table 6-9, Skin Tumors, p. 185, and Table 6-10, Benign and Malignant Nevi, p. 186.

Watch for any painful vesicular lesions in a dermatomal distribution.

Suspect *herpes zoster* from reactivation of latent varicella-zoster virus in the dorsal root ganglia. Risk increases with age and impaired cell-mediated immunity.[86]

In older bed-bound patients, especially when emaciated or neurologically impaired, inspect the skin thoroughly for damage or ulceration.

Pressure sores may develop from obliteration of arteriolar and capillary blood flow to the skin or from shear forces during movement across sheets or when lifted upright incorrectly. See Table 6-13, Pressure Ulcers, p. 191.

Head and Neck. Conduct a careful and thorough evaluation of the head and neck.

See Chapter 7, The Head and Neck, pp. 195–248.

Inspect the eyelids, the bony orbit, and the eye. The eye may appear recessed from atrophy of fat in the surrounding tissues. Observe any *senile ptosis* arising from weakening of the levator palpebrae, relaxation of the skin, and increased weight of the upper eyelid. Check the lower lids for *ectropion* or *entropion*. Note yellowing of the sclera, and *arcus senilis*, a benign whitish ring around the limbus.

See Table 7-6, Variations and Abnormalities of the Eyelids, p. 255, and Table 7-9, Opacities of the Cornea and Lens, p. 258.

Test visual acuity, using a pocket Snellen chart or wall-mounted chart. Note any *presbyopia*, the loss of near vision arising from decreased elasticity of the lens related to aging.

More than 40 million Americans have refractive errors.

The pupils should respond to light and near effort. Except for possible impairment in upward gaze, extraocular movements should remain intact.

Using your ophthalmoscope, carefully examine the lenses and fundi.

Cataracts, glaucoma, and macular degeneration all increase with aging.[87]

Inspect each lens carefully for any opacities. Do not depend on the flashlight alone because the lens may look clear superficially.

Cataracts are the world's leading cause of blindness. Risk factors include cigarette smoking, exposure to UV-B light, high alcohol intake, diabetes, medications (including steroids), and trauma. See Table 7-9, p. 258.

In older adults, the fundi lose their youthful shine and light reflections, and the arteries look narrowed, paler, straighter, and less brilliant. Assess the cup-to-disc ratio, usually 1:2 or less.

An increased cup-to-disc ratio suggests open angle *glaucoma,* caused by irreversible optic neuropathy and leading to loss of peripheral and central vision and blindness. Prevalence is three to four times higher in African-Americans than in the general population.[88]

Inspect the fundi for colloid bodies causing alterations in pigmentation, called *drusen*.

Macular degeneration causes poor central vision and blindness. Types include *dry atrophic* (more common but less severe) and *wet exudative,* or neovascular. Drusen may be hard and sharply defined, or soft and confluent with altered pigmentation, shown below and on p. 222.

Test hearing by occluding one ear and using the techniques for whispered voice or an audioscope. Be sure to inspect the ear canals for cerumen, because removal can quickly improve hearing.

See techniques for testing hearing, pp. 225–227. Screening by asking if hearing loss is present is effective. Patients who report hearing loss have an LR of 2.2 for impairment, with an LR of 0.13 if they report no hearing loss. Proceed to audiometry for those saying yes; check acuity to whispered voice for saying no (LR 6 if no acuity; LR 0.03 if acuity intact).[89, 90]

Examine the oral cavity for odor, appearance of the gingival mucosa, any caries, mobility of the teeth, and quantity of saliva. Inspect closely for lesions on any of the mucosal surfaces. Ask the patient to remove dentures so you can check the gums for denture sores.

Malodor may occur with poor oral hygiene or periodontitis, caries. *Gingivitis* may arise from periodontal disease. Dental plaque and cavitation may cause caries. Increased tooth mobility from abscesses or advanced caries warrants removal to prevent aspiration. Decreased salivation may develop from medications, radiation, Sjögren's syndrome, or dehydration. Lesions may arise from *oral tumors,* usually on the lateral borders of the tongue and floor of the mouth.[91]

Continue your usual examination of the thyroid gland and lymph nodes.

Thorax and Lungs.   Complete the usual examination, making note of subtle signs of changes in pulmonary function.

Increased anteroposterior diameter, purse-lipped breathing, and dyspnea with talking or minimal exertion suggest *chronic obstructive pulmonary disease.*

Cardiovascular System.   Review your findings from measurement of the blood pressure and heart rate.

Isolated systolic hypertension and a widened pulse pressure are cardiac risk factors, prompting a search for *left ventricular hypertrophy (LVH).*

As with younger adults, begin by inspecting the JVP, palpating the carotid upstrokes, and listening for any overlying carotid bruits.

A *tortuous atherosclerotic aorta* can raise pressure in the left jugular veins by impairing drainage into the right atrium. It may also cause kinking of the carotid artery low in the neck on the right, chiefly in women with hypertension, which can be mistaken for a carotid aneurysm.

Carotid bruits in the elderly warrant further investigation for possible carotid stenosis due to risk for ipsilateral stroke.

Assess the point of maximal impulse (PMI), then auscultate S_1 and S_2. Listen also for the extra sounds of S_3 and S_4.

Sustained PMI in LVH; diffuse PMI in congestive heart failure (see pp. 357–359)

In older adults an S_3 suggests dilatation of the left ventricle from congestive heart failure or cardiomyopathy; an S_4 often accompanies hypertension.

Beginning in the second right interspace, listen for cardiac murmurs in all areas of auscultation (see pp. 364–368). Describe the timing, shape, location of maximal intensity, radiation, intensity, pitch, and quality of each murmur you detect.

A systolic crescendo–decrescendo murmur in the second right interspace suggests aortic sclerosis or aortic stenosis, seen in approximately 30% and 2% of community-dwelling elders, respectively. Both carry increased risk for cardiovascular disease and death.[92]

For systolic murmurs over the clavicle, check for delay between the brachial and radial pulses.

Delay during simultaneous palpation (but not compression) of the brachial and radial pulses denotes aortic stenosis.[93]

A harsh holosystolic murmur at the apex suggests mitral regurgitation, also common in the elderly.

Breasts and Axillae. Palpate the breasts carefully for lumps or masses. Include palpation of the tail of Spence that extends into the axilla. Examine the axillae for lymphadenopathy.

Lumps or masses in older women, and rarely in older men, mandate further investigation for possible malignancy.

Abdomen. Continue your usual examination of the abdomen. Check for any bruits over the aorta, renal arteries, and femoral arteries. Inspect the upper abdomen; palpate to the left of the midline for any aortic pulsations. Try to assess the width of the aorta by pressing more deeply with one hand on each of its lateral margins (see p. 447).

Bruits in atherosclerotic vascular disease

Widened aorta and pulsatile mass in *abdominal aortic aneurysm*

Peripheral Vascular System. Auscultate the abdomen for aortic, renal, or femoral artery bruits.

Bruits over these vessels are found in *atherosclerotic disease.*

Assess the width of the abdominal aorta in the epigastric area and examine for a pulsatile mass.

Consider *abdominal aortic aneurysm* if aortic width is ≥ 3 cm or with a pulsatile mass, especially in older male smokers with coronary disease.

Palpate pulses carefully.

Diminished or absent pulses may indicate *arterial occlusion.* Consider confirmation with an office ankle–brachial index. Note that ≤33% of patients with peripheral vascular disease have symptoms of claudication.[94]

Female Genitalia and Pelvic Examination.[95–97] Take special care to explain the steps of the examination and allow time for careful positioning. Ask an assistant to help the older woman move onto the examining table, then into the lithotomy position. Raising the head of the table may make her more comfortable. For the woman with arthritis or spinal deformities who cannot flex her hips or knees, an assistant can gently raise and support the legs, or help the woman into the left lateral position.

Inspect the vulva for changes related to menopause such as thinning of the skin, loss of pubic hair, and decreased distensibility of the introitus. Identify any labial masses. Note that bluish swellings may be varicosities. Bulging of the anterior vaginal wall below the urethra may indicate a urethrocele or urethral diverticulum.

Benign masses include condylomata, fibromas, leiomyomas, and sebaceous cysts. See Table 14-2, Bulges and Swellings of the Vulva, Vagina, and Urethra, p. 547.

Look for any vulvar erythema.

Erythema with satellite lesions results from infection with *Candida;* erythema with ulceration or necrotic center is associated with *carcinoma.* Multifocal reddened lesions with white scaling plaques are consistent with *Paget's disease.*

Inspect the urethra for *caruncles,* or prolapse of fleshy erythematous mucosal tissue at the urethral meatus. Note any enlargement of the clitoris.

Clitoral enlargement may accompany *androgen-producing tumors* or use of androgen creams.

Spread the labia, press downward on the introitus to relax the levator muscles, and gently insert the speculum after moistening it with warm water or a water-soluble lubricant. If you find severe vaginal atrophy, a gaping introitus, or an introital stricture from estrogen loss, you will need to vary the size of the speculum.

Inspect the vaginal walls, which may be atrophic, and the cervix. Note any thin cervical mucus or vaginal or cervical discharge.

Estrogen-stimulated cervical mucus with ferning is seen with use of hormone replacement therapy, *endometrial hyperplasia,* and *estrogen-producing tumors.*

Discharge may accompany vaginitis or cervicitis. See Table 14-6, Vaginal Discharge, p. 550.

Use a wooden spatula or endocervical brush to obtain endocervical cells for the Pap smear. A blind swab may be indicated if the atrophic vagina is too small.

See Table 14-7, Positions of the Uterus, p. 551, and Table 14-8, Abnormalities of the Uterus, p. 552.

After removing the speculum, ask the patient to bear down to detect uterine prolapse, cystocele, urethrocele, or rectocele.

Perform the bimanual examination. Check for motion of the cervix and for any uterine or adnexal masses.

Mobility of the cervix is restricted with inflammation, malignancy, or surgical adhesion. Enlarging uterine fibroids, or leiomyomas, in *malignant leiomyosarcoma;* palpable ovaries in *ovarian cancer*

Perform the rectovaginal examination. Assess for uterine and adnexal irregularities through the anterior rectal wall, and for rectal masses. Change gloves first if blood from the bimanual examination is on the vaginal examining glove to obtain an accurate stool sample.

A uterus that is enlarged, fixed, or irregular may indicate adhesions or possible malignancy. Rectal masses are found in *colon cancer.*

Male Genitalia and Prostate.
Examine the penis, retracting the foreskin if present. Examine the scrotum, testes, and epididymis.

Findings include smegma, penile cancer, and scrotal hydroceles.

Proceed with the rectal examination, paying special attention to any rectal masses and any nodularity or masses of the prostate. Note that the anterior and median lobes of the prostate are inaccessible to rectal palpation, limiting the utility of the digital rectal examination for detecting prostate enlargement or possible malignancy.

Rectal masses are found in *colon cancer. Prostate hyperplasia* may be linked with enlargement; *prostate cancer* is possible with nodules or masses.

Musculoskeletal System.
Begin your evaluation with the 10-Minute Geriatric Screener (p. 914). If you find joint deformity, deficits in mobility, or pain with movement, conduct a more thorough examination. Review the techniques for examining individual joints in Chapter 16, The Musculoskeletal System.

Degenerative joint changes in *osteoarthritis;* joint inflammation in *rheumatoid* or *gouty arthritis.*

See Chapter 16, The Musculoskeletal System; see Tables 16-1 to 16-10, pp. 642–643.

Nervous System.
As with the musculoskeletal examination, begin your evaluation of the nervous system with the 10-Minute Geriatric Screener (p. 914).

Pursue further examination if you note any deficits. Focus especially on memory and affect.

Learn to distinguish delirium from depression and dementia (see Table 20-1). Careful search for underlying causes is warranted.[98] See Table 20-3, Screening for Dementia: The Mini-Cog, p. 932.

Also pay close attention to gait and balance, particularly standing balance; timed 8-foot walk; stride characteristics like width, pace, and length of stride; and careful turning.

Abnormalities of gait and balance, especially widening of base, slowing and lengthening of stride, and difficulty turning, are correlated with risk for falls.[99–101]

Note that standard neuromuscular tests have not been shown to predict impairments in mobility.[102] Further, although neurologic abnormalities are common in the older population, their prevalence without identifiable disease increases with age, ranging from 30% to 50%.[103] Examples of age-related abnormalities include unequal pupil size, decreased arm swing and spontaneous movements, increased leg rigidity and abnormal gait, presence of the snout and grasp reflexes, and decreased toe vibratory sense.

Search for evidence of tremor, rigidity, bradykinesia, micrographia, shuffling gait, and difficulty turning in bed, opening jars, and rising from a chair.

These findings are seen in *Parkinson's disease,* found in 1% of adults 65 years or older and 2% of those 85 years or older.[104,105] Tremor is of slow frequency and occurs at rest, with a "pill-rolling" quality. It is aggravated by stress and inhibited during sleep or movement. *Essential tremor* if bilateral and symmetric, with positive family history, and if diminished by alcohol.

Persistent blinking after glabellar tap and difficulty walking heel-to-toe in *Parkinson's disease* are also more common.

RECORDING YOUR FINDINGS

Note that initially you may use sentences to describe your findings; later you will use phrases. The style below contains phrases appropriate for most write-ups. As you read through this physical examination, you will notice some atypical findings. Try to test yourself. See if you can interpret these findings in the context of all you have learned about the examination of the older adult.

See Table 20-4, Managing Older Adults: The Siebens Domain Management Model, p. 933, for an alternative way to organize the record and patient care.

Recording the Physical Examination—The Older Adult

Mr. J is an older adult who appears healthy but underweight, with good muscle bulk. He is alert and interactive, with good recall of his life history. He is accompanied by his son.

Vital Signs: Ht (without shoes) 160 cm (5'). Wt (dressed) 65 kg (143 lbs). BMI 28. BP 145/88 right arm, supine; 154/94 left arm, supine. Heart rate (HR) 98 and regular. Respiratory rate (RR) 18. Temperature (oral) 98.6°F.

10-Minute Geriatric Screener   (see p. 914)

Vision: Patient reports difficulty reading. Visual acuity 20/60 on Snellen chart.

Needs further evaluation for glasses and possibly hearing aid.

Hearing: Cannot hear whispered voice in either ear. Cannot hear 1,000 or 2,000 Hz with audioscope in either ear.

Leg Mobility: Can walk 20 feet briskly, turn, walk back to chair, and sit down in 14 seconds.

Urinary Incontinence: Has lost urine and gotten wet on 20 separate days.

Needs further evaluation for incontinence, including "DIAPER" assessment (see p. 913), prostate examination, and postvoid residual, which is normally ≤ 50 ml (requires bladder catheterization).

Nutrition: Has lost 15 lbs over the past 6 months without trying.

Needs nutritional screen, p. 906.

Memory: Can remember three items after 1 minute.

Depression: Does not often feel sad or depressed.

Physical Disability: Can walk fast but cannot ride a bicycle. Can do moderate but not heavy work around the house. Can go shopping for groceries or clothes. Can get to places out of walking distance. Can bathe each day without difficulty. Can dress, including buttoning and zipping, and can put on shoes.

Consider exercise regimen with strength training.

(continued)

Physical Examination

Skin.   Warm and moist. Nails without clubbing or cyanosis. Hair thinning at crown.

Head, Eyes, Ears, Nose, Throat (HEENT).   Scalp without lesions. Skull NC/AT. Conjunctiva pink, sclera muddy. Pupils 2 mm constricting to 1 mm, round, regular, equally reactive to light and accommodation. Extraocular movements intact. Disc margins sharp, without hemorrhages or exudates. Mild arteriolar narrowing. TMs with good cone of light. Weber midline. AC ≥ BC. Nasal mucosa pink. No sinus tenderness. Oral mucosa pink. Dentition fair. Caries present. Tongue midline, slight beefy redness. Pharynx without exudates.

Neck.   Supple. Trachea midline. Thyroid lobes slightly enlarged, no nodules.

Lymph Nodes.   No cervical, axillary, epitrochlear, or inguinal lymph nodes.

Thorax and Lungs.   Thorax symmetric. Kyphosis noted. Lungs resonant with good excursion. Breath sounds vesicular. Diaphragms descend 4 cm bilaterally.

Cardiovascular.   JVP 6 cm above the left atrium. Carotid upstrokes brisk, without bruits. PMI tapping, in the 5th ICS, 9 cm lateral to the midsternal line. II/VI harsh holosystolic murmur at the apex, radiating to the axilla. No S_3, S_4, or other murmurs.

Abdomen.   Scaphoid, with active bowel sounds. Soft, nontender. No masses or hepatosplenomegaly. Liver span 7 cm in right midclavicular line; edge smooth and palpable at the RCM. No CVAT.

Genitourinary.   Circumcised male. No penile lesions. Testes descended bilaterally, smooth.

Rectal.   Rectal vault without masses. Stool brown, negative for occult blood.

Extremities.   Warm and without edema. Calves supple.

Peripheral Vascular.   Pulses 2+ and symmetric.

Musculoskeletal.   Mild degenerative changes at the knees, with quadriceps wasting. Good range of motion in all joints.

Neurological.   Oriented to person, place, and time. Mini-Mental State: score 29. Cranial Nerves II–XII intact. Motor: Decreased quadriceps bulk. Tone intact. Strength 4/5 throughout. RAMs, finger-to-nose intact. Gait with widened base. Sensation intact to pinprick, light touch, position, and vibration. Romberg negative. Reflexes 2+ and symmetric, with plantar response downgoing.

BIBLIOGRAPHY

CITATIONS

1. Administration on Aging, Department of Health and Human Services. Statistics: A Profile on Older Americans 2007. Available at: http://www.aoa.gov/prof/Statistics/profile/2007/3.asp. See also Statistics on Aging. Available at: http://agingstats.gov/agingstatsdotnet/Main_Site/Data/2006_Documents/Population.pdf. Accessed February 19, 2008.

2. Fries JF. Measuring and monitoring success in compressing morbidity. Ann Intern Med Suppl139(5):455, 2003.

3. Bodenheimer T, Wagner EH, Grumbach K. Improving primary care for patients with chronic illness. JAMA 288(14):1775–1779, 2002.

4. Geriatrics Interdisciplinary Advisory Group, American Geriatrics Society. Interdisciplinary care for older adults with complex needs: American Geriatrics Society Position Statement. J Am Geriatr Soc 54(5):849–852, 2006.

5. Perls TT. Understanding the determinants of exceptional longevity. Ann Intern Med Suppl 139(5):445, 2003.

6. Perls TT, Kunkel LM, Puca AA. The genetics of exceptional human longevity. J Am Geriatr Soc 50:359–368, 2002.

7. Rowe JW, Kahn RL. Human aging: usual and successful. Science 237:143–149, 1987.

8. Taffet GE. Physiology of aging. In: Cassel CK, Leipzig RM, Cohen HJ, et al., eds. Geriatric Medicine, 4th ed. New York: Springer, 2003:27–36.

9. Mulligan T, Saddiqi W. Changes in male sexuality. In: Cassel CK, Leipzig RM, Cohen HJ, et al., eds. Geriatric Medicine, 4th ed. New York: Springer, 2003: 719–726.

10. Kaiser FE. Sexual function and the older woman. In: Cassel CK, Leipzig RM, Cohen HJ, et al, eds. Geriatric Medicine, 4th ed. New York: Springer, 2003: 727–736.

11. DuBeau CE. Benign prostatic hyperplasia. In: Cassel CK, Leipzig RM, Cohen HJ, et al., eds. Geriatric Medicine, 4th ed. New York: Springer, 2003: 755–768.

12. Tangarorang GL, Kerins GJ, Besdine RW. Clinical approach to the older patient: an overview. In: Cassel CK, Leipzig RM, Cohen HJ, et al., eds. Geriatric Medicine, 4th ed. New York: Springer, 2003:149–162.

13. Bayer AJ, Chadna JS, Farag RR, et al. Changing presentation of myocardial infarction with increasing old age. J Am Geriatr Soc 34:263–266, 1986.

14. Trivalle C, Doucet J, Chassagrie P, et al. Differences in the signs and symptoms of hyperthyroidism in older and younger patients. J Am Geriatr Soc 44:50–53, 1996.

15. Doucet J, Trivalle C, Chassagrie P, et al. Does age play a role in clinical presentation of hypothyroidism? J Am Geriatr Soc 42:984–986, 1994.

16. Cigolle CT, Langa KM, Kabeto MU, et al. Geriatric conditions and disability: the health and retirement study. Ann Intern Med 147(3):156–164, 2007.

17. Tinetti ME, Williams CS, Gill TM. Dizziness among older adults: a possible geriatric syndrome. Ann Intern Med 132(5):337–344, 2000.

18. Fried LP, Sotrer DJ, King DE, et al. Diagnosis of illness presentation in the elderly. J Am Geriatr Soc 39:117–123, 1991.

19. Davis PB, Robins LN. History-taking in the elderly with and without cognitive impairment. J Am Geriatr Soc 37:249–255, 1989.

20. Ferraro KF, Su YP. Physician-evaluated and self-reported morbidity for predicting disability. Am J Public Health 90(1):103–108, 2000.

21. Kuczmarski MF, Kuczmarski RJ, Najjar M. Effects of age on validity of self-reported height, weight and body mass index: findings from the third National Health and Nutrition Examination Survey, 1988–1994. J Am Diet Assoc 101(1):28–34, 2001.

22. Lagaay AM, van der Meij JC, Hijmans W. Validation of medical history taking as part of a population based survey in subjects aged 85 and over. BMJ 304:1091–1092, 1992.

23. Kobylarz FA, Heath JM, Lide RC. The ETHNIC(S) mnemonic: a clinical tool for ethnogeriatric education. J Am Geriatr Soc 50(9):1582–1589, 2002.

24. Nunez GR. Culture, demographics, and critical care issues: an overview. Crit Care Clin 19:619–639, 2003.

25. Xakellis G, Brangman SA, Ladson H, et al. Curricular framework: core competencies in multicultural geriatric care. J Am Geriatr Soc 52(1):137–142, 2004.

26. Goldstein MZ, Griswold K. Practical geriatrics: cultural sensitivity and aging. Psychiatric Serv 49:769–771, 1998.

27. Lee SJ, Moody-Ayers SY, Landfeld CS, et al. The relationship between self-rated health and mortality in older black and white Americans. J Am Geriatr Soc 55(10):1624–1629, 2007.

28. Sudore RL, Mehta KM, Simonsick EM, et al. Limited literacy in older people and disparities in health and healthcare access. J Am Geriatr Soc 54(5):770–776, 2006.

29. Fick DM, Cooper JW, Wade WE, et al. Updating the Beers criteria for potentially inappropriate medication use in older adults: results of a US consensus panel of experts. Arch Intern Med 163:2716–2724, 2003.

30. Reuben DB, Herr KA, Pacala JT, et al. Geriatrics at Your Fingertips, 6th ed. Malden, MA: Blackwell Science, Inc., for the American Geriatrics Society, 2004:9–12.

31. Takahashi PY, Okhravi HR, Lim LS, et al. Preventive health care in the elderly population: a guide for practicing physicians. Mayo Clinic Proc 79:416–427, 2004.

32. Corti MC, Guralnik JM, Salive ME, et al. Serum albumin level and physical disability as predictors of mortality in older persons. JAMA 272(13):1036–1042, 1994.

33. Ferrell BA. Acute and chronic pain. In: Cassel CK, Leipzig RM, Cohen HJ, et al., eds. Geriatric Medicine, 4th ed. New York: Springer, 2003:323–342.

34. American Geriatrics Society Panel of Persistent Pain in Older Persons, American Geriatrics Society. The management of persistent pain in older persons. JAGS 50(6 Suppl):S205–S224, 2002. Available at: http://www.americangeriatrics.org/products/positionpapers/JGS5071.pdf. Accessed February 23, 2008.

35. Charlton JE, ed. Core Curriculum for Professional Education in Pain, 3rd ed. Seattle: International Association for the Study of Pain, 2005. Available at: http//www.iasp-pain.org/AM/

Template.cfm?Section=Publications&Template=/CM/HTMLDisplay.cfm&ContentID=2307#TOC. Accessed June 9, 2008.

36. American Medical Association. Pain Management Module 5: Assessing and Treating Pain in Older Adults. Available at: http://www.ama-cmeonline.com/pain_mgmt/module05/index.htm. Accessed February 23, 2008.

37. Jones TV, Lindsey BA, Yount P, et al. Alcoholism screening questionnaires: are they valid in elderly medical outpatients? J Gen Intern Med 8(12):674–678, 1993.

38. Callahan CM, Tierney WM. Health services use and mortality among older primary care patients with alcoholism. J Am Geriatr Soc 43(12):1378–1383, 1995.

39. American Geriatrics Society. Screening recommendation: clinical guidelines for alcohol use disorders in older adults. Available at: http://www.americangeriatrics.org/products/position papers/alcohol.shtml. Accessed February 23, 2008.

40. Tulsky JA. Doctor-patient communication issues. In: Cassel CK, Leipzig RM, Cohen HJ, et al., eds. Geriatric Medicine, 4th ed. New York: Springer, 2003:287–298.

41. Callahan D. The value of achieving a peaceful death. In: Cassel CK, Leipzig RM, Cohen HJ, et al., eds. Geriatric Medicine, 4th ed. New York: Springer, 2003:351–360.

42. Morrison RS, Meier DE. Clinical practice: palliative care. N Engl J Med 350(25):2582–2590, 2004.

43. Beck LH. Periodic health examination and screening tests in adults. Hosp Pract 15:121–126, 1999.

44. American Geriatrics Society Ethics Committee, American Geriatrics Society. Health screening decisions for older adults: AGS Position Paper. J Am Geriatr Soc 51(2):211–270, 2003. Available at http://www.americangeriatrics.org/products/positionpapers/stopscreening.shtml. Accessed February 23, 2008.

45. Bogardus ST, Yueh B, Shekelle PG. Screening and management of adult hearing loss in primary care: clinical applications. JAMA 289(15):1986–1990, 2003.

46. Nelson ME, Rejeski WJ, Blair SN, et al., American College of Sports Medicine, American Heart Association. Physical activity and public health in older adults: recommendation from the American College of Sports Medicine and the American Heart Association. Circulation 116(9):1094–1105, 2007.

47. Centers for Disease Control and Prevention (CDC). Recommended adult immunization schedule. October 2007–September 2008. http://www.cdc.gov/vaccines/recs/schedules/downloads/adult/07-08/adult-schedule-11x17.pdf. Accessed February 24, 2008.

48. Centers for Disease Control and Prevention (CDC). Vaccines and Immunizations. Recommendations and guidelines. Adult immunization schedule. Updated January 2008. Available at: http://www.cdc.gov/vaccines/recs/schedules/adult-schedule.htm#chgs. Accessed February 24, 2008.

49. Nichol KL, Nordin JD, Nelson DB, et al. Effectiveness of influenza vaccine in the community-dwelling elderly. N Engl J Med 357(14):1373–1381, 2007.

50. Oxman MN, Levin MJ, Johnson GR, et al. A vaccine to prevent herpes zoster and postherpetic neuralgia in older adults. N Engl J Med 352(22):2271–2284, 2005.

51. U.S. Consumer Product Safety Commission. Special Report: Emergency Room Injuries—Adults 65 and Older. 2002. Available at: http://www.nsc.org/public/issues/CPSCSafety Report.pdf. Accessed February 23, 2008.

52. Oddone EZ, Heflin MT, Feussner JR. Screening for cancer. In: Cassel CK, Leipzig RM, Cohen HJ, et al., eds. Geriatric Medicine, 4th ed. New York: Springer, 2003:375–392.

53. Unutzer J. Late-life depression. N Engl J Med 357(22):2269–2276, 2007.

54. U.S. Preventive Services Task Force. Screening for dementia: recommendations and rationale. June 2003. Rockville, MD: Agency for Healthcare Research and Quality. Available at: http://www.ahrq.gov/clinic/3rduspstf/dementia/dementrr.htm. Accessed February 23, 2008.

55. Cummings JL. Alzheimer's disease. N Engl J Med 351(1):56–67, 2004.

56. Small BJ, Gagnon E, Robinson B. Early identification of cognitive deficits: preclinical Alzheimer's disease and mild cognitive impairment. Geriatrics 62(4):19–23, 2007.

57. Karlawish JHT, Clark CM. Diagnostic evaluation of elderly patients with mild memory problems. Ann Intern Med 138(5):411–419, 2003.

58. Budson AE, Price BH. Memory dysfunction. N Engl J Med 352(7):692–699, 2005.

59. Tschanz JT, Weklsg-Bohmer KA, Lyketsos CG, et al. Conversion to dementia from mild cognitive disorder: the Cache County Study. Neurology 67(2):229–234, 2006.

60. Boyle PA, Wilson RS, Aggarwal NT, et al. Mild cognitive impairment: risk of Alzheimer's disease and rate of cognitive decline. Neurology 67(3):441–445, 2006.

61. Busse A, Hensel A, Guhne U, et al. Mild cognitive impairment: long-term course of four clinical subtypes. Neurology 67(12):2176–2185, 2006.

62. Dyer CB, Pickens S, Burnett J. Vulnerable elders: when it is no longer safe to live alone. JAMA 298(12):1448–1450, 2007.

63. Fulmer T, Guadagno L, Dyer CB, et al. Progress in elder abuse screening and assessment instruments. J Am Geriatr Soc 52:297–304, 2004.

64. Fulmer T, Hernandez M. Elder mistreatment. In: Cassel CK, Leipzig RM, Cohen HJ, et al., eds. Geriatric Medicine, 4th ed. New York: Springer, 2003:1057–1066.

65. Koretz B, Reuben DB. Instruments to assess functional status. Also see Reuben DB. Comprehensive geriatric assessment and systems approaches to geriatric care. In: Cassel CK, Leipzig RM, Cohen HJ, et al., eds. Geriatric Medicine, 4th ed. New York: Springer, 2003:185–204.

66. Moore AA, Siu AL. Screening for common problems in ambulatory elderly: clinical confirmation of a screening instrument. Am J Med 100:438–440, 1996.

67. Resnick NM. Urinary incontinence. In: Cassel CK, Leipzig RM, Cohen HJ, et al., eds. Geriatric Medicine, 4th ed. New York: Springer, 2003:931–956.

68. American Geriatrics Society. Urinary incontinence in older adults: management in primary practice. Contributors to incontinence. Available at: http://www.americangeriatrics.org/education/urinary_incontinence.shtml. Accessed February 23, 2008.

69. Ganz DA, Bao Y, Shekelle PG, et al. Will my patient fall? JAMA 297(1):77–86, 2007.

70. Montero-Odasso M, Schapira M, Soriano ER, et al. Simple gait velocity assessment predicts adverse events in healthy

seniors aged 75 years and older. J Gerontol A Biol Sci Med Sci 60(10):1304–1309, 2005.

71. Tinetti ME. Preventing falls in elderly persons. N Engl J Med 348(1):42–48, 2003.

72. Borson S, Scanlan J, Brush M, et al. The Mini-Cog: a cognitive "vital signs" measure for dementia screening in multi-lingual elderly. Int J Geriatric Psychiatry 15(11):1021–1027, 2000.

73. Borson S, Scanlan JM, Chen P, et al. The Mini-Cog as a screen for dementia: validation in a population-based sample. J Am Geriatr Soc 51(10):1451–1454, 2003.

74. Bulpitt CJ, Beckett NS, Cooke J, et al. Results of the pilot study for the hypertension in the very elderly trial. J Hypertens 21(12):2409–2417, 2003.

75. Oates DJ, Berlowitz DR, Glickman ME, et al. Blood pressure and survival in the oldest old. J Am Geriatr Soc 55(3):383–388, 2007.

76. Lloyd-Jones DM, Evans JC, Levy D. Hypertension in adults across the age spectrum: current outcomes and control in the community. JAMA 294(4):466–472, 2005.

77. Bobrie G, Genes N, Vaur L, et al. Is "isolated home" hypertension as opposed to "isolated office" hypertension a sign of greater cardiovascular risk? Arch Intern Med 161(18):2205–2211, 2001.

78. Chaudhry SI, Krumholz HM, Foody JM. Systolic hypertension in older persons. JAMA 292(9):1074–1080, 2004.

79. Papademetriou V. Comparative prognostic value of systolic, diastolic, and pulse pressure. Am J Cardiol 91(4):433–435, 2003.

80. Vaccarino V, Berger AK, et al. Pulse pressure and risk of cardiovascular events in the systolic hypertension in the elderly program. Am J Cardiol 88(9):980–986, 2001.

81. Carlson JE. Assessment of orthostatic blood pressure: measurement technique and clinical applications. South Med J 92(2):167–173, 1999.

82. Consensus Committee of the American Autonomic Society and the American Academy of Neurology. Consensus statement on the definition of orthostatic hypotension, pure autonomic failure, and multiple system atrophy. Neurology 46(5):1470, 1996.

83. McGee S, Abernethy WB, Simel DL. Is this patient hypovolemic? JAMA 281(11):1022–1029, 1999.

84. Ooi WL, Barrett S, Hossain M, et al. Patterns of orthostatic blood pressure change and their clinical correlates in a frail elderly population. JAMA 277(16):1299–1304, 1997.

85. Raiha I, Luntonen S, Piha J, et al. Prevalence, predisposing factors and prognostic importance of postural hypotension. Arch Intern Med 155(9):930–935, 1995.

86. Gnann JW, Whitely RJ. Herpes zoster. N Engl J Med 347(5):340–346, 2002.

87. Congdon NG, Friedman DS, Lietman T. Important causes of visual impairment in the world today. JAMA 290(15):2057–2060, 2003.

88. Freidman DS, Jampel HD, Munoz B, et al. The prevalence of open-angle glaucoma among blacks and whites 73 years and older: the Salisbury Eye Evaluation Glaucoma Study. Arch Ophthalmol 124(11):1625–1630, 2006.

89. Ragia A, Thavendiranathan P, Detsky AS. Does this patient have hearing impairment? JAMA 295(4):416–428, 2006.

90. Swan IRC, Browning GG. The whispered voice as a screening test for hearing impairment. J Royal Col Gen Pract 35:197, 1985.

91. Gordon SR, Jahnigen DW. Oral assessment of the dentulous elderly patient. J Am Geriatr Soc 34:276–281, 1986.

92. Otto CM, Lind BK, Kitzman DW, et al. Association of aortic-valve sclerosis with cardiovascular mortality and morbidity in the elderly. JAMA 341(3):142–147, 1999.

93. Leach RM, McBrien DJ. Brachiocardial delay: a new clinical indicator of the severity of aortic stenosis. Lancet 335(8699):1199–1201, 1990.

94. McDermott MM, Greenland P, Liu K, et al. The ankle brachial index is associated with leg function and physical activity: the walking and leg circulation study. Ann Intern Med 136(12):873–883, 2002.

95. Dumesic DA. Pelvic examination: what to focus on in menopausal women. Consultant 36:39–46, 1996.

96. American Geriatrics Society. Screening for cervical carcinoma in older women. J Am Geriatr Soc 49(5):655–657, 2001.

97. Hoffman MS, Cardosi RD, Roberts WS, et al. Accuracy of pelvic examination in the assessment of patients with operable cervical cancer. Am J Obstet Gynecol 190(4):986–993, 2004.

98. Holsinger T, Deveau J, Boustani M, et al. Does this patient have dementia? JAMA 297(21):2391–2404, 2007.

99. Baloh RW, Ying SH, Jacobson KM. A longitudinal study of gait and balance dysfunction in normal older people. Arch Neurol 60:835–839, 2003.

100. Guralnik JM, Ferrucci L, Simonsek E et al. Lower extremity function in persons over the age of 70 years as a predictor of subsequent disability. N Engl J Med 332(9):556–561, 1995.

101. Tinetti ME, Williams TF, Mayewski R. Fall risk index for elderly patients based on number of chronic disabilities. Am J Med 80(3):429–434, 1986.

102. Tinetti ME, Ginter SF. Identifying mobility dysfunctions in elderly patients. JAMA 259(8):1190–1193, 1988.

103. Odenheimer G, Funkenstein HH, Beckett L, et al. Comparison of neurologic changes in 'successfully aging' persons vs. the total aging population. Arch Neurol 51(6):573–580, 1994.

104. Rao G, Fisch L, Srinivasan S, et al. Does this patient have Parkinson disease? JAMA 289(3):347–353, 2003.

105. Nutt JG, Wooten GF. Diagnosis and initial management of Parkinson's disease. N Engl J Med 353(10):1021–1027, 2005.

ADDITIONAL REFERENCES

Ahmed A. Clinical manifestations, diagnostic assessment, and etiology of heart failure in older adults. Clin Geriatr Med 23:11–30, 2007.

American Geriatrics Society. Available at: http://www.american geriatrics.org. Accessed June 22, 2008.

American Geriatrics Society, Ethnogeriatrics Steering Committee. Doorway Thoughts: Cross-cultural Health Care for Older Adults. Sudbury, MA: Jones and Bartlett, 2004.

Amin SH, Kuhle CL, Fitzpatrick LA. Comprehensive evaluation of the older woman. Mayo Clin Proc 78(9):1157–1185, 2003.

Beckett NS, Peters R, Fletcher AE, et al., for the HYVET Study Group. Treatment of hypertension in patients 80 years of age or older. N Engl J Med 78(9):1887–1898, 2008.

Burks K. Osteoarthritis in older adults: current treatments. J Gerontol Nurs 31(5):11–19, 2005.

Cassel CK. Geriatric Medicine: An Evidence-based Approach, 4th ed. New York: Springer, 2003.

Carolan Doerflinger DM. How to try this: the mini-cog. Am J Nurs 107(12):62–71, 2007.

Chobanion AV. Isolated systolic hypertension in the elderly. N Engl J Med 357(80):789–796, 2007.

Clark CM, Karlawish JHT. Alzheimer disease: current concepts and emerging diagnostic and therapeutic strategies. Ann Intern Med 138(5):400–410, 2003.

Donowitz GR, Cox HL. Bacterial community-acquired pneumonia in older patients. Clin Geriatr Med 23(5):515–534, 2007.

Ene-Stroescu D, Gorbien MJ. Gouty arthritis: a primer on late-onset gout. Geriatrics 60(7):24–31, 2005.

Gupta V, Lipsitz LA. Orthostatic hypotension in the elderly: diagnosis and treatment. Am J Med 120(10):841–847, 2007.

Hazzard WR. Principles of Geriatric Medicine and Gerontology, 5th ed. New York: McGraw-Hill/Professional, 2003.

Inouye SK. Delirium in older persons. N Engl J Med 354(11):1157–1165, 2006.

Kales HC, Mellow AM. Race and depression: does race affect the diagnosis and treatment of late-life depression? Geriatrics 61(5):18–21, 2006.

Karlawish JHT, Clark CM. Diagnostic evaluation of elderly patients with mild memory problems. Ann Intern Med 138(5):411–419, 2003.

Kennedy-Malone L, Fletcher KR, Plank LR. Management Guidelines for Nurse Practitioners Working with Older Adults, 2nd ed. Philadelphia: FA Davis, 2004.

Khan AA, Hodsman AB, Papaioannou A, et al. Management of osteoporosis in men: an update and case example. CMAJ 176(3):345–348, 2007.

Kobylarz FA, Pomidor A, Heath JM. SPEAK: a mnemonic tool for addressing health literacy concerns in geriatric clinical encounters. Geriatrics 61(7):20–26, 2006.

Landefeld CS. Current Geriatric Diagnosis & Treatment. New York: Lange Medical Books–McGraw-Hill, 2004.

Meldon SW, Ma OJ, Woolard R, for American College of Emergency Physicians. Geriatric Emergency Medicine. New York: McGraw-Hill, 2004.

Moylan KC, Binder EF. Falls in older adults: risk assessment, management and prevention. Am J Med 120(6):493–497, 2007.

Morrison LJ, Morrison RS. Palliative care and pain management. Med Clin North Am 90(5):983–1004, 2006.

Nakasato YR, Carnes BA. Health promotion in older adults: promoting successful aging in primary care settings. Geriatrics 61(4):27–31, 2006.

Norton P, Brubaker L. Urinary incontinence in women. Lancet 367(9504):57–67, 2006.

Nusbaum MR, Lenahan P, Sadovsky R. Sexual health in aging men and women: addressing the physiologic and psychological sexual changes that occur with age. Geriatrics 60(9):18–23, 2005.

Scalf LA, Shenefelt PD. Contact dermatitis: diagnosing and treating skin conditions in the elderly. Geriatrics 62(6):14–19, 2007.

Small BJ, Gagnon E, Robinson B. Early identification of cognitive deficits: preclinical Alzheimer's disease and mild cognitive impairment. Geriatrics 62(4):19–23, 2007.

Springhouse Corporation, ed. Handbook of Geriatric Nursing Care, 2nd ed. Philadelphia: Lippincott Williams & Wilkins, 2002.

Staats DO. Preventing injury in older adults. Geriatrics 63(4):12–17, 2008.

Villareal DT, Apovian CM, Kushner RF, et al. Obesity in older adults: technical review and position statement of the American Society for Nutrition and NAASO, The Obesity Society. Am J Clin Nutr 82(5):923–934, 2005.

Vistamehr S, Shelsta HN, Pammisano PC, et al. Glaucoma screening in a high-risk population. J Glaucoma 15(6):534–540, 2006.

Walter LC, Lewis CL, Barton MB. Screening for colorectal, breast, and cervical cancer in the elderly: a review of the evidence. Am J Med 118(10):1078–1086, 2005.

Weiner DK. Office management of chronic pain in the elderly. Am J Med 120(4):306–315, 2007.

Wolkove N, Elkholy O, Baltzan M, et al. Sleep and aging: sleep disorders commonly found in older people. CMAJ 176(9):1299–1304, 2007.

The Bates' suite offers these additional resources to enhance learning and facilitate understanding of this chapter:

- Bates' Pocket Guide to Physical Examination and History Taking, 6th edition
- Bates' Nursing Online
- Bates' Visual Guide to Physical Examination, 4th edition
- thePoint online resources, http://thepoint.lww.com
- Student CD-ROM included with the book

TABLE
20-1

Minimum Geriatric Competencies*

Medication Management

1 Explain impact of age-related changes on drug selection and dose based on knowledge of age-related changes in renal and hepatic function, body composition, and Central Nervous System sensitivity.

2 Identify medications, including anticholinergic, psychoactive, anticoagulant, analgesic, hypoglycemic, and cardiovascular drugs that should be avoided or used with caution in older adults and explain the potential problems associated with each.

3 Document a patient's complete medication list, including prescribed, herbal and over-the-counter medications, and for each medication provide the dose, frequency, indication, benefit, side effects, and an assessment of adherence.

Cognitive and Behavioral Disorders

4 Define and distinguish among the clinical presentations of delirium, dementia, and depression.

5 Formulate a differential diagnosis and implement initial evaluation in a patient who exhibits cognitive impairment.

6 Urgently initiate a diagnostic workup to determine the root cause (etiology) of delirium in an older patient.

7 Perform and interpret a cognitive assessment in older patients for whom there are concerns regarding memory or function.

8 Develop an evaluation and nonpharmacologic management plan for agitated, demented, or delirious patients.

Self-Care Capacity

9 Assess and describe baseline and current functional abilities (instrumental activities of daily living, activities of daily living, and special senses) in an older patient by collecting historical data from multiple sources and performing a confirmatory physical examination.

10 Develop a preliminary management plan for patients presenting with functional deficits, including adaptive interventions and involvement of interdisciplinary team members from appropriate disciplines, such as social work, nursing, rehabilitation, nutrition, and pharmacy.

11 Identify and assess safety risks in the home environment, and make recommendations to mitigate these.

Falls, Balance, Gait Disorders

12 Ask all patients >65 years, or their caregivers, about falls in the last year, watch the patient rise from a chair and walk (or transfer), then record and interpret the findings.

13 For a patient who has fallen, construct a differential diagnosis and evaluation plan that addresses the multiple etiologies identified by history, physical examination, and functional assessment.

Health Care Planning and Promotion

14 Define and differentiate among types of code status, health care proxies, and advanced directives in the site where one is training.

15 Accurately identify clinical situations where life expectancy, functional status, patient preference, or goals of care should override standard recommendations for screening tests in older adults.

16 Accurately identify clinical situations where life expectancy, functional status, patient preference, or goals of care should override standard recommendations for treatment in older adults.

Atypical Presentation of Disease

17 Identify at least 3 physiologic changes of aging for each organ system and their impact on the patient, including their contribution to homeostenosis (the age-related narrowing or homeostatic reserve mechanisms).

18 Generate a differential diagnosis based on recognition of the unique presentations of common conditions in older adults, including acute coronary syndrome, dehydration, urinary tract infection, acute abdomen, and pneumonia.

Palliative Care

19 Assess and provide initial management of pain and key nonpain symptoms based on patient's goals of care.

20 Identify the psychological, social, and spiritual needs of patients with advanced illness and their family members, and link these identified needs with the appropriate interdisciplinary team members.

21 Present palliative care (including hospice) as a positive, active treatment option for a patient with advanced disease.

Hospital Care for Elders

22 Identify potential hazards of hospitalization for all older adult patients (including immobility, delirium, medication side effects, malnutrition, pressure ulcers, procedures, peri- and postoperative periods, and hospital acquired infections) and identify potential prevention strategies.

23 Explain the risks, indications, alternatives, and contraindications for indwelling (Foley) catheter use in the older adult patient.

24 Explain the risks, indications, alternatives, and contraindications for physical and pharmacologic restraint use.

25 Communicate the key components of a safe discharge plan (e.g., accurate medication list, plan for follow-up), including comparing/contrasting potential sites for discharge.

26 Conduct a surveillance examination of areas of the skin at high risk for pressure ulcers and describe existing ulcers.

---

* These pertain primarily to medical students but are generalizable to the health care team.

(Source: Association of American Medical Colleges/John A. Hartford Foundation, Inc. A Consensus Conference on Competencies in Geriatrics Education, October 5, 2007.)

TABLE
20-2

Delirium and Dementia

Delirium and dementia are common and very important disorders that affect multiple aspects of mental status. Both have many possible causes. Some clinical features of these two conditions and their effects on mental status are compared below. A delirium may be superimposed on dementia.

	Delirium	Dementia
Clinical Features		
Onset	Acute	Insidious
Course	Fluctuating, with lucid intervals; worse at night	Slowly progressive
Duration	Hours to weeks	Months to years
Sleep/Wake Cycle	Always disrupted	Sleep fragmented
General Medical Illness or Drug Toxicity	Either or both present	Often absent, especially in Alzheimer's disease
Mental Status		
Level of Consciousness	Disturbed. Person less clearly aware of the environment and less able to focus, sustain, or shift attention	Usually normal until late in the course of the illness
Behavior	Activity often abnormally decreased (somnolence) or increased (agitation, hypervigilance)	Normal to slow; may become inappropriate
Speech	May be hesitant, slow or rapid, incoherent	Difficulty in finding words, aphasia
Mood	Fluctuating, labile, from fearful or irritable to normal or depressed	Often flat, depressed
Thought Processes	Disorganized, may be incoherent	Impoverished. Speech gives little information.
Thought Content	Delusions common, often transient	Delusions may occur.
Perceptions	Illusions, hallucinations, most often visual	Hallucinations may occur.
Judgment	Impaired, often to a varying degree	Increasingly impaired over the course of the illness
Orientation	Usually disoriented, especially for time. A known place may seem unfamiliar.	Fairly well maintained, but becomes impaired in the later stages of illness
Attention	Fluctuates. Person easily distracted, unable to concentrate on selected tasks	Usually unaffected until late in the illness
Memory	Immediate and recent memory impaired	Recent memory and new learning especially impaired
Examples of Cause	Delirium tremens (due to withdrawal from alcohol) Uremia Acute hepatic failure Acute cerebral vasculitis Atropine poisoning	*Reversible:* Vitamin B_{12} deficiency, thyroid disorders *Irreversible:* Alzheimer's disease, vascular dementia (from multiple infarcts), dementia due to head trauma

Screening for Dementia: The Mini-Cog

Administration

The test is administered as follows:

1. Instruct the patient to listen carefully to and remember 3 unrelated words and then to repeat the words.

2. Instruct the patient to draw the face of a clock, either on a blank sheet of paper or on a sheet with the clock circle already drawn on the page. After the patient puts the numbers on the clock face, ask him or her to draw the hands of the clock to read a specific time.

3. Ask the patient to repeat the 3 previously stated words.

Scoring

Give 1 point for each recalled word after the clock drawing test (CDT) distractor.

Patients recalling none of the three words are classified as demented (Score = 0).

Patients recalling all three words are classified as nondemented (Score = 3).

Patients with intermediate word recall of 1–2 words are classified based on the CDT (Abnormal = demented; Normal = nondemented).

Note: The CDT is considered normal if all numbers are present in the correct sequence and position, and the hands readably display the requested time.

(From Borson S, Scanlan J, Brush M, et al. The Mini-Cog: a cognitive 'vital signs' measure for dementia screening in multi-lingual elderly. *Int J Geriatr Psychiatry* 15(11);1021–1027, 2000. Copyright John Wiley & Sons Limited. Reproduced with permission.)

TABLE 20-4

Managing Older Adults: The Siebens Domain Management Model

One framework to guide care of older adults is the Siebens Domain Management Model.[a,b] With practicality as a goal, the model organizes a patient's health-related problems and strengths into four domains: I. Medical/Surgical Issues; II. Mental Status/Emotions/Coping; III. Physical Function; and IV. Living Environment. Using these domain headings helps make care planning and documentation efficient and comprehensive and promotes interdisciplinary teamwork.

Format for Provider History & Physical Reports
(Modify as needed for Follow-Up Visits)
Revised with Siebens Domain Management Model (SDMM)[a]

Subjective[b]

Chief Concern or Reason for Visit (follow-up)

History of Present Illness
Symptoms/Workups to date/Patient's Perspective/Worries

Medications

Allergies

Past Medical History
Health maintenance

Family History

Social History
Education/functional health literacy
Marital status, Children, Pets
Nature of relationships (support/caregiver burden)
Alcohol/Tobacco/Drugs
Spirituality and Religious beliefs, practices
Health Power of Attorney/medical directive

Functional History
Prior level of function in Mobility,
Selfcare
Medication mgmt, paying bills
Work/Leisure/Fun activities

Review of Systems
Inclusive of sexuality

Objective[b]

Pertinent Physical Exam
Vital Signs and pertinent organ systems

Cognition, Affect
Mobility—moving in bed, getting out of bed or a chair, walking, etc.

Pertinent Labs
Electrolytes, renal function, CBC, alb, etc.

Assessment/Plan[b] (or Hospital Course)
(Note: Identified strengths and problems are best listed with assessment and plan together; each Domain must, ideally, be listed with selected categories as appropriate or else described as "no issues"; topics deemed important but not assessed can be listed with reminder "address tomorrow/next visit.")

I. Medical/Surgical Issues
Symptoms/Diseases/Prevention

II. Mental Status/Emotions/Coping
Cognition (preceded with Communication if any issues including a listing of vision/hearing/speech/language issues)
Emotions
Coping/Behavioral Symptoms
Spirituality
Patient Preferences—Advance Directives

III. Physical Function
Basic ADLs—(self care—dressing, bathing, home mobility, etc.)
Intermediate ADLs—(meals, medication and money management, etc.)
Advanced ADLs—(sexuality, work, parenting, leisure/fun, driving, general physical activity/exercise, etc.)

IV. Living Environment
A. Physical (home, adaptations, community)
B. Social (family supports/coping, social interactions, etc.)
C. Financial (health insurance, personal income, etc.) & Community Resources

---

[a] Siebens H. Applying the Domain Management Model in Treating Patients with Chronic Diseases Jt. Comm J Qual Improvement 2001;27:302–314.
[b] Note that information is also organized in the familiar SOAP format–Subjective, Objective, Assessment, Plan.
© Hilary C. Siebens, MD, 2005
Also available at: www.siebenspcc.com.

NOTE: Page numbers followed by b indicate in-chapter boxed material; those followed by t indicate end-of-chapter tables.

influences on, 333b
of leg, 473
physiology of, 333–334
recommended grading of, 482
Arteries
anatomy and physiology of, 471–473
of arm, 472
of leg, 473
Arteriovenous crossing, 263t
Arteritis, giant cell, headache due to, 250t–251t
Arthritis, 606
acromioclavicular, 647t
in ankle and feet, 635–637
of elbow, 648t
gonococcal, 578
gouty, 577
of feet, 652t
joint pain in, 644t–645t
in hands, 649t
of hip, 623–624
of knee, 628
in older adults, 923
osteoarthritis, 644t–645t
of hand, 604–605, 649t
posttraumatic, 605
psoriatic, 578, 605
rheumatoid, 577, 578, 583–584
acute, 649t
chronic, 649t
in feet, 635–636
hand deformities in, 604–605, 649t
joint pain in, 644t–645t
septic, acute, 577
of spine, 612
Articular capsule, of shoulder, 588, 590
Articular cartilage, 573
Articular disc, of temporomandibular joint, 586
Articular facets, 610, 610b
Articular processes, 610
Articular structures, 572
Articular tubercle, of temporomandibular joint, 586
Ascites, assessment of, 448–449, 465t
Assessment. *See also* Health history; Physical examination
clinical data and, 30–40
clustering data into single *vs.* multiple problems, 38–39
displaying, 43, 45–46, 48–49
integrating with clinical reasoning, 49–51
prevalence and predictive value of, 46, 46b–48b, 48–49
problem list, 37–38, 38b
quality of, 39–40, 40b
recording, 40–41, 41b–43b
sifting through, 39
clinical reasoning and, 27–30
clinical data integrating with, 49–51
steps in, 27–30, 27b
types of, 27
determining scope of, 4–6
objective data *vs.* subjective data in, 6
plan for care and, 25–26, 30. *See also* Clinical reasoning

example, 35b–37b
integrating, 49–51
overview, 25–26
Asteatosis, 917
Astereognosis, 693
Asterixis, 704
Asthma
in children, 821
dyspnea in, 314t–315t
hemoptysis in, 316t
physical findings in, 321t
Asymmetric tonic neck reflex, 794
Ataxia, 665, 688
cerebellar, 730t
sensory, 730t
Ataxic breathing, 134t
Atelectasis, physical findings in, 320t
Atheroma, 472
complex, 472
Atherosclerosis, 477, 485, 494t–495t
Athetosis, 721t
Atonic seizure, 719t
Atrial fibrillation, 375t, 376t
stroke and, 669b–670b
Atrial flutter, 375t, 376t
Atrial premature contraction, 376t, 778
Atrial septal defect, 866t
Atrioventricular node, 331
Atrioventricular valves, 325
Atrophy, muscular, 678
Attachment, in newborn, 749b
Attention, in mental status examination, 140, 141b, 152
Attention deficit/hyperactivity disorder (ADHD), 833
Auditory acuity, examination techniques for, 226
Auricle, 222, 225
Auricular lymph node, posterior, 239
Auscultation
of abdomen, 436–437
in infants, 783
defined, 18
of heart, 361–368
chest wall relations, 330
in children, 822–823
heart murmurs, 365–368, 366b
heart sounds, 361–365
in infants, 778–782
of lungs
in children, 820–821
in infants, 775–776
of thorax
anterior, 308
posterior, 302–305, 303b, 304b
Auscultatory gap, 116
Autonomic nervous system (ANS), eye, 210
Autonomy, in patient care, 92b
AV block, 375t
Avoidant personality disorder, 139
Axillae
examination techniques for, in older adults, 921
of older adults, 899
in physical examination, 20
Axillary lymph nodes, 389

Axillary temperature, 120
Axillary vein, 389
Axiohumeral muscle group, 590
Axioscapular muscle group, 589–590
Axons, 656

B

Babinski response, 701–702
in infants, 792
Back
movements of, 615–616
in physical examination, 20
Back pain
low, 642t
in health history, 575–576
lifting and biomechanics, 579
lumbosacral radiculopathy and, 703–704
during pregnancy, 875
Bacterial pneumonia, hemoptysis in, 316t
Bacterial vaginosis, 550t
Baker's cyst, 630
Balance
in older adults, 915, 915b, 923
risk of fall and, 915, 915b, 930t
Balanitis, 508
Ball-and-socket joints, 574
Ballard scoring system, for gestational age, 746, 748
Balloon sign, 630
Ballotting of the patella, 630
Barlow test, 787
Bartholin glands
anatomic considerations, 521–522
examination of, 536
Basal cell carcinoma, of skin, 165–166, 185t
of ear, 268t
in older adults, 917
Basal ganglia, 656
lesions of, 727t
Basal ganglia system, 661b
damage to, 662
Battered child syndrome, 861t
Beau's lines, 194t
Behavior
in mental status examination, 146–147
motor, 146
Bell, of stethoscope, 363
Bell's palsy, 676
Bending, lateral
of neck, 615
of spine, 616
Beneficence, in patient care, 92b
Benign prostatic hyperplasia (BPH), 558, 567t, 570t, 899–900
Bethesda system, for Pap smear classification, 530, 530b
Biceps muscle, tendon of the long head of the, 590–591
Biceps reflex, assessment of, 697
Biceps tendon, palpation of, 592
Bicipital groove, of humerus, 588–589
Bicipital tendinitis, 647t
Biliary colic, 454t–455t
Bilirubin, in jaundice, 425–426

Judgment, in mental status examination, 141b, 151
Jugular vein
  anatomic considerations
    external, 237, 334
    internal, 237, 334
    vs. carotid artery pulsations, 334, 350
Jugular venous pressure
  assessment of, 349–351, 349b–350b
  patient positioning, 334–335
  physiology of, 334–335
Jugular venous pulsations
  assessment of, 351–352
  physiology of, 336

K

Kaposi's sarcoma, 188t, 275t
Kappa *(k)* measurement of inter-observer agreement, 49, 49b
Kawasaki disease, skin conditions due to, 189t
Keloids, 181t, 268t
Keratosis
  actinic, 185t
  seborrheic, 185t
Kernig's sign, 703, 820
Kidneys
  anatomic considerations, 417
  enlargement of, 445–446
  examination techniques for, 445–446
  pain in, 428–429
Knee
  anatomy of, 625–627
  assessment of reflexes in, 699
    in older adults, 901
  examination techniques for, 627–632, 632b–634b
    for fluid detection, 630–631
    inspection, 627–628
    maneuvers for, 632, 632b–634b
    palpation, 628–631
  extension of, testing, 684–685
  flexion of, testing, 685
  movements of, 632
Knock-knee pattern, 830
Knock-knees, 627
Koplik's spots, 276t
Korotkoff sounds, 116, 121
  in children, 808

L

Labial frenulum, 231–232
Labial mucosa, 231–232
Labia majora, 521
Labia minora, 521
Labrum, 588
Labyrinth, equilibrium and, 224
Labyrinthitis, 252t
Lachman test, 633b
Lacrimal gland, 206
  examination techniques for, 214
Lacrimal puncta, 206
Lacrimal sac, 206
  examination techniques for, 214
  inflammation of, 256t

Lactose intolerance, 458t–459t
Lamina, 610b
Landau reflex, 795
Language, in mental status examination, 141b, 147–148
Language barriers, interviewing and, 78–79, 79b
Language development
  of children, 797–798
  of infants, 750
Lanugo, 760
LaPlace, law of, 473
Large for gestational age (LGA), 746–747
Laryngitis, hemoptysis in, 316t
Last menstrual period, 877
Lateral canthus, 205
Lateral collateral ligament (LCL), 625, 627, 633b
Lateral compartment, 629
Lateral condyle, of tibia, 625
Lateral epicondyle, 599
  of femur, 625
Lateral epicondylitis, 600, 648t
Lateral fornix, 522
Lateral lymph nodes, 392, 408
Lateral malleolus, 634
Lateral meniscus, 625–626
Latissimus dorsi muscle, 611
Law of LaPlace, 473
Lazy eye, 811
Learning ability, in mental status examination, 152–153
Left ventricle, 323–324
Left ventricular hypertrophy, 920
Left ventricular impulses. *See also* Point of maximum impulse (PMI)
  abnormalities of, 378t
Leg length discrepancy, 831, 846
Leg(s)
  arteries of, 473
  of children, 830–831
  in coordination assessment, 687
  edema of, 486–487
  of infant, 789
  length measurement, 637–638
  peripheral vascular system, examination techniques, 483–488
  venous system of, 473–474
Leg shortening, in children, 831
Lens of eye, 207
  examination techniques for, 215
  opacities of, 258t
Leopold's maneuvers, modified, 888–890
Lesser tubercle, of humerus, 588–589
Lethargy, 706
Leukemia, skin conditions due to, 189t
Leukonychia, 194t
Leukoplakia
  hairy, of tongue, 279t
  oral, 276t
  of tongue, 280t
Leukorrhea, 523
  during pregnancy, 875
Levator palpebrae, 206
Level of consciousness
  in comatose patient, 706

in general survey, 109
in mental status examination, 146
Lichenification, 181t, 188t
Lid lag, 216–217
Lid retraction, 255t
Lifestyle habits, in health history, 10
Lifestyle modifications, for cardiovascular disease, 345–347, 345b, 346b
Lifting, biomechanics and, 579
Ligaments
  of ankle and feet, 635
  defined, 572
  of knee, 625–627
  of spine, 610
Light, pupillary reactions to, 209, 215–216, 673
Lighting
  perpendicular, 14
  for physical examination, 14
  tangential, 14
Light reaction, pupillary, 209, 215–216
Likelihood ratio, 49, 49b
Limbus, 206
Linea nigra, 874
Lingual frenulum, 233
Lipoma, 464t
Lip(s)
  abnormalities of, 272t–273t
  carcinoma of, 273t
Listening, active, in interviewing, 69
Literacy, low, interviewing and, 79
Liver
  anatomic considerations, 416
  disease of
    risk factors for, 426–427
    skin conditions due to, 189t
  enlargement of, 469t
    in adolescents, 842
    in children, 824–825
  examination techniques for, 439–443
    in adolescents, 842
    in children, 824–825
    in infants, 784
    palpation, 441–443, 469t
    percussion, 439–440
  normal size of, 440
    in children, 824
  span of dullness, 439–440
Lobes
  of brain, 655–656
  of breast, 390
  of lung, 287
Lobule, 222
Longitudinal arch, 634
Loss, five stages of, 86
Loss of consciousness, in health history, 666
Low back pain, 642t
  in health history, 575–576
  lifting and biomechanics for, 579
  lumbosacral radiculopathy and, 703–704
Lower motor neurons, damage to, 662
Lubricant use, in pelvic or rectal examinations, 542b
Lumbar spinal stenosis, 642t
Lumbar vertebrae, anatomy of, 610b
Lumbosacral junction, 611

Migraine headache, 197, 269t
Milia, 763
Miliaria rubra, 762
Mini-Cog, screening for dementia, 932t
Minimum Geriatric Competencies, 930t
Miosis, 215
Mircocephaly, 766
Mitral regurgitation, 383t
  in older adults, 898
Mitral stenosis, 386t
  dyspnea in, 314t–315t
  hemoptysis in, 316t
Mitral valve, 325
MMSE (mini-mental state examination), 155, 155b
Modesty
  in adolescents, 837–838
  in children, 801
Molding, of newborn head, 765
Moles. *See also* Nevi
  detecting, 167, 167b, 171, 171b
Molluscum contagiosum, 858t
Mongolian spots, 764
Monoarticular joint pain, 576
Mononeuritis multiplex, 670
Mononeuropathy, peripheral nerve, 729t
Mons pubis, 521
Mood, in mental status examination, 140, 141b, 148–149
Mood disorders, 160t
Moro reflex, 794
Morton's neuroma, 636, 652t
Motion, limited, in joint pain, 577
Motor development
  of adolescents, 834–835
  of children, 797–798
  of infants, 750, 793, 796, 796b
Motor (efferent) fibers, 660
Motor function, 146
  in general survey, 111
  in newborn, 790
  in physical examination, 22
Motor neurons, 660
  damage to lower, 662
  damage to upper, 661–662
Motor pathways, 660–662, 660b–661b
Motor system
  examination of, 678–690
    body position, 678
    coordination, 686–690, 832
    involuntary movements, 678
    muscle bulk, 678–679
    muscle strength, 680–686, 680b
    muscle tone, 679
    recording findings for, 710
  of older adults, 901
Motor tone, in newborn, 790
Mouth
  abnormalities of, in children, 862t
  anatomy of, 231–234
  examination techniques for, 234–236
    in children, 816–819
    in infants, 771–772
  floor of, 235
  in health history, 201
  roof of, 235

Movements, involuntary
  in health history, 666
  motor assessment of, 678
  types of, 720t–721t
Mucopurulent cervicitis, 549t
Mucosal rings/webs, 456t
Mucous plug, 874
  loss of, 875
Murphy's sign, 451
Muscle(s). *See also specific muscle*
  of ankle and feet, 635
  of elbow, 599–600
  of eyes, 211, 216–218
  of hip, 618
  lesions of, 729t
  of mastication, 586–587
  motor assessment of
    bulk, 678–679
    strength, 680–686, 680b, 832
    tone, 679
  of neck, 236
  of shoulder, 589–590
  of spine, 611
  surrounding knee, 626
  of temporomandibular joint, 586–587
  of wrist and hand, 603
Muscle strength, motor assessment of, 680–686, 680b
  in children, 832
  grading system for, 680, 680b
Muscle tone
  assessment of, in comatose patient, 708–709
  disorders of, 726t
  motor assessment of, 679
  in newborn, 790
Muscle wasting
  hypothenar atrophy, 650t, 678
  of older adults, 901
  thenar atrophy, 650t, 678
Muscular atrophy, 678
Muscular dystrophy, 704–705, 832
  Duchenne, 678
Muscular hypertrophy, 678
Musculoskeletal system, 571–655. *See also* Joint(s); Muscle(s)
  anatomy of
    ankle and foot, 634–635
    elbow, 599–600
    hip, 618–619
    knee, 625–627
    shoulder, 588–591
    spine, 609–611
    temporomandibular joint (TMJ), 586
    wrist and hand, 601–603
  of children, abnormalities in, 868t
  common health complaints related to, 571
  examination techniques for
    in adolescents, 846–849
    ankle and foot, 635–637
    approach to, 583–585
    in children, 830–831
    elbow, 600–601
    hip, 619–624
    in infants, 786–790
    joint motion description, 638

knee, 627–632, 632b–634b
leg length measurement, 637–638
in older adults, 923
recording findings, 639
shoulder, 591–593, 593b–599b, 596
spine, 611–616, 613b
temporomandibular joint, 587
tips for successful, 583b–584b
wrist and hand, 603–609
in health history, 575–578
health promotion and counseling and, 578–582
of older adults, 900
in physical examination, 21
during pregnancy, 872
in review of systems, 12
Myasthenia gravis, 665
Mycosis fungoides, 177t
Mydriasis, 215
Mydriatic eye drops, 218
Myocardial contractility, 332
Myocardial infarction, chest pain in, 312t–313t
Myoclonus, 719t
Myomas, of uterus, 552t
Myopathy, 684
Myopia, 197, 211, 220
  in children, 812
Myringitis, bullous, 269t
Myxedema, facies in, 253t

N

Nabothian cyst, 548t
Naegele's rule, 877
Nail bed, 164
Nail plate, 164
Nail root, 164
Nail(s), finger
  abnormalities of, 193t–194t
  anatomy of, 164
  examination techniques, 170
  in older adults, 895
Narcissistic personality disorder, 139
Narrow-angle glaucoma, 215, 897
Nasal bone, 204
Nasal congestion, 200
Nasal flaring, in infants, 774
Nasal mucosa, 230
Nasal polyps, 816
Nasal septum, 228, 230
Nasolacrimal duct, 206
  obstruction of, 243
Nausea, 422
  during pregnancy, 875
Navicular bone, 635
Near reaction, pupillary, 210, 216, 674
Neck
  anatomy of, 236–238
  examination techniques for, 238–243
    in adolescents, 840
    in children, 819–820
    in infants, 773
    in older adults, 918–919
    during pregnancy, 883
  in health history, 201

Submandibular gland, 204
  ducts of, 233
Submandibular lymph nodes, 239
Submental lymph nodes, 239
Subscapularis muscle, 589
Subscapular lymph nodes, 392, 408
Substance abuse. *See also* Alcohol use
  screening for, 138b, 143–144
Subtalar (talocalcaneal) joint, 634, 637
Sudden infant death syndrome (SIDS), 774
Suicide risk
  question to ask, 148–149
  screening for, 143
Summarization, in interviewing, 73–74
Superficial veins, of leg, 473
Superior vena cava, 324–325, 473
Supination
  of elbow, 601
  of forearm, 598b
Supinator muscle, 599
Supinator reflex, assessment of, 698
Supine hypotensive syndrome, 881
Supraclavicular lymph nodes, 239
Supracondylar fracture, of elbow, 600–601
Suprapatellar pouch, 627, 629–630
Suprapubic pain, 419, 427
Supraspinatus muscle, 589, 591, 598b
Supraspinatus tendon, 591
Suprasternal notch, 283
Supraventricular premature contractions, 376t
Supraventricular tachycardia, in infants, 856t
Sutures, of skull, in infants, 765
Swallowing, assessment of, 676
Swan neck deformity, 649t
S wave, 331–332
Sweat glands, 165
Swelling
  in joint examination, 584b
  in joint pain, 577
Swinging flashlight test, 244
Swing phase, of gait, 619
Symphysis pubis, 415, 617, 620
Symptoms
  eliciting from older adults, 902–904, 904b
  in interview, 65–66, 65b
  overlap, 136–137
  seven attributes of, 8, 65, 65b
  unexplained and mental health disorders,
    136–137, 137b, 159t
Syncope, 716t–717t
  cardiac, 666
  cough, 716t–717t
  defined, 666
  in health history, 666
  micturition, 716t–717t
  in older adults, 895
  vasodepressor (vasovagal), 666, 716t–717t
Synovial cavity, 573
Synovial fluid, 573
Synovial joints
  bursae and, 574
  structure of, 573–574
  types of, 573
Synovial membrane, 573
Synovitis, 584

Syphilis, 531
  congenital, 860t
  on female genitalia, 546t
  on lip, 273t
  on male genitalia, 516t
  primary, 516t, 546t
  skin conditions due to, 190t
  on tongue, 280t
Systemic lupus erythematous (SLE), 577–578
  skin conditions due to, 190t
Systole
  defined, 326
  extra sounds in, 365, 381t
Systolic aortic murmur, 898
Systolic heart murmurs, 365–366, 369–370,
    384t–385t
Systolic pressure, 348

T

Tachycardia, 375t
  in infants, 774
  paroxysmal atrial, 778
  paroxysmal supraventricular, 758, 778
Tachypnea, 134t
  in infants, 759
  pneumonia and, in children, 810
Tactile fremitus, 318t
  assessment of, 298–299, 306
  asymmetric, 298
  in various disorders, 320t–321t
Talipes equinovarus, 789
Talkative patients, interviewing, 77
Talofibular ligament
  anterior, 635
  posterior, 635
Talus, 634
Tangential lighting, 14
Tanner stages for sexual maturity, 523
  in females
    breasts, 841–842, 842b
    genitalia, 845–846, 845b
  in males, 843–844
Tarsal plates, 206
Taste sensation, of older adults, 897
Tavistock principles, 94, 94b
Teeth
  abnormalities of, 278t
  adult, 232
  age of eruption, 817
  anatomy of, 232
  of children
    abnormalities of, 818, 863t
    dental caries in, 817
    examination techniques for, 816–817
    staining in, 817
  examination techniques for, 234–235
  Hutchinson's, 278t
  of older adults, 897, 919
Telangiectasia, 187t
  hereditary hemorrhagic, 273t
Temperature, body
  assessment of, 120–121
  in children, 810
  in infants, 759
  in older adults, 894

Temperature sensation
  assessment of, 675, 692
  sensory pathway for, 662
Temporal artery, superficial, 204
Temporal bone, 204, 586
Temporal lobe, 655–656
Temporal muscles, 587
Temporomandibular joint, 586–587
Tenderness
  abdominal, 467t–468t
  of breast, during pregnancy, 875
  elbow, 648t
  in joint examination, 584b
  rebound, 439
Tendinitis, 584
  Achilles, 631
  bicipital, 592, 647t
  calcific of shoulder, 646t
  rotator cuff, 646t
Tendon, defined, 573
Tenesmus, 424
10-minute Geriatric Screener, 910, 913–914,
    923
Tennis elbow, 600, 648t
Tenosynovitis, 605
  acute, 651t
  de Quervain's, 604–605, 607, 682
  gonococcal, 604
Tension headache, 197, 269t
Tension pneumothorax, needle insertion land-
    mark, 284
Teres major muscle, 611
Teres minor muscle, 589, 611
Terry's nails, 193t
Testes
  abnormalities of, 517t
  anatomy of, 501–502
  in boys, 825–826
  cancer of, 517t
  development of, Tanner stages for, 843–844
  palpation of, 510
  small, 517t
  undescended, 785, 826, 868t
Testicular self-examination, 507, 512–513, 512b
Testosterone, 502
Tetanus, 869t
Tetralogy of Fallot, 865t
Thalamus, 656
Thelarche, premature, 783
Thenar atrophy, 650t, 678
Thermometers, 120
Thoracentesis, insertion landmark, 285
Thoracic kyphosis, 613b
Thoracoabdominal paradox, 775
Thorax
  anatomical terms for locations on, 288
  anatomy of, 283–285
  anterior, examination of, 296, 305–309
    auscultation, 308
    inspection, 305
    palpation, 305–306
    percussion, 307–308
  examination techniques for
    in children, 820–821
    in infants, 773–776